A Manual of Orthopaedic Terminology

Eighth Edition

A Manual of Orthopaedic Terminology

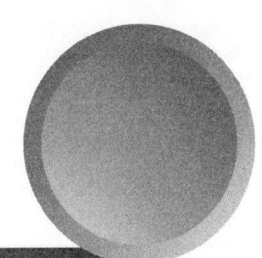

Fred R.T. Nelson, MD, FAAOS
Emeritus, Orthopaedics
Henry Ford Hospital
Detroit, Michigan

Carolyn Taliaferro Blauvelt
Formerly Writer-Editor, Medical-Dental Publications
Department of Orthopaedic Surgery
National Naval Medical Center and
Department of Surgery, Uniformed Services University
  of the Health Sciences
Bethesda, Maryland

1600 John F. Kennedy Blvd.
Ste 1800
Philadelphia, PA 19103-2899

A MANUAL OF ORTHOPAEDIC TERMINOLOGY,
EIGHTH EDITION   ISBN: 978-0-323-22158-0
Copyright © 2015 by Saunders, an imprint of Elsevier Inc.
Copyright © 2007, 1998, 1994, 1990, 1985, 1981, 1978 by Mosby, Inc., an affiliation of Elsevier, Inc.

All rights reserved. No part of this publication may be reproduced or transmitted in any form or by any means, electronic or mechanical, including photocopying, recording, or any information storage and retrieval system, without permission in writing from the publisher. Details on how to seek permission, further information about the Publisher's permissions policies and our arrangements with organizations such as the Copyright Clearance Center and the Copyright Licensing Agency, can be found at our website: www.elsevier.com/permissions.

This book and the individual contributions contained in it are protected under copyright by the Publisher (other than as may be noted herein).

Notices

Knowledge and best practice in this field are constantly changing. As new research and experience broaden our understanding, changes in research methods, professional practices, or medical treatment may become necessary.

Practitioners and researchers must always rely on their own experience and knowledge in evaluating and using any information, methods, compounds, or experiments described herein. In using such information or methods they should be mindful of their own safety and the safety of others, including parties for whom they have a professional responsibility.

With respect to any drug or pharmaceutical products identified, readers are advised to check the most current information provided (i) on procedures featured or (ii) by the manufacturer of each product to be administered, to verify the recommended dose or formula, the method and duration of administration, and contraindications. It is the responsibility of practitioners, relying on their own experience and knowledge of their patients, to make diagnoses, to determine dosages and the best treatment for each individual patient, and to take all appropriate safety precautions.

To the fullest extent of the law, neither the Publisher nor the authors, contributors, or editors, assume any liability for any injury and/or damage to persons or property as a matter of products liability, negligence or otherwise, or from any use or operation of any methods, products, instructions, or ideas contained in the material herein.

Library of Congress Cataloging-in-Publication Data

Nelson, Fred R. T., 1941- author.
 A manual of orthopaedic terminology / Fred R.T. Nelson, Carolyn Taliaferro Blauvelt. -- Eighth edition.
   p. ; cm.
 Includes index.
 ISBN 978-0-323-22158-0 (paperback : alk. paper)
 I. Blauvelt, Carolyn Taliaferro, 1933- author. II. Title.
 [DNLM: 1. Orthopedics--Terminology--English. WE 15]
 RD723
 616.7001'4--dc23
                                                            2014014681

Content Strategist: Delores Meloni
Content Development Specialist: Margaret Nelson
Publishing Services Manager: Catherine Jackson
Senior Project Manager: Mary Pohlman
Design Direction: Teresa McBryan

Printed in the United States

Last digit is the print number: 9 8 7 6 5 4 3 2 1

Foreword

Medical terminology is by necessity complex. Understanding the "jargon" of medicine takes extensive years of education and enculturation. Orthopaedic terminology is perhaps the most difficult of all because of the breadth of disease and injury that affects the musculoskeletal system. Terms related to anatomy, pathology, physiology, genetic injury descriptors, and syndromes require an intimate knowledge of the broad field of orthopaedics. Individuals other than those well versed in the terminology need resources to answer their inquiries and investigations. Practitioners in need of a lexicon include researchers, physicians in fields other than orthopaedics, the legal profession, and the universe of patients.

For 35 years, Nelson and Blauvelt have provided a wonderful resource to assist this population of consumers of orthopaedic information. They have periodically refined the manual to keep it up to date and comprehensive within the evolving universe of musculoskeletal medicine. This resource can guide individuals as they perform literature reviews, systematic reviews of that literature, meta-analyses, and other clinical investigations in the field of orthopaedics. This tool is straight-forward, easy to read, and comprehensive. It will continue to serve as the go-to reference for individuals needing to access orthopaedic information to serve their individual audiences.

Marc F. Swiontkowski, MD
Professor, Department of Orthopaedic Surgery
University of Minnesota
CEO, TRIA Orthopaedic Center

Preface

This manual was first published more than 35 years ago to encompass the vast terminology unique to orthopaedic surgery and its related allied health fields, (i.e., radiology, prosthetics, orthotics, and physical and occupational therapy). Scientific discoveries and technological advances led to new and updated editions and, during that time, the publishing industry merged and moved to the paperless electronic age of publishing.

The manual has continued to provide a reference source for medical students, interns, residents, orthopaedic nurses and technicians, and transcriptionists and office managers in hospital and doctors offices. Newcomers to orthopaedics, such as sales representatives for pharmaceutical and surgical devices, medical publishers, insurance adjustors, and attorneys, have also appreciated this reference source for better clarification of orthopaedic terminology. The format of this manual enables the layperson without a strong musculoskeletal background to understand why terms are not in A-Z order, but rather are placed in their proper context to facilitate understanding of both the words and their associations.

New procedures and devices have been developed that are rapidly replacing those found in former editions. However, some devices named have been retained because they may still be in use. Also, "jargon" not officially recognized by certifying organizations may continue to be found in legal reports and is retained here. ICD codes have been deleted from this edition because they can be found on the internet and other sources. The human genome project, DNA breakthroughs in cellular mechanisms, and changes in therapies have occurred at a rapid rate. This eighth edition reflects these new changes, and lots of new information has been updated.

From its inception, the authors have invited contributors with expertise in specific areas to review and update chapters to be current and accurate. The manual has continued to serve a need, and that is the goal of this eighth edition.

Fred R.T. Nelson
Carolyn Taliaferro Blauvelt

Contributors

No one can write a book on all areas of orthopaedics and keep it current without the help of many competent people. This manual is no exception. We have chosen contributors whose background and experience make them well qualified to assist in updating material for each edition and who work directly or indirectly in this specialty. These people have generously given their time, in view of other professional commitments, to improve the correctness and accuracy of information, provide an update, and give constructive criticism. We can share in the success of this manual with them, and we wish to express our appreciation and thanks to our past contributors, and to the following persons and organizations who participated in the revisions of the eighth edition.

Classifications of Fractures, Dislocations, and Sports-Related Injuries

Steven M. Kane, MD
Chairman and Program Director
Orthopaedic Surgery Residency
Atlanta Medical Center
Orthopaedic Residency Program
Atlanta, Georgia

Bruce H. Ziran, MD, FACS
Director of Orthopaedic Trauma
Gwinnett Orthopaedic Trauma
The Hughston Clinic at Gwinnett Medical Center
Lawrenceville, Georgia

Musculoskeletal Diseases and Related Terms

Sheila Ann Conway, MD
Associate Professor, Department of Orthopaedic Surgery
Program Director, Orthopaedic Surgery Residency Program
University of Miami/Jackson Memorial Medical Center
Miami, Florida

Robert J. Esther, MD
University of North Carolina
Department of Orthopaedics
Chapel Hill, North Carolina

Shawn R. Gilbert, MD
Associate Professor of Surgery
University of Alabama at Birmingham
Birmingham, Alabama

Craig S. Roberts, MD, MBA
K. Armand Fischer Professor and Chair
University of Louisville School of Medicine
Department of Orthopaedic Surgery
Louisville, Kentucky

Montri Daniel Wongworawat, MD
Department of Orthopaedic Surgery
Loma Linda University
Loma Linda, California

Imaging Techniques
Jean Jose, MD
Associate Professor of Radiology
Associate Chief, Musculoskeletal Radiology
Director, Imaging Sports Medicine
University of Miami Radiology Department
Miami, Florida

Orthopaedic Tests, Signs, and Maneuvers
J. Milo Sewards, MD
Director, Orthopaedic Surgery Residency
Temple University Hospital
Philadelphia, Pennsylvania

Laboratory Evaluations
Sudhaker D. Rao, MD, MB, BS, FACP, FACE
Section Head, Bone and Mineral Metabolism
Director, Bone and Mineral Research Laboratory
Henry Ford Hospital
Detroit, Michigan

Casts, Splints, Dressings, and Traction
Meagan Clark, CPO
Assistant Director of Clinical Education
Loma Linda University, el-MSOP Program
Loma Linda, California

Prosthetic and Orthotics
Meagan Clark, CPO
Assistant Director of Clinical Education
Loma Linda University, el-MSOP Program
Loma Linda, California

Anatomy and Orthopaedic Surgery
Sheila Ann Conway, MD
Associate Professor, Department of Orthopaedic Surgery
Program Director, Orthopaedic Surgery Residency Program
University of Miami/Jackson Memorial Medical Center
Miami, Florida

Robert J. Esther, MD
University of North Carolina
Department of Orthopaedics
Chapel Hill, North Carolina

Shawn R. Gilbert, MD
Associate Professor of Surgery
University of Alabama at Birmingham
Birmingham, Alabama

The Spine
Young Lu, BA
Icahn School of Medicine at Mount Sinai
Department of Orthopaedic Surgery
Mount Sinai Medical Center
New York, New York

Sheeraz Qureshi, MD, MBA
Associate Professor, Orthopaedic Surgery
Minimally Invasive Spinal Surgery
Mount Sinai Hospital
Icahn School of Medicine at Mount Sinai
Co-Director, Spinal Surgery Fellowship
New York, New York

The Hand and Wrist
Montri Daniel Wongworawat, MD
Department of Orthopaedic Surgery
Loma Linda University
Loma Linda, California

The Foot and Ankle
Anthony D. Watson, MD
Greater Pittsburgh Ortho Associates
Pittsburgh, Pennsylvania

Physical Medicine and Rehabilitation: Physical Therapy and Occupational Therapy
Eugene Bulkin, MD
Assistant Professor
Department of Orthopaedics
Mount Sinai School of Medicine
Port Washington, New York

Stacy Oster, MS, OTR/L, CHT
Senior Occupational Therapist
Certified Hand Therapist
Beth Israel Medical Center
Phillips Ambulatory Care Center
Department of Rehabilitation Medicine
New York, New York

Paul Zucker, MS, PT, LAc
Director of Ambulatory Services
PACC Administration
Department of Physical Medicine and Rehabilitation
Beth Israel Medical Center
New York, New York

The Research Enterprise
William Wu, PhD
Adjunct Associate Professor of Pharmacology
Wayne State Medical School
Detroit, Michigan

Introduction to the Orthopaedic Speciality

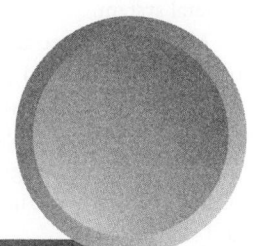

Orthopaedic (ortho-pae'dic) means correction or prevention of bony deformities (formerly, especially in children). The word comes from the Greek *orthos*, meaning "straight, upright, right, or true"—hence, also "correct" or "regular"—and from the Greek *pais*, meaning "child."

The scope of orthopaedic surgery includes the treatment, management, and rehabilitation of patients with musculoskeletal conditions affecting bones, muscles, joints, tendons, ligaments, cartilage, blood vessels, nerves, and related tissues through surgical, nonsurgical, and other medical measures. The nature of these conditions may involve congenital abnormalities, metabolic disease processes, metastatic (tumor) pathologic findings, or traumatic injuries (fractures) requiring the expertise of the orthopaedic specialty. When surgery is indicated, postoperative rehabilitation is equally important in the continued care and treatment plan.

The orthopaedic surgeon develops many skills and must possess a working knowledge of neurology, cardiopulmonary physiology, and bioengineering in the care of the orthopaedic patient. This expertise also includes electrical and magnetic bone stimulation, microsurgery, and knowledge of internal and external fixation devices. Orthopaedic medicine is continually changing, and the orthopaedic surgeon is challenged with the responsibility of keeping informed of new techniques through continued education in the field.

Nonoperative measures include everything from the application of casts for immobilization and management of fractures or scoliosis to the treatment of diseases and disabilities through conservative management. In the operating room, the orthopaedist is skilled in the repair and reconstruction of major skeletal defects, which include replacing diseased joints with plastic implants; inserting metallic rods and other devices for stability; or performing fusions, revisions, or amputations. Of a more delicate nature, he or she applies arthroscopic and microvascular techniques that include skin grafts, finger transplantations, nerve repairs, and similar difficult procedures.

The rheumatologist is an internist who specializes in rheumatic diseases that affect joints, muscles, and soft tissue. Often they work in collaboration with orthopaedic surgeons. The osteopathic physician specializes in orthopaedics with emphasis on body mechanics, or may specialize in rheumatology.

From a team approach, the orthopaedic specialty depends on many other disciplines in the treatment of patients. The immediate team members are the professional nurses who provide primary care of patients and who are assisted by orthopaedic technicians, both in the clinic and hospital setting. The second group of team members include the physical medicine and rehabilitation specialists called *physiatrists*. Physiatrists, physical therapists, and occupational therapists are directly involved in, and may be consulted for the development of a treatment plan in a patient's rehabilitation. The next group of team members include the prosthetists (artificial limbs) and orthotists (braces), who measure, fit, design, and fabricate expertly applied devices for the orthopaedic patient. The developers and manufacturers of internal orthopaedic appliances play an important role, as does the researcher who tests the biocompatibility of materials used in the musculoskeletal system.

All of these specialties are an integral part of the orthopaedic team and provide a combination of skills that benefit thousands of patients with musculoskeletal problems. Other disciplines that interface with orthopaedics include bioengineering, electrobiology, transplantation, diagnostic imaging, oncology, biochemistry, and similar areas.

Orthopaedic surgery has become so diverse that there is specialization within the specialty. In addition to general orthopaedics, a physician may specialize in diseases and surgery of the spine, soft tissues, the hand, the foot, major joints, trauma, sports medicine, or the ever-changing area of orthopaedic research. Many physicians are exposed to orthopaedic surgery during their training years, but only a select group actually pursue this difficult and diverse field to the point of certification.

The qualification for certification by the American Board of Orthopaedic Surgery is 5 or 6 years of postgraduate education after medical school. After graduation from an Accreditation Council for Graduate Medical Education–approved 5-year program, a candidate sits for Part 1, which is a written examination. After 22 months of practice in the same location, he or she may sit for Part 2, which is a practice-based examination reviewing cases and outcomes. The physician must complete all requirements to become board certified and a Diplomate of the Board. After completion of the certification requirements, an orthopaedic surgeon becomes eligible for Fellowship in the American Academy of Orthopaedic Surgeons, the national organization of the specialty. The admission to fellowship in the Academy requires board certification and recommendations from the community. This is typically 18 months following board certification. The Academy fellowship at present represents approximately 81% of the practicing orthopaedic surgeons in the United States. The national organization of the specialty developed the accepted definition of orthopaedics in 1952:

Orthopaedic Surgery is the medical specialty that includes the investigation, preservation, restoration, and development of the form and function of the extremities, spine, and associated structures by medical, surgical, and physical methods.

ORTHOPAEDIC ORGANIZATIONS OF NORTH AMERICA

American Academy for Cerebral Palsy and Developmental Medicine
American Association for Hand Surgery
American Association of Hip and Knee Surgeons
American Board of Orthopaedic Surgery, Inc.
American Orthopaedic Association
American Orthopaedic Foot and Ankle Society
American Orthopaedic Society for Sports Medicine
American Shoulder and Elbow Surgeons
American Society of Orthopaedic Physician's Assistants
American Society of Plastic Surgeons
American Society for Reconstructive Microsurgery
American Society for Surgery of the Hand
American Spinal Injury Association
Arthroscopy Association of North America
Association of Bone and Joint Surgeons
Association of Children's Prosthetic-Orthotic Clinics
Bones Society, Inc.
Cervical Spine Research Society
Clinical Orthopaedic Society
Clinical Orthopaedics and Related Research (journal)
Council of Musculoskeletal Specialty Societies
Eastern Orthopaedic Association
Federation of Spine Associations
Hip Society
International Cartilage Repair Society
International Society of Arthroscopy, Knee Surgery and Orthopaedic Sports Medicine
Irish American Orthopaedic Society
J. Robert Gladden Society
Knee Society
Limb Lengthening and Reconstruction Society
Mid-America Orthopaedic Association
Mid-Central States Orthopaedic Society, Inc.
Musculoskeletal Tumor Society
North American Spine Society
Orthopaedic Rehabilitation Association
Orthopaedic Research and Education Foundation
Orthopaedic Research Society

Orthopaedic Trauma Association
Osteoarthritis Research Society International
Pediatric Orthopaedic Society of North America
Ruth Jackson Orthopaedic Society
Scoliosis Research Society

SICOT Société Internationale de Chirurgie
  Orthopédique et de Traumatologie
Society of Military Orthopaedic Surgeons
Southern Orthopaedic Association
Western Orthopaedic Association

Contents

1 **Classifications of Fractures, Dislocations, and Sports-Related Injuries** 1
Terminology of Fractures and Dislocations 2
Classifications of Fractures 3
Classic and Descriptive Names (By Anatomic Location) 8
Contributing Factors 12
Degree and Nature of Healing 13
International Classification System and Trauma Registry System 13
Classification Systems by Grades, Types, and Mechanisms 14
The FEDS System for Classifying Glenohumeral Joint Instability 25
Dislocations 32
Subluxations 34
Strains and Sprains 35
Sports-Related Injuries 36
Trauma Scoring Systems and Associated Soft Tissue Injuries 39

2 **Musculoskeletal Diseases and Related Terms** 43
Bone Diseases 44
Infectious Bone Diseases 48
Tumors of Bone 49
Soft Tissue Tumors 53
Miscellaneous Bone Conditions 54
Eponymic Bone Diseases 59
Muscle Diseases 61
Cartilage Diseases 64
Diseases of (Specific) Soft Tissue 67
Ligament, Tendon, Bursa, and Fascia Diseases 69
Joint Diseases (Arthro-, Synovio-, Capsulo-, Ankylo-) 70
Vascular Diseases and Conditions 73
Neurologic Diseases 78
Metabolic Diseases 82
Diseases and Conditions by Anatomic Area 89
Congenital Limb Absences 94
Associated Disease Terminology 97

3 **Imaging Techniques** 105
General Radiologic Terms 106
Orthopaedic Radiographic Techniques and Procedures 107
Routine Radiographic Views 108
Radiographic Angles, Lines, Signs, and Methods 110
Invasive and Noninvasive Techniques 125
Vascular Diagnostic Studies 128
Radiation Therapy 130

4 **Orthopaedic Tests, Signs, and Maneuvers** 131
Tests, Signs, and Maneuvers 131
Neck 136
Back 138
Shoulder 140
Upper Limbs and Elbow 143
Hands 144
Hips 147
Lower Limbs 149
Knees 149

Feet and Ankles   154
Neurologic Examination   155
Metabolic Tests   157
General Observations   158
Gaits   158
Scales and Ratings   159
Other Physical Examinations   161

5 Laboratory Evaluations   163
Routine Evaluations   163
General Blood and Serum Tests   165
Serum and Urine Tests for Metabolic Disease   167
Bacteriologic Studies   168
Other Special Studies   169
Histologic and Pathologic Techniques   170
Laboratory Evaluations in Musculoskeletal Tumors   171
Blood Bank Procedures and Products   171
Routine Physiologic Parameters   174
Laboratory Abbreviations   174
Annotation of Units   175
Important Laboratory Notes   176

6 Casts, Splints, Dressings, and Traction   177
Cast Materials   178
Cast Immobilization   179
Devices Applied to Casts   181
Cast Complications   181
Splints and Accessories   182
Dressings   183
Suspensions, Tractions, and Frames   184
Emergency Stabilization   188

7 Prosthetics and Orthotics   189
Prosthetics   190
Orthoses   196
Shoe Modifications   205

8 Anatomy and Orthopaedic Surgery   209
Osteo- (Bone)   209
Arthro- (Joints)   226
Other Specific Tissues   230

Vascular (Blood Vessels) System   235
Specific Anatomy and Surgery by Location   240
Skin Grafts   272
Surgical Blocks   273
Surgical Approaches   273
Replantation Microsurgery   276
Treatment of Tumors   276
Amputations   277
Associated Surgical Terms   278

9 The Spine   283
General Anatomy of the Spine   283
Cervical Spine Anatomy   285
Thoracic Spine Anatomy   286
Lumbar and Lower Spine Anatomy   287
Diseases and Structural Anomalies   288
Surgery of the Spine   299

10 The Hand and Wrist   307
Anatomy of the Hand and Wrist   307
Diseases and Structural Anomalies   316
Surgery of the Hand and Wrist   330

11 The Foot and Ankle   343
Anatomy   343
Diseases and Conditions of the Foot and Ankle   351
Surgery   357

12 Physical Medicine and Rehabilitation: Physical Therapy and Occupational Therapy   365
Physical Medicine and Rehabilitation   365
Occupational Therapy   371

13 The Research Enterprise   377
The Research Proposal   377
Reporting the Results   378
General Research Terminology   378

Appendix

A Orthopaedic Abbreviations 395
Professional Organizations 403

B Anatomic Positions and Directions 405
Surface Location 405
Anatomic Planes 405
Specific Locations 406
Joint Motions 406
Anatomic Associated Terms 409

C Etymology of Orthopaedics 413

Bibliography 427

Suggested Readings 433

Classifications of Fractures, Dislocations, and Sports-Related Injuries

The musculoskeletal reaction to trauma can result in a variety of bone, muscle, and ligamentous disruptions; sometimes fracture and ligamentous injuries occur concurrently. The general types of musculoskeletal trauma are fractures, dislocations, subluxations, sprains, strains, and diastases.

This chapter defines fractures and dislocations by sections. The first part contains general terms that are easily understood by the nonspecialist, followed by classic, descriptive, and eponymic terms by anatomic location. The second section is a brief outline of the AO (Arbeitsgemeinschaft für Osteosynthesefragen) system and Orthopaedic Trauma Association Registry System of fracture classification. The third section defines the many eponymic classification systems by grades, types, and mechanisms. The last section covers the types of dislocations, subluxations, strains and sprains, and sports-related injuries. Many new terms have been added to this edition.

Most patients with musculoskeletal injuries present to an emergency room in an acute stage and are treated by the emergency room physician until it is determined that an orthopaedic specialist may be required. Good communication is essential when relating the assessment of acute injuries. A brief and accurate description is vital to the evaluation and immediate treatment of the injured, and familiarity with the classification systems that follow will help in understanding the importance of accurate communication. For example, an open, midshaft, comminuted, femur fracture gives a brief description but accurately relates a lot. To achieve this degree of accuracy, learning the classifications is an important tool to the end user.

A uniform descriptive system also allows accurate coding of specific diagnostic entities. The bony detail is described by the following:

- Open versus closed
- Portion of bone involved
- General appearance
- Alignment of fragments and position and alignment

Interestingly, fractures have specific terminology that varies from time of occurrence to healing. Fractures may be named for an anatomic location, a person, or a place. They are further defined in terms of how they occurred or reason for the break. As fractures begin to heal, the degree and nature of healing are described.

Contributing factors, such as tumors, infections, and repeated stress, are included in the descriptive terminology. This is important for diagnostic coding. The management of fractures is also clarified. *Closed* management (closed reduction) means that treatment is in the form of a manipulation, cast, splint–traction application, or some combination of the three. *Open* management (open reduction) requires a surgical incision to approximate the fracture fragments into normal position. Often, some form of internal fixation (*osteosynthesis*) is performed with open management of fractures. A *fracture of necessity* requires surgical fixation for reduction.

Many advances have been made in the management of fractures such as immobilization from casting to bracing, or a combination of both. The term *cast brace* has been applied to a form of treatment in which the brace design is incorporated into temporary standard cast materials. This method allows for limited motion in the brace during the early healing stage with controlled fracture movement. Its use has shown greater callus formation around the fracture site, improved ligamentous healing, and earlier recovery of joint mobility and muscle control.

Another method of fracture management employs magnetic and electrical bone stimulators, some with *surface electrodes* externally applied to a fracture site. Electromagnetic models use different modalities to effect an electric field that theoretically will induce piezoelectric microcurrents that help stimulate bone formation. Ultrasonic bone stimulation is also used and has recently been found to be more effective than previously thought.

An option of traumatic fracture management is the use of external fixation devices and frames, also called *fixateurs* or *fixators*. External fixation is a diverse system for managing loss of skeletal stability with various components placed in bone. Treatment methods and external skeletal fixation devices are discussed in Chapter 8. An external fixator is described procedurally as *monoplanar* or *multiplanar*. Fixators applied to an extremity are most commonly a combination of monoplanar devices. Two pins with a clamp or connecting bar between them on any given bone segment compose a monoplanar fixator. Several monoplanar segments can be applied and connected to each other for added stability. An example is a spanning knee frame, in which a monoplanar fixator to the femur and a monoplanar fixator to the tibia are connected to each other. Even though the construct is in more than one unique plane, the application is more that of monoplanar devices. Alternatively, the multiplanar fixator is typically that of the ring or Ilizarov type fixator. The planning and execution of ringed Ilizarov fixators is much more difficult and therefore considered separately.

Other changes to be noticed are the use of modern technologic terms for implants and procedures. Submuscular plating involves placing a plate underneath muscle using peripherally placed cutaneous incisions. Previously, *minimally invasive percutaneous plate osteosynthesis (MIPPO)* and *minimally invasive osteosynthesis (MIO)* were terms used to describe the same technique. Locked screws are another new and novel development described frequently. This technology allows for the connection of screw to plate through a threaded or interference interface. One may also hear the term *internal fixator*, which is a mechanical analogy to that of an external fixator that is "internalized." Thus a completely locked plate construct placed in a minimally invasive fashion has similar mechanical characteristics to that of an external fixator that is "internalized."

Terminology of Fractures and Dislocations

diastasis: may be one of two types: (1) disjointing of two bones parallel to one another, for example, radius and ulna, tibia and fibula complex; or (2) rupture of any solid joint, as in a diastasis of the symphysis pubis. Such an injury tends to occur in association with other fractures and is then called **fracture-diastasis**.

dislocation: (L., *luxatio*): complete displacement of bone from its normal position at the joint surface, disrupting the articulation of two or three bones at that junction and altering the alignment. This displacement affects the joint capsule and surrounding tissues (muscles, ligaments). Dislocation (**luxation**) may be traumatic (direct blow or injury), congenital (developmental defect), or pathologic (as in muscle imbalance, ligamentous tearing, rheumatoid arthritis, or infection).

fracture: (L., *fractura*): structural break in the continuity of a bone, epiphyseal plate, or cartilaginous joint surface, usually traumatic with disruption of osseous tissue.

fracture-dislocation: fracture of a bone that involves a dislocation of an adjacent articulation of that bone. Example: Shoulder fracture dislocation in which there is a proximal periarticular humerus fracture with an associated dislocation (not subluxation) of the humeral head.

sprain-ligament rupture: (L., *luxatio imperfecta*): stretching or tearing of ligaments (fibrous bands that bind bones together at a joint), varying in degrees from being partially torn (stretched) to being completely torn (ruptured), with the continuity of the ligament remaining intact. After a sprain, the fibrous capsule that encloses the joint may become inflamed, swollen, discolored, and extremely painful. Involuntary muscle spasm, and sometimes a fracture, may occur. Rest, elevation, and a restrictive bandage, splint, or cast are methods of treating these injuries until properly healed. When a ligament or tendon has been torn completely, dislocation may also occur. Surgical repair may be required in some cases.

strain: stretching or tearing of a muscle or its tendon (fibrous cord that attaches the muscle to the bone it moves) may result in bleeding into the damaged muscle area, which causes pain, swelling, stiffness, muscle spasm, and, subsequently, a bruise. A strain can be serious because muscle damage (scar tissue) may cause muscle shortening. With rest, strains will subside in 2-3 days, but symptoms may persist for months.

subluxation: incomplete or partial dislocation in that one bone forming a joint is displaced only partially from its normal position; also, a chronic tendency of a bone to become partially dislocated, in contrast to an outright dislocation, for example, shoulder, patella, and hip.

Classifications of Fractures

Open Versus Closed (Fig. 1-1)

closed f.: does not produce an open wound of the skin but does result in loss of continuity of bone subcutaneously; formerly called *simple f.*

open f.: one of the fragments has broken through the skin, and there is loss of continuity of bone internally; formerly called *compound f.*

Portion of Bone Involved

The portion of bone involved or the point of reference of a fracture may be referred to as the distal third (**D/3**), the middle third (**M/3**), and the proximal third (**P/3**).

FIG 1-1 Closed versus open fracture. *(From Schneider FR:* Handbook for the orthopaedic assistant, *ed 2, St Louis, 1976, The CV Mosby Co.)*

CLOSED FRACTURE OPEN FRACTURE
From within   From without

Middle third fractures are commonly called *midshaft fractures*. For specific anatomic locations, the following terms are commonly used.

apophyseal f.: avulsion of or fracture through an apophysis (bony prominence) where there is strong tendinous attachment.
articular f.: involves a joint surface; also called **joint f.** and **intraarticular f.**
cleavage f.: shelling off of cartilage with avulsion of a small fragment of bone such as the capitellum.
condylar f.: involves any round end of a hinge joint (see sections on femoral and distal humeral fractures).
cortical f.: involves cortex of bone.
diacondylar f.: transcondylar fracture (line across the condyles).
direct f.: results at specific point of injury and is due to the injury itself.
extracapsular f.: occurs near, but outside, the capsule of a joint, especially the hip; also called **extraarticular.**
intracapsular f.: occurs within the capsule of a joint; also called **intraarticular.**
nonphyseal f.: any childhood fracture that does not involve a growth plate.
periarticular f.: occurs near but not involving a joint.
transchondral f.: fracture through cartilage, which may not be apparent unless there is a bone fracture line into the joint; not to be confused with *transcondylar f.*
transcondylar f.: occurs transversely between the condyles of the elbow. This term is also used in fractures of the femur and bones with condyles; also called **diacondylar f.**
tuft f.: involves the distal phalanx (tuft) of any digit.

General Appearance (Fig. 1-2)

avulsion f.: tearing away of a part; a fragmentation of bone where the pull of a strong ligamentous or tendinous attachment tends to forcibly pull the fragment away from the rest of the bone. The fragment is usually at the articular surface.
bursting f.: multiple fragments, usually at the end of a bone; classically, f. of the first cervical vertebra or the body of the vertebra where there is typically displacement of bone into the spinal canal.
butterfly f.: a bone *fragment* shaped like a butterfly and part of a comminuted; usually involves high-energy force delivered to the bone.
chip f.: a small fragment, usually at the articular margin of a joint.
comminuted f.: more than two fragments; described by degree and quantity of pieces, any third fragment of bone will constitute some element of comminution. A butterfly segment is a type of comminution. Typically, comminution is used to describe multiple fracture fragments (highly comminuted) versus only an additional fragment or two (minimally comminuted); also called **splintered fracture** or **multifragmentary fracture.**
complete f.: the bone is completely broken through both cortices.
compression f.: crumbling or smashing of cancellous bone by forces acting parallel to the long axis of bone; applied particularly to vertebral body fractures.
depressed f.: typically an intraarticular depression of fragments, but may also be applied to depressed skull fractures.
double f.: segmental f. of a bone in two places.
epiphyseal f.: involves the portion of the bone that is distal to the physis, which is the growth plate.
fissure f.: crack in one cortex (surface) only of a long bone.
fragility fracture: fracture that occurs with minimal trauma; caused by osteoporosis.
greenstick f.: in children, incomplete, angulated fracture with a partial break; also called **incomplete f., interperiosteal f., hickory-stick f.,** and **willow f.**
hairline f.: nondisplaced fracture line (crack) in the cortex of bone.
impacted f.: fragments are compressed by force of original injury, driving one fragment of bone into adjacent bone.
incomplete f.: cortices of bone are buckled or cracked, but continuity is not destroyed; the cortex is broken on one side and only bent on the other. Microscopically, the fracture is present on bent side, and resorption and callus will occur on this side as well; types are **greenstick f., torus f.**

FIG 1-2 A, Midshaft fractures of the humerus. *1,* Comminuted. *2,* Transverse, undisplaced. *3,* Oblique, undisplaced. *4,* Spiral. *5,* Segmental. **B,** Apposition and alignment of midshaft fractures of the humerus, anteroposterior view. *1,* Perfect end-to-end apposition, perfect alignment. *2,* 50% end-to-end apposition, perfect alignment. *3,* Side-to-side (bayonet) apposition, slight shortening, perfect alignment. *4,* No apposition, approximately 30-degree angulation. *(From Mercier LR: Practical orthopaedics, ed 5, St Louis, 2000, Mosby.)*

infraction f.: small radiolucent line seen in pathologic fractures, most commonly resulting from metabolic problems.

insufficiency f.: a fracture that occurs because bone is made insufficient as a result of osteoporosis or a metabolic process.

linear f.: lengthwise fracture of bone straight line fracture; implies that there is no displacement.

multiple f.: two or more separate lines of fracture in the same bone.

oblique f.: slanted fracture of the shaft on long axis of bone.

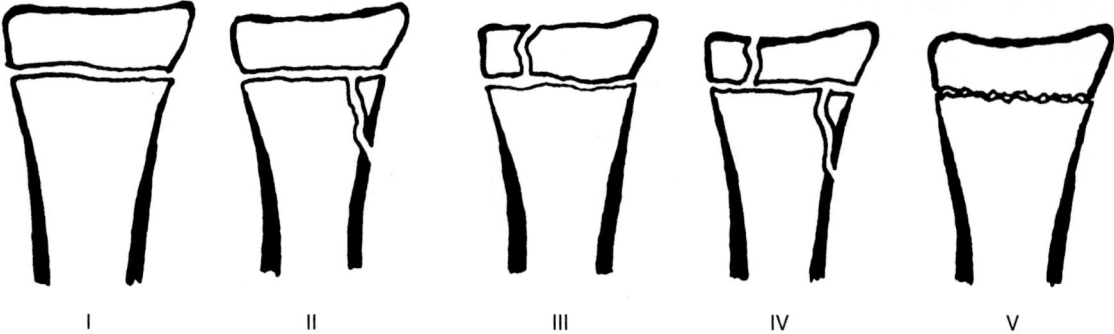

FIG 1-3 Epiphyseal fracture types classified by the Salter method.

occult f.: hidden fracture (undetectable on a radiograph), generally occurring in areas of the ribs, tibia, metatarsals, and navicula.

physeal f: one that involves the cartilaginous growth plate of a bone; also called **epiphyseal slip f., Salter f.,** and **Salter-Harris f.** (Fig. 1-3).

plastic bowing f.: curved deformity of a tubular bone without gross fracture; also called **bowing f., greenstick f.**

secondary f.: pathologic f. of bone weakened by disease.

segmental f.: several large fractures in the same bone shaft where the two principal fragments are not adjacent.

spiral f.: fracture line is spiral shaped, usually on shaft of long bones where the mechanism of injury is usually torsion.

stellate f.: numerous fissures radiate from central point of injury.

subperiosteal f.: bone but not its periosteal tube is broken; uncommon; usually the result of a direct blow.

torus f.: usually noticed in children; a stable, often incomplete f. in which one distal cortical surface appears to be wrinkled by compression forces, and the opposite cortex may or may not be infracted by tension forces.

transverse f.: line of fracture across the shaft at right angles to the long axis of a bone.

unstable f.: fracture that most often requires operative intervention because of the likelihood of recurrent deformity despite manipulation.

Position and Alignment of Fragments (Fig. 1-4)

The *position of a fragment* refers to any displacement of one bone fragment in reference to the next. Displacement, should it exist, can be in any plane. Alignment refers to rotatory or angular deviation of the distal fragment in relation to the proximal fragment. For example:

angulation: typically described by the apex of the deformity. An *apex anterior angulation* means that the "point" or apex of the fracture is pointed anteriorly. This could also be described as *antecurvatum*. An apex posterior angulation is therefore *recurvatum*.

bayonet position: the fragments touch and overlap, but there is good alignment. Internal and external rotation can also be stated in degrees.

bow: the two fragments form an angle where the apex is sometimes described as an anterior or posterior bow.

The descriptive radiographic interpretations of fractures are defined as follows. The *angulation* of the fracture is designated by the direction of the apex of the fracture points. *Fragments* themselves are designated as proximal and distal displacement, which is the amount of offset of the proximal to distal fragment as seen in an anterior to posterior or medial to lateral direction.

When broken ends of the principal fragments are touching, they are said to be in *apposition*. Accuracy or degree of apposition is defined in percentages, such as 50%, indicating at least one radiographic view shows 50% contact and other views may appear to be more.

FIG 1-4 Description of fracture deformity. *(From Schneider FR:* Handbook for the orthopaedic assistant, *ed 2, St Louis, 1976, The CV Mosby Co.)*

The *site* may be diaphyseal, metaphyseal, or epiphyseal portions of a specific bone or may be intraarticular. *Extent* may be described as *complete, incomplete, cracked, hairline, buckled,* or *greenstick*. The *configuration* may be *transverse, oblique,* or *spiral,* and is referred to as *comminuted* when more than two fragments are present. The *fracture fragments* may be *undisplaced* or *displaced*.

Thus a fracture is described radiographically by its site, bone name, extent, configuration, relationship of fragments to each other and to the external environment (open or closed), and the presence or absence of complications.

Classic and Descriptive Names (By Anatomic Location)

Shoulder Fractures (Proximal Humerus and Scapula)

anatomic neck f.: occurs in the area of tendinous attachments, the true neck of humeral metaphysis.
Bankart f.: detachment of a small piece of bone from the anteroinferior rim of the glenoid; seen with anterior shoulder dislocation, usually called a *Bankart fragment*. The cartilage rim may detach without a fracture and this is called a *Bankart lesion*.
coracoid f.: fracture of coracoid process of scapula.
greater tuberosity f.: fracture of bone prominence and attachment of supraspinatus.
lesser tuberosity f.: fracture of bone prominence for attachment of subscapularis.
Hill-Sachs f.: moderate compression f. or indentation f. of the humeral head usually seen after an anterior dislocation of the shoulder. In a classic Hill-Sachs lesion the anterior glenoid causes a dent or defect of the region near the greater tuberosity. A reverse Hill-Sachs is seen with posterior dislocations, and where the defect is in the region of the lesser tuberosity; also called **Hermodsson f.**
surgical neck f.: occurs in area below the anatomic neck of the humerus.

Arm and Elbow Fractures (Distal Humerus)

boxer's elbow: chip f. at the tip of the olecranon caused by a fast extension of the elbow in a missed jab (punch).
condylar f.: occurs at the medial or lateral articular process of the humerus at the elbow.
epicondylar f.: occurs through one of the two epicondyles, medial or lateral.
Holstein-Lewis f.: involves the humerus at the junction of the middle and distal thirds; associated with radial nerve paralysis because of nerve proximity to posterior septum and bone.
Kocher f.: semilunar chip f. of capitellum with displacement into joint.
Laugier f.: involves the trochlea of the humerus.
Malgaigne f.: extension mechanism supracondylar f. of humerus; name also applied to a vertically dissociated fracture dislocation of the pelvis and a proximal fibular fracture.
Posada f.: anteriorly angulated fracture of distal humerus associated with posterior dislocation of radius and ulna.
sideswipe f.: comminuted fracture of distal humerus and sometimes radius and ulna caused by direct blow against elbow.
supracondylar f.: occurs through the distal metaphysis of the humerus or femur.
T f.: intercondylar fracture shaped like a T.
Y f.: intercondylar fracture shaped like a Y.

Forearm and Wrist Fractures

Barton f.: an intraarticular fracture of the dorsal rim of the distal radius, usually resulting in subluxation of the radial carpal joint with the fracture site fragment.
chauffeur's f.: oblique fracture of the radial styloid caused by a twisting- or snapping-type injury; also called **backfire f., Hutchinson f.,** and **lorry driver's f.**
chisel f.: incomplete, usually involving medial head of radius, with fracture line extending distally.
Colles f.: named prior to x-ray technology; implies a fracture of the distal radius, either articular or nonarticular, with dorsal angulation of the distal fragment producing a silver fork deformity; generally associated with a fracture of the ulnar styloid.
corner f.: a small bucket-handle-appearing fracture in the distal metaphyseal corner in a young child, often associated with child abuse.
de Quervain f.: combination of a wrist scaphoid fracture with volar dislocation of scaphoid fragment and lunate.
dye-punch f.: an intraarticular fracture of the ulnar (volar) portion of the distal radius, usually caused by direct impaction of the lunate onto the lunate fossa of the distal radius.
Essex-Lopresti f.: a comminuted radial head fracture with an injury to the distal radioulnar joint caused by disruption of the interosseous membrane, which can cause a proximal migration of the radius if the radial head is excised secondarily.

Galeazzi f.: typically a displaced fracture of the distal third or quarter of the radius with disruption of the distal radioulnar joint; called **fracture of necessity** because surgical fixation is required for reduction; also called a **reverse Monteggia f., Dupuytren f.,** or **Piedmont f.**

Kocher f.: fracture of capitellum of distal humerus with possible displacement of fragment into joint.

Laugier f.: isolated fracture of the trochlea of the humerus at the elbow.

lead pipe f: typically in the forearm, a combination of greenstick fracture and torus fracture in the immature skeleton. Such fractures do not penetrate the entire shaft of the bone and have the appearance of a slightly bent lead pipe.

Lenteneur's f.: a distal radial fracture of the palmar rim, similar to Smith's type II fracture.

Monteggia f.: isolated fracture of proximal third of ulna, with posterior or anterior dislocation of radial head allowing angulation and overriding of ulnar fragments.

Moore f.: like a Colles f.; specifically, fracture of distal radius with dorsal displacement of ulnar styloid and impingement under annular ligament.

Mouchet f.: involves humeral capitellum.

nightstick f.: undisplaced fracture of the ulnar shaft caused by a direct blow.

Piedmont f.: oblique f. usually at the proximal portion of distal third of the radius; obliquity runs from proximal ulnar to distal radial aspect, allowing distal fragments to be pulled into the ulna by the pronator quadratus muscle; fracture of necessity requiring operative management.

radial head f.: involves the most proximal part of the radius, a dish-shaped portion of bone.

radial styloid f.: involves distal radial tip of radius.

reverse Barton f.: dorsal displacement of carpus on radius, with associated fracture of dorsal articular surface of radius. The mechanism and appearance of this fracture are similar to those of a Colles f.

Skillern f.: open f. of distal radius associated with greenstick f. of distal ulna.

Smith f.: fracture of the distal radius in which the distal fragment is displaced volarly; also called **reverse Colles f.** This fracture was defined before the advent of radiography, and, classically, there are three types:

Nonarticular
Intraarticular; also called **volar Barton f.**
Oblique nonarticular fracture near the joint line

Hand Fractures

Bennett f.: fracture of the base of the thumb metacarpal, usually leaving a volar ulnar fragment attached to a retaining ligament with radial subluxation of the metacarpal.

crush f.: term used for comminuted impaction of any bone, but for the finger is a distal phalanx fracture resulting from a crush injury.

mallet f.: avulsion f. of the extensor tendon from the dorsal base of the distal phalanx of any digit that includes insertion of extensor apparatus, thus allowing distal segment to drop into flexion; also called **baseball finger, drop finger,** and **mallet finger deformity.**

Rolando f.: an intraarticular comminuted fracture of the base of the thumb metacarpal resulting in a Y- or T-shaped fracture at the base of the metacarpal.

unciform f.: fracture of the hook of the hamate, usually caused by direct trauma that may or may not be associated with ulnar neuropathy.

Wilson f.: involves the proximal volar portion of the middle phalanx because of strong attachment of volar plate.

Spine Fractures

burst fracture: Involved a compressive fracture of the vertebra that can disrupt stability and cause retropulsion of bone into the spinal canal resulting in paralysis. Depending on severity and location, they can be treated by bracing or require extensive surgical intervention.

Chance f.: involves vertebra, with horizontal splitting of spinous process and neural arch with disruption through vertebral body; an unstable fracture.

compression fracture: most frequently a "wedge-shaped" compression fracture seen in older adults. They contribute to deformity of a "hunched" back commonly seen in older adults, and are mostly painful and do not risk neurologic compromise. They may be just as disabling and commonly caused by low-energy mechanisms (jolt or fall) with bone insufficiency resulting from osteoporosis.

clay shoveler's f.: involves spinous process(es) C-6, C-7, T-1, T-2, or T-3.

hangman's f.: posterior element (pedicles) fracture with anterior subluxation of the cervical neck of C-2 on C-3.

Jefferson f.: bursting f. of the ring of the first cervical vertebra (atlas).

posterior element f.: broad term used to describe any fracture of the spinous process, lamina, facets, pars interarticularis, or pedicle.

seatbelt f.: thoracic or lumbar spine fracture resulting from tensile stress that occurs on spine with forward motion of thorax with abdominal or thoracic restraint resulting in bony or ligament disruption. If only the bone is involved, the injury is called a **Chance f.**

sentinel f.: a cervical spine fracture characterized by fractures through the lamina on either side of the spinous process. A sentinel of potential instability.

slice f.: an unstable lumbar spine fracture caused by a flexion rotation injury that results in a fracture in the upper body of the lower vertebra and a dislocation of the articular process of the upper vertebra.

spondyloptosis: dislocation of one vertebra from another without any bone fracture.

teardrop f.: exists in two forms: (1) an isolated anteroinferior fracture of the cervical spine (unstable); or (2) a three-part, two-plane fracture of an anteroinferior corner of the vertebral body (the teardrop), a sagittal vertebral body, and the posterior neural arch.

vertebra plana f.: wafer-thin compression f. of a vertebral body resulting from an intrinsic pathologic condition of the bone.

wedge f.: anterior compression f. of any vertebra; most common in the dorsal thoracic spine.

Pelvis, Hip, and Proximal Femur Fractures

acetabular fracture: Any fracture that involves the acetabulum (socket).

basal neck f.: involves base of femoral neck at junction of trochanteric region **basicervical.**

bucket-handle f.: vertical shear fracture of anterior pubis and opposite ilium.

central f.: acetabular fracture, centrally displaced through inner wall of pelvis.

dashboard f.: posterior lip of acetabulum chips when femoral head is driven against it; often caused by a sudden jolt when knee hits dashboard.

dome f.: acetabular fracture involving weight-bearing surface of the acetabulum. This term can also be applied to a fracture of the superior surface of the talus.

Duverney f.: involves ilium just below the anterosuperior spine.

extracapsular f.: occurs outside of joint capsule of humerus or femur.

femoral neck f.: transcervical fracture through midportion of femoral neck.

hip f.: implies a fracture of the femoral neck or intertrochanteric area.

intracapsular f.: commonly used for high femoral neck fractures, but is also used for any fracture within a joint capsule.

intertrochanteric f.: the principal plane of the fracture disrupts the intertrochanteric line.

Malgaigne f.: occurs through wing of the ilium or sacrum with associated fractures through the ipsilateral pubic rami, allowing upward displacement of hemipelvis; often associated with internal injuries.

open book f: pelvis fracture with symphysis separation and disruption of the sacral pelvic ligaments to give appearance of opening a book.

pertrochanteric f.: involves proximal femur where the fracture line passes through both the lesser and greater trochanters.

ring f.: involves at least two parts of pelvic circumference.

shaft f.: occurs between subtrochanteric and supracondylar area.

sprinter's f.: involves anterosuperior or anteroinferior spine of ilium, with a fragment of bone being pulled forcibly by sudden muscular pull.

straddle f.: double f. or dislocation of the pubis usually caused by a straddling mechanism, for example, falling onto a rail with the point of contact between the legs.

subcapital f.: femoral fracture at head-neck junction.

subtrochanteric f.: transverse f. of femur just below lesser trochanter.

Waddell triad: femoral fracture associated with head and thorax injuries.

Walther f.: transverse ischioacetabular f. where the fracture line passes from ischial spine to acetabular cavity to ischiopubic junction.

Distal Femur, Knee, Tibia, and Fibula Fractures

bumper f.: involves the tibia or femur and is caused by a direct blow in area of the tibial tuberosity; commonly caused by a car bumper accident; may be bilateral.

cartwheel f.: fracture of the distal femoral epiphysis in a child, so named by mechanism of a leg caught in the spokes of a cartwheel.

clipping injury f.: fracture through growth plate of distal femur or proximal tibia caused by a strike from the lateral side of the knee when the foot is planted.

Hoffa f.: coronal fracture of medial femoral condyle.

patellar f.: involves kneecap.

pillion f.: T-shaped fracture of distal femur with displacement of the condyles posteriorly to femoral shaft, caused by severe blow to knee; so named for pillion back seat position of a motorcycle rider who sustains this injury. Not to be confused with pilon fracture, that is due to a vertical impaction of the distal tibia into the talus.

Segond f.: small avulsion f. of superolateral tibia caused by tension on the lateral capsule or ligament; usually associated with other severe ligamentous injuries leading to anterolateral knee instability; also called **lateral capsule sign.**

sleeve f.: involves a small chip of bone from the superior or inferior portion of the patella associated with loss of integrity of quadriceps extensor mechanism.

Stieda f.: avulsion f. of origin of medial collateral ligament on medial femoral condyle.

supracondylar f.: involves the distal shaft of bone above condyles of femur or humerus.

tibial plateau f.: involves proximal tibial articular surface.

toddler f.: nondisplaced fracture of the tibia seen in toddlers beginning to walk.

wagon wheel f.: involves distal femoral epiphysis in children; also called **cartwheel f.**

Y and T f.: combined supracondylar and intercondylar f. of the distal femur.

Ankle and Foot Fractures

ankle mortise diastasis: separation of tibia and fibula at ankle; often associated with a fracture or dislocation.

aviator's astragalus: denotes a talar neck fracture caused by sudden impaction of foot into ankle; may be associated with other fractures about the foot and ankle.

bimalleolar ankle f.: in which both the medial malleolus and distal fibula are fractured; also called **Pott f.**

bimalleolar equivalent: a fracture of the medial or lateral malleolus with ligamentous damage on the opposite side of an ankle.

boot-top f.: involves transverse, distal third of tibia, occurring at boot top of old-style ski boot; also called **skier's injury.**

Bosworth f.: fracture-dislocation of the ankle, with oblique fracture of the distal fibula and displacement of the proximal fibular fragment out of fibular groove to a place posterior and medial to the posterolateral ridge of the tibia.

bunkbed f.: intraarticular f. of the base of the first metatarsal in children.

Cedell f.: fracture of the posterior medial process of the talus; may be associated with tarsal tunnel syndrome.

Chaput f.: involves the anterior tubercle of distal tibia because of strong attachment of anterior tibiofibular ligament.

Conrad-Bugg trapping: incarceration of soft tissue, usually the posterior tibial tendon, between fragments of an ankle fracture. This produces an injury that usually is reduced by open methods.

Cotton f.: partial forward dislocation of the tibia to produce a fracture of the posterior inferior margin of the tibia, sometimes called the **posterior malleolus.** This is most commonly associated with a fibular fracture.

Descot f.: involves the posterior lip of tibia.

dome f.: involves the superior articular surface of talus or the weight-bearing portion of the acetabulum.

Dupuytren f.: spiral f. of the distal end of fibula; associated with ankle diastasis.

Gosselin f.: V-shaped fracture of the distal tibia into the tibiotalar joint.

Henderson f.: trimalleolar fracture of the ankle.

Jones f.: fracture of the base of the fifth metatarsal such that the fracture line extends from lateral to medial cortex in the shaft portion of the apophyseal tip. This term has been misapplied to fractures in the proximal apophyseal portion.

Kohler f.: involves the navicular and is associated with avascular necrosis; seen in children.

Lisfranc f.: usually a fracture-dislocation, with displacement of the proximal metatarsals.

Maisonneuve f.: spiral f. of proximal end of fibula, near the neck, associated with a tear of the anterior tibiofibular ligament and the potential for ankle diastasis.

march f.: stress f. of metatarsal caused by excessive marching; also called **fatigue f.**

midnight f.: open, oblique fracture of proximal phalanx of little toe caused by stubbing the toe on a solid object.

Montercaux f.: fracture of fibular neck with associated diastasis of ankle mortise.

paratrooper f.: involves posterior articular margin of tibia or lateral malleolus.

Pott f.: spiral oblique f. of distal fibula with associated rupture of the deltoid ligament; avulsion of the medial malleolus and lateral displacement of foot on tibia.

plafond f.: any fracture that involves the surface of the tibia that comes in contact with the dome of the talus.

Shepherd f.: involves posterior talus with sheared off piece of bone and, in some instances, a separate piece of bone (os trigonum).

Tillaux Kleiger f.: involves distal lateral tibia, vertically extending into the joint; sometimes associated with diastasis and other fractures about the ankle.

tongue f.: involves the posterosuperior portion of calcaneus.

trimalleolar f.: fracture of medial, lateral, and posterior malleolus.

triplane f.: involves the ankle in three planes: coronally through the posterior tibial metaphysis, transversely through the growth plate, and sagittally through the distal tibial epiphysis.

Volkmann f.: involves a triangular portion of the posterior lateral tibia into the joint, leaving a triangular bone fragment sometimes called **Volkmann's triangle**.

Wagstaffe f.: separation of a distal anterior fragment of the fibula, that is, the portion of attachment of the anterior tibiofibular ligament; also called **Le Fort f.**

Contributing Factors

Aside from a single obvious traumatic event, other factors contribute to fractures.

dyscrasic f.: results from weakening of bone by a disease process.

endocrine f.: occurs in bone weakened by an endocrine disorder.

fatigue f.: spontaneous fracture in healthy bone resulting from fatigue or stress produced by excessive physical activity in a short period; seen in fibulas and tibias of young long-distance runners, the hips and heels of young military recruits, and in the metatarsals; also called **stress f., march f.**

hoop stress f.: involves the medial or anteromedial femoral neck and occurs during broaching of the femoral canal for a prosthesis or during the actual impaction of the prosthesis.

inflammatory f.: occurs in association with inflammation secondary to an infection, such as syphilis.

insufficiency f.: stress f. that occurs in bone because of its diminished volume (i.e., osteopenia).

neoplastic f.: a form of pathologic f. Presence of a tumor in bone, whether originating in the bone or metastatic from elsewhere, causes sufficient weakening to allow it to fracture spontaneously or with less trauma than it would normally take to break a healthy bone.

neuropathic f.: fracture caused by overuse trauma to bone that occurs because of lack of pain perception.

pathologic f.: occurs with or without trauma where bone has been weakened by a local or systemic process. The most common causes are a tumor (benign or malignant), local infection, or bone cyst. This term is less widely applied to congenital disorders such as osteogenesis imperfecta, osteopetrosis, and neurofibromatosis. The term is applied more to congenital or acquired disorders such as osteomalacia, rickets, Paget disease, scurvy, and osteoporosis.

pseudofracture: radiographic finding of a line through bone that is due to abnormal mineralization that occurs in osteomalacia.

spontaneous f.: fracture that occurs without abnormal force. Usually caused by a pathologic condition of the bone or the cumulative overuse of a bone where the response to repeated stress is sufficient for a fracture to occur.

stress f.: crack in bone from overexertion placed on bone structure of limb or metatarsals and from pull of muscle on bone. Not noticeable on initial radiograph but is on later radiographs when callus formation has taken place at the site. A bone scan or magnetic resonance imaging will show the fracture; also called **march f., fatigue f.** More recently, the term **stress reaction to bone** has been used because fracture lines often do not appear and because the term more accurately describes the condition.

tension f.: bone fails at right angle to the direction of a tension force resulting in a transverse fracture.

Degree and Nature of Healing

The quality of bone healing is stated in terms of the solidity of adhesiveness of the bone fragments. As most fractures heal, a surrounding sleeve of bone, or **callus,** is formed. This new bone formation is composed of cartilage, bone, blood vessels, and fibrous tissue and is often referred to in discussing bone healing. If the bone is completely healed, the term **healed** is used. Anything less is considered a *state of healing,* unless there is *a failure of progression of healing with expectation of no further healing.* This is then considered a **nonunion.**

The absence of complete union is called **ununited,** but this term by some users implies an expectation of failure to unite. In **delayed union** the speed of callus formation (fracture healing) is slower than anticipated, but this does not imply expectancy of either total healing or nonunion. A **pseudoarthrosis** is the formation of a jointlike structure at the old fracture site and is a type of nonunion. It consists of fibrocartilaginous tissue and a synovial fluid sac. If a bone unites in an abnormal position or alignment, the term **malunion** is used. If two bones parallel to one another unite by osseous tissue, such as the tibia/fibula or ulna/radius complex, the result is a **crossunion,** or **synostosis.**

For example, in a simple fracture of the midshaft of the radius and ulna, assume that the radius adheres to the ulna at the distal fracture site and that the radius does not heal because of angulated healing of the ulna. Such a situation can be described as a **malunited fracture** of the **midshaft** of the ulna with a nonunion of the radius and crossunion of the distal radius and ulna. When the diagnoses are listed, they might be given as (1) malunion, fracture, closed, midshaft, ulna, right; or (2) nonunion, fracture, closed, midshaft, radius, right, associated with crossunion.

Secondary union has multiple meanings. It implies delayed healing either by the eventual adhesion of granulating surfaces of bone fragments or surgical intervention late in the course of fracture healing to promote union.

Nutritional support is important in bone healing to augment medical and surgical care. Bones need mineral and protein to heal, another consideration in treatment.

International Classification System and Trauma Registry System

AO/ASIF Long Bone Fractures

This is a scheme of fracture classification for research purposes and a more uniform description in the literature. The scheme has not been validated or used by all investigators. It tends to be cumbersome in some instances, but in certain locations, the first letter and number modifier is very useful in describing the extent and pattern of fracture. For example, a C3 distal femur fracture is notated as *33.C3.* This system is most commonly used in the distal femur, distal tibia, and distal humerus.

- The system defines bones by number (**1,** humerus; **2,** radius and ulna; **3,** femur; **4,** tibia and fibula; **5,** spine, jaw, clavicle, and scapula; **6,** pelvis and sacrum; **7,** hand; **8,** foot).
- Nature of fracture is identified by letter (**A,** simple involving at least 90% of the cortex or extraarticular; **B,** wedge with some contact between fragments or partial articular; **C,** complete with no contact between fragments or complete articular).

- Degree of comminution is identified by number (A: **1**, spiral; **2**, oblique; **3**, transverse less than 30 degrees. B: **1**, spiral wedge; **2**, bending wedge; **3**, fragmented wedge. C: **1**, spiral; **2**, segmental; **3**, irregular).
- The subgroups .1, .2, and .3 further define the complexity of each of the above groupings.
- Limitation: agreement among raters.*

AO/ASIF Soft Tissue Classification

For uniform description in the literature.

Integumentary Injury (I)
Closed (C)

IC1: no skin lesion
IC2: contusions but no skin laceration
IC3: circumscribed degloving
IC4: extensive closed degloving
IC5: necrosis from contusion

Open (O)

IO1: skin breakage from inside out
IO2: skin breakage from outside in < 5 cm, contusion at edges
IO3: skin breakage > 5 cm, increased contusion, devitalized edge
IO4: considerable full thickness contusion, abrasion, extensive open degloving, skin loss

Muscle/Tendon (MT) Injury

MT1: no muscle injury
MT2: circumscribed muscle injury, one compartment only
MT3: circumscribed muscle injury, two compartments
MT4: muscle defect, tendon laceration, extensive muscle contusion
MT5: compartment syndrome, crush syndrome with wide injury zone

Neurovascular (NV) Injury

NV1: no neurovascular injury
NV2: isolated nerve injury
NV3: isolated vascular injury
NV4: extensive segmental vascular injury
NV5: combined neurovascular injury, subtotal and total amputation.*

Classification Systems by Grades, Types, and Mechanisms

The trend toward standard classification of fractures and dislocations is certainly a step forward, but such a system is designed for computer storage and is sometimes difficult to apply when viewing a fracture for the first time. It should not be forgotten that most of these specific classification systems were developed to address a specific set of circumstances. Attempting to apply them to other areas frequently leads to misinterpretation and erroneous conclusions. The authors, therefore, feel that these systems should be interpreted as meant by the original authors. The reference is indicated in a footnote (see Bibliography for full reference citations).

Allman Classification for Clavicle Fractures[†]

To define location of most common sites of occurrence and of nonunion.

Group I: fractures of middle third
Group II: fractures distal to coracoclavicular ligament, nonunion frequent
Group III: fractures of proximal end; nonunion and displacement rare

Limitations: does not incorporate other factors such as degree of trauma.

Anderson and d'Alonzo Classification for Odontoid Fractures of the Second Cervical Vertebra[‡]

Based on location of fracture; to define fracture pattern likely to require surgery for healing.

Type I: avulsion fracture of tip of odontoid
Type II: fracture at junction of odontoid to body of vertebra

---

*Müller ME et al, 1991.

[†] Allman FL.
[‡] Anderson LD and D'Alonzo RT.

Type III: fracture line extends downward into cancellous bone of body of vertebra

Ashurst Classification for Ankle Sprains and Fractures*

Based on direction or mechanism of force.

External Rotation Injuries (Supination)

first degree: transsyndesmotic fracture of the fibula
alternate first degree: rupture of the anterior tibiofibular ligament with or without spiral fracture of the proximal fibula
second degree: rupture of the deltoid ligament
alternate second degree: avulsion of the medial malleolus
third degree: fracture of the entire lower end of the tibia and fibula with external rotation

Abduction Injuries (Pronation)

first degree: transverse fracture of the medial malleolus at or below its base
second degree: rupture of the deltoid ligament or fracture of the medial malleolus followed by a fracture of the distal fibula
third degree: fracture of both lower tibia and medial malleolus lateral displacement

Adduction Injuries (Supination)

first degree: avulsion of the fibular malleolus at or below its base
second degree: avulsion of the fibular malleolus at or below its base with medial malleolus below plafond, a shear vertically into tibial shaft
third degree: supramalleolar fracture in both the tibia and fibula with medial displacement

Fracture by Compression in Long Axis of Leg

first degree: isolated marginal fracture of the distal weight-bearing plate of the tibia
second degree: comminution of the tibial plafond
third degree: T or Y fractures (V fracture of Gosselin)

Limitations: fracture patterns overlap.

Badelon Classification for Lateral Condylar Fractures of the Humerus in Children*

Roentgenographic basis for stability versus displacement, which requires surgical reduction.

Type I: nondisplaced fracture that can be seen only on one view
Type II: visible fracture line with minimal displacement
Type III: displacement of more than 2 mm on all views
Type IV: severe displacement with complete separation of fracture edges

Bado Classification for Fractured Ulna with Dislocation of the Radial Head [Monteggia]†

Based on mechanism of injury; to help define management.

Type 1: fracture of any portion of the ulna diaphysis with anterior angulation and anterior dislocation of the radial head
Type 2: fracture of the ulnar diaphysis with posterior angulation and posterior or posterolateral dislocation of the radial head
Type 3: fracture of the ulnar metaphysis with lateral or anterolateral dislocation of the radial head
Type 4: proximal fracture of both bones at the same level with anterior dislocation of the radial head

Limitations: some controversy as to relationship to treatment; types I and II have equivalents that involve dislocation radial head only (type 1) and fractured radial head.

Bohn and Durbin Classification for Epiphyseal Fractures of the Distal Femur and Proximal Tibia Resulting in a "Floating Knee"‡

Too complicated for inclusion, a complex system based on angulation, dislocation, and associated injury. See Arslan H et al.

---

*Ashurst APC.

*Badelon O et al.
†Bado JL.
‡Arslan H et al.

Brendt and Harty Modified Classification for Fractures or Development of Osteochondritis Dissecans of the Dome of the Talus*

To define stages of osteochondritis of bone.

Stage I: normal x-ray but positive bone scan or change seen on magnetic resonance imaging (repeated minitrauma)
Stage II: incomplete separation of subchondral fragment (single injury event)
Stage IIA: cyst formation (repeated minitrauma)
Stage III: complete separation of fragment, which is in anatomic position (single injury event)
Stage IV: separation of fragment (single injury event)

Boyd and Griffin Classification for Extracapsular Fractures of Proximal Femur from Neck to 5 cm Distal to Lesser Trochanter†

To define surgical approach and prognosis for fractures near and around the femoral neck.

Type 1: intertrochanteric f., simple to reduce and maintain
Type 2: intertrochanteric f. with comminution and additional coronal seen from lateral
Type 3: subtrochanteric f. with at least one fracture line passing just distal to or through lesser trochanter
Type 4: fractures of the trochanteric region and proximal shaft and fracture in two planes requiring two-plane fixation

Limitations: crosses over from subtrochanteric fracture type to intertrochanteric and neck fractures.

Bryan and Morrey Classification for Capitellar Fractures

To define shape and direction of elbow capitellar fractures.

Type 1: shear fracture in plane of capitellum involving none or little of the trochlea
Type 2: a variable amount of the cartilage of the capitellum with minimal attached subchondral bone
Type 3: comminuted or compression fracture of the capitellum

Canale-Kelly Classification for Talar Fractures*

Based on location of fracture and association with displacement and effect on blood supply; to define prognosis for long-term outcome with particular reference to avascular necrosis.

Type I: minimal displacement, only one source of blood supply might be disrupted
Type II: subtalar subluxation or dislocation, two or three sources of blood supply might be affected
Type III: body of talus dislocated from the ankle and the subtalar joint
Type IV: fracture of talar neck associated with dislocation of the body from the ankle, or subtalar joint and additional subluxation or dislocation of the head of the talus from the talonavicular joint

Cervical Spine Injury Score System

Four columns: anterior, right pillar, left pillar, and posterior.

For each column, an analogue scale using fracture displacement and ligament disruption is given:

Fracture nondisplaced with mild ligamentous 1–3 mm (analogue scale 0–1)
Fracture displaced 1–3 mm, mild ligamentous 1–3 mm (analogue scale 1–2)
Fracture displaced 1–3 mm, moderate ligamentous 3–5 mm (analogue scale 2–3)
Fracture displaced 3–5 mm (analogue scale 3–4)
Fracture displaced > 5 mm, severe ligamentous > 5 mm (analogue scale 4–5)

Chadwick and Bentley Classification for Distal Tibia Fractures Affecting Epiphysis in Children†

Based on x-ray analysis; reflects the mechanism of type IV Salter fractures of the distal tibia and fibula and helps predict retardation of growth.

---

*Anderson IF.
†Boyd HR and Griffin LL.

*Canale ST and Kelly FB.
†Chadwick CJ and Bentley G.

Group I: epiphysis not fractured
  Group 1a: abduction injury with fracture of the distal fibular shaft and lateral displacement
  Group 1b: supination/hyperplantar flexion injury with posterior metaphyseal fragment of the tibia and posterior displacement
  Group 1c: supination/external rotation injury with large anteromedial metaphyseal component, tibia, and posterior displacement
  Group 1d: adduction injury (rare), posteromedial metaphyseal fragment of the tibia with fracture of the distal fibular shaft and medial displacement
Group II: vertical fracture through epiphysis with shift of lateral fragment
Group III: adduction injury, Salter type I or II fibular slip with type IV medial malleolar fracture

Colonna (Delbet) Classification for Hip Fractures in Children*

Attributes classification to Delbet; no purpose given.

Type I: transepiphyseal separations with or without dislocation of femoral head
Type II: transcervical fractures, displaced and nondisplaced
Type III: cervicotrochanteric fractures, displaced and nondisplaced
Type IV: intertrochanteric fractures

Colton Classification for Olecranon Fractures†

To define treatment.

Avulsion group: transverse fracture line separating a small fragment of olecranon with or without displacement
Oblique group: primary failure being an oblique line from the trochlear notch to the distal outer ulnar shaft, degree of comminution staged a to d
  Stage a: single fracture line, displaced and nondisplaced
  Stage b: nondisplaced single central large V-shaped fragment
  Stage c: displaced single central large V-shaped fragment
  Stage d: highly comminuted central pieces of bone with displacement
Fracture dislocation (Monteggia group): fracture line at or slightly proximal to coronoid, which may result in anterior fracture or dislocation of the elbow
Unclassified group: high energy, highly comminuted fractures not matching previous descriptions

Denis Classification for Sacral Fractures

Denis 1: Lateral to foramen
Denis 2: Through or involving foramen
Denis 3: Medial to foramen

Dias-Tachdjian Classification for Ankle Fractures in Children*

Uses Lauge-Hansen guidelines, foot position, and direction of force in correlation with the Salter-Harris classification to plan surgical and other treatment approaches.

Supination-inversion: inversion force applied to supinated foot
  Grade I: Salter-Harris type I or II of distal fibular epiphysis
  Grade II: grade I with Salter-Harris type III or IV of tibial epiphysis
Supination-plantar flexion: plantar flexion force on supinated foot
  Grade I: Salter-Harris type I or II of distal tibia, usually with posterior displacement
Supination-external rotation: external rotation ankle force on fully supinated foot
  Grade I: Salter-Harris type II of distal tibia with long spiral fracture of distal tibia
  Grade II: grade I with spiral fracture of fibula
Pronation-eversion-external rotation: a combination of eversion and external rotation force on pronated foot
  Grade I: posterolateral displacement of Salter-Harris type II tibial fracture with short oblique fibular fracture above physis

Limitations: fractures not covered under this system include Salter-Harris type III distal tibia and triplane fracture (as described by author).

---

*Colonna PC.
†Colton CL.

*Dias LS and Tachdjian MO.

Essex-Lopresti Classification for Os Calcis Fractures*

Based on direction of injury force (A–C superior to inferior, and D–F anterosuperior to posteroinferior); helps define method of closed and open management.

Type A: nondisplaced fracture inferior to lateral process of talus and through lateral cortex
Type B: type A with shearing of sustentaculum tali along with one-third to one-half of the posterior facet
Type C: type B with depression of joint and superior posterior displacement of distal portion
Type D: affects lateral half or two thirds of subtalar joint and fracture of the lateral cortex without displacement
Type E: type D with superior displacement of anterior portion of calcaneus
Type F: type E with displacement of posterior facet of calcaneus and further superior migration of anterior portion

Evans-Wales Classification for Intertrochanteric Fractures of Femur†

Grouped by stable or unstable and expected response to treatment.

Type I: fracture line extends upward and outward from lesser trochanter:
Undisplaced stable
Displaced reduced with stable medial apposition
Displaced unreduced with no medial apposition
Comminuted unstable with no medial apposition
Type II: reversed obliquity with line from lesser trochanter to inferior lateral cortex

Limitations: directed at open versus closed management, which is no longer used.

Ferkel-Cheng Arthroscopic Classification of Osteochondral Lesions of the Talus‡

To define stages of appearance and attachment of lesion to subchondral bone.

Stage A: smooth, intact, but soft or ballottable
Stage B: rough surface
Stage C: fibrillations or fissures
Stage D: flap present or bone exposed
Stage E: loose, nondisplaced fragment
Stage F: displaced fragment

Ferkel-Sgaglione Classification for CT Classification of Osteochondral Lesions of the Talus)*

To define stages of attachment of subchondral bone.

Stage I: cystic lesion within dome of talus
Stage IIA: cystic lesion with communication to talar dome surface
Stage IIB: open articular surface lesion with overlying nondisplaced fragment
Stage III: nondisplaced lesion with lucency
Stage IV: displaced fragment

Fielding-Magliato Classification for Subtrochanteric Fractures of Femur†

Based on distance from lesser trochanter for selection of method of surgical fixation.

Type 1: at level of lesser trochanter
Type 2: between 2.5 and 5 cm below lesser trochanter
Type 3: 5–7.5 cm below lesser trochanter

Limitations: oblique and comminuted fractures involve more than one level, newer appliances cover a wider spectrum of conditions.

FRAX Fracture Risk Assessment Tool

For assessment of fracture risk using a copyright computer-based algorithm that employs bone density, age, and a number of clinical risk factors to help patients and their doctors predict the likelihood of having a fracture in the next 10 years.

---

*Essex-Lopresti P.
†Evans EM and Wales SS.
‡Ferkel RD et al, 1995.

*Ferkel RD et al, 1990.
†Fielding JW and Magliato HJ.

Frykman Classification for Distal Radial and Ulnar Fractures*

Based on radial joint involvement with and without ulnar styloid fractures to define method of fixation.

Type I: radial extraarticular without ulnar styloid fracture
Type II: radial extraarticular with ulnar styloid fracture
Type III: radiocarpal joint only without ulnar styloid fracture
Type IV: radiocarpal joint only with ulnar styloid fracture
Type V: distal radioulnar joint only without ulnar styloid fracture
Type VI: distal radioulnar joint only with ulnar styloid fracture
Type VII: both radiocarpal and distal radioulnar joint without ulnar styloid fracture
Type VIII: both radiocarpal and distal radioulnar joint with ulnar styloid fracture

Garden Classification for Subcapital Fractures of Femoral Neck†

Based on anteroposterior (AP) and lateral radiographic guidelines for reduction and likelihood of avascular necrosis.

Stage 1: incomplete, impacted, head tilted in posterolateral direction
Stage 2: complete but undisplaced
Stage 3: complete, displaced, but fragments remain in contact
Stage 4: fracture fragments completely displaced, no contact between fragments

Gartland Classification for Supracondylar Fractures of the Humerus in Children‡

Based on displacement; to define surgical treatment.

Type I: undisplaced
Type II: displaced and difficult to hold with cast immobilization
Type III: posteromedial or posterolateral displacement with difficult reduction that is hard to maintain due to periosteal stripping

Gerber Classification for Proximal Humerus Fractures*

Too complicated for inclusion, a complex system based on size, location, and displacement. See Zuix JM et al.

Gustilo Classification for Open Fractures†

Based on intraoperative assessment of size of wound and soft tissue involvement; to determine fixation types and limb salvage.

Type I: clean wound < 1 cm minimal contamination
Type II: laceration > 1 cm without extensive soft tissue damage, flaps, or avulsions
Type IIIA: despite extensive soft tissue damage or high-energy trauma, soft tissue coverage of the bone is adequate. Also includes segmental or highly comminuted fractures regardless of size of wound
Type IIIB: extensive soft tissue laceration with periosteal stripping, exposed bone, usually massively contaminated, requiring soft tissue coverage
Type IIIC: arterial injury, requires repair regardless of size of wound. An arterial injury that does not require repair for limb salvage is not a IIIC

Limitations: types II and III have interobserver variation.

Hawkins Classification for Talar Neck Fractures‡

Based on location of fracture and association with displacement and effect on blood supply; prognosis for long-term outcome with particular reference to avascular necrosis.

Type I: minimal displacement, only one source of blood supply might be disrupted
Type II: subtalar subluxation or dislocation, two or three sources of blood supply might be affected

---

*Frykman G.
†Garden RS.
‡Gartland JJ.

*Zuix JM et al.
†Gustilo RB et al, 1990.
‡Hawkins LG.

Type III: body of talus dislocated from the ankle and the subtalar joint

Herbert and Fisher Classification for Wrist Scaphoid Fractures*

To differentiate between fractures that are likely to unite in 6 to 8 weeks and those that would not; to define need for surgery.

Type A1: nondisplaced tubercle hairline fracture
Type A2: nondisplaced hairline wrist fracture
Type B1: oblique fracture of distal third
Type B2: displaced middle wrist fracture
Type B3: proximal pole fracture
Type B4: fracture dislocation of carpus
Type B5: comminuted fractures
Type C: delayed union
Type D1: fibrous union
Type D2: sclerotic nonunion (pseudoarthrosis)

Limitations: type B5 and C have been deleted; D2 changed to pseudoarthrosis; D3 sclerotic pseudoarthrosis; D4 avascular necrosis.

Hohl-Moore Classification for Tibial Plateau Fractures†

Based on pattern; designed for surgical planning.

Type 1: minimally displaced
Type 2: local compression
Type 3: split compression
Type 4: total condyle
Type 5: both condyles

Limitations: does not take into account ligament injury.

Ideberg Classification for Glenoid Fractures of the Scapula‡

To define mechanism and to compare surgical and nonsurgical treatment.

Type I: avulsion of the anterior margin
Type II: transverse fracture through glenoid fossa with inferior triangular fragment displaced with the humeral head
Type III: oblique fracture through the glenoid exiting on the midsuperior border of the scapula; often associated with acromioclavicular fracture or dislocation
Type IV: horizontal, exiting through medial border of the blade
Type V: type IV with a separation of the inferior half of the glenoid

Isler Classification for Sacral Fractures Involving Lumbosacral Junction

Type I: fracture through foramen of lateral sacrum and transverse process L5
Type II: fracture through foramen of lateral sacrum, superior sacral facet, and transverse process L5
Type III: fracture through foramen of lateral sacrum extending medially at superior margin and transverse process L5

Jensen Classification for Intertrochanteric Femur Fractures*

Modified Evans system to determine possibility of stable reduction and secondary fracture displacement.

Type I: single fracture line, nondisplaced, stable on fixation
Type II: single fracture line, displaced, stable on fixation
Type III: comminuted, not involving the lesser trochanter; risk of loss of reduction
Type Gartland IV: unstable, lesser trochanteric fragment, portion of greater trochanter attached to neck; greater risk of loss of reduction
Type V: unstable lesser and greater trochanteric fragments; greatest risk of loss of reduction

Johansson Classification for Femoral Fractures Following Total Hip Replacement†

To define fracture pattern that is likely to require surgery for healing.

---

*Filan SL and Herber TJ, 1996.
†Hohl M and Moore TM.
‡Ideberg R.

*Jensen JS.
†Johansson JE et al.

Type I: fracture proximal to tip of the prosthesis
Type II: fracture extends from proximal shaft to point distal to tip of prosthesis
Type III: fracture lines entirely below distal tip of prosthesis

Key and Conwell Classification for Pelvic Fractures*

Based on stability and location; to define need for stabilization.

I: fractures without break in pelvic ring
   A. avulsion fractures
      1: anterosuperior spine
      2: anteroinferior spine
      3: ischial tuberosity
II: single break in pelvic ring
   A: fracture of two ipsilateral rami
   B: fracture near or subluxation of symphysis pubis
   C: fracture near or subluxation of the sacroiliac joint
III: double break in pelvic ring
   A: double vertical fractures or dislocation of pubis (straddle)
   B: double vertical fractures or dislocation (Malgaigne)
   C: severe multiple fractures
IV: fractures of the acetabulum
   A: small fragment with dislocated hip
   B: linear fracture associated with nondisplaced pelvic fracture
   C: linear fracture associated with hip joint instability
   D: fracture secondary to central dislocation of the acetabulum

Kilfoyle Classification for Medial Condylar Fractures of the Humerus in Children[†]

To define need for closed (first two types) versus open treatment (type III).

Type I: greenstick impacted fracture on medial condylar apophyseal region, stable
Type II: fracture through the medial condyle into the joint with little or no displacement
Type III: intraarticular fracture of medial epicondyle with displacement and rotation

Kyle Classification for Femoral Trochanteric Fractures*

Based on stability and displacement; to define nail-type management.

Type I: stable, undisplaced intertrochanteric fractures
Type II: stable, displaced varus deformity with fracture of the lesser trochanter
Type III: unstable, displaced fracture of greater trochanter with posteromedial comminution and varus deformity
Type IV: type III with subtrochanteric component

Limitations: designed to compare sliding versus rigid nail; other devices now available.

Lauge-Hansen Classification for Ankle Fractures[†]

Patterns that describe the position of the foot and the forces across the ankle that produced the fracture; to identify surgical and other treatment approaches.

supination-eversion: external or lateral rotation
supination-adduction
pronation-abduction
pronation-adduction

Limitations: interobserver disagreement; eversion a misnomer—it should be external rotation or lateral rotation; mechanism not consistent in producing specific injury.

Letournel and Judet Classification for Acetabular Fractures (Fig. 1-5)[‡]

Based on division into five basic groups (fractures of the posterior wall, posterior column, anterior wall, anterior

---

* Key JA and Conwell HE.
[†] Kilfoyle RM.

* Kyle RF et al.
[†] Lauge-Hansen N.
[‡] Judet R et al.

FIG 1-5 Acetabular fractures. **A,** Fracture of posterior wall. Repair with plate and lag screw. **B,** Fracture of posterior column. Repair with plate and lag screws. **C,** Wedge fracture of anterior wall. Repair with lag screws. **D,** Fracture of anterior column. Repair with plate and long screws. **E,** Transverse fracture. Repair with plate and lag screws. **F,** Posterior column/posterior wall. **G,** Transverse/posterior wall. **H,** T-shaped fracture. Repair with plate and lag screws. **I,** Anterior column/posterior hemitransverse **J,** Both columns. *(Modified from Guyton JL and Perez EA: Fractures of acetabulum and pelvis. In Canale ST, Beaty JH, editors: Campbell's operative orthopaedics, ed 12, Philadelphia, 2013, Elsevier, Fig. 56-17.)*

column, and transverse fractures) to define best surgical approach for reduction.

Elementary

PW: posterior wall
PC: posterior column
AW: anterior wall
AC: anterior column
Tx: transverse

Associated

PC/PW: posterior column and posterior wall
Tx/Pw: transverse and posterior wall
T: T-shaped
APHT: anterior and posterior hemitransverse
ABC: complete, both columns

The transverse component of the fracture in transverse and T-type fractures is commonly further classified based on the location of the transverse fracture relative to the dome or tectum of the acetabulum.

Transtectal: through the superior weight-bearing area (delineated by the sclerotic line above the acetabulum, commonly called the sourcil [eyebrow])
Juxtatectal: Just below the superior region or tectum, and above the cotyloid fossa
Infratectal: Below the cotyloid fossa

Anterior column fractures are divided into three variants:

Low anterior column: exiting at or below the iliopectineal eminence

Middle anterior column: exiting above the acetabulum and below the anterior superior iliac spine (ASIS)

High anterior column: exiting above the ASIS through the iliac crest

The stem of the T fracture is further classified based on its anterior to posterior location.

Anterior, central, or posterior stems: By definition, the stem has to exit into the obturator fossa and out the ischial or pubic ramus. A *transischial* T is a fracture that has its stem contained mostly within the posterior column.

Letts-Vincent-Gouw Classification for Floating Knee Fracture in Children Involving Both Femur and Tibia*

For descriptive purposes.

Type A: both bones diaphyseal closed
Type B: one bone metaphyseal and other diaphyseal closed
Type C: epiphyseal and diaphyseal closed
Type D: one open fracture
Type E: two open fractures with major soft tissue injury

Levine-Edwards Classification for Axis Fracture[†]

Treatment based on location, displacement, and mechanism of injury.

Type I: through neural arch, no angulation, displacement to 3 mm
Type II: through neural arch, angulation, and translation
Type IIa: through neural arch, slight, or no translation but very severe angulation
Type III: severe angulation and displacement with concomitant unilateral or bilateral facet dislocation at second and third cervical vertebrae

Mallory Classification for Femoral Shaft Fractures Occurring during Total Hip Replacement Surgery*

Based on location, prognosis, and degree of internal and external fixation required for healing.

Type I: fracture includes areas of lesser trochanter and calcar.
Type II: fracture extends beyond lesser trochanter to a point up to 4 cm proximal to the prosthetic tip.
Type III: fracture line extends below a point 4 cm above prosthetic tip.

Mason Classification for Radial Head Fractures[†]

Prognosis based on displacement and comminution.

Type I: undisplaced marginal fracture
Type II: displaced segmental
Type III: comminuted
Type IV: comminuted with posterior elbow dislocation

Mast-Spiegel-Pappas Classification for Distal Tibial Fractures Affecting Tibial Plafond, Pilon[‡]

Based on mechanism of deforming load to help define a clear prognosis.

Type I: essentially malleolar fracture with large posterior plafond fragment
Type II: spiral extension mechanism includes a spiral shaft fracture with no comminution plafond
Type III: central compression with impaction of talus into distal tibia, graded A to C per Rüedi and Allgöwer:
  Type IIIA: cleavage fracture of articular surface without displacement
  Type IIIB: significant fracture and dislocation of articular surface without comminution
  Type IIIC: type IIIB with significant comminution and impaction

---

*Letts M et al.
[†]Levine AM and Edwards CC.

*Mallory TH et al.
[†]Mason ML.
[‡]Mast JW et al.

Limitations: the word *pilon* implies impaction into a surface, which is more a posterior or rotatory displacement in types I and II.

Mayo Classification for Olecranon Fractures*

Surgical and closed management based on location, comminution, and stability.

Type I: undisplaced
    IA: noncomminuted
    IB: comminuted
Type II: displaced, stable
    IIA: noncomminuted
    IIB: comminuted
Type III: unstable
    IA: noncomminuted
    IB: comminuted

Meyers-McKeever Classification for Intercondylar Eminence Fractures of the Tibia in Children†

For surgical planning.

Type I: nondisplaced avulsion
Type II: anterior one-third to one-half lifted with posterior rim intact
Type III: completely displaced

Milch Classification for Medial and Lateral Condylar Fractures of the Humerus in Children‡

To define closed versus open treatment.

Type 1: fracture line from trochlear groove to lateral superior or trochlear sulcus to medial superior; more stable on reduction (compression fracture mechanism)
Type 2: fracture line from trochlear sulcus to lateral superior or trochlear groove to medial superior; more unstable (compression fracture-dislocation mechanism)

Monteggia Classification for Fracture of Ulna with Dislocation of Radial Head

Type I: volar bow of ulnar fracture with superior radial head dislocation
Type II: dorsal bow ulnar fracture with inferior radial head dislocation
Type III: lateral bow ulnar fracture with lateral radial head dislocation
Type IV: midshaft radius and ulnar fractures with radial head dislocation

Myerson Classification for Lisfranc Joint Fracture of the Foot

Type A: total incongruity; can be either medially or laterally displaced
Type B1: partial incongruity medial
Type B2: partial incongruity lateral
Type C1: partial divergent displacement
Type C2: total divergent displacement

Neer Classification for Stability of Distal Clavicle Fractures

Type I: interligamentous and stable with proximal and distal fragments stabilized by coracoclavicular ligaments
Type IIA: medial to coracoclavicular ligaments with conoid and trapezoid remaining attached to distal fragment
Type IIB: medial to coracoclavicular ligaments with either the conoid or both the conoid and trapezoid torn
Type III: intraarticular extension into acromioclavicular joint with no ligamentous injury and are stable

Neer Classification for Humeral Head Fractures*

Based on location and number of fragments; to define method of treatment. Note: a part is not a part unless it is separated by 1 cm or more or there is 40 degrees of angulation.

One-part fractures are fractures that do not meet the angulation or displacement criteria.

Two-part fractures have two parts that meet displacement or angulation criteria. Note that there may

---

*Cabenela ME and Morrey B.
†Meyers MH and McKeever FM.
‡Milch H.

*Neer CSI.

be a fracture of greater and lesser tuberosities from the shaft that constitute three parts, but only the components that meet displacement criteria are included in the classification. Thus a fracture with three parts, one of which is undisplaced, may be called a *two-part fracture*.

Three-part fractures have three fracture components that meet displacement and angulation criteria.

Four-part fractures have all parts displaced and angulated that meet criteria.

anatomic neck: two-part (neck and shaft only)
surgical neck: below tuberosity; considered two-part even if comminuted
greater tuberosity: may be two-part, three-part with anatomic neck, or four-part with anatomic neck and lesser tuberosity
lesser tuberosity: may be two-part, three-part with anatomic neck, or four-part with anatomic neck and greater tuberosity
fracture-dislocation, anterior: two-part with greater tuberosity, three-part with anatomic neck and greater tuberosity, four-part with lesser tuberosity
fracture-dislocation, posterior: two-part with lesser tuberosity, three-part with anatomic neck, four-part with greater tuberosity

Limitations: interobserver disagreement on x-ray interpretation.

Neer-Horowitz Classification for Proximal Humeral Physeal Fractures in Children*

Based on location.

Grade I: < 5 mm displacement
Grade II: displaced up to one-third the width of the shaft
Grade III: displaced from one- to two-thirds the width of the shaft
Grade IV: displaced more than two-thirds the width of the shaft

The FEDS System for Classifying Glenohumeral Joint Instability

System based on frequency, etiology, and direction.
Frequency
    Solitary 1 episode
    Occasional 2 -5 episodes
    Frequent >5 episodes
Etiology
    Traumatic
    Atraumatic
Direction
    Anterior
    Inferior
    Posterior
The direction is confirmed at the time of the physical examination using provocative tests to determine directions most closely reproduces symptoms.
Severity
    Subluxation
    Dislocation

O'Driscoll Classification for Coronoid Fractures of the Ulna

Type 1: fractures involve the tip of the coronoid process and are divided into two subtypes based on size of the fracture: subtype I fractures, smaller than 2 mm, and subtype II fractures, larger than 2 mm.
Type 2: fractures involve the anteromedial facet and are divided, based on anatomic location, into three subtypes: subtype I, involving the rim; subtype II, involving the rim and the tip; and subtype III, involving the rim and the sublime tubercle with or without the tip.
Type 3: basal coronoid fractures involving at least 50% of the height of the coronoid; divided into two subtypes, depending on whether the fracture involves the base of the olecranon.

Ogden Classification for Fractures with Injury to All Bone and Cartilage Components that May Affect Growth*

To better define effects on growth, including nonphyseal growth areas.

Type 1: entirely through physis

---

*Neer CSI and Horowitz BS.

*Ogden JA.

1A: undulates through provisional calcification of hypertrophic zone; no effect on growth
1B: more into degenerative cartilage zone and primary spongiosa; no effect on growth
1C: affects a portion of germinal layer of physis leading to bridging bar
Type 2: through provisional calcification and hypertrophic zone with piece of metaphysis
2A: attached metaphyseal fragment
2B: comminuted metaphyseal fragment
2C: shorter metaphyseal fragment that traverses most of metaphysis
2D: similar to type 1C; affects germinal layer of physis with growth effect
Type 3: fracture extends from articular surface through epiphysis up to, but not across, physis
3A: transverse fracture line entirely through physis
3B: transverse fracture line through spongiosa, leaving small portion of metaphysis with epiphysis
3C: local compression of physis
3D: nonarticular epiphysis such as ischial tuberosity
Type 4: fracture extends from articular surface, through epiphysis and past physis to metaphysis
4A: basic transepiphyseal physeal fracture
4B: with line across portion of physis, similar to type 3
4C: involves nonarticular cartilaginous region such as proximal femur
Type 5: affects germinal layer without bony fracture
Type 6: involves zone of Ranvier (ring of cells at margin of physis from local contusion)
Type 7: completely intraepiphyseal
7A: involves both articular cartilage and bone of secondary ossification center
7B: injury to cartilage growth surface on articular surface of epiphysis
Type 8: injury to metaphyseal growth and remodeling mechanism
Type 9: selective injury to diaphyseal growth mechanism, appositional

Limitations: complexity.

Ogden Classification for Disruption of Proximal Tibiofibular Joint

Type A: subluxation laterally, medially, anteriorly and posteriorly
Type B: anterolateral dislocation
Type C: posteromedial dislocation
Type D: superior dislocation with some lateralization.

Ogden Classification for Tibial Tuberosity Fractures in Children*

Need for surgical reduction and fixation.

Type 1: injury to most distal part of tuberosity
1A: mild displacement, relatively stable, possible propagation into main ossification center
1B: separation of fragment from metaphysis with or without separation from rest of the secondary ossification center
Type 2: separation of entire ossification center of tuberosity with possible propagation into main ossification center of proximal end of tibia; fracture of tuberosity segment at juncture of main ossification centers of tibia and tuberosity
2A: without communication of ossification center
2B: with communication of ossification center
Type 3: more severe separation of fragments; propagation of fracture through main proximal tibial epiphysis into joint; disruption of articular surface under anterior attachments of medial or lateral meniscus or both
3A: single displaced fragment
3B: comminuted displaced fragments

Olecranon Classification for Fractures (No Eponym)†

Type I: involves only proximal third of articular surface or no articular surface
Type II: involves middle third of articular surface
Type III: may occur in conjunction with anterior displacement of the radius

Orthopaedic Trauma Association (OTA) Classification for Fractures

Skin

1. Laceration with edges that can be approximated
2. Laceration with edges that do not approximate
3. Laceration associated with extensive degloving

---

* Ogden JA et al.
† Crenshaw AH.

Muscle

1. No muscle in area, no appreciable muscle necrosis, no muscle injury with intact muscle function.
2. Loss of muscle but the muscle remains functional, some localized necrosis in the zone of injury that requires excision; intact muscle-tendon unit.
3. Dead muscle, loss of muscle function, partial or complete compartment excision, complete disruption of a muscle-tendon; muscle defect does not approximate.

Arterial

1. No major vessel disruption
2. Vessel injury without ischemia
3. Vessel injury with distal ischemia

Contamination

1. None or minimal contamination
2. Surface contamination (easily removed, not embedded in bone or deep soft tissue)
3. Contaminant embedded in bone or deep soft tissues, or high-risk environmental conditions (barnyard, fecal matter, dirty water, etc.).

Bone loss

1. None
2. Bone missing or devascularized but still some contact between proximal and distal fragments
3. Segmental bone loss

Pauwels Classification for Femoral Neck Fractures*

Based on angle of fracture to define stability of fracture in management.

Type I: angle of fracture line is 30 degrees from the horizontal.
Type II: angle of fracture line is 50 degrees from the horizontal.
Type III: angle of fracture line is 70 degrees from the horizontal.

Pipkin Classification for Hip Dislocations with Femoral Head Fracture*

Based on location of fracture head and neck when associated with a posterior hip dislocation (type V Epstein Thompson); to determine prognosis for long-term outcome.

Type I: posterior dislocation of the hip with fracture of the femoral head caudad to fovea centralis
Type II: posterior dislocation of the hip with fracture of the femoral head cephalad to fovea centralis
Type III: type I or II with femoral neck fracture
Type IV: type I, II, or III with associated acetabular fracture

Poland Classification for Childhood Fractures Involving Epiphysis†

Entirely descriptive, written at time of development of radiographs.

Type I: separation across physis only
Type II: separation across physis with fragment metaphysis
Type III: separation of portion of epiphysis across physis
Type IV: separation of both portions of epiphysis from physis

Quénu and Küss Modified Classification for Fractures and Dislocations of Tarsometatarsal Articulation‡

To determine the magnitude of soft tissue injury, displacement plane, prognosis, and treatment.

Type A: total incongruity; all five metatarsals displaced in same direction
Type B: partial incongruity:
  medial dislocation
  lateral dislocation
Type C: divergent usually between first and second ray:
  total—all five rays involved
  partial—some lateral rays intact

---

*Pauwels F.

*Pipkin G.
†Poland J.
‡Hardcastle PH et al.

Riseborough and Radin Classification for Distal Humeral Intercondylar T Fractures*

Based on roentgenographic analysis to compare closed versus open treatment.

Type 1: undisplaced fracture between capitellum and trochlea

Type 2: nondisplaced T or Y fracture, with fracture exiting from groove proximally between condyle and then dividing transversely or obliquely across the shaft separating the condyles from each other and the shaft; no appreciable separation or rotation on anteroposterior roentgenogram

Type 3: significant separation with rotational displacement of condyles

Type 4: severe comminution of articular surface and wide condylar separation

Rockwood Classification for Acromioclavicular Separations[†]

To determine degree of injury or need for surgical intervention.

Type I: neither acromioclavicular nor coracoclavicular ligament torn

Type II: acromioclavicular ligament torn but coracoclavicular ligament intact

Type III: both acromioclavicular and coracoclavicular ligaments torn

Type IV: both ligaments torn and clavicle displaced posteriorly through trapezius

Type V: both ligaments torn and wide superior separation of the clavicle

Type VI: both ligaments torn and distal clavicle caught inferior to coracoid and posterior to conjoined tendon

Rowe and Lowell Classification for Central Fracture Dislocations of Acetabulum[‡]

To define surgical planning and risk of complications.

---

* Riseborough EJ and Radin EL.
† Rockwood CA.
‡ Rowe CR and Lowell JD.

Type I: undisplaced (single line or stellate)
Type II: inner wall fractures
  Type IIA: femoral head reduced under acetabular dome initially
  Type IIB: femoral head out, reduced under acetabular dome initially
Type III: superior dome fractures
  Type IIIA: acetabulum generally congruent with femoral head
  Type IIIB: acetabulum incongruent with femoral head
Type IV: bursting fracture (all elements of acetabulum involved)
  Type IVA: fractures with congruity between femoral head and acetabular dome
  Type IVB: fractures with incongruity between femoral head and acetabular dome

Rüedi and Allgöwer Classification for Distal Tibial Pilon Fractures*

Degree of comminution and displacement of articular fragments; to define nature of management of pilon fractures of the distal tibia.

Type A: cleavage fracture of the articular surface without major dislocation of the fragments

Type B: significant fracture and dislocation of the articular surface without comminution

Type C: severe comminution and impaction of tibial articular surface

Russell-Taylor Classification for High Proximal Femoral Fractures[†]

To predict effectiveness of closed nailing techniques.

Group I: does not involve piriformis fossa.
  Group Ia: comminution and fracture line extends from below lesser trochanter to femoral isthmus.
  Group Ib: fracture line and comminution involving area from lesser trochanter to femoral isthmus.
Group II: involvement of piriformis fossa.
  Group IIa: fracture extends from lesser trochanter to isthmus with involvement of piriformis fossa (seen on lateral roentgenogram).

---

* Rüedi T and Allgöwer M.
† Russell TA.

Group IIb: fracture extends into the piriformis fossa (seen on lateral roentgenogram) with significant medial comminution and loss of lesser trochanteric continuity.

Salter-Harris Classification for Fractures Involving the Physis in Children*

To predict growth disturbance and need for exact reduction.

Type I: fracture line across physis only
Type II: fracture line across physis with portion through metaphysis
Type III: fracture through physis and portion of epiphysis
Type IV: fracture line through epiphysis, crosses physis, and out metaphysis
Type V: crush injury to physis

Samilson-Preito Classification for Degenerative Change Associated with Shoulder Dislocation†

Relating degenerative change to timing of treatment.

mild: inferior exostosis of humeral head or glenoid < 3 mm in size on anteroposterior radiograph
moderate: inferior exostosis of humeral head or glenoid between 3 and 7 mm in size with slight joint irregularity
severe: > 8 mm osteophyte with joint narrowing and sclerosis

Schatzker Classification for Tibial Plateau and Proximal Tibial Fracture Patterns‡

Based on pathoanatomic factors, etiologic factors, and therapeutic features; to determine treatment of fracture of the tibial plateau and proximal tibia.

Type I: pure cleavage
Type II: cleavage combined with depression
Type III: pure central depression
Type IV: fracture of medial condyle
Type V: bicondylar fractures
Type VI: plateau fracture with dissociation of tibial metaphysis and diaphysis

Limitations: type V could be divided into axial, laterally tilted, and medially tilted.

Seinsheimer Classification for Femoral Intertrochanteric and Subtrochanteric Fractures*

Based on number of fragments and the location and configuration of fracture lines; to select method of surgical fixation.

Type I: nondisplaced or < 1 mm displacement
Type II: two-part fractures
   Type IIA: transverse
   Type IIB: spiral with lesser trochanter attached to proximal fragment
   Type IIC: spiral with lesser trochanter attached to distal fragment
Type III: three-part fractures
   Type IIIA: spiral with lesser trochanter a part of the proximal fragment
   Type IIIB: spiral with lesser trochanter a butterfly fragment
Type IV: comminuted with four or more fragments
Type V: subtrochanteric-intertrochanteric configuration

Limitations: lesser trochanteric continuity and involvement of piriformis fossa a major factor of stability.

Stewart and Milford Classification for Hip Dislocation with Associated Acetabular and Femoral Head Fracture†

For prognosis.

Grade I: simple dislocation without acetabular fracture
Grade II: dislocation with one or more large acetabular fractures but stable after reduction

---

* Salter RB and Harris WR.
† Samilson RL and Preito V.
‡ Schatzker J et al.

* Seinsheimer FI.
† Stewart MJ and Milford LW.

Grade III: explosive or blast fracture with disintegration of acetabular rim, unstable after reduction

Grade IV: dislocation with fracture of head or neck of femur

Stress Injury to Bone Classification for Stress Fractures

To grade relative state or level of effect on bone.

Grade 0: positive bone scan in an asymptomatic subject with negative radiographs; seen only in research surveys

Grade I: local symptoms associated with a positive bone scan and negative radiographs

Grade II: local symptoms with a positive bone scan and minimal findings on radiographs

Grade III: local symptoms with a positive bone scan and clear evidence of bone absorption on radiographs

Grade IV: local symptoms with a positive bone scan and actual bone fracture

Thompson and Epstein Classification for Hip Dislocation with Acetabular Fracture*

Based on size and stability of associated fractures to determine outcome of treatment.

Type I: with or without minor fracture

Type II: with a large single posterior acetabular rim fracture

Type III: with comminution of the posterior rim with or without a major fragment

Type IV: with fracture of the acetabular floor

Type V: with fracture of the femoral head

Limitations: does not take into account size and place of femoral head fragment (see Pipkin classification).

Tile Classification for Pelvic Fractures†

Numbers used by the AO group based on mechanism and letters based on vertical and rotational stability (A, stable; B, rotationally unstable and vertically stable; C, rotationally and vertically unstable) to determine if surgical or closed treatment is indicated.

Type A1: does not involve pelvic ring such as avulsion fracture and fractured ilium

Type A2: stable pelvic ring such as low energy fall in older adults; minimal displacement

Type B1: open book or anterior compression injury

Type B2: lateral compression force with ipsilateral fracture

Type B3: lateral compression force with contralateral fractures

Type C1: unilateral fracture with both anterior and posterior complex

Type C2: bilateral injuries

Type C3: vertical shear fracture with fractured acetabulum

Torode and Zieg Classification for Pelvic Fractures in Children*

Type I: avulsion of the bony elements of the pelvis

Type II: iliac wing fractures

Type III: simple ring fracture including pubic rami or disruption of pubic symphysis

Type IV: unstable ring fracture including straddle (bilateral pubic rami) fractures, pubic rami or symphysis with posterior elements or sacroiliac joint disruption, anterior fracture with acetabular fracture

Tronzo Classification for Intertrochanteric Fractures†

Based on reduction potential.

Type I: incomplete trochanteric fracture reduced anatomically with traction

Type II: uncomminuted fracture of both trochanters, with or without displacement, reduced with traction; anatomic reduction usually achieved

Type III: comminuted fracture with large lesser trochanteric fragment, posterior wall exploded; fracture line makes beak of inferior femoral neck unstable

Type IV: comminuted and unstable disengaged trochanteric fractures with explosion of posterior wall and medial displacement of femoral neck spike

---

*Thompson VP and Epstein HC.
†Tile M.

*Torode I and Zieg S.
†Tronzo RG.

Type V: trochanteric fracture with reverse obliquity (downward from a medial to lateral direction)

Tscherne Classification for Closed Fractures with Associated Soft Tissue Injury*

To define risk of surgical management.

Grade C0: simple fracture configuration with little or no soft tissue injury

Grade CI: superficial abrasion, mild to moderately severe fracture configuration

Grade CII: deep contaminated abrasion with local damage to skin or muscle, moderately severe to severe fracture configuration

Grade CIII: extensive contusion or crushing of the skin or destruction of the muscle, severe fracture

Limitations: definition of severity is lacking, no vascular annotation.

Vancouver Classification for Periprosthetic Fracture Hip

Type A: around the trochanter
  AG: greater trochanter
  AL: lesser trochanter
Type B: around or just distal to prosthetic stem
  B1: stable stem
  B2: loose stem
  B3: loose implant with substantial bone loss
Type C: well below the implant

Watson-Jones Classification for Tibial Tuberosity Fractures in Children[†]

To determine need for surgical reduction and fixation.

Type I: small fragment displaced superiorly
Type II: larger fragment hinged upward involving secondary center of ossification
Type III: displaced fracture passes posteriorly and proximally across epiphyseal plate

Limitations: does not account for potential entry of type II into knee joint.

---

*Oestern HH and Tscherne H.
[†]Watson-Jones R.

Weber Classification for Ankle Fractures (Danis-Weber)[†]

Based on the appearance of the fibular fracture; to define direction of causative and thus reducing forces.

Type A: caused by internal rotation and adduction; produces a transverse fracture of the lateral malleolus below the plafond.

Type B: caused by external rotation resulting in an oblique fracture of the lateral malleolus.

Type C-1: abduction injury with oblique fracture of fibula proximal to disrupted tibiofibular ligament (medial malleolus or deltoid ligament may be affected).

Type C-2: abduction-external rotation injury with more proximal fracture of fibula and more extensive disruption of interosseous membrane (medial malleolus or deltoid ligament may be affected).

Winquist-Hansen Classification for Femoral Shaft Fractures[†]

Based on comminution and stability; to determine if static locking nail is necessary.

Grade O: transverse
Grade I: comminuted with small piece not affecting stability
Grade II: comminuted with 50% abutting major cortex sufficient to prevent rotation and shortening with good proximal and distal nail purchase
Grade III: < 50% major cortex contact allowing rotation or shortening; requires proximal and distal cross-fixation
Grade IV: no fixed contact between major proximal and distal fragment; requires proximal and distal cross-fixation

Young-Burgess Classification for Pelvic Fractures (Fig. 1-6)[‡]

Radiologic assessment based on probable mechanism to recognize pattern at high risk for hemorrhage or related injury in acute setting.

---

*Weber BG.
[†]Winquist RA and Hansen ST.
[‡]Young JW et al.

APC: symphyseal diastasis or longitudinal rami fractures
  I: slight widening of pubic symphysis and/or anterior sacroiliac (SI) joint; stretched but intact SI, sacrotuberous, and sacrospinous ligaments; intact posterior SI ligaments
  II: widened anterior SI joint; disrupted anterior SI, sacrotuberous, and sacrospinous ligaments; intact SI posterior ligaments
  III: complete SI joint disruption with lateral displacement; disrupted anterior SI, sacrotuberous, sacrospinous ligaments; disrupted posterior SI ligaments
  VS (vertical shear): symphyseal diastasis or vertical displacement anteriorly and posteriorly, usually through the SI joint, occasionally through the iliac wing or sacrum
  CM (combination): combination of other injury patterns, LC/VS being the most common

Zickle Classification for Subtrochanteric Fractures*

To define a method of fixation.

Type IA: short oblique fracture from above the lesser trochanter to the lower lateral shaft
Type IB: long oblique fracture from above the lesser trochanter to the lower lateral shaft; comminution may be present
Type IC: transverse fracture just below lesser trochanter to a point near the isthmus

Dislocations

This section is divided into two parts: The first is a general list of terms applied to all joints, and the second is a list by specific anatomic location. Posttraumatic arthritis, recurrent dislocation, limitation of joint motion, joint mice, instability, or avascular necrosis may accompany various dislocation types. Hand and wrist dislocations are complicated and are discussed separately in Chapter 10.

FIG 1-6 Young and Burgess classification of pelvic fractures. **A,** Lateral compression force. **B,** Anteroposterior compression. **C,** Vertical shear. (From Islam A: Fractures of the pelvis and acetabulum. In Eastman AL: The Parkland trauma handbook, ed 3, Philadelphia, 2009, Elsevier, Fig. 38-1.)

LC: transverse fracture of pubic rami, ipsilateral, or posterolateral to posterior injury
  I: sacral compression on side of impact
  II: crescent (iliac wing) fracture on side of impact
  III: LC-I or LC-II injury on side of impact: contralateral open-book anterior-posterior compression (APC) injury

*Zickle RE.

General Dislocations

closed d.: one in which the skin is not broken; formerly called **simple d.**
complete d.: one that completely separates the joint surfaces.
complicated d.: associated with surrounding tissue injuries.
consecutive d.: the luxated bone has changed its position since its first displacement.
developmental dysplasia: exists in infancy with or without dislocation of the hips; formerly called **congenital d.**
frank d.: a complete dislocation in any area.
habitual d.: one that repeatedly recurs; usually congenital.
incomplete d.: subluxation with only slight displacement.
old d.: inflammatory changes have occurred.
open d.: one in which the skin is broken; formerly called **compound d.**
partial d.: incomplete dislocation.
pathologic d.: results from paralysis or disease in the joint or surrounding area.
primitive d.: bones remain as originally displaced.
recent d.: there is no complicating inflammation.
recurrent d.: repetitive dislocation with or without adequate trauma.
traumatic d.: caused by serious injury.
voluntary d.: dislocation that is caused by will of the person and can be reduced as well by the will of the person.

Specific Dislocations (By Anatomy)

Cervical Dislocation

Bell-Dally d.: nontraumatic dislocation of the first cervical vertebra (atlas)

Shoulder Dislocations

A/C joint separation: acromioclavicular joint disruption and separation
anterior shoulder d.: involves the glenohumeral joint with the humeral head displaced anteriorly and inferiorly; may be associated with one of the following:
  Bankhart lesion: seen surgically as detachment of the glenoid labrum and sometimes a bone fragment from the glenoid; also called **Perthes-Bankhart lesion**
  Hill-Sachs lesion: seen radiographically as an indentation of the posteromedial humeral head, which occurred at the time of the dislocation; also called **hatchet head deformity**
locked scapula: rare scapulothoracic dissociation with entrapment of scapula into chest wall or with anterior displacement; usually associated with severe neurovascular injury.
luxatio erecta: dislocation of shoulder so that the arm stands straight up over the head with humerus locked in 110 to 160 degrees abduction.
multidirectional instability: shoulder that is unstable in multiple planes, commonly anterior inferior and posterior inferior.
posterior shoulder d.: involves the glenohumeral joint with the humeral head displaced posteriorly.
reverse Bankhart lesion: seen surgically as a detachment of the rim of the posterior labrum from the glenoid rim.
reverse Hill-Sachs lesion: defect of anteromedial humeral head; may be seen on radiographs or at surgery
sternoclavicular joint separation: disruption of the sternoclavicular joint.
subcoracoid d.: glenohumeral dislocation with the humeral head displaced medially.
subglenoid d.: glenohumeral dislocation with the humeral head displaced inferiorly.

Elbow Dislocations

direct injury d.: posterior displacement of the olecranon
divergent d.: ulna and radius are dislocated separately
milkmaid's d.: a very common problem in young children, the radiocapitellar joint slips out after a relatively gentle pull with dislocation of radial head superiorly and anteriorly (e.g., when a child walking with an adult is helped by lifting the child up by one arm); also called **superior radial head d., milkmaid's elbow, nursemaid's elbow**

Monteggia f.-d.: fracture of the ulna with a radial head dislocation

Spine Dislocations

spondylolisthesis: not a true dislocation, because it rarely occurs as a result of trauma or muscle imbalance, but is a forward displacement of one vertebral body over another; usually occurs as a result of a defect in the pars interarticularis.

spondylolysis: acute (traumatic) dissociation of pars interarticularis or posterior elements (lamina) with or without spondylolisthesis.

unilateral facet subluxation: dislocation of one of the two facets at any level; most common in the cervical region.

Hip Dislocations

anterior d.: involves the femoral head anteriorly.

central d.: one in which the femur jams into the acetabulum; also called **bursting d.**

developmental dysplasia of the hip (DDH): formerly called **congenital dysplasia of the hip (CDH), congenital d., luxatio coxae congenita.**

luxatio perinealis: dislocation of femoral head into the perineum.

Monteggia d.: involves femoral head to near the anterosuperior spine of the ilium; hip joint dislocation.

Otto pelvis: gradual central displacement of the femur by unknown causes.

posterior d.: femoral head slips posteriorly; more common than anterior d. Also called **dashboard d.**

posterior f.-d.: chip f. of the acetabulum with a posterior d. of the femoral head.

Patella (Dislocation vs. Subluxation)

One of the most common dislocations is a patellar dislocation, erroneously called a *dislocated knee*. The dislocated patella simply goes out of the femoral groove. A subluxation is a tendency for the patella to move partially out of the groove. The most common direction is lateral, but may be medial.

Knee Dislocations

horseback rider's knee: dislocation of fibular head; injury associated with rider hitting leg against a post.

knee d.: slippage of the femur off the tibia; commonly called a **true knee d.** to distinguish it from a dislocated patella.

parachute jumper's d.: anterior dislocation of proximal fibula.

Ankle and Foot Dislocations

Chopart d.: navicula and cuboid dislocate across talus and calcaneus (Chopart joint).

fracture-dislocation of ankle: any combination of tibial and fibular fractures resulting in a displaced talus.

Lisfranc d.: tarsometatarsal dislocation; not to be confused with a **frank dislocation,** which denotes a complete dislocation in any area.

medial swivel d.: navicula is displaced medially on a fracture of the midtalus, but the calcaneocuboid joint stays intact and the subtalar joint is not dislocated. The calcaneus rotates on the intact interosseous talocalcaneal ligament.

metatarsophalangeal joint d.: occurs at the base of the toe.

Nélaton d.: dislocation of the ankle in which the talus is forced between the end of the tibia and fibula.

Smith d.: upward and backward dislocation of the metatarsals and medial cuneiform bone.

subastragalar d.: separation of the calcaneus and navicular bone from the talus.

tarsal d.: usually an ankle dislocation associated with a fracture of the neck of the talus; commonly an open injury. This term may also denote other tarsal bone dislocations, such as of the cuneiform and cuboid.

Subluxations

Subluxations are categorized by anatomic location as there are no eponymic terms.

facet s.: malalignment of opposing facet, allowing one cervical body to rotate around another.

patellar s.: most commonly in a lateral direction.

radioulnar s.: involves the distal ulnar radial joint.

sacroiliac s.: involves the sacroiliac joint; usually associated with a pelvic fracture and other dissociations of the pelvic ring.

shoulder s.: involves the glenohumeral joint (as opposed to the acromioclavicular joint).

wrist s.: involves the proximal carpal bones on the radius and ulna.

Strains and Sprains

The term **strain** applies to an injury of muscle or its tendon. The term **sprain** applies to ligamentous injury. However, the term *strain* is often interchanged with the word *sprain*. In part, this is because both injuries can occur at the same time, such as a low-back strain. It is clear at the time of injury that there is an acute tear or stretching of a back muscle, but there can also be a concurrent injury to the ligaments or disk tissue. If the symptoms continue, the sprain component becomes more apparent because the muscle normally recovers very rapidly.

Strains are often associated with injury to muscle caused by strenuous exercise without preconditioning and are usually referred to the back region. **Sprains** and ruptures of ligaments occur in the knee, ankle joints, and, sometimes, shoulder. At the ankle, a sudden twisting motion with full weight on the side of the foot can cause a sprain. A fracture may occur as well. There are many terms for muscle, tendon, and ligament injuries as follows.

Shoulder Sprain

acromioclavicular s.: stretching of the ligaments of the acromioclavicular joint or the coracoclavicular ligaments. The grades are from I to VI. When there is separation (grades II to VI), it is termed a **shoulder separation.** Often the term **shoulder sprain** implies this specific condition, as opposed to an effect on the glenohumeral joint.
   Type I: no disruption of acromioclavicular joint
   Type II: less than joint height separation of acromioclavicular joint
   Type III: joint height separation of acromioclavicular joint
   Type IV: posteriorly displaced incarceration of clavicle into trapezial muscle
   Type V: very wide superior separation of clavicle from acromion
   Type VI: inferior incarceration of clavicle under acromion
floating shoulder: disruption of combination of the glenoid, coracoid process, coracoclavicular ligaments (conoid and trapezoid), distal part of the clavicle, acromioclavicular joint, and acromion process; resulting in separation of the glenohumeral joint from the scapula.

Knee Sprains

anterior cruciate s.: commonly associated with a medial collateral ligament tear, dislocated patella, or torn meniscus; may occur as an isolated injury; allows the femur to slide backward on the tibia (tibia slides forward on the femur).
lateral collateral s.: isolated injury that may be associated with rupture of the biceps femoris tendon, anterior or posterior cruciate ligament, and iliotibial tract; allows the joint to open laterally, and with some associated injuries allows the lateral femur to slide backward on the tibia (tibia slides forward on the femur). Also, the peroneal nerve, fabellarfibular ligament, popliteus, and popliteal-fibular ligament may be at risk in a posterolateral complex injury.
medial collateral s.: occurs as a result of a clipping injury; may be associated with a cruciate ligament tear, patellar dislocation, or torn medial meniscus; allows the joint to open medially, and with some associated injuries allows the medial femur to slide backward on the tibia (tibia slides forward on the femur).
posterior cruciate s.: allows the tibia to slide backward on the femur; often seen alone; allows the femur to slide forward on the tibia (tibia slides backward on the femur).
posterior oblique ligament s.: part of the medial collateral ligament s. or rupture complex; allows the medial femur to slide backward on the tibia (medial tibia slides forward on the femur).

Ankle Sprains

deltoid s.: commonly occurs with a fibular fracture; rarely an isolated rupture.
fibular collateral s.: general term for sprain or rupture of one or more of three ligaments on the lateral side of the ankle.
   anterior talofibular s.: most common sprain or rupture of the ankle ligaments.
   calcaneofibular s.: sprain or rupture of middle of three lateral ankle ligaments, usually associated with other injuries.

tibiofibular s.: without rupture, there is no spreading of the tibia and fibula; with rupture, a diastasis occurs; syndesmotic sprain, high ankle sprain.

Sports-Related Injuries

Injuries from vocational and avocational sports activities have greatly increased over the years. In the United States, more than 2 million sports-related injuries occur annually. So much time and effort have been devoted to the more immediate identification and treatment of these athletic injuries that the development of the subspecialty of sports medicine became an integral part of orthopaedics.

Sports medicine has had a dramatic effect on the activities themselves. Exercise as a science has opened new dimensions in health care. Improved sports equipment and design have been developed through the combined efforts of engineers and medical support personnel, and rule changes are often made in consideration of the safety of the players.

Many sports injuries are a result of muscle and tendon overuse rather than a specific sprain or strain. Some of these conditions are so common in certain sports that they are named after the sport, for example, *baseball finger*.

This terminology applies to the nonathletic population, as well, who experience similar conditions. This may be the result of an increase in activity from a previously sedentary, nonactive lifestyle, or other factors such as degenerative joint disease. The classic example is that of tennis elbow. Many people with this problem cannot attribute it to a change in activity, such as painting or tennis, but have a condition of the cervical spine that causes the muscle of the forearm to tighten, resulting in overuse of the tendon.

The following terms are related mostly to athletic injuries of the soft tissues. Fracture-related sports injuries are listed in the preceding section.

ALPSA lesion: anterior labrum of the glenoid tears during anterior shoulder dislocation and strips the glenoid periosteum, leaving labrum attached to periosteum. This gives the shoulder the arthroscopic appearance of an intact labrum (ALPSA: *a*nterior *l*abrum *p*osterior *s*uperior to *a*nterior).

archer's shoulder: recurrent posterior dislocation or subluxation of the shoulder.

backpack palsy: similar to Erb palsy, a brachial plexus compression caused by a heavy pack with shoulder straps, resulting in palsy of the fifth and sixth cervical nerve muscle distribution.

BAGHL: *b*ony *a*vulsion of *g*leno*h*umeral *l*igament.

baseball elbow: condition of baseball pitchers in which overstress on the medial side of the elbow causes medial collateral ligament bone spurs, myositis, ulnar nerve injuries, or posterior compartment loose bodies; also called **javelin thrower's elbow, thrower's elbow, posteromedial impingement, baseball thrower's humerus, grenade arm.**

baseball finger: acute rupture of the terminal end of the distal extensor tendon. This may be either intratendinous or bony and is a result of a direct axial blow to the digit. The injury causes an inability to extend the distal interphalangeal joint (extensor lag). There is usually full passive movement of the digit; also called **mallet finger.**

basketball foot: subtalar dislocation of the foot.

bicycle spoke injury: bruising, swelling, and sometime necrosis seen in ankle 24–48 hours after foot and ankle get caught in spoke of a bicycle tire.

BIL lesion: *b*iceps *i*nterval *l*esion seen in rotator cuff at biceps tendon and subscapularis muscle. Pain and swelling occur over intertubercular groove.

black-dot heel: small dark spot on the heel fat pad caused by blood under the skin on the lateral side where there is repeated trauma to heel in athletic activity or shear stress in running; also called **black heel syndrome.**

bowler's thumb: irritation of the flexor tendon of the thumb with increased nerve sensation on the lateral side caused by the repeated grasping of a large bowling ball.

boxer's f.: fracture of the fifth metacarpal head with volar angulation. This is usually caused by punching a wall or hard object.

breaststroker's knee: irritation of the medial capsule of the knee, tibial collateral ligament, or patellar cartilage caused by repeated thrusts of the limbs by a breaststroke swimmer.

charley horse: cramping, stiffness of quadriceps muscles caused by muscle overuse, contusion, or direct blow to the thigh as in a sports injury.

coach's finger: proximal interphalangeal joint dislocation in finger.

coracoid impingement syndrome: specific impingement of the rotator cuff and lesser tuberosity by the coracoid process.

cross-over syndrome: extensor tendon inflammation at the wrist seen in kayak and canoe sports enthusiasts.

flexor origin syndrome: tendonitis originating at the flexor wad of five at the medial elbow; also called **medial epicondylitis, reverse tennis elbow, golfer's elbow.**

football ankle: area of ill-localized pain in superior part of the ankle above malleoli. X-ray changes show exostosis or loose bodies.

football finger: avulsion of the deep flexor tendon of the distal phalanx of the ring finger; often occurs when trying to tackle an opponent by hooking the finger over the pants belt line; also called **rugger jersey finger.**

gamekeeper's thumb: a traumatic rupture of the ulnar collateral ligament of the metacarpophalangeal joint of the thumb; usually a hyperabduction injury; also called **skier's thumb.**

gobies: rock-induced skin abrasions that are observed on the fingers and dorsal surfaces of hands in rock climbers; also called **bouldering** and **face climbing.**

golfer's elbow: inflammation at the origin of the wrist and finger flexor muscles of the inner elbow; also called **thrower's elbow, medial epicondylitis,** and **reverse tennis elbow.**

gymnast's wrist: widening of the distal radius physis associated with repeated impact forces on the wrist.

HAGL: *h*umeral *a*vulsion of *g*lenohumeral *l*igament.

handlebar palsy: palsy of the muscles of the hand innervated by the ulnar nerve, caused by pressure against bicycle handlebar.

heel spur: ossification in area of inflammation of the proximal attachment of the plantar fascia; usually involves the median tubercle of the plantar surface of the calcaneus; often seen in runners and commonly the result of excessive joint pronation. Anything that causes stress on the plantar fascia (weakened feet, structural deformity, or excessive pronation of the subtalar joint) will encourage the development of a heel spur.

hip pointer: very painful irritation of the insertion of abdominal muscles along the superior iliac crest. Pain localized here can also represent the pull of a thigh muscle in that region.

hockey player's hip: painful bone bruise of the greater trochanter caused by landing on the ice.

horseback rider's knee: a posterior dislocation of the proximal fibula on the tibia.

iliotibial band syndrome: condition seen in distance runners and other endurance athletes; pain on the lateral side of the knee just anterior to the lateral collateral ligaments caused by swelling in a bursa or thickening of the distal expansion of the iliotibial band.

impingement syndrome: alludes to symptomatic compression on the rotator cuff by overhanging acromioclavicular structures, the anterolateral acromion, and acromioclavicular ligament; graded according to the **Neer staging system.**
  Stage I: inflammation and edema of the rotator cuff
  Stage II: degenerative fibrosis
  Stage III: partial or full-thickness tear

jersey finger: an injury to the ring finger seen commonly in football and rugby players. This is a closed rupture of the flexor digitorum profundus (FDP); also called **rugger jersey finger.** There are three types:
  1. FDP retracts to the palm with total loss of blood supply.
  2. FDP retracts to the proximal interphalangeal joint with partial loss of blood supply.
  3. FDP retracts to the A4 pulley with a large bone fragment; blood supply is usually intact.

jogger's heel: irritation of the fibrous and fatty tissue covering the heel caused by striking the ground surface when jogging.

jogger's toe: dark nail that develops in some distance runners, caused by impaction of the nail into the shoe with long distance running and blood under nail.

jumper's knee: infrapatellar tendonitis or quadriceps tendonitis, often seen in athletes who jump as part of that sport, for example, basketball, skiing, and volleyball.

linebacker's arm (tackler's arm): a myositis ossificans reaction in the lateral brachial muscle; usually seen in the midarm of tacklers.

Lisfranc injury: low-velocity injury of tarsometatarsal joints (Lisfranc joint) resulting from forced plantar flexion in rotation with or without abduction, as seen in runners and basketball players. The injury was first described as one sustained during a fall from a horse while the foot is caught in the stirrup. The injuries may be severe enough to include fractures or dislocations as opposed to a lesser sprain.

little leaguer's elbow: in children, a traction injury of the elbow on the medial epicondyle caused by prolonged pitching or throwing. Serious in that it may lead to fragmentation of the bone and disturbance of growth.

little leaguer's shoulder: traction injury to the shoulder in the growth plate of the proximal humerus that may lead to a painful shoulder and eventual deformity if throwing is continued.

muscle cramps: a sudden cramp in the hamstring and calf muscles usually during athletic activities. Occurs often in athletes because of overuse of an undertrained muscle or inadequate salt or water intake during hot weather. This term is used diversely to specify a hamstring and calf muscle spasm or a contusion to the quadriceps.

PASTA: *p*artial *a*rticular *s*ide *t*endon *a*vulsion.

RHAGL: *r*everse *h*umeral *a*vulsion of *g*lenohumeral *l*igament injury.

ring man shoulder: bony resorption or sclerosis at the insertion of the pectoralis major muscle of upper arm; seen in gymnasts who use rings.

rotator cuff injury: inflammation or rupture of one or more of the tendons that lie deep in the shoulder and bridge the glenohumeral joint. This type of injury is inhibiting in pitchers and tennis players, in particular, and can be caused by excessive use (repetitive microtrauma), direct blow, or stretch injury.

runner's bump: prominence of the posterior heel at the point of insertion of the Achilles tendon; associated with distance running.

runner's knee: tight and tense condition of quadriceps muscle of thigh that directs pain to anterior knee.

sailboarder's injury: stirrup-type injury that occurs when surfer falls from board with foot caught in strap, causing a forced equinus position with disruption of dorsal stabilizers at Lisfranc joint; also found in horseback riders.

shin splints: pain in the anterior lower limbs (shins) that follows repeated stress such as running or walking long distances without conditioning; describes a painful condition rather than a specific anatomic lesion. The most common causes are posterior tibial tendonitis, stress fracture of tibia, muscle strain, periostitis, periosteal avulsion, fascial hernia, stress fracture, and anterior tibial compartment syndrome with the inability of blood to reach the muscle (ischemia) because of compartmental swelling during increased activity; also called **medial tibial stress syndrome.**

shoulder apprehension: apprehension of the patient during shoulder abduction and external rotation caused by glenohumeral subluxation (usually in patients with a previous shoulder dislocation).

shoulder pointer: a tearing of the anterior deltoid muscle leading to a distinct point of discomfort at the origin (immediate vicinity of the acromioclavicular joint) of the deltoid muscle.

SLAP lesion: *s*uperior *l*abrum from *a*nterior to *p*osterior tear that occurs along a line from biceps tendon attachment to superior labrum; condition causes shoulder pain with throwing motion.

spear tackler's spine: cervical spine injury in contact sports (e.g., football) where an individual spear tackles opponent head-on (with top of helmet); findings may include cervical cord or brachial plexus neuropraxia or preexisting posttraumatic abnormalities; condition may lead to posttraumatic arthritis.

sportman's hernia: insidious groin pain primarily affecting young males undertaking sports activities with frequent kicking and twisting. Possible causes are a weakening of the posterior inguinal wall or injuries of the fascias of the muscles and insertions of tendons at the pubic bone.

surfer's knots: lower limb and foot nodular swelling with possible bony changes caused by trauma and pressure from using a surfboard.

swimmer's shoulder: overuse of rotator cuff muscle usually caused by training errors in swimming training.

tennis elbow: inflammation of the wrist and finger extensor muscles near their origin at the elbow; also called **lateral epicondylitis.**

tennis leg: tear of the medial head of the gastrocnemius or plantaris muscle; often seen in tennis players.

tennis toe: subungual hematoma causing a black toenail; usually painless and requires no treatment; also called **marathoner's toe.**

turf-toe: an acute injury of the first metatarsal phalangeal joint as a result of hyperextension leading to separation of the medial and lateral sesamoid occurs.

This is classically described in football players on artificial turf, but it can occur in any sport where sudden push-off on the foot and great toe occur.

weight-lifter's shoulder: osteolysis of the lateral aspect of the clavicle as seen in weight lifters.

whiplash: a stretch injury to the neck that includes the muscles, ligaments, and disks of the cervical spine; caused by an acceleration (forward movement) or deceleration (backward movement) of the head as in a vehicular accident. A direct head injury may also cause a whiplash because of the resultant forces on the neck. Damage may involve minor neck ligament sprain, rupture, or subluxation (partial dislocation). This term denotes a complex of symptoms including pain and stiffness and is sometimes biomechanically inaccurate because there are many mechanisms that can produce these symptoms.

wryneck: torticollis; stiff condition of the neck caused by spastic muscle contractions.

Trauma Scoring Systems and Associated Soft Tissue Injuries

Injury Scales and Scores

Limb Salvage Index

To assess the likely success of attempts at limb salvage in severe injury.

Artery

    0: Contusion, intimal tear, partial laceration or avulsion (pseudoaneurysm) with no distal thrombus and palpable pedal pulses; complete occlusion of one of three shank vessels or profunda

    1: Occlusion of two or more shank vessels, complete laceration, avulsion or thrombus of femoral or popliteal vessels without palpable pulses

    2: Complete occlusion of femoral, popliteal, or three of shank vessels with no distal runoff available

Nerve

    0: Contusion or stretch injury; minimal clean laceration of femoral, peroneal, or tibial nerve

    1: Partial transaction or avulsion of sciatic nerve; complete or partial transaction of femoral, peroneal, or tibial nerve

    2: Complete transaction or avulsion of sciatic nerve; complete transaction or avulsion of both peroneal and tibial nerves

Bone

    0: Closed fracture one or two sites; open fracture without comminution or with minimal displacement; closed dislocation without fracture; open joint without foreign body; fibula fracture

    1: Closed fracture at three or more sites on same extremity; open fracture with communication or moderate to large displacement; segmental fracture; fracture dislocation; open joint with foreign body; bone loss < 3 cm

    2: Bone loss > 3 cm; type III-B or II-C fracture (open fracture with periosteal stripping, gross contamination, extensive soft tissue injury-loss)

Skin

    0: Clean laceration; single or multiple, small avulsion injuries, all with primary repair; first-degree burn

    1: Delayed tissue closure resulting from contamination; large avulsion requiring split thickness skin graft or flap closure; second- and third-degree burns

Muscle

    0: Laceration or avulsion involving a single compartment or single tendon

    1: Laceration or avulsion involving two or more compartments; complete laceration or avulsion of two or more tendons

    2: Crush injury

Deep vein

    0: Contusion, partial laceration or avulsion; complete laceration or avulsion if alternate route of venous return is intact, superficial vein injury

    1: Complete laceration, avulsion, or thrombosis with no alternate route or venous return

Warm ischemia time

    0: < 6 hours

    1: 6–9 hours

2: 9–12 hours
3: 12–15 hours
4: > 15 hours

Mangled Extremity Severity Score (Degree of Injury to Soft and Hard Tissue of a Limb)*

The mangled extremity severity score (MESS) assesses the prognostic effects of injury, ischemia, shock, and age.

Skeletal and Soft Tissue

Group 1: low-energy stab wounds, low caliber gun shot, simple fractures—1 point
Group 2: medium-energy, open, or multiple-level fractures, moderate crush injury—2 points
Group 3: high-energy, close-range shotgun blast, or high-velocity gunshot wound—3 points
Group 4: massive crush injury, industrial accident—4 points

Shock Group

Group 1: normotensive; blood pressure stable at scene and during surgery—0 points
Group 2: transient hypotension; unstable blood pressure at scene but stable when given intravenous drugs—1 point
Group 3: prolonged hypotension; systolic blood pressure < 90 mm Hg with recovery in operating room only

Ischemia Group

Group 1: none; no signs of ischemia, pulses intact—0 points
Group 2: mild; diminished pulses without ischemia—1 point
Group 3: moderate; no pulse by Doppler, sluggish capillary refill and other activity, paresthesias—2 points
Group 4: advanced; no pulse, cool, no capillary refill—3 points

Age

Group 1: < 30 years—0 points
Group 2: > 30 to < 50 years—1 point
Group 3: > 50 years—2 points

---
* Helfet DL et al.

Predictive Salvage Index

System predictive of amputation based on arterial, bone, muscle, and skin injury.

Level of arterial injury
    Suprapopliteal 1
    Popliteal 2
    Infrapopliteal 3
Degree of bone injury
    Mild 1
    Moderate 2
    Severe 3
Degree of muscle injury
    Mild 1
    Moderate 2
    Severe 3
Interval from injury to arrival in the operating room
    < 6 hours 0
    6–12 hours 2
    > 12 hours 4
    A + B + C + D = predictive salvage index

NISSSA Score

System predictive of amputation based on *n*erve, *i*schemia, *s*oft tissue, *s*keletal injury, as well as *s*hock and *a*ge.

Nerve injury
    Sensate 0
    Dorsal 1
    Plantar partial 2
    Plantar complete 3
Ischemia
    None 0
    Mild 1
    Moderate 2
    Severe 3
Soft tissue/contamination
    Low 0
    Medium 1
    High 2
    Severe 3
Skeletal
    Low energy 0
    Medium energy 1

High energy 2
Severe energy 3
Shock
    Normotensive 0
    Transient hypotension 1
    Persistent hypotension 2
Age
    < 30 years 0
    30–50 years 1
    > 50 years 2

Associated Soft Tissue Injuries

degloving: term applied to stripping or loss of skin and subcutaneous tissue from site of injury to point distal to the injury site.

Morel-Lavallée lesion: seen usually with severe pelvic fractures where there is a closed soft tissue degloving injury, where the skin and soft tissue around the area of the pelvis is separated from the underlying fascia. This may be seen in other locations such as lower limbs of football players.

Musculoskeletal Diseases and Related Terms

One hundred years ago, the nomenclature of musculoskeletal (MS) disorders was based on a specific affected anatomic part, organ, tissue, or gross appearance of the individual. This nomenclature persists, and in many instances, terms have been supplemented or replaced with biochemical or genetic terminology. More dramatically, over the past decade, the understanding of MS diseases has undergone dramatic change as reflected in the eighth edition of this chapter. We continue to use our previous descriptive terminology, but in many instances, have inserted the biologic mechanism of the disorder.

Many MS tumors are associated with changes in chromosome architecture, making accurate diagnoses more possible. We now have microchip tests that allow for detection of thousands of single nucleotide polymorphisms (SNPs), which, depending on location, can have mild to lethal effects. To avoid repetition, the science of our understanding of disease is discussed in Chapter 5, "Laboratory Evaluations."

With all of the forces and biologic assaults, the MS system reacts with changes in integrity, shape, and function. Knowledge of the chemistry and biomechanics of these changes has produced many new terms. The varied responses to repetitive force, infection, and inflammation are now better understood and add new meanings to terminology. These include joints that become arthritic; bursae that are inflamed; muscles, ligaments, and tendons that are strained, stretched, weakened, or torn; muscles that spasm or atrophy; cartilage that may degenerate; disks that become compressed and rigid; and vascular and metabolic changes that may affect both bone and soft tissue. All of these areas of the MS system can be affected temporarily or permanently.

The terms *disease* and *syndrome* are sometimes used interchangeably, but to be precise, they have different meanings.

A **disease** is a specific result of a pathologic condition that presents as a group of symptoms associated with physical or psychologic changes. A disease may be classified *acute* or *chronic, congenital* or *acquired, focal* or *systemic, malignant* or *benign,* and *contagious* or *noninfectious.* Diseases may also be characterized as *hereditary, inflammatory, metabolic, degenerative,* or *idiopathic.*

A **syndrome** is a group of symptoms that occur together and are associated with any morbid condition that constitutes the scenario for a specific disease.

Many diseases of the musculoskeletal system overlap into other specialties, such as neurology, neurosurgery, and vascular surgery, and the patient's symptoms often present as an orthopaedic problem. Therefore terminology of other specialties is included as it relates to orthopaedics.

Both soft tissue and skeletal disorders can be associated with **referred pain,** which means that the pain is felt at a site other than its origin. Pain is a perception, and as with all perceptions, illusions are possible. For example, pain can originate at the lumbar region but be felt at some point in the lower limb. Referred pain can also occur with direct pressure on a spinal nerve root in the back (a form of sciatica). In most cases of a back disorder with pain perceived to be in the lower limb, actual pressure is not on a spinal nerve root. Pain in the distribution of the muscles supplied by a specific spinal nerve is called **sclerotomal** pain. Pain in the sensory distribution of a spinal nerve is called **dermatomal** pain. The distinction is important in that a dermatomic distribution of pain tends to be more distinctive of actual nerve root irritation.

The goal in the treatment of musculoskeletal diseases and conditions is to help the patient become functional and productive as quickly as possible through a conservative approach, surgery, or other measures. The musculoskeletal diseases are defined here by tissue type and anatomic location.

Bone Diseases

Osteo-, the Greek root for "bone," can be used in various combinations that include more than one root, for example, osteochondral (bone and cartilage), or in terms in which *osteo-* is preceded by other terms, for example, *polyostotic fibrous dysplasia*. The *os* terms relate to small bones (**ossicles**), especially those in the foot, and are named in Chapter 11.

Bone disease types are grouped together for purposes of identifying similar or related processes by anatomic or eponymic terms. However, eponyms that are used more often than the common (Greek or Latin) terms are listed separately. The bone diseases are divided as follows: *osteo-* root diseases, infectious bone diseases, tumors of bone, miscellaneous Latin and English terms, and eponymic bone diseases.

Osteo- Root Diseases

hyperosteoidosis: excess osteoid tissue caused by defective mineralization (osteomalacia) and to normal but delayed mineralization; also called **hyperparathyroidism, hyperthyroidism, Paget d.**
ostealgia: pain within bone. (archaic)
osteitis: nonspecific term indicating inflammation of bone with enlargement, tenderness, dull aching; many varieties.
osteitis condensans: idiopathic increase in bone density, can be seen in clavicle, ilium, pubis. Ilium form also called **piriform sclerosis ilium.**
osteitis deformans: disease of unknown origin resulting in bowing of long bones and deformation of flat bones; also called **Paget d.**
osteitis fibrosa cystica: bone disease caused by hyperfunction of parathyroid gland; also called **osteoplastica.**
osteitis ossificans: an older general term denoting an inflammatory process in bone that results in increased bone density. (archaic)
osteitis pubis: increased bone density seen at symphysis pubis; may be associated with pain or increased physical activity.
ostemia: abnormal congestion of blood in bone. (archaic)
ostempyesis: suppuration (pus) within bone. (archaic)
osteoaneurysm: aneurysm in bone.
osteoarthritis: Osteoarthritic diseases (OA) are a result of both mechanical and biologic events that destabilize the normal coupling of degradation and synthesis of articular cartilage chondrocytes and extracellular matrix, and subchondral bone. Although they may be initiated by multiple factors, including genetic, developmental, metabolic, and traumatic, OA diseases involve all of the tissues of the diarthrodial joint. Ultimately, OA diseases are manifested by morphologic, biochemical, molecular, and biomechanical changes of both cells and matrix, which lead to a softening, fibrillation, ulceration, loss of articular cartilage, sclerosis, and eburnation of subchondral bone osteophytes and subchondral cysts. When clinically evident, OA diseases are characterized by joint pain, tenderness, limitation of movement, crepitus, occasional effusion, and variable degrees of inflammation without systemic effects.
osteoarthropathy: a condition of increased bone formation at the joints; sometimes used to refer to osteoarthritis. Variations of osteoarthropathy are hypertrophic, hypertrophic pulmonary, pulmonary trophic, and secondary hypertrophic.
osteoarthrosis: same as the term **arthrosis**; a heterogeneous group of conditions that lead to joint symptoms and signs associated with defective integrity of

FIG 2-1 Surface of tibia following excision for total knee replacement. Joint surfaces are rough with loss of cartilage and formation of new bone and cartilage at margin (osteophytes). *(Courtesy Orthopaedic Research Laboratory, Good Samaritan Medical Center, West Palm Beach, FL.)*

Pressure Epiphyses
Blount d.: epiphyseal plate of tibia
Avascular Necrosis Types
Brailsford d.: radial head
Burns d.: humeral trochlea
Freiberg d.: second metatarsal head
Haas d.: head of humerus
Kienböck d.: lunate
Köhler d.: midpatella
Köhler d.: tarsal navicular
Konig d.: femoral condyle
Legg-Calvé-Perthes d.: femoral head
Mauclair d.: metacarpal heads
Panner d.: capitellum
Scheuermann d.: epiphysitis of vertebral body
Thiemann d.: proximal phalanx

articular cartilage, in addition to related changes to the underlying bone at the joint margins* (Fig. 2-1).

osteoarticular: pertaining to or affecting bones and joints.

osteocachexia: chronic disease of bone resulting in the wasting of bone. (archaic)

osteochondritis: inflammation of bone. Formerly called **osteochondrosis**. Osteochondritis applies to a number of conditions in which the pathologic findings and cause may vary. In children, the disease affects the ossification centers at the *pressure epiphysis* (joints) or *traction epiphysis* (e.g., the patellar tendon to the tibia or the Achilles tendon attachment to the heel). In a pressure epiphysis, an area of avascular necrosis or similar process can occur. In the absence of a clear etiologic relationship or consistent pathologic findings, the osteochondritis diseases (as specified by areas affected) can be separated into traction and pressure epiphyses as follows:

Traction Epiphyses
Osgood-Schlatter d.: patellar tendon to tibia
Sever d.: Achilles tendon to calcaneus
Sindig-Larsen-Johansson d.: patellar tendon to patella

---

*Altman R et al, 1990.

osteochondrodesmodysplasia: a mucopolysaccharide disorder associated with multiple deformities of bone, joints, and tendons; also called **Rotter-Erb syndrome**.

osteochondrodystrophy: dwarfing disease mainly affecting spine and hips with little or no mental disturbance; also called **Morquio syndrome**.

osteochondrofibroma: tumor containing elements of osteoma, chondroma, and fibroma.

osteochondrolysis: osteochondritis dissecans.

osteochondromatosis: Transformation of synovial villi into bone and cartilage masses, causing loose bodies in the joint. This condition occurs in joints affected by trauma or other degenerative diseases. A condition specifically called **synovial osteochondromatosis** and **Henderson-Jones chondromatosis**.

osteochondropathy: condition affecting bone and cartilage; marked by abnormal enchondral ossification.

osteochondrophyte: an archaic term synonymous with osteochondroma.

osteochondrosis: term being replaced by **osteochondritis**; condition in children that affects the epiphyseal and apophyseal regions where increased stress occurs.

osteochondrosis dissecans: formation of a separate center of bone and cartilage on an epiphyseal surface. The osteochondral fragment may remain in place, be absorbed and replaced slowly, or break loose and become a loose body. Multiple etiologic factors probably exist. This was originally believed to be an inflammatory lesion, but there is no clear evidence for this; hence the change of the term from *osteochondritis* to *osteochondrosis*. Another probable etiologic factor is a demarcation of an area of avascular necrosis; also called **osteochondritis dissecans**.

osteoclasia: breaking down and absorption of bone tissue.

osteocope: syphilitic bone disease with severe pain within bone. (archaic)

osteocystoma: cystic tumor in bone. (archaic)

osteodiastasis: abnormal separation of bones.

osteodynia: pain in bones. (archaic)

osteodystrophy: defective bone formation.

osteofibrochondrosarcoma: malignant tumor containing bone and fibrous and cartilaginous tissue.

osteofibroma: tumor containing both osseous and fibrous elements.

osteofibromatosis: formation of multiple osteofibromas.

osteofibrous dysplasia: lesion that has a histologic appearance similar to fibrous dysplasia, except that the bone is being formed by osteocytes rather than by fibrocyte-like cells; also called **campanacci lesion, ossifying fibroma of long bones**.

osteogenesis imperfecta: condition in which bones are abnormally brittle and subject to fractures; inherited and usually is a function of abnormal type I collagen. There are a few rare osteogenesis imperfecta disorders not associated with type I collagen. Classifications are based on physical appearance and not the type of mutation. Also called **osteitis fragilitans, fragilitas ossium congenita, osteopsathyrosis idiopathica,** and **brittle bones**.

Shapiro Classification System
congenita A: fractures at birth, bones radiographically abnormal
congenita B: fractures at birth, bones radiographically normal
tarda A: first fracture before or at walking stage, bones narrow and osteopenic
tarda B: first fracture before or at walking stage, bones radiographically normal

Sillence Classification System (Modified)
Type IA: mild, dominant inherited, associated with blue sclerae and no skeletal deformity
Type IB: mild, dominant inherited, associated with blue sclerae, no skeletal deformity, and dentinogenesis imperfecta
Type II: lethal, recessive inherited, associated with multiple fractures and a short; survival; **Bauze:** Lethal osteogenesis imperfecta
Type III: severe, recessive inherited, associated with progressive deformity, white or blue sclerae, and nonambulatory status; **Bauze:** Severe osteogenesis imperfecta
Type IVA: moderate, inherited dominant new mutation, associated with some deformity and white sclerae in adults; **Bauze:** Mild osteogenesis
Type IVB: moderate, new mutation, associated with some deformity, white sclerae in adults, and dentinogenesis imperfecta

These groups were formerly called:

osteogenesis imperfecta congenita: severe form of brittle bone disease and deformity expressing itself in infancy or even at birth; can be fatal.

osteogenesis imperfecta tarda: brittle bone disease expressing itself when child begins to walk; also called **Lobstein d.** or **Lobstein syndrome**.

osteohalisteresis: loss or deficiency of mineral elements of bones, producing softening.

osteolipochondroma: cartilage tumor with bone and fatty elements.

osteolipoma: fatty tumor containing osseous elements.

osteolysis: dissolution of bone.

  familial expansile osteolysis: an autosomal dominant bone dysplasia with general and focal skeletal changes occurring in the second decade of life. There is usually pain, osteoclastic resorption, bowing, and a tendency toward pathologic fracture. Deafness and early loss of teeth may also occur.

  massive osteolysis: rare condition characterized by prevalent monostotic unilateral, localized, concentric osteolysis. Also called **Gorham d., phantom bone d., vanishing bone d., disappearing bone d., hemangiomatosis, lymphangiomatosis,** and **hemolymphangiomatosis**.

  pubic osteolysis: in adults, a worrisome-appearing lesion that may be mistaken for chondrosarcoma of the pubic bone area. Characterized by progressively destructive radiographic changes, soft tissue mass with calcification, histologic features of metaplastic cartilage, bone formation, and granulation tissue with myxoid and angiomatoid patterns.

osteomalacia: a reduction of physical strength of bone caused by decreased mineralization of osteoid; may result from a deficiency of vitamin D, calcium, or phosphorous with or without renal disease. Osteomalacia in the child is associated with the growth deformities of rickets.

osteomesopyknosis: autosomal dominant disorder characterized by osteosclerosis similar to that in pyknodysostosis but localized to the axial spine, pelvis, and proximal part of the long bones.

osteomyelitis: inflammation of bone marrow, cortex, tissue, and periosteum; can be caused by any organism, but usually bacteria. (See "Infectious Bone Diseases" later in this chapter.)

osteomyelodysplasia: thinning of osseous tissue of bone with increase in size of marrow cavities, accompanied by leukopenia (low white blood cell count) and fever.

osteonecrosis: death of bone tissue, usually of vascular origin.

osteoneuralgia: nerve pain in bone. (archaic)

osteopathia striata: affection of bone giving distinct striped appearance on radiographs; lesions characterized by multiple condensation of cancellous bone tissue, sometimes said to be in association with osteopetrosis; also called **Voorhoeve d.**

osteopathy: any disease process of bone.

osteopenia: any state in which bone mass is reduced below normal. This includes osteoporosis and osteomalacia. The World Health Organization redefined this to mean that bone density is significantly diminished (< −0.1 standard deviation below normal but greater than −2.5 standard deviation below normal). The term **low bone mass** is preferred instead of the term *osteopenia*.

osteoperiostitis: inflammation of bone and periosteum.

osteopetrorickets: the association of rickets and osteopetrosis in children characterized by hypophosphatemia, hypocalcemia, widened growth plates, and increased skeletal mass.

osteopetrosis: areas of condensed bone within bone caused by a variety of gene disorders, which include an autosomal recessive disorder of macrophage colony-stimulating factor, an autosomal recessive disorder of carbonic anhydrase receptor in a malignant infantile form, an autosomal dominant disorder of the carbonic anhydrase receptor in a less severe form, and an autosomal recessive disorder of beta 3 integrin. Also called **Albers-Schönberg d., osteosclerosis fragilis.**

osteophlebitis: inflammation of the veins in bone.

osteophyte: bony excrescence or osseous outgrowth, usually found around the joint area of bone. Around margins of arthritic joints, osteophytes are formed by new cartilage and bone. Around the spine and at strong ligamentous attachments, a portion of the ligament may turn to bone.

osteoplastica: inflammatory bone changes seen in cystic fibrosis.

osteopoikilosis: presence of multiple sclerotic foci in ends of long bones and scattered stippling in round and flat bones; usually without symptoms but noted on radiographs.

osteoporosis: the current definition by the National Osteoporosis Foundation is a systemic disorder characterized by decreased bone mass, microarchitectural deterioration, and increased susceptibility to fracture in the absence of other recognizable causes. Primary osteoporosis is an age-related disorder characterized by decreased bone mass and increased susceptibility to fractures in the absence of other recognizable causes of bone loss. The secondary cause of osteoporosis is most commonly immobilization, such as casting. The World Health Organization (WHO) definition is bone density −2.5 standard deviations below normal.

osteoradionecrosis: necrosis (death) of bone following irradiation.

osteosclerosis: hardening or abnormal denseness of bone.

osteosis: formation of bone tissue with infiltration of connective tissue within bone.

osteospongioma: spongy tumor of bone. (archaic)

osteosynovitis: inflammation of synovial membranes and neighboring bones.

osteotabes: condition in which bone marrow cells are destroyed and marrow disappears; usually in infants. (archaic)

osteothrombophlebitis: inflammation through intact bone by progressive thrombophlebitis of small venules.

osteothrombosis: blood clots or plugging of veins of bone.

parosteitis: inflammation of tissues around a bone.

parosteosis: ossification of the tissue outside the periosteum.

Infectious Bone Diseases

Osteomyelitis (Fig. 2-2) may be caused by bacteria or fungi. (Viruses have been suggested as a cause, but this has not been proved.)

Bacteria associated with osteomyelitis:
  Staphylococcus aureus
  Streptococcus organisms
  Escherichia coli
  Pseudomonas organisms
  Klebsiella organisms
  Salmonella organisms
  Neisseria gonorrhoeae
  Mycobacterium tuberculosis
Fungal types (rare):
  Actinomycosis
  Blastomycosis
  Histoplasmosis

Terms Related to Osteomyelitis (Bone Infection)

acute o.: possibly up to 6 weeks, radiographs may be negative for first 2 weeks.

chronic o.: more than 6 weeks; may last for years.

chronic recurrent multifocal o. (CRMO): multiple foci of bone inflammation, which tend to be episodic. These are thought to be inflammatory in nature rather than true infections.

chronic sclerosing o. of Garré: minimally symptomatic, long-term osteomyelitis associated with radiographic findings of densely scarred bone but not the usual abscess formation.

cloacae: in osteomyelitis, these are the openings in the infected sequestra of bone.

FIG 2-2 Different radiographic presentations of subacute osteomyelitis with classification scheme. Growth plate (physis) is below joint surface. Type IA is a punched out lucency suggestive of eosinophilic granuloma. Type IB has a sclerotic margin (not depicted) as seen in a more chronic form called *Brodie's abscess.* Type II has loss of metaphyseal cortical bone. Type III has loss of diaphyseal cortical bone. Type IV has onion skin layering of subperiosteal bone. Type V has an epiphyseal lesion. Type VI is an osteomyelitic lesion of the vertebral body. *(© 1994 American Academy of Orthopaedic Surgeons. Reprinted from the* Journal of the American Academy of Orthopaedic Surgeons, *Volume 2(6), pp. 333-341 with permission.)*

cystic o.: the radiographic appearance of an aborted osteomyelitis where a fluid-filled cystic cavity remains in the bone.

Gledhill classification: for subacute hematogenous osteomyelitis.

iatrogenic o.: an infection brought about by surgery or other treatment.

involucrum: bone formation around infected cortical bone.

mastocytosis: rare condition associated with accumulation of histamine-producing cells called *mastocytes* or *mast cells*. Painless, sclerotic bone lesions can occur.

nonsuppurative o.: term applied to tuberculosis of bone.

primary subacute o.: osteomyelitis that presents as localized, progressive bone pain with periods of remission. There is usually little or no systemic illness and no temperature elevation. Radiographic changes are identifiable on the first visit.

sequestrum: detached piece of dead bone from sound, healthy bone during process of necrosis.

sinus: drainage tract extending from an area of infected bone to skin.

suppurative o.: infection of bone with active production of pus; may be acute or chronic.

synovitis-acne-pustulosis-hyperostosis osteomyelitis (SAPHO) syndrome: related to the pustulotic arthrosteitis syndrome.

Tumors of Bone (Fig. 2-3)

A staging system for musculoskeletal tumors has gained wide acceptance and is applied to both bone and soft connective tissue. It has been adopted by the Musculoskeletal Tumor Society and may be referred to as the **Musculoskeletal Tumor Society Grading System.** The system is based on the relationship of the following factors: grade (G), site (T), and metaphysis (M).

Histologic grade:
  G_1: low-grade—few mitoses and uniform cell type
  G_2: high-grade—many mitoses and atypical cells

Benign

Stages 1-3. Histologically benign (G_0); variable clinical course and biologic behavior

Stage 1. Remains static or heals spontaneously with indolent clinical course. Well encapsulated

Stage 2. Active; progressive, symptomatic growth. Remains intracapsular. Limited by natural boundaries but may often deform them

Stage 3. Aggressive; locally aggressive but not limited by capsule or natural boundaries. May penetrate cortex or compartment boundaries. Higher rate of recurrence

Malignant

Stage I. Histologically low grade (G_1); well differentiated; few mitoses; moderate nuclear atypia. Tends to recur locally. Radioisotope uptake moderate

IA - Intraosseous or intracompartmental
IB - Extraosseous or extracompartmental; penetrates cortex or compartment boundaries

Stage II. Histologically high grade (G_2); poorly differentiated; high cell-to-matrix ratio; many mitoses; much nuclear atypia, necrosis, neovascularity; permeative. Radioisotope uptake intense. Higher incidence of metastases

IIA - Intraosseous or intracompartmental
IIB - Extraosseous or extracompartmental; penetrates cortex or compartment boundaries

Stage III. Metastases; regional or remote (visceral, lymphatic, or osseous)

FIG 2-3 Staging of the musculoskeletal tumors. *(Netter illustration from www.netterimages.com. © Elsevier Inc. All rights reserved.)*

TABLE 2-1 American Joint Committee on Cancer Staging System

Stage	T Tumor size	Nodes Spread to Lymph Nodes?	Metastasis?	Histologic Grade
IA	T1 (< 8 cm)	N0 (No)	M0 (none)	G1-2 (low)
IB	(T2 ≥8 cm) or T3 (multiple sites)	N0	M0	G1-2
IIA	T1	N0	M0	G3-4 (High)
IIB	T2	N0	M0	G3-4
III	T3	N0	M0	G3-4
IVA	T1-3	N0	Yes (lungs)	G1-4
IVB	T1-3	N1 (yes)	Yes (other)	G1-4

Site:
  T_1: lesion confined within a compartment
  T_2: lesion has spread beyond compartment
Metastasis
  M_0: no metastasis
  M_1: metastasis

There are three grades, each divided into *a* and *b* subgrades.

Ia: low grade intracompartmental (G_1, T_1, M_0)
Ib: high grade extracompartmental (G_1, T_2, M_0)
IIa: low grade intracompartmental (G_2, T_1, M_0)
IIb: high grade extracompartmental (G_2, T_2, M_0)
IIIa: intracompartmental, metatstatic (G_{1-2}, T_1, M_1)
IIIb: extracompartmental, metastatic (G_{1-2}, T_1, M_1)

The American Joint Committee on Cancer (AJCC) Staging System (Table 2-1): increasingly used as an alternative or adjunct to the Enneking-Musculoskeletal Tumor Society staging system and is recommended for communication with oncologists and for central registry data entry. It is based on tumor size, spread to lymph nodes, metastasis, and histologic grade. For treatment purposes, bone cancers are grouped into localized (I–III) and metastatic (IV).

The term *osteogenic sarcoma* formerly defined all the bone sarcomas (e.g., osteosarcoma, chondrosarcoma, and fibrosarcoma). Currently, more specific terms are preferred.

Benign tumors of bone are classified by the type of neoplastic tissue within the lesion. Nine general categories of tumors are described in the classification system of the WHO.

I. Bone-forming tumors
  1. osteoma
  2. osteoid osteoma
  3. osteoblastoma

II. Cartilage-forming tumors
  1. chondroma
  2. osteochondroma
  3. chondroblastoma
  4. chondromyxoid fibroma

III. Marrow tumors (none)

IV. Vascular tumors
  1. hemangioma
  2. lymphangioma
  3. glomus tumor

V. Other connective tissue tumors
  1. desmoplastic fibroma
  2. lipoma
  3. fibrous histiocytoma

VI. Other tumors
  1. neurilemmoma
  2. neurofibroma

VII. Unclassified tumors (none)
  1. giant cell tumors

VIII. Tumor-like lesions
  1. solitary bone cyst
  2. aneurysmal bone cyst
  3. metaphyseal fibrous defect
  4. eosinophilic granuloma
  5. fibrous dysplasia
  6. osteofibrous dysplasia
  7. myositis ossificans
  8. brown tumor of hyperparathyroidism
  9. intraosseous epidermoid cyst
  10. giant cell (reparative) granuloma

TABLE 2-2 Mirels Scoring System

Variable	Score 1	Score 2	Score 3
Site	Upper	Lower	Peritrochanteric
Pain	Mild	Moderate	Functional
Lesion	Blastic	Mixed	Lytic
Size	<1/3 diameter	1/3–2/3 diameter	>2/3 diameter

Mirels Scoring System (Table 2-2): for metastatic bone tumors, a weighted scoring system to estimate the risk of sustaining a pathologic fracture through a lesion in a long bone. Using this system, a score of 8 or higher represents a high risk of pathologic fracture and consideration for prophylactic internal fixation.

General Terms

tumor capsule: a layer of compressed normal tissue surrounding a tumor

tumor pseudo-capsule: a layer of compressed normal tissue and neoplastic tissue surrounding a tumor

Bone Tumors

osteoblastoma: a benign, locally aggressive tumor composed mostly of osteoblasts, occasional giant cells, fibrovascular tissue, and new bone formation; generally located in the spine or diaphysis of long bones.

osteoid osteoma: a benign vascular tumor characterized by a small nidus of fibrovascular neoplastic cells and abundant surrounding reactive bone, often seen as a thick sclerotic border radiographically and histologically. Typically located in the cortex of long bones.

osteoma: benign tumor characterized by dense bone production; usually located in the skull.

osteosarcoma: a high-grade malignant bone tumor (sarcoma) characterized by osteoid production by malignant stromal cells with variable morphologic characteristics. Typically generally located in the medullary cavity of the metaphyseal region of the distal femur, proximal tibia, and proximal humerus. It is characterized by osteoid production by malignant osteoblasts, with variable amounts of cartilage being present.

parosteal osteosarcoma: a low-grade malignant bone tumor characterized by osteoid formation by malignant stromal cells. This tumor is located on the outer surface of the periosteum, without involvement of the medullary cavity. Posterior cortex of the distal femur is a common location.

periosteal osteosarcoma: an intermediate-grade malignant bone tumor located beneath the periosteum but outside the cortex characterized by osteoid production by malignant stromal cells. Histologically, these osteosarcomas frequently contain cartilaginous elements.

secondary osteosarcoma: osteosarcoma that arises in preexisting pathologic bone, such as in Paget disease or following irradiation treatment.

telangiectatic osteosarcoma: intramedullary high-grade osteosarcoma characterized by abundant vascular changes and mesenchymal tissue in conjunction with sparse malignant osteoid production; also called **osteotelangiectasia.**

Cartilage Tumors

chondroblastoma: benign tumor composed of chondroblasts (immature chondrocytes), giant cells, and sparse chondroid material. Calcification often appreciated surrounding the chondroblasts (chicken-wire calcification). This tumor generally is located in the epiphysis in the skeletally immature; also called **Codman tumor.**

chondroma: an extraosseous benign tumor that contains mature chondrocytes in a cartilage matrix often surrounded by a rim of reactive bones. Varying degrees of calcification can be appreciated on radiographs and histologic examination.

chondromyxoid fibroma: a benign, locally aggressive tumor composed of cartilage and myxomatous and fibrous components; commonly located in the proximal tibia.

chondrosarcoma: a malignant tumor characterized by cartilage production by malignant stromal cells.

clear cell chondrosarcoma: malignant cartilage tumor that histologically is characterized by clear, vacuolated cells and frequently is located in the epiphysis.

dedifferentiated chondrosarcoma: malignant tumor in which a well-differentiated low-grade cartilaginous component is associated with a poorly differentiated noncartilagenous neoplasm of higher grade.

enchondroma: an intraosseous benign cartilage tumor; similar both radiographically and histologically to a chondroma with mature chondrocytes and cartilage matrix.

enchondromatosis: proliferation of multiple benign cartilaginous neoplasms within the metaphysis of several bones. It can result in thinning of the overlying cortices and distortion of length in growth. Higher risk of malignant transformation into secondary chondrosarcoma than a single enchondroma **(Ollier d.)**, and when associated with phleboliths **(Maffucci's d.)**.

epiphyseal osteochondroma: development of intraosseous cartilage lesion within the epiphysis with occasional extension beyond epiphyseal margins. May occur from infancy to adulthood. Formerly called **osteomatosis, epiphyseal exostosis, intraarticular osteochondroma, epiarticular osteochondroma, dysplasia epiphysealis hemimelica,** and **epiarticular osteochondromatous dysplasia.**

mesenchymal chondrosarcoma: tumor with a well-differentiated cartilaginous component associated with high-grade malignant round or spindle cell component.

multiple osteochondromatosis: multiple osteochondromas located in the metaphysis of long bones and pelvis resulting in growth abnormalities, with an autosomal dominant inheritance pattern; also called **multiple hereditary exostosis.**

osteochondroma: a cartilage-capped cortically based benign tumor demonstrating continuity of the cortex and medullary canal with underlying bone; generally located in the distal femur, proximal tibia, or proximal humerus. Can be pedunculated (with a stalk) or sessile (no stalk visualized); also called **exostosis.**

parosteal chondrosarcoma: malignant, cartilage-producing tumor arising from the surface of the bone.

periosteal chondroma: a cortically based benign cartilage tumor located between the periosteum and bone cortex characterized by cartilage and active chondrocytes.

secondary chondrosarcoma: cartilage malignancy occurring in a previously benign cartilage tumor, such as an osteochondroma or enchondroma.

Round Cell Tumors

eosinophilic granuloma (formerly histiocytosis X): term used to describe what is now called **Langerhans cell histiocytosis.**

Ewing's sarcoma: high-grade malignant tumor commonly presenting in children; characterized by monotonous sheets of small round cells.

Hand-Schüller-Christian d.: one of the so-called histiocytosis X group of diseases; a complex of bony tumors caused by either accumulation of cholesterol, metabolic error, or neoplasm; characterized by eosinophilic granuloma, exophthalmos, and diabetes insipidus.

Hodgkin tumor: low-grade malignant process involving the lymphatic system, with rare 13% bone involvement characterized by Reed-Sternberg cells.

Langerhans cell histiocytosis: formerly called *histiocytosis X* and *eosinophilic granuloma*; a nonneoplastic condition characterized by monocyte-macrophage lineage cell infiltration of multiple organs, including bone. Histologically composed of masses of histiocytes (Langerhans cell), cholesterol, and eosinophils. Common locations include the pelvis, scapula, and diaphysis of long bones in children. Associated with cranial disorder, diabetes insipidus, and exophthalmositis. **Hand-Schüller-Christian d.** is the most severe form; it can be fatal in infancy and is called **Letterer-Siwe d.**

lymphoma: a general term for neoplastic growth of a single cell lineage of the lymphatic system. Many types exist and are classified by neoplastic cell type (B lymphocyte, T cell lymphocyte, etc.).

multiple myeloma: common malignant tumor characterized by multiple lytic lesions of bone and caused by a neoplastic proliferation of plasma cells.

myeloblastoma: benign tumor of bone marrow.

myeloproliferative disease: any bone marrow condition resulting in abnormal increase in the number of specific bone marrow cells.

plasmacytoma: uncommon malignant tumor characterized by a single lytic focus of neoplastic plasma cells in a bone. Often progresses to multiple myeloma.

primary lymphoma of bone: a rare variant of malignant lymphoma that occurs in bone, without involvement of the lymphatic system or the typical systemic presentation of lymphomas. Characterized by multiple malignant lymphocytes in bone.

Fibrous Tumors

Campanacci disease: combination of nonossifying fibromata, café-au-lait spots, mental retardation, hypogonadism or cryptorchidism, and ocular and cardiovascular malformations.

desmoplastic fibroma of bone: an aggressive but benign fibrous tumor characterized by spindle cells and dense fibrous (collagenous) matrix.

fibrosarcoma: a malignant tumor characterized by malignant fibroblastic cells and no significant matrix production, with a herringbone pattern histologic appearance.

malignant fibrous histiocytoma: malignant tumor consisting of pleomorphic fibrous and histiocytic cell proliferation without osteoid or chondroid production; also called an **undifferentiated pleomorphic sarcoma.**

nonossifying fibroma: common benign fibrous tumor presenting in childhood; located in the metaphysis of long bones. Characterized by whorling patterns of spindle cells, fibrous tissue, numerous xanthoma cells, and occasionally giant cells; also called **fibroxanthoma, cortical desmoid,** and **metaphyseal fibrous defect.**

Other Tumors

adamantinoma: a malignant epithelial tumor of bone characterized by epithelial and sarcomatous components, typically located in the anterior cortex of the tibia.

chordoma: a malignant tumor commonly located in the sacrum or cervical spine; arises from residual notochord tissue with the characteristic physaliferous cells noted on histologic examination.

giant cell tumor: benign aggressive lesion consisting of osteoclast-like giant cells located in the metaphysis and epiphysis of long bones, frequently extending to subchondral bone. Lytic and expansile on radiographs without any reactive bone formation. Also called **osteoclastoma.**

Nora tumor: an unusual surface tumor of bone, synonymous with bizarre parosteal osteochondromatous proliferation. Also called **bizarre parosteal osteochondromatous proliferation (BPOP).**

Soft Tissue Tumors

Soft tissue tumors can be benign or malignant (sarcomas) and are generally characterized by the tissue they most resemble histologically. This classification process is often augmented by additional pathologic testing, including immunohistochemistry and translocation studies. The staging of soft tissue sarcomas is determined by the tumor size and depth, histologic grade, and whether the tumor has spread to lymph nodes or distant sites (frequently the lungs).

The 2010 **AJCC staging system** for soft tissue sarcomas system is summarized in Table 2-3.

angiosarcoma: malignant soft tissue tumor arising from blood vessels (hemangiosarcoma) or lymphatics (lymphangiosarcoma).

chondrofibroma: benign fibromatous soft tissue tumor with cartilaginous elements.

chondrolipoangioma: a well-circumscribed tumor in which there is a predominance of mature cartilage, mature blood vessels, and mature fat.

chondrolipoma: fatty soft tissue tumor containing cartilaginous elements.

chondromyoma: benign soft tissue tumor characterized by muscle and cartilaginous elements.

clear cell sarcoma: soft tissue sarcoma characterized by clear, vacuated-appearing cells; commonly occurs in the foot.

dermatofibrosarcoma protuberans (DFSP): low-grade, slow-growing malignant tumor that frequently occurs

TABLE 2-3 American Joint Committee on Cancer Staging System

Stage	Grade	Size	Nodal Disease	Metastasis
IA	G1	T1a, T1b	N0	M0
IB	G1	T2a, T2b	N0	M0
IIA	G2, G3	T1a, T1b	N0	M0
IIB	G2	T2a, T2b	N0	M0
III	G3	T2a, T2b	N0	M0
	Any G	Any T	N1	M0
IV	Any G	Any T	Any N	M1

Grade: G1 (low grade), G2 (intermediate grade), G3 (high grade)
Tumor: T1 (less than 5 cm), T2 (greater than 5 cm), a (superficial), b (deep/subfascial)
Nodes: N0 (no detectable node metastasis); N1 (regional lymph node metastasis)
Metastasis: M0 (no distant mets); M1 (distant mets)

in a subcutaneous location with fibroblasts and collagenous stroma.

elastofibroma: benign tumor usually seen in a subscapular location. It is a slow-growing, firm, mass that microscopically contains collagen and elastin fibers with few fibroblasts.

epithelioid sarcoma: soft tissue tumor composed of epithelial-like cells and sarcomatous cells, frequently occurring in the hand.

extraabdominal desmoid: a soft tissue tumor characterized by dense collagen; can be locally aggressive with a high local recurrence rate; also called **aggressive fibromatosis, extraabdominal fibromatosis.**

fibroma: benign fibroblastic soft tissue tumor.

fibromatosis: term used for a variety of conditions including plantar and palmar fibromatosis, neurofibromatosis, and a more aggressive and locally invasive fibromatosis called **aggressive fibromatosis** or **extraabdominal fibromatosis**).

hemangioendothelioma: rare, well-differentiated (low-grade), soft tissue sarcoma composed mostly of endothelial cells.

hemangioma: benign soft tissue tumor of dilated blood vessels; when occurring near the skin, may cause patchy discoloration; can also occur intramuscularly.

hemangiopericytoma: soft tissue tumor composed of perivascular tissue, spindle cell tumor which arises from pericytes. This soft tissue tumor may be benign or malignant; also called **solitary fibrous tumor.**

hemangiosarcoma: malignant blood vessel tumor; also called **angiosarcoma.**

hibernoma: benign lipomatous soft tissue tumor in which the fat cells resemble vestigial brown fat.

high-grade pleomorphic undifferentiated sarcoma (HGPUS): soft tissue sarcoma that histologically does not resemble any recognizable tissue type and cannot be otherwise classified; a diagnosis by exclusion.

leiomyoma: benign soft tissue tumor histologically resembling smooth muscle.

leiomyosarcoma: malignant soft tissue tumor with histologic characteristics resembling smooth muscle cells.

lipoblastoma: benign soft tissue tumor characterized by immature fat cells.

lipofibroma: benign soft tissue tumor of fibrous and fatty tissue.

lipoma: fatty tumor; tumor made up of benign fat cells.

liposarcoma: malignant soft tissue tumor composed of lipoblasts and malignant stromal cells.

malignant fibrous histiocytoma: term previously used to describe a group of malignant soft tissue tumors; terminology has changed and this is no longer an accepted subtype of soft tissue sarcoma. Also called **malignant fibrous xanthoma, fibroxanthosarcoma,** and **malignant giant cell tumor of soft tissue.**

myoblastoma: tumor of striated muscle consisting of groups of granular-appearing cells resembling primitive myoblasts.

myocytoma: benign muscle tumor.

myofibroma: muscular and fibrous tumor; fibroma containing muscular elements.

myolipoma: fatty tumor of muscle.

myxoma: benign soft tissue tumor containing myxoid cells.

myxofibrosarcoma: soft tissue sarcoma with myxoid and fibrous histologic features.

neurofibroma: abnormal proliferation of nerve sheath cells; also called **Schwann tumor** and **schwannoma.**

neurofibrosarcoma: malignant tumor of nerve sheath tissue; also called **malignant peripheral nerve sheath tumor (MPNST)** and **malignant Schwannoma.**

rhabdomyosarcoma: a high-grade sarcoma with histologic characteristic resembling skeletal muscle, with many histologic subtypes, including alveolar, embryonal, and pleomorphic.

synovial cell sarcoma: a malignant tumor composed of spindle cells; histologic architecture often resembles a growth pattern that resembles the appearance of synovium.

synovioma: a benign tumor of the synovial membrane.

Miscellaneous Bone Conditions

acroosteolysis: resorption of bone that involves the distal regions of the limbs but most commonly the phalanges of the fingers.

algodystrophy syndrome: association of pain and dystrophic changes in bone.

aneurysmal bone cyst: single or multiple benign, blood-filled cysts of bone.

apophysitis: inflammation of an apophysis. Depending on the location, specific types may be referred to as:
Iselin d.: base of the fifth metatarsal
Osgood-Schlatter d.: tibial apophysis at the insertion of the patellar tendon
Sever d.: apophysitis of the heel bone at the insertion of the Achilles tendon
Scheuermann d.: osteochondrosis of the vertebral epiphysis in juveniles
aseptic necrosis: osteonecrosis (bone death) caused by vascular insult, usually at the end of a bone. In adults, the most common symptom producing aseptic necrosis occurs in the femoral head (avascular necrosis). In children, aseptic necrosis is called **epiphyseal ischemic necrosis** or **epiphyseal aseptic necrosis.** The precise pathologic condition of these diseases is debatable; therefore the term is used here in reference to epiphyseal osteochondritis or by area:
Assmann d.: head of first metatarsal
Buchman d.: medial cuneiform
Freiberg d.: second metatarsal head
Iselins d.: base of the fifth metatarsal
Kappis d.: talus
Kienböck d.: lunate bone of wrist
Köhler d.: tarsal navicular; sometimes of the patella
Kümmell disease: vertebral body
Lance d.: cuboid
Legg-Calvé-Perthes d.: femoral head; also called **Legg-Perthes d., Perthes d.,** and **coxa plana**
Panner d.: capitellum of the humerus
Silfverskiöld d.: calcaneus
Thiemann d.: proximal phalanges
Wagner d.: base of the first metatarsal

Aseptic necrosis is also called **avascular necrosis.** The following are classification systems for aseptic necrosis.

International Classification for Osteonecrosis of the Femoral Head

Stage 0: bone biopsy results consistent with avascular necrosis; normal findings in all other tests.

Stage I: positive scintiscan or magnetic resonance image (MRI); lesions subdivided into medial, central, or lateral depending on location and involvement of femoral head.
  I-A: < 15% involvement of femoral head
  I-B: 15%–30% involvement of femoral head
  I-C: > 30% involvement of femoral head

Stage II: radiographic abnormalities (mottled appearance of femoral head, osteosclerosis, cyst formation, and osteopenia); no signs of collapse of femoral head on radiographs or computerized tomography scan; positive scintiscan and MRI; no changes in acetabulum; lesions subdivided into medial, central, or lateral depending on location of involvement of femoral head.
  II-A: < 15% involvement of femoral head
  II-B: 15%–30% involvement of femoral head
  II-C: > 30% involvement of femoral head

Stage III: crescent sign; lesions subdivided into medial, central, or lateral depending on location of involvement of femoral head.
  III-A: < 15% crescent sign or < 2-mm depression of femoral head
  III-B: 15%–30% crescent sign or 2- to 4-mm depression of femoral head
  III-C: > 30% crescent sign or 4-mm depression of femoral head

Stage IV: Articular surface flattened radiographically and joint space shows narrowing; change in acetabulum with evidence of osteosclerosis, cyst formation, and marginal osteophytes.

Lichtman Classification for Osteonecrosis of the Lunate in the Wrist

Stage I: linear line possibly seen across lunate or no radiographic finding.

Stage II: definite density changes in lunate compared with other carpal bones.

Stage III: lunate collapse with proximal migration of capitate.

Stage IV: Stage III plus degenerative changes in the carpus.

Pittsburgh for Osteonecrosis of the Femoral Head

To review this complex magnetic resonance imaging–based classification system, see Babis et al., 2011.

Steinberg Classification for Osteonecrosis of the Hip (Fig. 2-4)

Stage 0: normal radiograph, bone scan, and MRI

Stage I: normal radiograph; abnormal bone scan or MRI

Stage II: sclerosis or cyst formation in femoral head
  A: mild (15% of head)
  B: moderate (15%–30%)
  C: severe (> 30%)

Stage III: subchondral collapse (crescent sign) without flattening
  A: mild (15% of surface)
  B: moderate (15%–30%)
  C: severe (> 30%)

Stage IV: flattening of femoral head without joint narrowing or acetabular involvement
  A: mild (15% of surface and < 2-cm depression)
  B: moderate (15%–30% of surface and 2- to 4-mm depression)
  C: severe (> 30% of surface or > 4-mm depression)

FIG 2-4 Steinberg classification. **A,** Very early osteonecrosis of the femoral head (Steinberg stage 2). The femoral head shows sclerotic and radiolucent areas. **B,** Early osteonecrosis of the femoral head (Steinberg stage 3). There is a short break in the cortical line of the superolateral segment of the femoral head. **C,** Osteonecrosis of the femoral head (Steinberg stage 4). Mild flattening of the superolateral part of the femoral head despite long-standing disease. **D,** Advanced osteonecrosis of the femoral head (Steinberg stages 5–6). Gross destruction and remodeling of the femoral head. Osteoarthritic changes are significant. *(From Hagley K, De Ceulaer K: Joint and bone lesions in hemoglobinopathies. In Hochberg MC et al, editors: Rheumatology, ed 6. Philadelphia, 2011, Elsevier, Figs. 191-5 to 8.)*

Stage V: flattening of head with joint narrowing or acetabular involvement

  A: mild (15% of surface and < 2-cm depression)
  B: moderate (15%–30% of surface and 2- to 4-mm depression)
  C: severe (> 30% of surface or > 4-mm depression)

Stage VI: advanced degenerative changes

bone infarct: area of bone where blood supply is interrupted.

bone island: small areas of compact but microscopically normal bone that appear as 0.5- to 1-cm areas on radiographs.

bone spur: ossification of ligamentous or muscular attachment to bone. Generally applied to any bony excrescence seen on radiographs, but specifically refers to a portion of ligament or tendon that has turned to bone at the attachment to bone. The most common areas include the heel, patella, humeral epicondyles, and vertebral body margins.

brown tumor: brown-appearing lesion in bone secondary to hyperparathyroidism; also called **osteoclastoma**.

caisson disease: avascular necrosis of bone (and soft tissue) caused by sudden increase and release in air pressure causing infarct; also called **diver's disease**.

cleidocranial dysostosis: autosomal dominant defect of a core binding protein (**cfba-1, RUNX2**) resulting in failure to form collarbones and portions of the skull.

condensing osteitis of the clavicle: rare and benign disorder of unknown origin affecting the medial clavicle, characteristically in women of late childbearing age. The level of discomfort varies, and radiographs reveal a slight expansion of the medial one third of the clavicle.

congenital pseudarthrosis: inborn propensity for breakdown of integrity of midshaft of tibia with formation of a false joint. There are six types:
  Type I: congenital anterior bowing and defect in tibia. There may be other congenital deformities.
  Type II: congenital anterior bowing and hourglass deformity of tibia. Fracture occurs usually before 2 years of age.
  Type III: bone cyst forms first, then bowing or fracture.
  Type IV: sclerotic bone, then fracture occurs.
  Type V: dysplastic fibula may develop pseudarthrosis of tibia or fibula.
  Type VI: intraosseous neurofibroma or schwannoma may develop, but usually does not result in pseudarthrosis.

cortical fibrous dysplasia: benign anomaly of bone cortex, usually found in children and characterized by a cystic-appearing lesion on radiographs. Microscopically, this lesion is characterized by a fibrous replacement of cortex with some trabecular bone; also called **ossifying fibroma of long bone, intracortical fibrous dysplasia**.

exostosis: excess bone formation, usually near a joint.
  hypertrophic exostosis: sometimes used to describe excess bone formation in osteoarthritis.
  multiple hereditary exostoses: autosomal dominant disorder of **EXT** or **EXT2** genes resulting in multiple bony excrescences growing from cortical surfaces. May be pedunculated or sessile. Also called **Jaffe d.** and **Beggel-Hansen d.**

fibrodysplasia ossificans progressiva: autosomal dominant disease of BMP 4 and autosomal recessive disorder of **BMP 1 receptor type 1A (ACVR1)** resulting in connective tissue disease in which soft tissue ossification leads to skeletal malformation and disability; also called **myositis ossificans progressiva, hyperplasia fascialis ossificans progressiva, myositis fibrosa generalisata,** and **fibrositis ossificans progressiva**.

fibrogenesis imperfecta ossium: rare inherited disorder in which bone in adults is replaced with collagen-deficient tissue throughout the skeleton, resulting in multiple fractures.

giant cell reparative granuloma: common benign lesion of the jaw characterized by a fibrous background within which there are scattered multinucleated giant cells. A multicentric form is seen in the small bones of the hands and feet.

heterotopic ossification: formation of normal bone at ectopic soft tissue locations. In the acquired form, abnormal bone formation usually follows trauma, burns, or surgery, and will sometimes occur around joints after a closed head injury. Two rare heritable and developmental forms are fibrodysplasia ossificans and progressive osseous heteroplasia.

Brooker Classification for Heterotopic Ossification

Class I: islands of bone within the soft tissues about the hip.

Class II: bone spurs from the pelvis or proximal end of the femur, leaving at least 1 cm between opposing bone surfaces.

Class III: bone spurs from the pelvis or proximal end of the femur, reducing the space between opposing bone surfaces to less than 1 cm.

Class IV: apparent bone ankylosis of the hip.

Hamblen Classification of Heterotopic Ossification

Grade 0: no ossification.

Grade I: formation of new bone involving less than one third of the area of the hip occupied by the femoral head and capsule.

Grade II: formation of new bone involving between one- and two-thirds of the same area of the hip.

Grade III: formation of new bone involving more than two-thirds of that area of the hip.

hypophosphatasia: rare (1 in 100,000) usually autosomal-recessive bone disorder resulting from deficient alkaline phosphatase activity, characterized by defective mineralization of the skeletal and dental structures leading to an appearance of rickets and very low alkaline phosphatase. There are four types based on the severity of alkaline phosphatase abnormality: **perinatal hypophosphatasia** with neonatal death, **infantile hypophosphatasia** presenting in the first year of life with severe skeletal fractures, **childhood hypophosphatasia** with rickets appearance and abnormal teeth, and **adult hypophosphatasia** with osteoporosis and fractures.

infantile cortical hyperostosis: painful hyperostosis with involvement of long bones and the mandible. This usually occurs in infants 5 months of age and younger, and is associated with irritability, fever, and soft tissue swelling; also called **Caffey d.**

intraosseous lipoma: rare condition of benign fatty tumor that develops in the medullary canal of a long bone.

intraosseous lipomatosis: very rare disorder of progressive systemic development of leg and foot lipomas in medullary canals, producing bone pain and pathologic fractures.

intraosseous pneumatocyst: rare benign small pocket of air that appears usually in iliac bone. No treatment is required.

longitudinal epiphyseal bracket: ossification anomaly in which an abnormal arcuate or C-shaped secondary ossification center brackets a tubular bone in the hand or foot.

malacoplakia: disease that usually involves the gut and has a probable infectious cause. Histiocytes respond with the formation of Michaelis-Gutmann bodies. Bone lesions are rare and can be destructive.

melorheostosis: form of osteosclerosis or hyperostosis (dense bone); linear longitudinal thickenings of the shaft of long bones, very rare, resulting in a candle wax (dripping) appearance of the bone.

milk-alkali disease: excess calcium in tissue resulting from heavy ingestion of milk and certain antacids.

myelofibrosis: replacement of bone marrow by fibrous tissue.

ochronosis: hereditary error of protein metabolism marked by accumulation of **homogentisic acid** resulting in degenerative arthritis and a characteristic blackening of cartilage.

ossifying fibroma of the jaw: fibroma of the jaw with histologic appearance of small areas of ossification. This is in distinction to the rare ossifying fibroma of long bones.

pachydysostosis: enlargement of fibular length resulting in bowing of the leg.

periostitis: inflammation of bone covering (periosteum); usually the result of an infection such as syphilis.

progressive diaphyseal dysplasia: neuromuscular dystrophy associated with general wasting; abnormally formed shafts of long bones; also called **Engelmann d.**

progressive osseous heteroplasia: heritable disease characterized by focal dermal ossification with progression to intramembranous ossification of subcutaneous fat and deeper tissues leading to ankylosis. **Hemimelic progressive osseous heteroplasia** is a very rare condition in which only one side of the body is involved.

pulmonary osteodystrophy: hypertrophic cortical bone changes occurring near joints in the long bones of patients with chronic lung disease.

pyknodysostosis: condition marked by patchy areas of thickening of the cortex of bone.

regional migratory osteoporosis: most often seen in middle-aged men; characterized by arthralgias of lower limb joints, severe intercurrent osteoporosis, with symptoms lasting 6 to 9 months with recovery.

rickets: failure of deposition of bone salts within the organic matrix of cartilage and bone associated with stunting of growth and bone deformities.

Rothmund-Thomson syndrome (RTS): characterized by growth retardation, thin eyebrows and lashes, juvenile cataracts, sunlight sensitivity, hypogonadism, and teeth abnormalities. This is associated with an increased risk for cancer, such as cutaneous epitheliomas (basal, squamous), gastric adenocarcinoma, fibrosarcoma, and osteosarcoma.

skeletal amyloidosis: deposition of **amyloid β-microglobulin** material in bone that produces bubbly appearing lesions on radiographs. Condition is associated with plasma cell dyscrasias, primary systemic amyloidosis, focal amyloidosis, and those undergoing hemodialysis for chronic renal insufficiency.

slipped capital femoral epiphysis (SCFE): gradual or sudden movement of the femoral head toward a posterior and medial direction; usually occurs in preteenage children. In the United States, the acronym *SCFE* is so common that the slang word "skiffy" is used.

solitary fibromatosis of bone: similar to generalized fibromatosis, except bone lesion is isolated to one location. Systemic symptoms do not occur.

subperiosteal giant-cell reparative granuloma: self-limited condition seen in older adults characterized by subperiosteal bony lesions located in cortical bone of the diaphysis with giant cells and reparative cells with bone formation; also called **subperiosteal ABC, periostitis ossificans, florid reactive periostitis,** and **pseudomalignant fibroosseous tumors.**

transient osteopenia: decreased bone mass usually following immobilization or injury. Most often, bone mass is recovered. It may be seen as a spontaneous event in the juvenile hip.

uncommitted metaphyseal lesion: benign but radiologically aggressive-appearing lesion seen in the proximal metaphysis of children, microscopically characterized by whorls of fibrous tissue, new bone, giant cells, and vascular components.

unicameral bone cyst: benign bone anomaly in which a fluid-filled cavity is seen in the metaphysis of a long bone of a child. Microscopically, the cavity is lined with fibrous stroma, curlicues of trabecular bone similar to fibrous dysplasia, and cholesterol clefts.

weaver's bottom: ischial gluteal bursitis often seen in patients with a sedentary occupation.

Eponymic Bone Diseases

Albers-Schönberg d.: osteopetrosis affecting the ends of bone; also called **chalk bones** and **marble bones.**

Albright syndrome: spontaneous mutation of gene for **GS alpha protein for adenylate cyclase (GNAS-1)** resulting in hypophosphatemic precocious puberty associated with bone deformities resulting from fibrous dysplasia; also called **polyostotic fibrous dysplasia, Albright-McCune-Sternberg syndrome,** and **McCune-Albright syndrome.**

Apert d.: autosomal dominant disease caused by **fibroblast growth factor receptor 2** disorder that results in early fusion of the skull (craniosynostosis) and fusion of the digits, multiple deformities, and mental retardation; also called **acrocephalosyndactylism.**

Assmann d.: avascular necrosis of the head of the first metatarsal.

Blount d.: lesion of the medial proximal tibial epiphysis causing valgus (lateral bowing) deformity of the tibia; also called **osteochondrosis deformans tibia** and **tibia vara** (Fig. 2-5).

Boeck sarcoid: condition usually affecting small bones of hands and feet with granulomatous inflammatory reaction in lymph nodes, spleen, lungs, and liver.

Bouchard nodes: cartilaginous and bony enlargement of the proximal interphalangeal joints of fingers in degenerative joint disease.

Brailsford d.: avascular necrosis of the radial head seen in children.

Brodie abscess: chronic infection of bone resulting in a characteristic coin-sized sclerotic lesion with a lucent center.

FIG 2-5 Blount disease.

Buchman d.: avascular necrosis of the medial cuneiform.

Burns d.: avascular necrosis of the humeral trochlea head seen in children.

Caffey d.: subperiosteal cortical defect; infantile cortical hyperostosis; self-limited process of excess bone formation seen in newborns to 2-year-olds.

Camurati-Engelmann Disease (CED): a very rare autosomal dominant disorder, often involving the **TGF β2 receptor**. Bones are thickened, possibly affecting the nerve passages and resulting in hearing and visual loss. Hearing loss may also be due to changes in the middle ear ossicles.

Crouzon d.: autosomal dominant disease caused by **fibroblast growth factor receptor 2** disorder that results in early fusion of the skull (craniosynostosis) and facial deformities that vary widely in severity.

Engelmann d.: a rare autosomal dominant disorder often involving the TGF β2 receptor, leading to alteration of intramembranous ossification that usually affects the cortex of long bones and the skull with less frequent effects on the face. Bones are thickened, possibly affecting the nerve passages and resulting in hearing and visual loss. Hearing loss may also be due to changes in the middle ear ossicles. Also called **Camurati-Engelmann dysplasia**.

Freiberg d.: aseptic (avascular) necrosis of the second metatarsal head.

Fröhlich adiposogenital dystrophy: slipped capital femoral epiphysis; also called **Babinski-Fröhlich syndrome**.

Gardner syndrome: multiple osteomas concurrent with intestinal polyps, fibromas, and epidermal cysts.

Gaucher d.: autosomal dominant bone disorder resulting from lipid storage disease that is due to an absence of glucocerebrosidase. Excessive production of histiocytes with interference of marrow function and destruction of bone occurs; also called **cerebroside reticulocytosis**.

   Type 1: Adult—chronic, nonneuronopathic form associated with enlarged liver and spleen, bone lesions, no brain defect, skin pigmentation, and pingueculae.

   Type 2: Infantile—acute neuronopathic form manifested in infancy; is associated with severe neuronal abnormalities and early demise resulting from severe liver and brain disorder.

   Type 3: Juvenile—subacute neuronopathic form that has the features of the adult form but with neurologic symptoms that develop in the first decade of life with seizures; the liver and spleen are sometimes affected.

Gorham d.: rare condition characterized by localized, concentric osteolysis that most commonly affects the pelvis, shoulder girdle, humerus, or skull. Proliferation of vascular tissue within bone is the hallmark.

Haas d.: avascular necrosis of the head of the humerus seen in children.

Hajdu-Cheney syndrome: rare syndrome of resorption of bone of the distal part of the limbs with associated skeletal dysplasias.

Heberden nodes: cartilaginous and bony enlargement of the distal interphalangeal joints in osteoarthritis.

Iselins d.: apophysitis of the base of the fifth metatarsal.

Jaffe-Campanacci d.: osteoid ostcoma; hereditary multiple exostosis. Also called **Jaffe-Lichtenstein d.**

Kappis d.: avascular necrosis of the talus.

Kienböck d.: aseptic necrosis affecting lunate or ilium.

Klippel-Feil syndrome: congenital bone abnormalities of neck associated with dental, scapular, and other abnormalities.

Köhler d.: aseptic necrosis of tarsal navicular (scaphoiditis) or patella.

König d.: osteochondrosis dissecans of the knee; a separate formation of bone and cartilage segment at the joint surface.

Kümmell disease: avascular necrosis of the vertebral body usually following a trivial spinal trauma. Also called **posttraumatic vertebral osteonecrosis; vertebral pseudarthrosis; intervertebral vacuum, cleft, or gas; delayed vertebral collapse;** and **nonunion of a vertebral compression fracture**.

Lance d.: avascular necrosis of the cuboid.

turret exostosis, traction exostosis: dome-shaped extracortical mass on dorsum of middle or proximal phalanx of the hand caused by laceration of the deep extensor mechanism.

Legg-Calvé-Perthes d.: aseptic epiphyseal ischemic necrosis of the capital femoral epiphysis in children; also called **coxa plana, Perthes d.,** and **Legg-Perthes d.**

Lateral Pillar (Herring) Classification
A. The lateral pillar of the femoral head is intact.
B. The lateral pillar of the femoral head is less than 50% collapsed B/C. Border: The lateral pillar of the femoral head is thin or poorly ossified or has collapsed exactly 50%.
C. The lateral pillar of the femoral head is more than 50% collapsed.

Letterer-Siwe d.: histiocyte tumor of bone, usually fatal in infants and small children; also called **eosinophilic granuloma**.

Marie-Bamberger d.: hypertrophied joints resulting from lung disease.

Mauclair d.: avascular necrosis of the metacarpal heads seen in children.

Milkman syndrome: bone disease in which multiple transparent stripes are seen on radiograph.

nail-patella syndrome: autosomal dominant disorder characterized by hypoplastic patella, deformed fingernails, elbow deformities, and pelvic horns.

Niemann-Pick d.: fatal fat storage disease affecting bone marrow in infancy, marked by absence of sphingomyelinase.

Ollier d.: enchondromatosis.

Osgood-Schlatter d.: osteochondritis affecting anterior tibial tuberosity.

Paget d.: disease of excess bone removal and replacement with deformity; seen in older people; also called **osteitis deformans**.

Panner d.: aseptic necrosis; osteochondritis dissecans of capitellum of humerus.

Perthes d.: aseptic necrosis of the hips in children.

Pott d.: osteomyelitis; tuberculosis of the spine.

Ribbing d: rare bone dysplasia associated with painful long bone central sclerosis after skeletal maturity; often resolves spontaneously.

Scheuermann d.: osteochondritis affecting anterior vertebral body apophysis.

shepherd's crook deformity: characteristic deformity of proximal femur seen in fibrous dysplasia. The deformity has the appearance of a shepherd's crook.

Silfverskiöld d.: avascular necrosis of the calcaneus.

Sinding-Larsen-Johansson d.: apophysitis of the inferior pole of patella.

Stewart-Morel syndrome: hyperostosis of frontal bone; also called **Morel syndrome**.

Thiemann d.: avascular necrosis of proximal phalanges.

Tietze syndrome: chronic inflammation of the costochondral junction of a rib or ribs, causing pain; also called **chondropathia tuberosa**.

Van Neck d.: nonspecific ischiopubic osteochondritis.

Volkmann deformity: congenital dislocation of the ankle caused by absent or defective fibula; not to be confused with *Volkmann ischemic contracture*.

von Recklinghausen d.: autosomal dominant disorder of nuclear factor neurofibromin (NF1) resulting in fatty tumors, peripheral nerve tumors, areas of skin pigment changes, and other disorders; also called **neurofibromatosis**.

Voorhoeve d.: osteopathia striata.

Wagner d.: avascular necrosis of the base of the first metatarsal.

Waldenström d.: osteochondrosis of distal humerus at the radial site of elbow (capitellum).

Muscle Diseases

Myo- (Gr. *mys*) is a combining form denoting relationship to muscle. The *myo-* root diseases are followed by miscellaneous muscle diseases, the muscular dystrophies (listed together for comparison), and other muscle disorders. Eponymic terms are included.

Myo- Root Diseases

myasthenia: lack of muscle strength; also called **amyosthenia**.

myasthenia gravis: syndrome of attacks of muscle weakness that are episodic and reversible; also called **Erb-Goldflam d.**

myatrophy: muscle wasting.

myobradia: sluggish muscle reaction to electric stimuli.

myocele: herniation and protrusion of muscle through its ruptured muscle sheath.

myocelialgia: pain in abdominal muscles.

myocelitis: inflammation of abdominal muscles.

myocellulitis: myositis with cellulitis.

myocerosis: waxy-appearing degeneration of muscle.

myoclonus: any disorder in which rapid rigidity and relaxation alternate; also called **myoclonia**.

myocoele: the cavity within a myotome.

myocytoma: benign muscle tumor.
myodegeneration: muscle degeneration.
myodemia: fatty degeneration of muscle. (archaic)
myodiastasis: separation of muscle that may be congenital or traumatic.
myodynia: pain in the muscles; also called **myalgia, myosalgia.**
myodystonia: disorder of muscle tone.
myoedema: edema, muscle swelling. (archaic)
myofascitis: inflammation of muscle and its fascia, particularly of fascial insertion of muscle into bone.
myofibrosis: replacement of muscle tissue by fibrous tissue.
myogelosis: area of hardening in a muscle. (archaic)
myoglobinuria: protein myoglobin that appears in urine after vigorous activity; may lead to renal shutdown.
myohypertrophia: muscular hypertrophy.
myoischemia: local deficiency of blood supply in muscle.
myokerosis: waxy degeneration of muscle tissue; also called **myocerosis.**
myolipoma: fatty tumor of muscle.
myolysis: disintegration of degeneration of muscle tissue.
myoma: tumor made up of muscular elements.
myomalacia: pathogenic softening of muscle. (archaic)
myomatosis: formation of multiple muscle tumors.
myomelanosis: black pigmentation of a portion of muscle.
myoneuralgia: muscular nerve pain.
myoneurasthenia: relaxed state of the muscular system in neurasthenia (lack of strength caused by muscle nerve supply loss).
myoneuroma: nerve tumor containing muscle tissue.
myoneurosis: any abnormal nerve condition of the muscles. (archaic)
myopachynsis: hypertrophy of muscle; thickening. (archaic)
myopalmus: muscle twitching. (archaic)
myoparalysis: paralysis of muscle; also called **myoparesis.**
myopathy: any disease of the muscles.
myophagism: atrophy or wasting away of muscle tissue, with removal of tissue by inflammatory cells. (archaic)
myopsychopathy: any muscular nerve affection associated with mental weakness or disorder.
myorrhexis: muscle rupture.
myosclerosis: hardening of muscle. (archaic)
myoseism: jerky, irregular muscle contractions. (archaic)
myositis: inflammation of a voluntary muscle.
myositis ossificans: ossification of muscle in response to trauma. To distinguish the traumatic form of myositis ossificans from the generalized form, the terms **myositis ossificans circumscripta** and **proliferative myositis** are sometimes used.
myospasia: clonic contraction of muscle. (archaic)
myospasm: muscle spasm. (archaic)
myospasmia: disease characterized by uncontrolled muscle spasms. (archaic)
myosteoma: bony tumor in muscle. (archaic)
myosynizesis: adhesions of muscle. (archaic)
myotenositis: inflammation of muscle and its tendon insertion.
myotonia: increased muscular irritability and contractility with decreased power of relaxation; tension and tonic spasm of muscle.

Miscellaneous Muscle Diseases and Conditions

amyoplasia congenita: disorder of fascia and muscle resulting in contracted joints during growth; a specific form of arthrogryposis.
amyotonia congenita: muscle disorder of the newborn, usually fatal; characterized by muscle degeneration with failure of replacement (**congenital hypotonia, Oppenheim d.**); several types including **Werdnig-Hoffmann d.** (central nervous system origin), rod d. (microscopic rods forming within muscle cells), and central core d., which is not fatal.
ataxia: defective muscular coordination (lack of order) when voluntary muscular movements are attempted. Many types (e.g., locomotor, autonomic, sensory, spinal).
congenital myotonia: disorder found at birth, in which initiation and cessation of voluntary movement are delayed; also called **Thomsen d.**
delayed-onset muscle soreness (DOMS): muscle weakness, restricted range of motion, and tenderness on palpation that occurs 24 to 48 hours after intense or prolonged muscle activity.

Emery-Dreifuss muscular dystrophy: rare muscular disease with mixed patterns of inheritance affecting both skeletal and heart muscle. Contractures are common.

eosinophilia-myalgia syndrome: severe myalgia associated with elevated eosinophile count in blood in the absence of any infection. It has been believed to be associated with high doses of tryptophan.

familial periodic paralysis: disorder of muscle metabolism in which periods of partial to nearly complete paralysis occur; also called **myotonia intermittens.**

mitochondrial myopathy: slowly progressive muscular weakness associated with abnormal mitochondria, a cell structural component important in oxygen metabolism. The onset of symptoms is usually between birth and 10 years of age, but the disorder may not appear until adulthood.

monoplegia: in cerebral palsy an isolated paralysis of one limb.

muscle atrophy: general loss of muscle from various causes; also called **muscle wasting.**

muscle contracture: condition of fixed high resistance to passive stretch of a muscle resulting from fibrosis of the tissues supporting the muscles or the joints, or from disorders of the muscle fibers such as trauma or a congenital disorder.
  ischemic c.: contracture and degeneration of muscle caused by interference with circulation from pressure, as by a tight bandage or from injury or cold.
  organic c.: contracture that is permanent and continuous.
  postpoliomyelitic c.: any distortion of joint motion following an earlier attack of poliomyelitis.

muscle cramps: uncontrolled contraction of muscle; one common example is a **charley horse,** the cause of which is often unknown.

muscle guarding: involuntary contraction of muscle in effort to avoid pain that would be produced by moving the body part.

muscle ischemia: decreased blood supply to a muscle; can be spontaneously reversible; if not, ischemic contracture may develop.

muscle spasm: sudden contraction of muscle, usually in reflexive response to stimulus from external source, for example, back spasm caused by a herniated disk.

muscular dystrophy: group of degenerative disorders of muscle resulting in atrophy and weakness; also called **Erb d.**
  dystrophinopathy muscular dystrophy: autosomal recessive form of muscular dystrophy resulting from failure of formation of **dystrophin,** resulting in a severe form; also called **Duchenne muscular dystrophy,** or a less severe form, **Becker muscular dystrophy.**
  pseudohypertrophic muscular dystrophy: dystrophy of shoulder girdle and sometimes pelvic girdle muscles, beginning with hypertrophy in childhood, followed by atrophy; also called **Erb paralysis.**
  fascioscapulohumeral muscular dystrophy: marked atrophy of face, shoulder girdle, and arm muscles with autosomal dominant inheritance; also called **Landouzy-Dejerine disease.**
  limb girdle muscular dystrophy: slow, progressive dystrophy, affecting mostly the back and pelvic muscles. There are a number of types, including **type I:** autosomal dominant; **type IIA:** autosomal recessive with lack of calcium-activated neutral protease-3 (calpain-3); **type IIB:** autosomal recessive; **type IIC and D:** autosomal recessive lack of gamma-sarcoglycan; and **type IIE:** autosomal with lack of beta-sarcoglycan.
  distal dystrophy muscular dystrophy: dystrophy affecting mostly the distal muscles of the extremities and usually slowly progressive proximally.
  ocular muscular dystrophy: dystrophy usually confined to the levator and other facial muscles; also called **progressive dystrophic ophthalmoplegia.**
  myotonic muscular dystrophy: myotonia followed eventually by atrophy of face and neck muscles, ultimately extending to muscles of trunk and extremities caused by autosomal dominant lack of myotonin-protein kinase.

oculopharyngeal muscular dystrophy: seen after age 40, a progressive drooping of eyelids and weakness of the eye muscles, followed by difficulty swallowing and proximal limb weakness.

Poland syndrome: a rare birth defect with absence of the chest muscle on one side and usually webbing of the fingers on the same side.

pyomyositis: infection of muscle in which an abscess forms.

rhabdomyolysis: destruction of muscle following excessive activity, crush, or compartment syndrome. It can cause renal failure caused by high levels of myoglobulin in blood.

Stewart-Morel syndrome: intermittent progressive muscular rigidity; **stiff man syndrome.**

trigger points: this term has several different meanings. In general, these are specific points of muscle or muscle attachment that are very tender and related to muscle spasm. Pressure on these points may cause pain referred distal to those points. These point areas may be the result of chronic spinal disorders or caused by overuse of specific muscle groups.

Cartilage Diseases

Chondro- (Gr. *chondros,* gristle or cartilage) refers to cartilage, which serves a very important function in the growing process and joint motion. Healthy cartilage is essential for normal growth.

A growth plate called the *epiphysis,* a cartilage layer near or outside the joint, is essential to most of the longitudinal growth of bone during childhood. Disorders of this structure can lead to dwarfism or deformity. Cartilage is not apparent on radiographs, and many cartilage diseases are not detected until sufficient degeneration to cause joint narrowing takes place. Often a disorder that affects cartilage affects bone as well, such as *osteo-/-chondr-/-itis* (inflammation of bone and cartilage) or *osteo-/-chondr-/-oma* (bone and cartilage tumor).

Because diseased cartilage cells affect the combined function of bones and joints, many cartilage disease terms are found in the sections on bone tumors and joint diseases. The cartilage-related diseases are categorized in this section as follows:

1. *Chondro-* root diseases
2. Miscellaneous cartilage diseases
3. Abnormalities of the epiphyses
4. Mucopolysaccharidoses (proteoglycan abnormalities)

Chondro- Root Diseases

chondralgia: pain in cartilage; also called **chondrodynia.** (archaic)

chondritis: although the term implies inflammation of cartilage, it alludes to pain from a cartilage bone interface such as ribs, costochondritis, where inflammation may not be present.

chondrodysplasia: hereditary deforming abnormal cartilage formation; also called **dyschondroplasia.**

chondrodysplasia punctata: X-linked dominant or recessive disorder.

chondrodystrophia: rare condition of nutritional abnormality of cartilage development.

chondroepiphysitis: inflammation of epiphyseal cartilage.

chondrofibroma: fibroma with cartilaginous elements.

chondrolipoangioma: a well-circumscribed tumor in which there is a predominance of mature cartilage, mature blood vessels, and mature fat.

chondrolipoma: fatty tumor containing cartilaginous elements.

chondrolysis: degeneration of cartilage cells, ending in cell death.

chondromalacia: softening of cartilage, as of the patella.

chondromatosis: multiple formation of chondromas.

chondrometaplasia: condition in which cells that would normally form cartilage function abnormally.

chondromyoma: muscle tumor with cartilaginous elements.

chondromyxoma: mucous tumor of bone with cartilaginous elements.

chondronecrosis: necrosis (death) of cartilage.

chondroosteodystrophy: nutritional abnormality of bone and cartilage.

chondropathology: diseased state of cartilage.

chondropathy: disease of cartilage.

chondrophyte: excess cartilaginous growth at bone ends, at the margins of a joint.

chondroporosis: normal growth process in childhood; in adults, the formation of empty space in cartilage is a part of a disease process. (archaic)

chondrosarcomatosis: multiple chondrosarcomas; abnormal tumor cartilage.

chondrosteoma: tumor made up of bone and cartilaginous tissue.

Miscellaneous Cartilage Diseases

achondroplasia: autosomal dominant disorder affecting fibroblast growth factor-3; resulting in congenital dwarfism associated with deformed long bones and misshapen epiphyses; also called **achondroplastic dwarfism** and **chondrodystrophia fetalis**.

cartilage-hair hypoplasia: autosomal recessive mutation in **RMRP**, a non-encoding RNA resulting in short stature and abnormal facial appearance; also called **McKusick-type metaphyseal chondrodysplasia**.

diastrophic dwarfism: autosomal recessive dwarfism with flattening subluxation of various epiphyses caused by defect in sulfate transporter; also called **diastrophic dysplasia**.

Henderson-Jones chondromatosis: synovial formation of multiple loose pieces of cartilage within a joint, often associated with pain and swelling. The condition can spontaneously resolve with absorption of the cartilage bodies.

hypochondrodysplasia: autosomal dominant condition caused by mutation of fibroblast growth factor-3, resulting in milder dwarfing than achondroplasia and normal facial appearance.

Jansen d.: autosomal dominant disease of parathyroid hormone-related peptide receptor associated with mental retardation, short-limb dwarfism, exophthalmia, hypercalcemia, and long bone bowing; also called **metaphyseal chondrodysplasia**.

Maffucci syndrome: dyschondroplasia with hemangiomas, some of which have calcified walls as seen on radiographs.

Ollier d.: multiple enchondromatosis, usually benign cartilage tumors of bone.

precocious osteoarthritis: degenerative arthritis that develops at a very young age, often a genetic defect such as type II collagen.

Schmid d.: autosomal disorder affecting type X collagen and characterized by short stature, bowed lower extremities, coxa vara, flared metaphyses, and a waddling gait; also called **metaphyseal chondrodysplasia** and **Schmid type**.

Stickler syndrome: autosomal dominant disorder of type II collagen associated with small lower jaw, nearsightedness, thin limbs, mild scoliosis, and early degenerative arthritis. In another form, type XI collagen is affected and there is no eye disorder.

synchondrosis: joint formed by union of two bones with hyaline or fibro cartilage (e.g., skull sutures). Often converted to bone at skeletal maturity. This may be a disease state or a normal maturation process, depending on the location.

synoviochondromatosis: process in which the joint lining forms small nodules of cartilage, which may break loose and be free in the joint. Also called **synovial osteochondromatosis, osteochondromatosis**.

Abnormalities of the Epiphyses (Fig. 2-6)

The epiphyses are the cartilaginous layers at the end of long bones at the joints responsible for growth. Any dysfunction of metabolic origin or injury can cause deformity or dwarfism such as the following.

dysplasia epiphysealis hemimelia: osteochondroma arising from an epiphysis and projecting from the articular surface. This usually interferes with joint function.

epiphyseal hyperplasia: condition in which the epiphyses form from multiple centers and become enlarged and misshapen.

epiphysiodesis: premature fusion of the epiphysis to diaphysis. This can be due to injury or surgical intent.

epiphysiolysis: separation of an epiphysis from the shaft of the bone.

epiphysiopathy: any disease of the epiphyses.

epiphysitis: inflammation of joint cartilage or epiphyses in contrast to the rest of the bone.

hatchet head shoulder: flattening of humerus seen in multiple epiphyseal dysplasia. Not to be confused with hatchet head deformity seen after an anterior shoulder dislocation.

multiple epiphyseal dysplasia: multiple irregular epiphyseal ossification centers causing enlargement and flaring. Type I multiple epiphyseal dysplasia is due to an autosomal dominant disorder affecting **oligomeric protein of cartilage (cartilage oligomeric matrix protein [COMP])**, and type II–IV multiple epiphyseal dysplasia is due to an autosomal dominant disorder affecting **type IX collagen** (A1, A2, and A3). Type V is caused by autosomal dominant disorder of **matrilin 3**. There are additional dominant and recessive forms. Also called **dysplasia epiphyseal multiplex congenita**.

FIG 2-6 Disease conditions that affect the epiphysis often also affect the physis, which is the growth plate or epiphyseal plate. *(Netter illustration from www.netterimages.com. © Elsevier Inc. All rights reserved.)*

physeal bar: usually caused by a fracture bridging the growth plate; bone replaces the growth plate cartilage, typically resulting in bone growth abnormalities.

slipped epiphysis: subluxation or dislocation of the epiphysis from the shaft of the bone. This may not necessarily be a single traumatic event, but may occur gradually.

spondyloepiphyseal dysplasia: autosomal dominant and recessive disorders of type II collagen causing a spectrum of changes including inability to ossify normal epiphyseal centers, resulting in dwarfing or precocious osteoarthritis, primarily in spine and hips. There are four forms: **spondyloepiphyseal dysplasia congenita** (autosomal dominant); **spondyloepiphyseal dysplasia tarda** (autosomal recessive); dominant X-linked resulting from a defect in sedlin; and **Kniest dysplasia** (autosomal dominant).

spondyloepiphyseal dysplasia of Maroteaux: disorder of development of vertebrae and hips but without associated biochemical and eye changes seen in Morquio syndrome.

stippled epiphysis: radiologic sign of chondrodystrophia calcificans, a disease associated with multiple calcifications of epiphyseal cartilage. A mild form of the condition may be called **epiphyseal dysplasia**.

Mucopolysaccharidoses (Metabolic Effects)

The mucopolysaccharidoses (MPSs) are a variety of hereditable metabolic disorders of mucopolysaccharides presently called *proteoglycans*. Glycosaminoglycan chains are sugars that contain amino and sulfate components, are attached to a protein core molecule, and are formed by posttranslational pathways in the cell. Specific enzymatic failures are responsible for the accumulation of specific chemicals. *Muco-* originally signified the gelatinous appearance of the pure aggregate of these molecules. Most disorders of mucopolysaccharide metabolism are autosomal recessive. For many types, the eponymic designations are preferred because the metabolic nomenclature is complex.

Hunter s.: similar to Hurler syndrome, but less severely deforming; sex-linked dominant inheritance affecting **sulfoiduronate sulfatase, MPS II**. There are severe and mild forms of the disease.

Hunter-Scheie s.: condition that has mixed clinical appearance of Hunter and Scheie s.; also called **MPS I H/S**.

Hurler s.: autosomal recessive severely deforming condition associated with blindness, mental retardation, and early death; caused by a deficiency of **alpha-L-iduronidase**; **MPS I H**. Formerly called **gargoylism** and **lipochondrodystrophy**.

Maroteaux-Lamy s.: growth retardation, lumbar kyphosis, sternal protrusion; no mental retardation; also called **MPS VI**.

McArdle s: autosomal recessive disorder caused by deficiency of muscle **glycogen phosphorylase** leading to muscle weakness, cramps, and muscle pain on exercise.

Morquio s.: dwarfing disease affecting mostly the spine and hips; little or no mental retardation. There are two forms that have similar clinical appearance—**MPS IV A** and **MPS IV B**; **chondroosteodystrophy**. Both types are autosomal recessive inherited disorders caused by defects in galaxtosamine-6-sulphate sulfatase and a defect in beta-galactosidase.

Sanfilippo s.: four forms of this autosomal recessive disease resulting in accumulation of heparan sulfate exist and all have profound mental retardation, hyperactivity, and relatively mild somatic manifestations—**MPS III A, MPS III B, MPS III C,** and **MPS III D**.

Scheie s.: autosomal recessive disorder resulting from dysfunction of **alpha-1-iduronidase** with no mental impairment but noted corneal clouding, aortic disease, and stiff joints; also called **MPS I S**.

Sly s.: autosomal recessive disorder of **glucuronidase,** which causes multiple long bone growth abnormalities associated with liver and spleen enlargement; wide spectrum of severity; also called **MPS VII**.

Diseases of (Specific) Soft Tissue

In addition to bone, muscle, and cartilage, other tissues surround a joint. The root terms for these tissues (*fibro-, lipo-, myxo-, muco-*) denote the relationship to certain disease processes and disorders.

Fibro- Root Diseases

Fibro- (L. *fibra*, fiber) is a combining form indicating fibrous tissue such as tendons and ligaments. Such tissue contains collagen, which is the major supportive protein of bone, tendon, cartilage, and connective tissue. Fibrouslike tissues and structures can arise in a number of places.

fibrosis: proliferation of fibrous tissue as a result of reaction to a reparative process.
fibrositis: inflammation of fibrous tissue.
fibrous histiocytoma: benign tumor of bone containing fibrous stroma, xanthomatous cells, and a round and spindle cell component. There is a malignant form called **malignant fibrous histiocytoma.**
Garrod fibromatosis (Garrod pads): thickening of the skin almost always confined to the dorsal aspects of the proximal interphalangeal joints of the hand.
juvenile hyaline fibromatosis: disease that develops in early childhood and is characterized by multiple fibromatous lesions of the skin, muscle, bone, and ligaments, possibly leading to joint contractures. It is not necessarily progressive; histologically, it is characterized by multiple spindle cells with an amorphous matrix or collagenous tissue.
monostotic fibrous dysplasia: disease of bony remodeling, causing deformity of only one bone.
polyostotic fibrous dysplasia: disease caused by a defect in **GS alpha protein of adenylate cyclase (GNAS-1)** marked by fibrous tissue replacement of bone with resultant deformities and clinical appearance of café-au-lait skin pigmentation and precocious puberty; also called **Albright syndrome.**
neurofibroma: abnormal proliferation of nerve sheath cells; also called **Schwann tumor.**
periarticular fibrositis: inflammatory condition of fibrous tissue surrounding a joint.
periosteal fibroma: fibrous tumor of bone-covering tissue.
pseudosarcomatous fibromatosis: disease of extensive subcutaneous fibroma formation; also called **subcutaneous pseudosarcomatous fibromatosis, proliferative fasciitis.**

Lipo- Root Diseases

Lipo- (Gr. *lipos*, fat) is a combining form denoting relationship to fat and fatty tissue. Several disease processes are based on this root.

lipochondrodystrophy: lipodystrophy as it affects cartilage.
lipodystrophy: defective metabolism of fat that results in the absence of subcutaneous fat, either partial or total. May be congenital or acquired.

Myxo- Root Diseases

Myxo- (Gr. *myxa*, mucus) is a combining form denoting relationship to mucus. Myxomatous cells contain mucous material that is clear in appearance. These cells are naturally found in the intervertebral disks, but when seen elsewhere they usually represent an abnormality. Myxomatous cells contain the mucopolysaccharide (proteoglycan) material, which could rupture, causing mucous cysts to form. Terms containing *myxo-* indicate the presence of this type of cell and are found in the "Soft Tissue Tumor" section earlier in this chapter.

Muco- Root Diseases

The Latin word *mucus,* for the purposes of orthopaedics, does not imply secretions but rather the association of tissues that contain certain chemicals called *mucopolysaccharides,* which, when sufficient collection of material occurs, are in the form of a clear jelly and seen in certain cysts. Elsewhere in medicine, the terms *mucus* and *mucous* relate particularly to the gut and respiratory tract.

ganglion cyst: a sac, usually 1 mm to more than 5 cm in size, commonly near a joint; contains a mix of collagen, proteoglycans, and other proteins with water such that the content appears clear and gelatinous. Ganglion cysts may occur anywhere, including within bone (intraosseous ganglion) and just under the periosteum (periosteal ganglion).
mucopolysaccharidosis: any of a variety of heritable disease states resulting from abnormalities in mucopolysaccharide (sugars containing SO_4, COOH, and NH_2) metabolism. These mainly affect cartilage in terms of orthopaedic diseases and cause stunted growth.
mucous cyst: in orthopaedics, a benign cyst under the fingernail.

Ligament, Tendon, Bursa, and Fascia Diseases

Desmo- Root Diseases

Desmo- (Gr. *desmos*, ligament) is a combining form denoting relationship to a band, bond, or ligament. Ligaments are composed of fibrous tissue that binds the joints together. Desmogenous dysfunctions and diseases may be any of the following.

desmectasis: stretching of a ligament. (archaic)
desmitis: inflammation of a ligament. (archaic)
desmocytoma: now called **fibrosarcoma**. (archaic)
desmodynia: pain in a ligament; also called **desmalgia**. (archaic)
desmoid: collection of fibrous tissue occurring at the insertion of a tendon (cortical desmoid) or arising from soft tissue of an extremity. The latter is a true tumor, recurrent but not malignant; also called **periosteal desmoid** and **extraabdominal desmoid**.
desmoma: a fibroma; a benign fibrous tumor.
desmopathy: any pathologic disease of a ligament.
desmoplasia: formation and development of fibrous tissue.
desmoplastic: producing or forming adhesions.
desmorrhexis: rupture of a ligament.
desmosis: disease of connective tissue. (archaic)

Eponymic Ligamentous Diseases

Duplay d.: capsulitis of the glenohumeral joint area; also called **frozen shoulder**.
MGHL cord: pattern in which the *m*iddle *g*leno*h*umeral *l*igament is cordlike and enlarged.
Pellegrini-Stieda d.: ligamentous calcification of the medial collateral ligament of the knee following trauma.

Tendo-/Teno- Root Diseases

Tendo- and *teno-* (L. *tendo*; Gr. *tenōn*) are combining forms denoting relationship to a tendon. A tendon is a fibrous cord of connective tissue in which the fibers of a muscle end and by which the muscle is attached to bone.

tendonitis: although this term implies an inflammation of tendons or of tendon-muscle attachments, it is now clear that many tendons that have focal swelling and soreness do not have evidence of the increased blood supply seen with inflammation. The biologic effects to the tendon that creates the symptoms in these cases has no apparent effect on the blood supply; also called **tenontitis, tenonitis,** and **tenositis**.
  bicipital t.: inflammation of a biceps muscle at tendon insertion of shoulder.
  calcific t.: inflammation associated with calcium deposits in the tendon or bursa (i.e., subacromial or subdeltoid bursa) producing pain and tenderness and limiting motion of shoulder.
  tendonitis ossificans traumatica: development of ossification in areas of tendons caused by trauma.
tenodynia: pain in a tendon; tenontodynia.
tenontagra: gouty affection of tendons. (archaic)
tenontophyma: tumorous growth in tendon. (archaic)
tenontothecitis: inflammation of a tendon sheath. (archaic)
tenoperiostitis: inflammation of muscle-tendon attachment to bone, for example, tennis elbow and golfer's elbow.
tenophyte: growth or concretion in tendon.
tenositis: inflammation of a tendon.
tenostosis: ossification of a tendon.
tenosynovitis: inflammation of a tendon sheath and synovial sac; tendosynovitis.

Other Tendon-Related Diseases

acute calcific tendonitis: rapid onset of pain and occasionally fever associated with swelling and redness. Most commonly confused with infection. Radiographs reveal subtle soft tissue calcification. Seen most commonly in the hands and wrist but may be seen in the shoulder, elbow, hip, or knee. It is rarely seen in the small, deep anterior neck muscles. This condition may be called **acute calcific retropharyngeal tendonitis,** and is important to orthopaedics because it is a rare but benign cause of severe neck pain.
Albert achillodynia: discomfort felt around terminal segment of heel cord; also called **achillodynia, achillobursitis**.
de Quervain d.: tenosynovitis of the abductor pollicis longus and extensor pollicis brevis of the hand.

enthesopathy: degenerative disorders of ligaments, muscles, and tendon attachments to bone, the central structure in the disease process. **Enthesis** is the site of a tendon, ligament, or muscle attachment to bone. However, the term is more specifically applied to certain degenerative disorders of tendons such as supraspinatus and Achilles tendonitis. Because a neighboring bursa may be involved, it is sometimes called a **bursitis.**

enthesitis: inflammation resulting from stress on muscle or tendon that is attached to bone. There is a strong tendency toward fibrosis, calcification, and even rupture.

epicondylitis: inflammation of the tendon origins on the medial epicondyle **(golfer's elbow, thrower's elbow)** or the lateral epicondyle **(tennis elbow).**

Bursa-Related Diseases

Bursae (pl.) are closed sacs of fibrous tissue lined with synovial membrane, filled with viscid fluid, and situated in places in tissue where friction would otherwise inhibit function, such as near joints. Most disorders of bursae are part of another disease process.

bursitis: inflammation of a bursa at site of bony prominences between muscles or tendons.
  calcific bursitis: deposition of calcium in a bursa, usually associated with inflammation; can often be seen on a radiograph.
bursolith: calculus or concretion in a bursa.
bursopathy: any pathologic condition of bursae.

Fascia-Related Diseases

Fasciae (L. *fascia*, band) are bands of fibrous tissue that lie deep to the skin and form an investment for muscles and various organs of the body. *Retinacula* (*retinaculum*, sing.) are also thickened bands that bind muscles and tendons of distal portion of limbs into position. Several processes are disease related.

Dupuytren contracture: thickening and shortening of the palmar fascia of the hand resulting in flexion contractures of the fingers.
fasciitis: inflammation of fascia. Usually an anatomic structure is named when describing the location of the fasciitis, for example, plantar fasciitis, inflammation of the fascia of the sole of the foot.

necrotizing fasciitis: severe, life-threatening bacterial infection of the soft tissues that spreads rapidly along fascial planes. Most commonly caused by group A *Streptococcus*, but may be caused by other bacteria as well.
nodular fasciitis: fasciitis resulting in the formation of nodules.

Joint Diseases (Arthro-, Synovio-, Capsulo-, Ankylo-)

The joint (*arthro-*) has a smooth inner lining or fluid sac (synovium) and a strong fibrous outer connective tissue enclosure (*capsulo-*). Affections of the joint cartilage, synovium, and capsule may result in transient or permanent functional changes. When motion is severely or completely lost, **ankylosis** (an abnormal fusion of a joint) is the result. The terms in this section relate to loss of joint function or a change in appearance of the joint. Joint function depends on its surrounding tissue. Diseases or dysfunctions affecting the joint spaces are presented here.

Arthro- Root Diseases

Arthro- (Gr. *Arthron,* joint) is a combining form denoting relationship to a joint, the junction where two bones meet and articulate with one another. *Articulatio* (Latin) is a general term for joint. The *arthro-* root diseases are as follows.

arthralgia: pain in a joint; arthrodynia.
arthrempyesis: infection in a joint; arthroempyesis.
arthritis: pathologic inflammation of a joint; may be crippling; can become a degenerative joint disease. Various types are **osteoarthritis, gouty a., rheumatoid a., septic a., traumatic a., infectious a., allergenic a.,** and **hemophilic a.**
arthrocace: infected cavity of a joint; caries. (archaic)
arthrocele: swollen joint. (archaic)
arthrochalasis: abnormal relaxation or flaccidity of a joint. (archaic)
arthrochondritis: inflammation of the cartilages of a joint. (archaic)
arthrodysplasia: deformity of various joints; hereditary condition. (archaic)

arthrogryposis: resulting from a variety of sex-linked recessive and autosomal recessive disorders that lead to decreased fetal movement and subsequent soft tissue contractures affecting two or more joints.

arthrokatadysis: limitation of motion of the hip resulting from protrusio acetabuli (deep-shelled acetabulum).

arthrokleisis: ankylosis of a joint. (archaic)

arthrolith: deposit of calculus in a joint. (archaic)

arthromeningitis: synovitis; inflammation of the membranous lining of a joint. (archaic)

arthroncus: joint swelling; arthrophyma. (archaic)

arthroneuralgia: nerve pain in a joint. (archaic)

arthronosos: disease of joints. (archaic)

arthropathy: any joint disease.

arthrophyte: abnormal growth in a joint cavity.

arthropyosis: suppuration, or formation of pus, in a joint cavity.

arthrorheumatism: articular rheumatism. (archaic)

arthrosclerosis: hardening or stiffening of a joint. (archaic)

arthrosis: disease or abnormal condition of a joint.

arthrosteitis: inflammation of any bony joint structure. (archaic)

arthrosynovitis: inflammation of the synovial membrane of a joint. (archaic)

arthroxerosis: chronic osteoarthritis. (archaic)

Other Joint Diseases and Conditions

constriction ring syndrome (Streeter bands): congenital constriction bands with an unknown cause in which intrauterine bands or rings create deep grooves in distal limbs, particularly fingers and toes.

cystic arthrosis: development of large cysts just under the bony surface of a joint. It is not clear whether this is due to cystic degeneration within the bone that leaves the articular cartilage intact or to synovial invasion from the joint. Condition progresses to degenerative arthritis. This condition is probably separate from ganglions that form within the bone and are not associated with arthritic progression.

diffuse idiopathic sclerosing hyperostosis (DISH): excess bone formation at the margins of large joints, particularly the lumbar spine and hips.

flail joint: complete loss of ligamentous stability.

frozen shoulder: severe loss of motion in the shoulder joint resulting from inflammation of the capsule.

hemarthrosis: extravasation of blood into a joint or synovial cavity.

hydrarthrosis: accumulation of watery fluid in the joint cavity.

hypertrophic arthritis: increased bone formation around the joint, as seen on radiographs; **osteoarthritis.**

internal derangement of joint: commonly named internal knee injuries, particularly when the precise nature of the injury is unknown.

joint mice: loose pieces of cartilage or other organic material in the joint.

pannus: growth of blood vessels onto margin of articular cartilage surface.

pauciarticular: involving a few joints as opposed to many joints.

polyarthritis: inflammation of many joints.

pseudoarthrosis: false joints that result from nonunion of a fracture or from a pathologic bone condition.

pustulotic osteoarthropathy: pain, swelling, and radiographic findings of hypertrophy and sclerotic changes involving the sternum, ribs, and clavicle associated with the skin condition pustulosis palmaris et plantaris. The sacrum, spine, and peripheral joints may also show radiographic changes. The cause is unknown.

rice bodies: small, glistening, soft, loose bodies either in joints or bursae; loose fibrocartilage tissue.

sporotrichosis (Rose gardener's disease): fungal disease of skin in which joint disorders can occur.

suppurative arthritis: bacterial infection causing pain, swelling, tenderness, redness, and effusion; **pyarthrosis.**

synarthrosis: ankylosis and contracture; usually caused by arthritic joint disease.

villous lipomatous proliferation: rare disorder of synovial joint lining in which there is fatty proliferation with the formation of numerous villous formations. The term **lipoma arborescens** was applied to this condition. Because it is not a neoplasm, the term *villous lipomatous proliferation* is preferred.

Eponymic Joint Diseases

Behçet syndrome: disease of undetermined cause that may produce joint complaints predominantly in young people in the third decade of life. Marked by oral and genital ulcerations and eye and skin lesions. Often arthritis, thrombophlebitis, gastrointestinal lesions, and central nervous system lesions also occur.

Kawasaki d.: mucocutaneous lymph node syndrome in children characterized by fever, exanthematous skin disease, and sometimes arthritis (30%–40%).

Lyme d.: inflammatory arthritis involving usually a few joints, particularly the knees, caused by an organism that is transmitted by a tick.

Reiter syndrome: arthritis of various joints, usually associated with one or more of the triad of urethral drip, conjunctivitis, and oral mucosal lesions.

Synovio-Related Diseases

Synovial fluid, or synovia, is an alkaline viscid transparent fluid resembling egg white that is found in joint cavities, tendon sheaths, and bursae, and is responsible for lubrication and nourishment of these joint structures. Synovial membrane is the inner lining of a joint, which is a two-layer membrane on a bed of fat composed of certain cells that produce synovial fluid; other cells act as phagocytes. Related disease processes are the following.

synovial cyst: accumulation of fluid in any bursa forming a firm cystic structure. The fluid often becomes gelatinous as seen in a ganglion. The contents and structures of these cysts are often indistinguishable from a ganglion. Some can communicate with a joint or tendon sheath.
  popliteal cyst: seen behind the knee, this cyst usually involves the gastrocnemius-semimembranosus bursa.
  antefemoral cyst: located in the suprapatellar area.
  anteromedial cyst: found in association with the pes anserinus bursa below the anteromedial joint line.
  tibiofibular cyst: associated with the tibiofibular joint, which in 10% of people communicates with the knee.

synovial osteochondromatosis: formation by the synovium of cartilage bodies, which develop into bone.

synoviochondromatosis: synovial formation of cartilage bodies.

synovitis: inflammation of synovial membrane, which may be associated with swelling.

Miscellaneous Synovial Diseases

pigmented villonodular synovitis: inflammation of synovium with production of pigment, giant cells, and other characteristic cell types.

villous synovitis: inflammation of joint lining, resulting in long fronds of synovium.

Capsulo-Related Diseases

The capsule is the thick, fibrous tissue enclosing the cavity of the synovial joint and defines the limits of the joint; it may be referred to as *joint capsule* or *synovial capsule*. There are two related dysfunctions.

adhesive capsulitis: adhesive inflammation between joint capsule and the peripheral articular cartilage of the shoulder, obscuring the subdeltoid bursa. It produces a painful shoulder, stiffness, and may result in limited joint motion; also called **frozen shoulder** and **adhesive bursitis**.

capsulitis: inflammation of the capsule.

Ankylo-Root Diseases

The combining form *ankylo-* means "bent" or "deformed." It was originally used to describe untreated deforming loss of joint function. Now such terms apply to joints fused congenitally or those that are aligned normally because of a surgical process. Therefore the implication of *ankylo-* is not necessarily "bent" or "deformed," but rather "complete fusion" or "restricted motion" of a joint.

ankylodactylia: adhesions of fingers or toes to one another.

ankylosis: consolidation and abnormal immobility of a joint caused by fibrous or bone tissue bridging the joint space.
  bony a.: abnormal union of bones at joint site; also called **true ankylosis.**
  extracapsular a.: caused by rigidity of structure exterior to joint capsule, usually a surgically implanted piece of bone.

false a.: results from other causes not related to the abnormal union of bones composing the joint.
fibrous a.: caused by formation of fibrous bands within the joint.
intracapsular a.: caused by undue rigidity of structure within the joint capsule.
ligamentous a.: results from rigidity of ligaments.
spurious a.: false ankylosis.

Vascular Diseases and Conditions

Blood Vessels

All tissues of the body are supplied with nutrients and oxygen by blood vessels. These vessels are subject to an assortment of disease processes. The larger named arteries are sometimes impaired by arteriosclerosis or trauma, whereas the larger named veins may be impaired by trauma or thrombosis, and the smaller unnamed vessels (on either side of the circulation) can be injured by arteriosclerosis, trauma, or systemic degenerative disorders (e.g., collagen vascular diseases). In addition to these, the heart itself can be afflicted by diseases of the arteries that feed the heart muscle, causing deterioration of the muscle (cardiomyopathy).

Trauma and arteriosclerosis (hardening of the arteries) are the two most frequent arterial conditions that are seen by the orthopaedic surgeon. However, the orthopaedist often sees a host of other vascular disorders or symptoms that influence the treatment of a musculoskeletal problem. Often, patients with these specific disease entities are referred to the peripheral vascular surgeon, and a combined effort is made to restore function. The venous and arterial disorders, collagen vascular disorders, and blood vessel tumors are considered here.

Venous Disorders

deep venous thrombosis (DVT): blood clots in the deep venous circulation usually of the lower extremity, in the calf, thigh, or pelvis. Portions of these clots may break off and lodge in the lungs, causing pulmonary emboli. These clots in the veins eventually destroy the valves of the veins and can cause chronic problems related to venous insufficiency.
phlebitis: inflammation of a vein; may be a result of infection, inflammation, or trauma, and is usually associated with thrombus in that vein (thrombophlebitis).
phlebothrombosis: clot in a vein; phlebitis with secondary thrombosis.
postphlebitic syndrome: chronic venous insufficiency of lower limbs resulting from deep venous thrombosis. Develops with loss of function of valves in veins, allowing blood to pool and cause swelling, pain, leg ulceration, and varicose veins. Also the result of scar-thickened deep veins.
pulmonary embolism (PE): acute obstruction to circulation in lungs as a result of a clot that has migrated from the pelvic or leg veins and lodged in the lung. A life-threatening problem requiring anticoagulant, thrombolytic therapy, and sometimes surgery.
thrombophlebitis: inflammation of a vein associated with thrombosis (blood clots) usually in the lower limbs. The clot can also become infected, becoming septic thrombophlebitis.
thrombosis: formation of a clot (thrombus) within a blood vessel that results in occlusion or stenosis of the vessel, which may cause infarction of tissue supplied by that vessel.
varices (*sing.* -ix): enlarged and tortuous (twisted) veins or lymphatic vessels, usually of the lower limbs.
varicose veins: a degenerative condition of veins whereby the muscle fibers in the walls of the vessel become stretched out and baggy, losing elasticity. The valves become incompetent and blood falls back the wrong way creating a reflux and further wall failure. Return flow becomes inefficient, producing pain, tenderness, and swelling.
venous insufficiency (reflux): malfunction of venous valves that allow blood to flow in a retrograde (backward) direction; also called **postphlebitic syndrome.**

Arterial Disorders

aneurysm: thin-walled, dilated segment of a vessel wall that may be caused by degeneration from arteriosclerosis, congenital abnormality, or trauma. Complications of aneurysms include rupture, thrombosis, or break-off of a blood clot that has collected in the aneurysm.
arterial insufficiency: inadequate blood flow to an organ or extremity often caused by arteriosclerotic

narrowing or occlusion of the blood vessel restricting blood flow. In severe cases, necrosis and gangrene may develop, requiring amputation of a limb.

arterial occlusive disease: hardening of the arteries; also called **arteriosclerosis.**

arteriosclerosis: name for degenerative process that affects most blood vessels in most people (in varying degrees) and begins in early teens. Its progression is related in part to genetics, diet, smoking, and high blood pressure. It can be exacerbated by injuries such as trauma or surgery; it causes narrowing and irregular surfaces in blood vessels, where fatty plaque forms on vessel walls and occludes the blood supply, which leads to ischemia. It is the most frequent problem in arteries; also called **atherosclerosis.**

arteriovenous fistula (AVF): abnormal communication between an artery and a vein; also called **AV fistula.** May be the result of trauma or may be created intentionally for dialysis access.

arteriovenous malformation (AVM): congenital arteriovenous connection often resulting in disfigurement or malfunction. Often seen as a discolored area on the skin, but may represent a much larger diversion of blood such that it interferes with organ function. Its continuing presence may interfere with the heart because of the large alteration in flow that it creates.

atheroma: localized collection of arteriosclerosis (thickened arterial intima—plaque) that has degenerated.

blue toe syndrome: bluish or black tender and painful discoloration of a toe. It is the result of a localized acute ischemia of the toe caused by distal embolization of platelet aggregates or arteriosclerotic plaque, which then occludes the small end vessels. This represents a proximal emboligenic source, for example, aneurysm or significant arteriosclerotic plaque.

Buerger disease: thromboangiitis obliterans: an inflammation of the arteries (and veins) in an extremity causing severe ischemia; occurs usually in young smokers and is a pathologic variant of arteriosclerosis.

cerebrovascular accident (CVA): an outdated term; see *stroke*.

chilblains: breakdown of skin and swelling of the hands and feet from overexposure to cold moisture; also called **thermal injuries.**

claudication: inadequate blood flow to large muscle groups of lower limbs resulting from hardening of the arteries, causing pain, numbness, or heaviness in muscle groups brought on by exercise and relieved promptly by rest; may produce similar symptoms in the upper limbs after prolonged use; also called **intermittent claudication.**

compartment syndrome: compromise of circulation and function of tissue within a closed space caused by increased pressure within that space, with diminished oxygenated blood supply; may be due to overexertion of leg muscles, a tight bandage, or trauma. The syndrome may self-correct or progress, with eventual muscle necrosis (ischemia), loss of arterial blood supply, nerve palsy, or loss of limb. The most commonly affected compartments are the anterior leg **(anterior compartment syndrome),** volar forearm (leading to Volkmann ischemic contracture), and anterior thigh **(rectus femoris syndrome).**

diabetic foot disease: blood flow can be limited by thickened blood vessels and arteriosclerosis producing relative ischemia predominantly to the foot. The neurologic response is blunted, creating sensory deficit and decreased shunting of blood to the affected area. Additionally, altered anatomy, such as tightened tendons, bony changes, dry skin, and deformed nails can create a foot susceptible to infection, ulceration, osteomyelitis, and progression to limb loss.

embolus (*pl.* emboli): blood clot or piece of atheromatous debris that blocks an artery or vein. It can also be made up of an air bubble, fat, portion of tumor, or piece of prosthetic material. An embolus may cause a heart attack if in the heart, a stroke if in the brain, and acute ischemia if in the lower limbs.

fibromuscular dysplasia (FMD): uncommon degenerative disease of the arteries often affecting the renal arteries of young females. The problem causes narrowing of the vessel with weblike deformities that appear as a string of beads on an arteriogram. It can also cause aneurysm.

fistula: abnormal communication between any two structures that normally do not communicate; can be the result of trauma, arteriosclerosis, or surgical procedure.

An arteriovenous fistula may be created and used for hemodialysis. (See *arteriovenous fistula [AVF]*.)

frostbite: damage to tissue resulting from exposure to cold; may lower blood supply sufficiently to cause permanent sensory loss, chronic pain, or partial limb loss.

gangrene: sign of substantial ischemia involving death of tissue. May be dry (not infected) or wet (infected).

Hollenhorst plaque: cholesterol emboli in a small retinal eye artery. Usually indicative of carotid arteriosclerosis. May represent a transient ischemic attack or warning for a stroke.

infarct: area of ischemic necrosis resulting from acute interruption of blood supply. This term is often applied to areas of the brain or heart.

ischemia: acute or chronic decreased blood flow (perfusion) to organ or limb caused by obstruction of inflow of arterial blood or by vasoconstriction. Acutely, the symptoms include the six *P*s: pain, pallor, pulselessness, paresthesias, paralysis, and poikilothermia (coldness).

kinking: bending of an artery, causing pain; result of trauma or body position.

pallor: loss of color of skin representing a marked decrease in blood flow, either acute or chronic; may be present only with the elevation of the extremity.

peripheral arterial occlusion (PAO): results from buildup of atherosclerosis (fatty tissue) that can cut off blood supply to the limbs and feet.

popliteal artery cyst: degeneration of the wall of the popliteal artery resulting in a cysticlike structure within the wall of the artery that can partially or completely obstruct the artery. Not to be confused with the more common synovial or ganglion type.

popliteal entrapment: partial or complete obstruction of popliteal artery as a result of abnormal location of adjacent medial head of the gastrocnemius muscle. It may include an artery, vein, or nerve.

pseudoaneurysm: an aneurysm that does not include all three layers of the blood vessel wall. True aneurysms contain all three layers. Pseudoaneurysms can be the result of a traumatic partial disruption of a blood vessel wall, or the result of an infection that allows a surgical anastomosis to come apart slowly. An infected prosthetic graft is a typical example.

rest pain: distal foot pain caused by acute or chronic arterial ischemia representing a significant decrease in blood flow, usually from hardening of the arteries. The pain is burning and sharp in nature. Symptoms may be relieved temporarily by a dependent position.

rubor (dependent): dark purplish-red color to foot when foot is hung over the edge of bed. It represents maximally dilated capillary beds that are responding to decreased arterial inflow and their subsequent fill by gravity.

stroke: ischemia of a portion of the brain as a result of an occluded blood vessel from an embolus arising from the heart or great vessels of the neck; often the result of hardening of the arteries, a rupture of the blood vessel in the brain, or a tumor. (Formerly called a *cerebrovascular accident [CVA]*.)

Sudeck atrophy: vascular reflex in a limb, caused by trauma, resulting in a red, stiff, and severely painful limb; referred to as **chronic regional pain syndrome** when caused by trauma involving a large area or affecting a large nerve.

subclavian steal syndrome: reversed blood flow down the vertebral or carotid artery neck vessels away from the brain. Produced by arm activity in the face of a blocked subclavian artery. Flow is stolen down these vessels to meet the needs of the arm muscles, producing dizziness, syncope, or visual symptoms because of transient decreased blood flow.

transient ischemic attack (TIA): transient neurologic deficit that clears within 24 hours. Usually the result of decreased blood flow to the portion of brain from a blood clot from either the heart or extracranial carotid vessels. Usually from hardening of the arteries—atheromatous plaque breaks off and lodges in the vessels of the brain or eye.

venous thromboembolic d.: a clot in the venous system, usually the legs or lungs, caused by stasis, endothelial injury, or hypercoagulable state.

Volkmann contracture: final state of an unrelieved forearm compartment syndrome; decreased blood supply to forearm muscles resulting in muscle death, contractures of tendons to wrist and hand, and a claw-hand deformity. This usually starts out as a compartment syndrome that develops after an elbow or forearm fracture.

Collagen Vascular Disorders

Collagen vascular diseases are a series of disorders relating to the basic building blocks of the body, that is, collagen. The walls of blood vessels are made up of collagen, a type of protein seen in all connective tissue such as bone, cartilage, and tendon. Certain diseases affect the collagen, particularly in scattered blood vessels.

Through a variety of mechanisms, the immune system of the body begins to attack, thereby causing degeneration in small blood vessels and parts of the bony anatomy (joint capsule, synovial fluid of joint and synovium). The systemic inflammatory condition that results can be mildly inconvenient or severely disabling, or can result in death. Certain diseases such as rheumatoid arthritis affect this collagen and, as a result, interfere with the function of bones, joints, and blood vessels. The term **inflammatory joint disease** is often used to describe gout, pseudogout, and some other systemic causes of arthritis.

Dyscollagenosis and **systemic connectivitis** are older terms specifically related to the collagen vascular disorders that are due to immune processes such as rheumatoid arthritis, systemic lupus erythematosus, Sjögren syndrome, progressive systemic sclerosis, polyarteritis nodosa, polymyositis, dermatomyositis, and eosinophilic fasciitis. This spectrum of disorders represents the effects on the different collagens of the joint lining and vascular walls.

The treatment of these disorders is often complicated and frustrating for both patient and physician. Medication often involves corticosteroids (antiinflammatory drugs) and nonsteroidal antiinflammatory drugs (ibuprofen, aspirin), and often drugs that directly interfere with the immune mechanism of the body (antimetabolites). **Rheumatology** is the specialty devoted to the diagnosis and treatment of these systemic conditions. A **rheumatologist** is an internal medical specialist. Although rheumatologists often deal with nonsystemic joint diseases, specialty training in this field equips them with the pharmacologic knowledge required to diagnose the broad spectrum of autoimmune, collagen vascular, and metabolic joint disorders.

Terms associated with these various conditions are discussed here along with a series of other miscellaneous disorders.

acrosclerosis: thickening of the skin and other soft tissues of the distal part of a limb. This is usually a part of a larger disease complex such as scleroderma or CREST syndrome.

ankylosing spondylitis: inflammatory joint disease mainly affecting the spine, hips, and pelvis. Seen most commonly in young men, this can lead to fusion of the spine with deformity, depending on the position of the spine during the fusion process. Seen in the child, the disorder is called Marie-Strümpell disease or rheumatoid spondylitis.

arteritis: inflammation of small arteries.

calcinosis circumscripta: quadrad of calcium deposits in the skin (calcinosis cutis), Raynaud phenomenon, scleroderma, and telangiectasia is seen in this collagen disease that has been considered a variant of scleroderma.

CREST syndrome (limited scleroderma): complex of *c*alcinosis of articular tissue associated with *R*aynaud phenomenon, *e*sophageal dysmotility, *s*clerodactyly, and *t*elangiectasia. This condition appears to be less aggressive than scleroderma.

dermatomyositis: idiopathic, autoimmune, inflammatory myopathy characterized by proximal limb and neck weakness. Muscles may become painful, weak, and stiff. A rash can appear on the knees, knuckles, and elbows. The pathologic findings are muscle necrosis and regeneration.

ergotism: acute or chronic effects of ergot alkaloids on the blood flow to an organ such as the brain or limbs. Ergot alkaloids are in some plants and medicines that are taken for headaches.

Felty syndrome: a combination of chronic rheumatoid arthritis, enlarged spleen, and a reduced number of granulocytes in the white blood count.

focal scleroderma: disease of unknown cause characterized by circumscribed areas of fibrosis of the skin, subcutaneous fat, fascia, and muscle into bone. It is usually restricted to a limb and usually occurs in children and young adults; also called **Addison's keloid.**

intermittent hydrarthrosis: rare disorder characterized by recurrent swelling in joints with no associated problems or deformity.

Jaccoud syndrome: deformity of hands and feet as a result of recurrent episodes of rheumatic fever or lupus synovitis. It is often mistaken for rheumatoid arthritis.

lupus erythematosus: disease affecting not only the joints but also heart, heart lining, and circulation in bone. It is life threatening, although a protracted mild course is possible. This disease may be called **systemic lupus erythematosus** to distinguish it from discoid lupus, a more benign process.

Marie-Strümpell d.: begins in childhood, similar to rheumatoid arthritis, usually resulting in ankylosis of the spine and involvement of the liver and spleen; also called **rheumatoid spondylitis** or **ankylosing spondylitis**.

Mönckeberg sclerosis: calcification of the middle coat of small and medium-sized muscular arteries; **medial arteriosclerosis**.

palindromic rheumatism: recurrent acute arthritis and periarthritis with symptom-free intervals of days to months. A number of patients with this disorder develop rheumatoid arthritis.

polyarteritis nodosa: disease-causing nodules in small arteries with some microscopic clotting, resulting in muscle cramps and eventual loss of muscle tone; can be severe.

polymyalgia rheumatica: a syndrome of pain or stiffness affecting the muscles, with some associated with an inflammatory condition of blood vessels. It is typically treated with oral corticosteroids and usually goes away in several years.

progressive systemic sclerosis: spectrum of disorders characterized by fibrosis and degenerative changes in the skin. This includes scleroderma and CREST syndrome.

polymyositis: seen in adults with muscle weakness in the proximal upper and lower limbs. Weakness is usually progressive and associated with an autoimmune process.

pyoderma gangrenosum: rare, destructive cutaneous lesion that starts as a painful, rapidly enlarging ulcer leading to a chronic, draining wound. This is often associated with inflammatory bowel disease, rheumatoid arthritis, seronegative arthritides, hematologic malignancies, and monoclonal gammopathies.

Raynaud d. or phenomenon: small arterioles of upper limbs, particularly of the fingertips, become extremely sensitive to cold, and the vessels undergo segmental spasm, interrupting blood flow to tissue; occasionally progresses to necrosis and dry gangrene in fingertips.

rheumatoid arthritis: generalized inflammatory joint disease. In children, it is called **juvenile idiopathic arthritis** and **Still disease.** The disease may result in mild, lifelong discomfort, or it may become severely crippling; in some cases, there is associated skin nodularity. Certain laboratory studies support the diagnosis (positive rheumatoid factor).

scleroderma: disease causing a waxy thickening of the skin and classically affecting swallowing; tends to be severely progressive.

Sjögren syndrome: a group of conditions including keratoconjunctivitis sicca (dry eyes), arthritis, dry mouth, and enlargement of the parotid glands.

vasoconstriction: narrowing of vessel lumen caused by contraction of muscular vessel walls.

vasodilatation: enlargement of vessel lumen caused by relaxing of muscular vessel wall.

vasospastic: localized intermittent contraction of a blood vessel.

Blood Vessel Disorders

port wine hemangioma: a birth mark that occurs most often in the face and persists for life. This may occasionally be a part of a congenital disease.

Associated Vascular Conditions

acrocyanosis: mottling of the skin of the extremity not produced by major vascular occlusions. It may be related to an emotional change or temperature.

atrophy: reduction in size of an anatomic structure, often related to disuse or decreased blood supply.

arrhythmia: abnormal rhythm of the heart.

bradycardia: abnormal slowing of heart rate, usually less than 60 beats/minute.

bruit: abnormal sound on mediate auscultation over a blood vessel or the heart that indicates turbulence.

congestive heart failure: condition in which heart is unable to pump out venous blood returning to it, resulting in pooling of venous blood and accumulation of fluid in various parts of the body (lungs, legs, etc.).

cyanosis: bluish-purple discoloration of the skin or nail beds; represents decreased blood flow to that area.

hypercholesterolemia: elevated blood cholesterol level; also called **hypercholesteremia** and **hypercholesterinemia.**

hypertension: elevated blood pressure, either temporary or permanent; may be an elevation of the systolic or diastolic blood vessels or pressure.

hypotension: blood pressure below normal.

hypovolemia: loss of normal amount of circulating blood volume; could be the result of hemorrhage from trauma, or from an ulcer.

hypoxia: decreased amount of oxygen in any given tissue.

myocardial infarction (MI): acute or chronic blockage of blood vessels to the heart, resulting in localized area of ischemia (heart attack).

necrosis: pathologic definition of death of tissues caused by lack of blood supply to that part.

normotensive: referring to normal blood pressure.

occlusion: closed or shut, such as an occluded artery or vein.

palpitation: sensation either by patient or examiner of irregular heartbeat.

phlegmasia cerulea dolens: an acute, rare condition that includes a nonpitting edema (swelling that cannot be indented with pressure) in the legs associated with a cyanotic mottled appearance and high muscle compartment pressures. This has been associated with the use of vena cava filters.

stasis: decrease or absence of blood flow in the venous circulation.

stenosis: narrowing of lumen of blood vessel; a stricture.

tachycardia: abnormal increase in heart rate, usually more than 100 beats/minute in an adult.

Neurologic Diseases

Neuro- (Gr. *neuron*, nerve) is a combining form denoting the relationship to a nerve or nerves, or to the nervous system in general. Of all the specialties in medicine, neurology interrelates with orthopaedics more often than any other. The presenting symptoms of certain neurologic disorders may be quite similar to those of some orthopaedic disorders or diseases in that they result in muscular loss, altered function, and possible deformities, particularly in growing individuals.

In orthopaedic diagnoses, the nervous system is considered in two portions, the central and the peripheral. The central portion is composed of the brain and spinal cord and their covering soft tissues. The peripheral portion is composed of all the nerves in the body. Because some diseases affect both the central and peripheral nervous systems simultaneously, discussion of both is presented in an alphabetic listing of nerve disorders, except for some eponymic terms that belong to a specific category. The same term may be defined several times in this chapter to avoid cross-referencing.

General Neurologic Diseases

amyotrophic lateral sclerosis (ALS): disease seen in adult life affecting the spinal cord, with loss of motor control and eventual death; also called **Charcot d.** and **Lou Gehrig d.**

apraxia: inability to perform purposeful movements although there is no sensory or motor impairment; also called **kinetic apraxia** and **motor apraxia.**

arachnoiditis: inflammatory disease of the covering, spider web–like membrane of the spinal cord and nerves. In the lumbar spine, this condition can lead to fibrosis that will bind the roots of the cauda equina.

atonia: lack of tone or tension; relaxation, flaccidity.

autonomic dysreflexia: syndrome marked by muscle spasms, low blood pressure, headache, sweating, goose bumps, and other signs of autonomic nervous system instability. It can be associated with spontaneous joint dislocation.

axonotmesis: disruption of nerve plasma without disruption of the axon sheath, resulting in a recovery of nerve function during a period of up to 3 years.

Barre-Lieou syndrome: degenerative or arthritic changes of C3, C4, and intervertebral disks, often involving the fifth and sixth cervical nerves. Affects mainly middle-aged and older patients, many of whom have associated complaints of dizziness, nausea, headaches, transitory deafness, blurred vision, and loss of balance because of presumed involvement of the cervical sympathetic nervous system and the vertebral artery.

cerebral palsy (CP): general term applied to nonprogressive central nervous system disorders caused by an insult to the developing brain before or during birth or in infancy. Impaired motor control results in physical disability with a broad spectrum of patterns and severity of involvement. Frequently described by pattern and type of involvement (e.g., *spastic diplegia*).

Types
spastic CP: most common form; increased resting tone or tension in muscles.
ataxic CP: additional elements of incoordination.
athetoid CP: uncontrolled writhing movements.
flaccid CP: very severe form in which muscle contractions cannot be initiated.

Patterns
diplegic: involving lower extremities to much greater extent than upper extremities.
hemiplegic: involving one side of the body (typically results from discrete insult to one side of brain.
quadriplegic or total body involvement: most severe pattern; involves upper and lower extremities as well as affecting head and trunk control, swallowing, and speech.

chorea: continuing uncontrolled jerking motions caused by brain disease; may occur as a result of rheumatic fever or other diseases. The inherited form is called **Huntington chorea;** also called **St. Vitus dance.**

complex regional pain syndrome: severe regional pain, usually in a stocking or glove distribution in a limb. This is often associated with a lesion of a peripheral nerve, crush injury, fracture, infection, or vascular inflammation. Symptoms include burning pain, hypersensitivity, and paresthesias in the limb. The terms **reflex sympathetic dystrophy, posttraumatic reflex dystrophy, Sudeck atrophy, causalgia, mimocausalgia,** and **algodystrophy** are used for those disorders.

dysautonomia: an often familial condition characterized by labile blood pressure, insensitivity to pain, abnormal gastrointestinal motility, ataxia, and spinal deformity.

dural ectasia: often seen with neurofibromatosis, thickening of the dural tissues may occur. This can lead to dissolution of the spinal elements and eventual spinal instability.

entrapment syndrome: symptoms caused by entrapment of a nerve in soft or hard tissue, for example, occipital nerve entrapment syndrome, a chronic muscle irritation of the neck, causing impingement on occipital nerve.

epilepsy: disorder of nervous system characterized by seizures in which there may be clonic and tonic muscular contractions and loss of consciousness.
grand mal epilepsy: epilepsy marked by major convulsions, usually first tonic then clonic, oscillating eyeballs, feeble pulse, stupor, and unconsciousness.
petit mal epilepsy: mild or minor attack (small seizures) of epilepsy without convulsions other than slight twitching of muscles of the face or extremities.
Jacksonian epilepsy: recurrent episodes of localized convulsive seizures or spasms limited to a part of the body, without loss of consciousness.

epineural fibrosis: scarring of the covering of a nerve, usually following trauma.

familial dysautonomia: autosomal recessive disorder of autonomic system causing loss of control of multiple organs including bowel, bladder, heart, and lungs.

ganglioneuroma: tumor made up of ganglion cells.

glioma: tumor arising from specialized connective tissue found in brain and spinal cord.

glomus tumor: benign tumor consisting of nerve and small-vessel components. These small lesions often produce severe pain and local vascular effects. They are often found near the tips of digits of the hands and feet.

Gross Motor Function Classification System (GMFCS)

This classification system is for cerebral palsy function based on self-initiated movement with emphasis on function.

Level I: Walk indoors and outdoors and climb stairs without limitation. With running and sports, speed and balance are impaired.

Level II: Walk indoors and outdoors and climb stairs holding onto a railing, but have limitation with uneven walking, inclines, crowds, and confined spaces.

Level III: Walk indoors or outdoors on a level surface with an assistive mobility devise. May climb stairs holding onto a railing. May propel a wheelchair manually be transported when traveling for long distances, outdoors, or on uneven terrain.

Level IV: May walk for short distance on a walker or rely more on wheeled mobility at home, school, and community.

Level V: Unable to maintain antigravity head and trunk postures. No independent mobility.

hemiplegia: paralysis of one side of the body.

intraneural fibrosis: scarring of the internal fibers of a nerve, usually following trauma.

Klumpke palsy (lower obstetrical palsy): palsy of the lower cervical nerve roots C8 and T1; usually seen following an infant delivery but may be seen in adult life after trauma.

locomotor ataxia: severe progressive disease of the central nervous system, caused by syphilis and characterized by demyelination of the dorsal columns of the spinal cord; **tabes dorsalis.**

lumbar thecoperitoneal shunt syndrome: occurs after a thecoperitoneal shunt for idiopathic communicating hydrocephalus; characterized by severe, rigid, and progressive lumbar lordosis, severe bilateral restriction of straight leg raising, and abnormalities of stance and gait.

meralgia: pain in the thigh, usually caused by irritation of lateral cutaneous nerve of the thigh.

mononeuritis multiplex: impairment of sensation, usually in the foot, where there is increased or decreased sensitivity associated with a vasculitis, usually seen in rheumatoid vasculitis.

monoplegia: in cerebral palsy an isolated paralysis of one limb.

motor neuron d.: any disease caused by destruction of the nerve cells involved in voluntary muscle function.

  upper motor neuron d.: any brain disorder that affects the normal pathways leading to voluntary muscle function.

  lower motor neuron d.: disorder of the cells in the spinal cord, resulting in loss of motor function.

multiple sclerosis: a slowly progressive central nervous system disease characterized by degeneration of the myelin (nerve) sheaths in the spinal cord, resulting in multiple and varied neurologic symptoms; usually with remission and exacerbation.

myopathy hand: characteristic hand dysfunction caused by spinal cord injury. A loss of adduction power, extension of the ulnar two or three fingers, and an inability to grip and release rapidly with these fingers distinguishes this hand weakness from other hand dysfunctions caused by peripheral nerve disorders.

neural tube defect: group of malformations of the brain and spinal cord that originate at various times during fetal development, resulting in failure of the neural tube to close. The most common kind is meningomyelocele in which the spinal cord and its covering (meninges) are exposed outside the skin. Also called **spina bifida.**

neuralgia: pain along the course of a nerve or nerves.

neuritis: inflammation of any nerve; usually painful.

neurogenic: originating from nervous tissue; resulting from nervous impulses. In orthopaedics the term is used to define a neurologic cause of a disorder such as a deformity arising from nerve imbalance.

neurologic d.: any disease of the nervous system.

neurolysis: dissolution of the nerve tissue in disease process.

neuroma: this condition is not an actual tumor but is due to a tumescence in the nerve caused by hypertrophy of the cells covering the inside and outside of the nerve.

  traumatic neuroma: neuroma caused by a complete cutting of the nerve or by sufficient injury to cause excess scarring in the nerve.

  amputation neuroma: a traumatic neuroma occurring after an amputation.

neuropathy: a symptom complex rather than a disease entity that occurs outside the brain and spinal cord.

neuropraxia: contusion of a nerve resulting in transient disruption of nerve function; less severe than axonotmesis or neurotmesis.

neurotmesis: complete transection of a nerve, resulting in cell death.

paralysis: loss or impairment of voluntary muscle function; palsy.

paralysis agitans: chronic nervous disease in later life marked by muscular tremor or by a shuffling gait; also called **Parkinson disease.**

paraplegia: paralysis of lower part of body or lower extremities.

paresis: incomplete loss of voluntary muscle function.

paresthesia: abnormal sensations such as numbness, burning, tickling, and crawling caused by central or peripheral nerve system lesions such as multiple sclerosis or locomotor ataxia.

pellagra: vitamin B_6 deficiency disease manifested by disorders of skin, alimentary tract, and nervous system.

peripheral neuropathy: any disorder of nerve function resulting in abnormal conduction of impulses resulting in loss of sensation or muscle control.

poliomyelitis: inflammation of gray matter of spinal cord; may result in loss of voluntary muscle control.

polyneuritis: inflammation of multiple nerves.

quadriplegia: loss of voluntary muscle function in both arms and legs.

radial tunnel syndrome (supinator syndrome): peripheral nerve syndrome caused by compression of radial nerve as it passes through the region between the radial head and the arcade of Frohse.

radiculitis: inflammation of intradural portion of a spinal nerve root before its entrance into the intervertebral foramen, or of the portion between that foramen and the nerve plexus.

radiculoneuritis: inflammation of nerve root and nerve.

Rett syndrome: genetically determined disorder of the extrapyramidal system manifested by scoliosis, hip dislocation, and lower-limb contractures. It expresses itself in the second year of life in girls.

syringomyelia: disorder of spinal cord, marked by abnormal cavities filled with liquid.

tabes dorsalis: severe progressive disease of the central nervous system, caused by syphilis and characterized by demyelination of the dorsal columns of the spinal cord; also called **locomotor ataxia** and **Duchenne d.**

taboparesis: condition in which symptoms of tabes dorsalis and general paresis are associated; also called **neurosyphilis.**

tic: involuntary and usually quick, repetitious contractions of a muscle or muscle groups; repeated twitching.

tic douloureux: painful affliction (neuralgia) involving the trigeminal nerve.

tremor: involuntary trembling or quivering; shaking.

vertigo: loss of equilibrium.

Eponymic Neurologic Diseases

allodynia: a condition in which nonpainful stimuli, such as touch or light pressure, cause pain.

Bell palsy: loss of function of the facial nerves.

Brown-Séquard syndrome: injury to only one side of the spinal cord, resulting in loss of motion on one side of the body and loss of sensation on the opposite side.

Charcot joint d.: joint destruction caused by loss of normal sensation. This is a **neurogenic arthropathy** that is due to the interference of both normal nerve activity as well as vascular control. The result is a rapid dissolution of the joint with subsequent severe deformity in some cases; typically seen in diabetic neuropathy.

Charcot-Marie-Tooth d.: spontaneous degeneration of the neuromuscular complex, most commonly peroneal nerve, but also ulnar nerve, generally starting in childhood; also called **Marie-Charcot-Tooth d.**

  type I motor and sensory neuropathy: a slowly progressive peripheral neurologic condition of childhood that can result in recurrent dislocation of the patella, peroneal muscle atrophy, high-arched/turned-in foot, and scoliosis. This is autosomally inherited and results from a failure of normal peripheral **myelin protein 22** (type 1A), a failure of **myelin protein 0** (type 1B), unknown defect (type 1C), and **early growth response gene EGR2** (type 1D).

  type II motor and sensory neuropathy: a neuronal disorder associated with peroneal muscular atrophy. Type IIA is inherited as an autosomal dominant. Other types being defined include type 2, an autosomal recessive, and two x-linked, one of which is associated with a disorder of **connexin-32.**

Dejerine d.: spontaneous local hypertrophic interstitial neuropathy of a peripheral nerve, cause unknown.

Dejerine-Sottas syndrome (familial interstitial hypertrophic neuritis): familial neuritis associated with high-arched feet and marked sensory changes in all limbs.

double crush syndrome: peripheral nerve compression on the same nerve bundle such as cervical nerve root compression, concurrent with carpal tunnel compression at the wrist.

Erb palsy (upper obstetrical palsy): to be distinguished from Erb paralysis (form of muscular dystrophy). Palsy affects muscles supplied by upper cervical nerve roots C5 and C6; usually caused by a distraction injury, such as a difficult infant delivery, but may occur in adult life after trauma.

Friedreich ataxia: autosomally recessive inherited disease caused by lack of frataxin in mitochondria, resulting in oxidative stress leading to sclerosis of the dorsal and lateral columns of the spinal cord, attended by loss of coordination; usually apparent in early childhood; can be fatal.

Guillain-Barré syndrome: viral disorder involving spinal cord, peripheral nerves, and nerve roots; recovery of lost voluntary muscle function usually occurs, but the disease can be fatal.

modified Mallet classification: for birth brachial plexus palsies using five categories graded 0 to 5. The five categories assess overall upper extremity limb function based on global shoulder abduction and external rotation, hand to neck and mouth, and hand on the spine.

Naffziger syndrome: scalenus anticus syndrome; pain in brachial plexus distribution, caused by muscle impingement.

Parkinson d.: chronic nervous disease in later life marked by muscular tremor or by a shuffling gait; also called **paralysis agitans**.

Parrot pseudoparalysis: decreased movement of the extremity caused by syphilitic bone covering inflammation (periostitis) in infants.

Parsonage-Andrew-Turner syndrome: condition of the brachial plexus resulting in sudden onset of pain and muscle weakness in upper limbs that may lead to muscle wasting (atrophy). Pain may occur simultaneously or after several weeks, and last 1 to 4 weeks or persist for 18 months. Cause unknown. Also called **neuralgic amyotrophy**.

Pott paraplegia: lower limb paralysis caused by spinal cord compression, caused by an abscess, a caseous mass such as tuberculosis, or by harder tissue such as a sequestrated disk.

Refsum syndrome: hypertrophic neuropathy that begins in childhood and progresses with repeated remissions and reactivation consisting mostly of distal sensory and motor loss.

Roussy-Lévy syndrome (hereditary areflexic dystasia): disease of peripheral nerves associated with a tremor that becomes arrested at puberty.

schwannoma: neoplasm of a nerve sheath.

Seddon Classification

The Seddon classification system is for peripheral nerve injury to determine treatment and prognosis.

Neurapraxia: the nerve remains intact but signaling is decreased with expectation of full return. An example is a contusion to a nerve. The endoneurium, perineurium, and the epineurium are intact and there is no wallerian degeneration.

Axonotmesis: the axon is damaged but the surrounding connecting tissue remains intact. Wallerian degeneration occurs below the site of injury.

neurotmesis: severing of the nerve with axon and connective tissue damage.

Sunderland Classification

The Sunderland classification system is for peripheral nerve injury to determine treatment and prognosis.

First-degree: segmental demyelination; neurapraxia.

Second-degree: severed axon but intact endoneurium; axonotmesis.

Third-degree: discontinuous axon and endoneurial tube, with preserved perineurium and fascicular arrangement; axonotmesis.

Fourth-degree: discontinuous axon, endoneurial tube, perineurium, and fasciculi, with intact epineurium; neuroma in continuity; axonotmesis.

Fifth-degree: complete nerve transection; neurotmesis.

---

von Recklinghausen disease: multiple neurofibromatosis.

Metabolic Diseases

There are thousands of chemicals in the body. Most of them are being rapidly destroyed and replaced as part of the essential chain of events that supplies energy, growth, and normal tissue replacement. There are conditions in which some of these chemicals may accumulate or be produced in inadequate quantity for normal function. Not all metabolic diseases can be identified at birth.

Gout is a disease in which uric acid accumulates in the soft tissues and joint spaces; it usually does not occur until middle adult life. **Sickle cell anemia** is the result of production of the wrong kind of chemical, causing changes in the shape of red cells and a subsequent decreased oxygen supply; this disorder is usually detected in infancy.

Many such disorders of chemical production and destruction (metabolism) have been defined elsewhere in this text because of certain characteristic tissues or extremity appearances. Some terms are redefined here, with greater emphasis placed on the metabolic aspects.

Osteopenia is a term that defines abnormally diminished bone content. It may occur regionally after immobilization or be due to a systemic effect involving the entire skeleton. The term does not define the quality of the bone, but simply states that there is less of it. The WHO definition of osteopenia refers to T scores between –1.0 and –2.5. Normal bone density is present if the T score is greater than –1.

Osteoporosis is a condition in which the mineral and organic content is normal, but there is less bone. The most common generalized osteoporosis is associated with aging *(senile osteoporosis)*. Some metabolic conditions such as the postmenopausal state and abnormal gastrointestinal absorption are associated with a generalized osteoporosis. If no specific cause is found, the condition is often referred to as **idiopathic osteoporosis**. In children it is called **juvenile osteoporosis**. The WHO Working Group defines osteoporosis according to measurements of bone mineral density (BMD) using dual-energy x-ray absorptiometry (DEXA). They define osteoporosis as a bone density T score at or below 2.5 standard deviations (T score) below normal peak values for young adults. One or more fragility fractures in conjunction with a T score less than –2.5 is called *established* or *severe osteoporosis*. The WHO definition of osteoporosis only takes into consideration measurement of bone density, with no component of bone quality. The National Institutes of Health Consensus Development Panel on Osteoporosis in 2001 defined osteoporosis as a skeletal disorder characterized by compromised bone strength predisposing a person to an increased risk of fracture. This definition takes into consideration that there are other factors that influence bone quality such as the microarchitecture of bone.

Osteomalacia describes softening of bone, resulting from vitamin D deficiency or kidney disease. Milk allergy, liver disease, excision of the ovaries, kidney disorders, and chronic intestinal problems may interfere with vitamin D metabolism, absorption of calcium, or other processes, resulting in abnormal bone formation and mineralization.

Diseases Associated with Osteomalacia

autosomal dominant hypophosphatemic rickets: autosomal dominant disorder caused by a dysfunction in **fibroblast growth factor 23 receptor (FGFR23)** with a range of disorders present in childhood with limb deformity to adult-onset bone pain caused by osteomalacia secondary to renal phosphate loss.

Fanconi syndrome: severe form of vitamin D–resistant rickets, often fatal, and characterized by the presence of glucose, amino acids, and other chemicals in the urine.

hyperparathyroidism: abnormal increase in the level of parathyroid hormone, resulting in loss of calcium from bones.

hypoparathyroidism: abnormal decrease in the level of parathyroid hormone, either congenital or acquired, resulting in decreased bone formation and lowered serum calcium.

hypophosphatasia: autosomal recessive inherited disease characterized by severe skeletal defects resulting from a failure of calcification of bone.

milk-alkali syndrome: osteoporosis and/or osteomalacia, usually resulting from excessive intake of milk and alkali to treat ulcer disease; changes in therapy have reduced the prevalence of this disorder.

pseudohypoparathyroidism (PHPT): deficient hormone action caused by target tissue resistance. Associated with short stature, shortened metacarpals and metatarsals (particularly the fourth), obesity and rounded face, reduced intelligence, subcutaneous calcification and ossifications, and some less common bone abnormalities; also called **Albright hereditary osteodystrophy.** Specific forms include PHPT as a result of guanine nucleotide deficiency, parathyroid hormone (PTH) receptor abnormality, and circulating antagonists to PTH action type II with normal bone responsiveness (hypo- and hyperparathyroidism).

renal osteodystrophy: descriptive of a specific bone resorptive pattern seen in children and adults who have chronic kidney disease.

rickets: deficiency of bone mineralization in children; refers to the specific appearance of stunted growth, prominent rib cartilage (rachitic rosary), skull deformity (hot cross bun skull), and bowlegs; these are characteristic of a variety of disorders that lead to a failure of normal calcification of bone; may be due to inadequate dietary intake of vitamin D or to kidney problems that produce a bone salt loss.

vitamin D–resistant rickets (VDDR1): rickets caused by an autosomal recessively inherited deficiency of the **vitamin D enzyme 25-α-hydroxycholicaliferol-1-hydroxylase**, resulting in severe rickets; also called **pseudo deficiency rickets.**

vitamin D–resistant rickets (VDRR2): autosomal recessive disease caused by dysfunction of **25-α-hydroxycholecaliferol receptor** resulting in rickets marked by normal-appearing kidneys that excrete excessive phosphorus into the urine; resistant to usual vitamin D therapy but responds to very high doses of vitamin D; also called **pseudo deficiency rickets.**

x-linked hypophosphatemic rickets: sex-linked dominant disorder caused by a disorder of intracellular signaling of a **phosphate endopeptidase homolog (PHEX)** leading to postnatal rickets with growth retardation and dental abnormalities.

Diseases Associated with Osteoporosis

Cushing d.: disease caused by increase in corticosteroids from the adrenal glands or medication; may result in a characteristic vertebral body appearance and generalized osteoporosis.

hyperthyroidism: increased thyroid hormone production and increased general metabolism; may result in osteoporosis.

hypothyroidism: decreased thyroid hormone; may result in less bone production and osteoporosis.

Other Metabolic Genetic Conditions

(Table 2-4)

acrocapitofemoral dysplasia: rare autosomal recessive condition caused by abnormality of **Indian hedgehog (IHH)** function, characterized by short stature and short limbs. Radiographs show cone-shaped epiphyses mainly in hands and hips.

Angelman syndrome: Failure of production of **UBE3A**, a component of this ubiquitin pathway, a protein that helps degrade proteins in the brain. This results in a stiff, jerky gait, absent speech, excessive laughter, and seizures.

beta$_2$-microglobulin amyloidosis: intraosseous and soft tissue deposition of beta$_2$-microglobulin seen in long-term hemodialysis patients.

calcific periarthritis: a painful condition of soft tissue immediately surrounding joints caused by the deposition of calcium phosphate crystals with a white cell inflammatory response.

Coffin-Lowry syndrome: heritable disorder characterized by pronounced mental retardation, peculiar facies, short stature, and a clumsy, broad-based gait. There are multiple skeletal abnormalities.

diabetes: disorder of insulin and sugar metabolism (diabetes mellitus), resulting in high blood glucose levels. Does not necessarily cause bone disorders, but in later life causes vascular compromise to the legs and feet, possibly leading to amputation (diabetic foot d.).

Down syndrome: mongolism; the condition is produced by chromosomal abnormality; also called **trisomy 21.**

dyssegmental dysplasia: rare lethal form of short-limbed dwarfism with different abnormal shapes of the vertebral bodies.

Ehlers-Danlos syndrome (EDS): spectrum of disorders marked by laxity of joints, velvety skin that is soft and hyperextensible, and vessel fragility. Some of these have known specific collagen defects. Because of an improved understanding of the consequence of the various genetic defects, the classification system has been reorganized to incorporate related conditions and reassign others:

New Classification

Classic type (EDS I & II): (I) autosomal dominant, easy bruising, mitral valve prolapse, premature rupture of the fetal membranes, or premature birth, type V collagen disorder. (II) autosomal dominant, similar to type 1, but the effects are milder; type V collagen disorder.

Hypermobility type (EDS III): autosomal dominant, striking joint hypermobility and minimal skin changes, multiple gene; type III collagen being one.

Vascular type (EDS IV): autosomal dominant, vascular/ecchymotic form, prominent venous markings, which are readily visible through the skin. Patients are subject to spontaneous rupture of the bowel, the medium-sized arterial structures, or both; type III collagen disorder.

Kyphoscoliosis type (EDS VI): autosomal recessive, retinal detachments, microcornea, myopia, scoliosis, and neonatal hypotonia caused by deficiency of lysine hydroxylase effect on collagen.

Arthrochalasia type (EDS VIIB): both types VIIA and VIIB, autosomal dominant, multiplex congenita (overflaccidity of the joints without hyperelasticity of the skin), short stature, and micrognathia. Dermatosparaxis (EDS VIIC) is autosomal recessive, multiplex congenita overflaccidity of the joints without hyperelasticity of the skin, short stature, and micrognathia.

> **Types not included in new scheme include the following:**
>
> **EDS type V:** a sex-linked recessive form described only in a single family somewhat similar to type 2 EDS.
>
> **EDS type VIII:** classic type with periodontitis, autosomal dominant. Multiple skin striae and significant dental problems, including early tooth loss, periodontitis, and alveolar bone loss.
>
> **EDS type IX:** allelic to Menkes syndrome X-linked recessive. Occipital exostoses, bladder diverticula or rupture, bony dysplasias, and decreased copper and ceruloplasmin. The gene is related to a condition termed *cutis laxa* or occipital horn syndrome, caused by failure of the activity of lysyl oxidase, a copper-dependent enzyme involved in cross-link formation in collagen.
>
> **EDS type X:** Described in one family; autosomal recessive, fibronectin-1 disorder. Patients exhibit poor wound healing, petechiae, and a platelet aggregation defect, which can be corrected by fibronectin supplementation.

gout: disease process in which uric acid crystals are deposited into the joint lining or inflammatory cells within the joint and soft tissue. The most common form is urate (monosodium urate monohydrate). Other forms include pyrophosphate (calcium pyrophosphate dihydrate), apatite (various calcium crystals), cholesterol, and oxalate (calcium oxalate monohydrate and dihydrate).

gouty arthritis: inflammatory joint changes associated with gout; may be associated with tophi.

gouty node: collection of uric acid crystals near joints.

hemophilia: inherited disorder of coagulation; sex-linked; repeated hemorrhages may result in bone and joint deformity.

TABLE 2-4 Genetic Musculoskeletal Disorders

Musculoskeletal Disorder	Mutation	Site	Inheritance	Notes
Osteogenesis imperfecta	Type I collagen	Protein product in matrix	Most autosomal dominant	COL1A1 or COL1A2
Type IA; IB (teeth affected, more severe)	Type I collagen	Protein product in matrix	Autosomal dominant	IA mild to moderate, blue sclera
Type II Lethal	Type I collagen	Protein product in matrix	Autosomal dominant	
Type III	Type I collagen	Protein product in matrix	Autosomal dominant	Early child hood fx, dentinogenesis
Type IV	Type I collagen	Protein product in matrix	Autosomal dominant	Later childhood, sclera normal or pale blue
Ehler-Danlos type I	Type V or Type I	Protein product in matrix	Autosomal dominant	
Ehler-Danlos type 2	Type V or Type I	Protein product in matrix	Autosomal dominant	
Ehler-Danlos type 3	Type III collagen or tenascin X	Protein product in matrix	Autosomal dominant	
Ehler-Danlos type 4	Type III collagen	Protein product in matrix	Autosomal dominant	
Ehler-Danlos VI	Type I collagen (lysyl hydroxylase)	Protein product in matrix	Autosomal recessive	
Ehler-Danlos 7IA and B	Type I collagen (amino propeptidase)	Protein product in matrix	Autosomal dominant	
Ehler-Danlos 7C	Type I collagen ADAMTS 2	Protein product in matrix	Autosomal recessive	
Kneist dysplasia	Type II collagen	Protein product in matrix	Autosomal dominant	
Stickler dysplasia	Type II collagen	Protein product in matrix	Autosomal dominant	
Stickler dysplasia without involvement of eyes	Type XI collagen	Protein product in matrix	Autosomal dominant	Minor collagen associated with fibrillar assembly
Precocious osteoarthritis	Type II collagen	Protein product in matrix	Autosomal dominant	
Spondyloepiphyseal dysplasia, congenita	Type II collagen	Protein product in matrix	Autosomal dominant	
Spondyloepiphyseal dysplasia, tarda	Type II collagen	Protein product in matrix	Autosomal recessive	

Continued

TABLE 2-4 Genetic Musculoskeletal Disorders—cont'd

Musculoskeletal Disorder	Mutation	Site	Inheritance	Notes
Multiple epiphyseal dysplasia	Type IXA1,2,3 COMP, matrilin 3	Protein product in matrix	Autosomal dominant	
Schmid metaphyseal dysplasia	Type X collagen	Protein product in matrix	Autosomal dominant	
Spondyloepiphyseal dysplasia, x-linked	Sedlin	Protein product in matrix	X-linked dominant	
Marfan	Fibrillin 1	Protein product in matrix	Autosomal dominant	Not all are fibrillin
Marfan-like	Fibrillin 2	Protein product in matrix	Autosomal dominant	Contracture fingers
Pseudoachondroplasia	COMP, matrilin	Protein product in matrix	Autosomal dominant	
Ehler-Danlos X	Fibronectin-1	Protein product in matrix	Autosomal dominant	
Hypophosphatasia: neonatal, infantile, childhood, adult	Decreased alkaline phosphatase	Protein product in matrix	Autosomal recessive	
Neurofibromatosis	Neurofibrilin	Protein product in matrix	Autosomal dominant	
Type I Hurler	Alpha-1-iduronidase	Posttranslation in matrix	Autosomal recessive	Enlarged heart
Type II Hunter	iduronate-2-sulfatase	Posttranslation in matrix	X dominant	
Type III Sanfilippo	accumulation of heparan sulfate	Posttranslation in matrix	Autosomal recessive	
Type IVA Morquios A	Galactosamine 6 sulphate sulfatase	Posttranslation in matrix	Autosomal recessive	
Type IVB Morquios B	Galactosidase	Posttranslation in matrix	Autosomal recessive	
Type V Scheie (MP 1S)	Alpha-l-iduronidase	Posttranslation in matrix	Autosomal recessive	
Type VII Sly	Beta-glucuronidase	Posttranslation in matrix	Autosomal recessive	
Mcardle	Glycogen phosphorylase	Posttranslation in matrix	Autosomal recessive	
Gaucher type I, II, and III	Glucocerebrosidase, and others	Posttranslation in matrix	Autosomal recessive	
Diastrophic dysplasia	Sulfate transporter	Posttranslation in matrix	Autosomal recessive	
Alkaptonuria	Homogentisic acid oxidase	Posttranslation in matrix	Autosomal recessive	
Ehler Danlos progenoid form	Glactosyltransferase 1	Posttranslation in matrix	Autosomal recessive	
Homocystinuria	Cystathionine beta-synthase	Posttranslation in matrix	Autosomal recessive	
Pfeiffer	FGF receptor 1 fibroblast growth factor	Cell surface receptor	Autosomal dominant	
Apert syndrome	FGF receptor 2 fibroblast growth factor	Cell surface receptor	Autosomal dominant	Type 1 acrocephalosyndactyly
Crouzon syndrome	FGF receptor 2 fibroblast growth factor	Cell surface receptor	Autosomal dominant	
achondroplasia	FGF receptor 3 fibroblast growth factor	Cell surface receptor	Autosomal dominant	
Thanatophoric dysplasia	FGF receptor 3 fibroblast growth factor	Cell surface receptor	Spontaneous mutation	
Hypochondrodysplasia	FGF receptor 3 fibroblast growth factor	Cell surface receptor	Autosomal dominant	

TABLE 2-4 Genetic Musculoskeletal Disorders—cont'd

Musculoskeletal Disorder	Mutation	Site	Inheritance	Notes
Vitamin D resistant rickets (VDDR2)	25-α-hydroxycholicaliferol receptor	Cell surface receptor	Autosomal recessive	
Osteopetrosis	Carbonic anhydrase type II	Cell surface receptor	Autosomal dominant	
Proton pump in humans			Autosomal recessive in malignant infantile form	
Jansen metaphyseal chondrodysplasia	PTH/PTHrP receptor	Cell surface receptor	Autosomal dominant	
Osteopetrosis	Beta-3 integrin	Cell surface receptor	Autosomal recessive	
Fibrodysplasia ossificans progressiva	Activin receptor type IA (ACVRI)	Cell surface receptor	Autosomal dominant	
Autosomal dominant hypophosphatemic rickets	FGF23	Cell surface receptor	Autosomal dominant	
McCune-Albright polyostotic fibrous	GS alpha protein of adenylate	Intracellular signaling	Mosaic spontaneous	
Dysplasia	Cyclase (GNAS-1)	Intracellular signaling		
Duchenne muscular dystrophy	Dystrophin	Intracellular signaling	X-linked recessive	
Autosomal limb girdle dystrophy	Part of dystrophin-glycoprotein complex	Intracellular signaling	Autosomal recessive	
Multiple hereditary exostosis	EXT, EXT2 genes	Intracellular signaling	Autosomal dominant	
Vitamin D resistant rickets (VDDR1)	25-α-hydroxycholicaliferol-1-hydroxylase	Intracellular peptidase	Autosomal recessive	
Neurofibromatosis	NF-1 (neurofibromin)	Nucleus	Autosomal dominant	
Acheiropodia	C7orf2 gene affects DNA transcription	Nucleus	Autosomal recessive	
Bone dysplasia sclerosteosis	a novel cystine knot-containing protein	Nucleus	Autosomal recessive	
Camptomelic dysplasia	SOX 9	Nucleus	Autosomal dominant	
Camurati-Engelmann disease	TGF-Beta 1	Nucleus	Autosomal dominant	
Cleidocranial dysostosis	cbfa1 (core binding protein) (RUNX 2)	Nuclear	Autosomal dominant	
McKusick metaphyseal chondrodysplasia	mutations in RMRP, a nonencoding RNA	Nuclear	Autosomal recessive	
Nail-patella syndrome	LMX1b finger protein	Nuclear	Autosomal dominant	
X-linked hypophosphatemic rickets	PEX, a Zn-metallopeptidase	Nuclear	X-linked dominant	
Osteopetrosis	MCSF	Paracrine factor	Autosomal recessive	
Fibrodysplasia ossificans progressiva	BMP-4	Paracrine factor	Autosomal recessive	
Acrocapitofemoral dysplasia	IHH (Indian Hedge Hog)+B42	Paracrine factor	Autosomal recessive	
Fredrich's ataxia	Frataxin	Microsome	Autosomal recessive	

Continued

TABLE 2-4 Genetic Musculoskeletal Disorders—cont'd

Musculoskeletal Disorder	Mutation	Site	Inheritance	Notes
Angelman syndrome	UBE3A:ubiquitin protein ligase E3A		Autosomal recessive	
Prader-Willi	?		Spontaneous	
Trichorhinophalangeal syndrome	?		Autosomal dominant	Combined nose, hair, joint affect
Charcot-Marie-Tooth				
Type I	Types 1a–1f, 1x, different proteins	Myelin wrapping	Autosomal dominant	PMP 22 gene, etc.
Type 2	Types 2a–2e, axonal proteins	Axonal transmission	Autosomal dominant	
Type 3	Myelin protein	Myelin deterioration	Autosomal recessive	
Type 4	Not clear	Rare	Autosomal recessive	

COMP, *Cartilage oligomeric matrix protein*; FGF, *fibroblast growth factor*; fx, *fracture*.

infantile hypophosphatasia: autosomal recessive disorder affecting alkaline phosphatase affecting bone formation seen in infants.

Kashin-Beck disease: endemic in eastern Siberia and northern China and Korea; abnormalities in enchondral bone growth leading to osteoarthrosis.

Klinefelter syndrome: failure of full sexual development in males, with development of some female characteristics; results from the fertilized egg receiving both female X chromosomes and the male Y chromosome.

lipid storage disease: inherited disorder resulting in multiple problems; bone disorders are secondary to displacement of the marrow by abnormal cells, resulting in avascular necrosis of the hip or irregular patterns on radiographs; also called **lipid reticuloendotheliosis.**

lipocalcinogranulomatosis: probable metabolic-based disorder with lipid-filled histiocytes and associated tumoral calcinosis.

Marfan syndrome: autosomal dominant disorder of **fibrillin-1** resulting in elastic inherited defect in elastic tissue resulting in ligamentous laxity and spiderlike fingers, with joint and vessel disorders.

Marfan-like syndrome: autosomal dominant disorder of **fibrillin-2** resulting in elastic inherited defect in elastic tissue resulting in ligamentous laxity and spiderlike fingers, with joint and vessel disorders.

Menkes kinky-hair syndrome: X-linked recessive disorder that is fatal in infancy or early childhood; associated with depigmented and kinky hair, hypertrophic gingiva, loose joints, vascular tortuosity, seizures, and severe mental retardation. Similar to types V and IX Ehlers-Danlos syndrome.

metachondromatosis: autosomal dominant disorder characterized by multiple osteochondromas of the hand and feet associated with paraosseous calcification or ossifications, and metaphyseal osteochondromas in long bones and iliac crest. These may progress or regress unpredictably.

metallosis: in orthopaedics, the term is applied to conditions resulting from very tiny microscopic particles that come from internal prosthetic devices.

Milroy d.: swelling of distal parts caused by a congenital disorder in which there is a retention of lymph fluid; also called **familial lymphedema.**

Pfeiffer syndrome: an autosomal dominant disorder of **fibroblast growth factor receptors 1 and 2 (FGFR 1 & FGFR 2)** resulting in early fusion of the skull (craniosynostosis), dental problems caused by crowded teeth, often a high palate, poor vision, and hearing loss in approximately 50% of children.

prune belly syndrome: undescended testicles, urinary tract obstructions, and hypoplastic abdominal muscles that result in a prune belly appearance and assorted musculoskeletal abnormalities; also called **Eagle-Barrett syndrome.**

pseudoachondroplasia: autosomal dominant condition caused by defect in **collagen oligomeric matrix protein (COMP)** affecting major joints with deformity and short stature.

pseudogout: more appropriately called **calcium pyrophosphate deposition disease (CPPD)**. Usually occurs after age 60. Joint symptoms are consistent with degenerative arthritis development and x-rays reveal deposition of calcium within the cartilage. Can be, but not necessarily is, associated with mineral metabolic disorders such as renal disease or hyperparathyroidism.

Shwachman syndrome: pancreatic exocrine insufficiency associated with cyclical low white blood cell production in children. Orthopaedic conditions include profound short stature.

sickle cell anemia: autosomal recessive inherited disease that affects the shape of red cells (oat-shaped erythrocytes); the results that most concerns orthopaedists are bone infections (sometimes caused by *salmonella*), which is a very rare cause of bone infection in normal children, and bone infarcts in adolescents and adults, particularly of the hip.

thalassemia: autosomal recessive inherited disease of red cell structure; may result in skeletal deformity.

thanatophoric dysplasia: autosomal dominant mutations in the **fibroblast growth factor receptor 3** gene (**FGFR3**), the most common form of skeletal dysplasia that is lethal in the neonatal period because of respiratory insufficiency and compression of the brainstem. TD type 1 (TD1, TD I) has a normally shaped skull and curved long bones. TD type 2 (TD2, TD II) has a cloverleaf-shaped skull and straight femurs.

trichorhinophalangeal syndrome: There are two types: TRPSI and TRPSII.
  TRPSI Sugio-Kajii syndrome: characterized by unique facial features, cone-shaped epiphysis, and mild growth retardation.
  TRPSII Langer Giedion syndrome: similar to TRPSI with exostosis and redundant skin.

tumoral calcinosis: probable metabolic disorder in which there is massive accumulation of calcium phosphates, pyrophosphates, or calcium carbonates in the soft tissues, particularly around joints.

Turner syndrome: failure of development of some female characteristics in girls; results from failure of the fertilized egg to receive both female X chromosomes.

Ullrich congenital muscular dystrophy (UCMD): a form of congenital muscular dystrophy in which children are often double jointed in their hands and feet and may have some tightness in other joints such as the hips. They have stiffness of the spine and may have respiratory problems leading to the need for respiratory support at night.

Diseases and Conditions by Anatomic Area

The back and neck disease section is found in Chapter 9, The Spine.

Miscellaneous Shoulder and Elbow Conditions

Buford complex: shoulder joint anatomic variance consisting of a cordlike middle glenohumeral ligament that blends with a loosely attached superior labrum. The third variance is a large sublabral hole.

effort thrombosis: thrombosis of upper limb sometimes associated with limb activities such as weight lifting or throwing; also called **Paget-Schroetter syndrome.**

Hamada Fukuda Classification

The Hamada Fukuda classification system is for shoulder osteoarthritis and rotator cuff combinations

Grade 1: the acromiohumeral distance (AHD) is greater than 6 mm

Grade 2: the AHD is 6 mm or less

Grade 3: acetabulization, defined as a concave deformity of the acromion under the surface, is added to the grade 2 characteristics

Grade 4: narrowing of the glenohumeral joint is added to the grade 3 features

Grade 5: humeral head collapse is present, which is characteristic of the cuff tear arthropathy

---

hooked acromion: hooked appearance of the anterolateral acromion sometimes associated with impingement of the underlying rotator cuff. This is a condition that develops in adult life. The appearance has been categorized into three types seen on radiographs:
  type I acromion: normal flat appearance of undersurface of acromion

type II acromion: slight hooked or roughened undersurface of acromion

type III acromion: markedly curved appearance of undersurface of acromion

impingement syndrome: when used in reference to the shoulder, this term denotes symptoms that are related to the bursa or rotator cuff changes that result in pain in the acromial, subacromial, and lateral arm produced by abducted positions where bursal impingement occurs.

Milwaukee shoulder syndrome: destructive arthritis of the shoulder characterized by rotator cuff loss.

painful arc syndrome: pain in the acromioclavicular (A/C) area on active shoulder abduction; a sign of arthritis of the A/C joint.

patella cubiti: compatible with good function, a rare developmental variant in which the proximal part of the olecranon appears like a patella separate from the remaining olecranon.

quadrilateral space syndrome: weakness of shoulder muscle supplied by axillary nerve resulting from sports or surgical injury at point that the axillary nerve exits the quadrilateral space.

snapping scapula: grinding sensation felt by the patient on specific motions of the scapula; may be a sign of a prominent rib or an osteochondroma of the scapula.

spinoglenoid cyst: fluid-filled cyst resulting from degenerative changes in the glenohumeral joint. The cyst forms near the scapular notch where the supraspinatus nerve crosses.

Steindler effect: in attempting to replace the lost biceps function, a transfer of the flexor wad proximally results in unwanted finger flexion while trying to flex elbow.

student's elbow: term used for posterior elbow bursitis; also called **olecranon bursitis.**

superior labrum anterior to posterior (SLAP) lesions:
  Type I: partial tear and degeneration to the superior labrum, in which the edges are rough and fray along the free margin, but the labrum is not completely detached.
  Type II: commonest type in which the superior labrum is completely torn off the glenoid.
  Type III: a bucket-handle shaped tear of the labrum in which the torn labrum hangs into the joint and causes symptoms of catching with solder motion.
  Type IV: tear of the labrum extends into the long head of biceps tendon.

winged scapula: winging of scapula and prominence of interior angle at rest or on active range of motion. It may be a sign of muscle paralysis, particularly palsy of the long thoracic nerve.

Hip (Coxa) Diseases

The Latin term *coxa* refers to the part of the skeleton lateral to and including the hip joint. (Do not confuse coxa [hip] with coccyx [tailbone].) The most common adult problems of the hip are osteoarthritis, other arthropathies, and avascular necrosis. These are defined in the sections dealing with bone, cartilage, and joint disease.

acetabular rim syndrome: pain and impaired function that precede osteoarthritis in hips that are congenitally dysplastic or have superior lateral trauma to the limbus or bony rim.

arthrokatadysis: deep hip socket formed as a part of degenerative arthritis.

cam impingement: ellipsoid shape of femoral head causes impingement on acetabulum, leading to osteoarthritis.

Campanacci disease: combination of nonossifying fibromata, café-au-lait spots, mental retardation, hypogonadism or cryptorchidism, and ocular and cardiovascular malformations.

Charnley Hip Arthroplasty Classification

The Charnley hip arthroplasty classification system is for assessment of the severity of disability in potential hip-replacement recipients.

Class A: patients with only one affected hip prior to replacement and no other function affecting mobility

Class B: patients with both hips affected prior to replacement and no other function affecting mobility

Class C: patients with some factors that contribute to decreased locomotion, such as multiple joint involvement, cardiac, inflammatory or other disease

---

They can be further subdivided into (a) anterior (b) posterior, and (c) combined anterior-posterior lesions.

coxa breva: short femoral neck with a small femoral head caused by premature closure of the epiphysis.

coxa magna: enlarged femoral head.

coxa plana: flat femoral head (osteochondrosis) of the capitular epiphysis of the femur; also called **Legg-Perthes d.**

coxa saltans: snapping of the hip because of tightness of the iliotibial tract over the greater trochanter, snapping of the musculotendinous iliopsoas over structures deep to it, or lesions within the hip joint, such as a labral tear; also called **snapping hip.**

coxa senilis: degenerative hip disease concomitant with old age; also called **malum coxae senilis.** (archaic)

coxa valga: hip deformity in which the angle of axis of the head and neck of the femur and the axis of its shaft (neck shaft angle) is increased.

coxa vara: reduced neck shaft angle, usually caused by failure of normal bone growth; also called **coxa adducta.**

coxa vara luxans: fissure of neck of femur, with dislocation of the head. (archaic)

coxalgia: hip pain. (archaic)

coxarthrocace: fungal disease of the hip joint. (archaic)

coxarthropathy: any hip joint disease.

coxarthrosis: degenerative joint disease or osteoarthritis of the hip joint.

coxitis: inflammation of the hip joint; also called **coxarthria** and **coxarthritis.** (archaic)

coxotuberculosis: tuberculosis of the hip joint. (archaic)

developmental dysplasia of the hip (DDH): spectrum of disorders of the hip associated with deficient development of the acetabulum. This is usually apparent at birth and may start as or progress to subluxation or dislocation of the hip. This term is now replacing the older terms **congenital hip disease, congenital hip dysplasia,** and **congenital hip dislocation.**

Crowe Classification for Percent of Hip Subluxation
Grade I: < 50%
Grade II: 50%–75%
Grade III: 75%–100%
Grade IV: more than 100%

femoral acetabular impingement (FAI): impingement of the femoral neck on the acetabulum caused by a cam-shaped hip, deep-seated femoral head, or an acetabular deformity that leads to impingement.

Acetabular Labral Tear Classification
Stage 1: free margin with intact cartilage
Stage 2: labral tear with femoral head chondromalacia
Stage 3A: labral tears with acetabular cartilage lesion smaller that 1 cm.
Stage 3B: labral tears with acetabular cartilage lesion larger that 1 cm.
Stage 4: labral tear with diffuse degenerative joint disease

Meyer dysplasia: developmental anomaly that simulates Perthes d. of the hip, but presents at an earlier age, and does not have the progression of hip changes seen with Perthes d.; also called **dysplasia epiphysealis capitis femoris.**

Namaqualand hip dysplasia: autosomal dominant condition seen in African children from 3 to 20 years of age. There is a failure of growth in the femoral epiphysis, resulting in pain associated with an early degenerative arthritis of the hip.

observation hip: group of symptoms referred to the hip that includes a limp, pain, and limited motion of the hip joint with normal radiographs. The condition is a diagnostic dilemma in that it may be due to toxic synovitis, infection, or an early avascular necrosis.

pincer impingement: deep-seated femoral head leading to increased acetabular wear and osteoarthritis.

protrusio acetabuli: arthritic development of hip socket into a deep, egg-shaped appearance.

proximal focal femoral deficiency (PFFD): failure of normal formation of the thigh side of the hip; varies in severity. The new term for this condition is **longitudinal deficiency of the femur, partial (LDFP).**

windswept hips: condition seen in individuals with cerebral palsy with pelvic obliquity, scoliosis, and one hip held in adduction and the opposite hip in abduction.

Deficiencies of the Acetabulum and Femur

The Committee on the Hip, American Academy of Orthopaedic Surgeons, has developed the following classification for bone deficiencies of the acetabulum and femur as relates to total hip arthroplasty.

Acetabular Classification for Congenital Deficiencies

1. Segmental
   • Peripheral (rim)
      a. Anterior
      b. Posterior
      c. Superior
   • Central
2. Cavitary
      a. Anterior
      b. Posterior
      c. Superior
      d. Medial (protrusion with intact medial wall)
3. Combined segmental and cavitary
      a. Superior segmental, superior cavitary
      b. Medial segmental, medial cavitary (protrusion with deficient medial wall)
      c. Posterior segmental, posterior cavitary
4. Pelvic discontinuity
5. Fusion

Femoral Classification for Congenital Deficiencies
segmental defect: any loss of bone in the outer cortical shell of the femur. **cavitary defect:** excavation of cancellous or cortical bone from within, the outer cortical shell remaining unviolated. **ectasia:** dilatation or expansion of the outer cortical shell without perforation. **intercalary:** segmental defect with intact bone above and below (cortical window).

Level of Defect

Level I: proximal to the lesser inferior trochanter
Level II: inferior lesser trochanter to 10 cm distal
Level III: below level II

Knee Disorders

Genu is a Latin term for knee (pl. *genua*). It is also a general term denoting any anatomic structure that is bent like a knee. Specifically, it is the site of articulation between the femur and tibia. Knee-related problems are divided into three sections:

1. Old genu descriptive terms
2. Joint injury
3. Other terms specifically related to the knee but not to a specific injury

FIG 2-7 A, Normal meniscus. **B,** Longitudinal, or bucket-handle, tear. **C,** Tear of the posterior horn. *(From Mercier LR:* Practical Orthopaedics, *ed 5, St Louis, 2000, Mosby.)*

Genu Terms

genu recurvatum: ability of the knee to bend backward; caused by trauma or general joint laxity; also called **back-knee.**
genu valgum: deformity in which knees are close together, with ankle space increased; also called **knock-knee.**
genu varum: deformity in which knees are bowed out and ankles are close in; may be associated with internal tibial torsion.

Outcome of Joint Injury

The knee is an unusual joint because it contains *ligaments* within the joint. There are also medial and lateral *menisci* (crescent-shaped cartilages) that can be damaged. Finally, the normal motions of the knee are very complex, including two planes of rotation; therefore it is very common to see multiple injuries.

A sprained knee is often a benign injury involving only mild damage to the ligament. However, a tear of the meniscus can occur in association with a sprain (Fig. 2-7). A **meniscus tear** or **torn meniscus** is commonly described by its appearance, such as a **parrot-beak tear** or a **bucket-handle tear.** In the young person, a tear is usually vertical and longitudinal to the diameter of the meniscus. In degenerative tears that appear in older people, the tear is horizontal and may not be apparent on the superior surface of the meniscus. When the meniscus becomes fragmented, the condition is often termed a **degenerative tear** of the meniscus. The location of tears may be used to define a specific meniscus injury, for example, *posterior horn* or *anterior horn*. Meniscus injury commonly occurs as a result of a rotational injury. *Rotational instability* (rotatory or angular) is produced by rupture of specific anatomic structures. A meniscal rim can regenerate from the margin of a completely, or nearly completely, resected meniscus resulting in what is referred to as a **regenerated meniscus**. The normal up-and-down gliding mechanism of a patella may be disrupted, and the patella has a tendency to move out of its groove laterally *(subluxing patella)*. A subluxing patella need not be caused by injury but does commonly occur with rotational injury. All these disorders can result in a chronic reaction in the knee, similar to the eyes' response to a foreign body. The lining of the knee becomes inflamed and may allow fluid *(effusion)* to collect. If the effusion is persistent, a *pouch*, called a *Baker cyst*, may form behind the knee.

Another outcome of knee injury is the formation of loose fragments *(loose bodies)* of meniscal cartilage or other tissue, causing inflammation *(synovitis* or *meniscitis)*. The cartilage of the kneecap may become frayed *(chondromalacia patellae)*. However, not all cases of chondromalacia result from injury. If the inflammation persists long enough, the patient will eventually develop *degenerative arthritis*. Often the examiner is not sure of the exact problem of the knee but suspects that something is functionally incorrect. The general term then used is *internal derangement of the knee (IDK)*.

Other Conditions of the Knee

anterolateral rotatory instability (ALRI): the most common instability of the knee characterized by abnormal anterior displacement or subluxation of the lateral tibial plateau. It results from a tear of the anterior cruciate ligament or the mid-third of the lateral capsular ligament, and is determined by the Lachman test, anterior drawer sign, and flexion-rotation drawer test.

Baker cyst: sac of usually clear fluid specifically in the popliteal fossa of the knee. In the adult, it is a synovial fluid cystic extension caused by intraarticular disease that results in a new synovial-lined sac in the popliteal fossa. In a child, the cyst is usually a ganglion arising from one of the tendons in the popliteal area.

bipartite patella: patella that has bony maturation occurring from two centers rather than one center, usually congenital, causing no symptoms, but may be mistaken for a fracture.

congenital dislocation: progressive anterior dislocation of the tibia caused by abnormal tissue remodeling; seen in infancy.

discoid meniscus: meniscus that is less crescentic and more D shaped. Often leads to symptoms in young adult life.

Watanabe Classification for Discoid Meniscus
Type I: complete, extending across entire lateral tibial plateau.
Type II: meniscus wider than normal, but some articular cartilage exposed.
Type III (Wrisberg-ligament type): deficiency of posterior tibial meniscal attachment that allows meniscus to move abnormally back and forth in joint.

flexion contracture: formation of fibrous bands that prevent complete extension of the knee.

focal fibrocartilaginous dysplasia: rare cause of unilateral genu varum (bowleg), which appears before 18 months with a cortical lucency in the proximal tibia and surrounding sclerosis. Condition is usually self-limited and resolves by age 4.

hamstrung knee: tight hamstrings during growth resulting in a slight knee flexion gait with subsequent synovitis and chondromalacia.

housemaid's knee: prepatellar bursitis: inflammation of the bursa in front of the patella.

jockey cap patella: chronic subluxating patella resulting in lateral spurring deformity.

jumper's knee: tenderness in the area of the inferior pole of the patella; usually seen in volleyball and basketball players.

lateral patella tendon conflict: combination of patella alta and lateral patella alignment results in impingement of the patella tendon (ligament) on the lateral femoral condyle causing focal tenderness.

megahorn meniscus: a congenitally enlarged part of either the anterior or posterior portion of the meniscus of the knee, usually the lateral side, usually associated with a variety of discoid menisci.

meniscal flounce: a normal wavy or folded pattern of the meniscus seen during arthroscopic inspection.

Parson's third tubercle: in knee arthritis, formation of an osteophyte anterior to the anterior tibial spine resulting in a loss of terminal extension.

patella alta: a patella that is located more superior than expected, usually considered by the ratio of the length of the patella tendon to the height of the patella being greater than 1.25; also called **high-riding patella.**

patella baja: low-riding patella with a relatively shortened patellar tendon, usually associated with knee pain.

patella clunk syndrome: a patellar snap that occurs in total joint replacement (knees) when going from flexion to extension; caused by the catching of scar tissue immediately above the patella.

patellofemoral syndrome: patellar and peripatellar pain often ascribed to chondromalacia patellae, but which may be due to other disorders such as patellar malalignment.

plica syndrome: pain or snapping in knee caused by inflammation or enlargement of a band of tissue that is present at birth and may become symptomatic in association with other conditions. There are four common plicas:

ligamentum mucosum: in front of the anterior cruciate ligament

suprapatellar plica: in the suprapatellar area

medial shelf/medial plica: from the infrapatellar fat pad to the medial wall of the knee

lateral plica: from the lateral infrapatellar fat pad to the lateral synovium of the knee

popliteal cyst: any ganglion or synovial cyst behind the knee. In adults, this is usually an outpouching of the posterior knee joint area and is a sign of chronic inflammation in the knee. In children and young adults, this may be a ganglion cyst arising from one of the tendons around the knee. Not to be confused with popliteal arterial cyst.

popliteal pterygium syndrome: severe flexion of the knee and equinus deformity of the foot associated with popliteal web extending from the ischium to the heel. Other concurrent deformities include toenail dysplasia and oral cavity abnormalities such as cleft palate or lip pits.

small-patella syndrome: autosomal disorder with small patellae, pelvic girdle hypoplasia, and other skeletal anomalies.

snapping knee syndrome: the combination of dramatic popping and often intermittent locking is most commonly associated with discoid meniscus, but may also be due to other intraarticular abnormalities of the knee such as meniscal tears and enlarged bands of tissue.

snowstorm knee: formation of hundreds of brilliant, white loose bodies within the knee, usually following an earlier traumatic event.

squinting patella: patella that appears to point inward when the person is standing or walking forward. It is usually a sign of femoral anteversion.

tethered patellar tendon syndrome: condition seen after total knee replacement. A large fibrous band develops behind the patella, causes pain, and interferes with joint motion.

Type I: band oriented medial to lateral in suprapatellar region

Type II: band oriented vertically

Type III: band oriented from anterior fat pad to posterior notch

thigh atrophy: loss of muscle tone of the quadriceps, causing dynamic instability.

Congenital Limb Absences

The International Organization for Standardization adopted a limb absence classification system designed to eliminate terms such as *ectromelia, peromelia,* and *dysmelia.* This system has two basic categories: transverse losses in which all structures for that segment are absent; and longitudinal, in which only a part of the longitudinal part of the segment is absent. This is based on radiologic appearance as opposed to specific reference to embryologic factors, etiologic factors, or epidemiologic factors.* It is presented first. However, given the variance in practice throughout the orthopaedic world, two systems are in this edition. A former standard classification divided congenital deficiency based on the end of a limb (terminal) or somewhere in the middle (intercalary). In addition, transverse or longitudinal deficiencies were defined the same way.†

Frantz-O'Rahilly classification: complex classification system for congenital limb deficiency. See Hall et al. (1966).

---

*International Organization for Standardization, 1989.
†Frantz CH et al, 1961.

International Organization for Standardization for Limb Deficiencies (IOS)

For both transverse and longitudinal absences.

1. Name the bone(s) affected from proximal to distal. Any bone not named is presumed normal (this defines intercalary defects).
2. State if each affected bone is totally or partially absent.
3. If partial, state the fraction and position of the absent part.
4. For the rays in hands and feet, the number of the digit starting from the radial or tibial side is stated.
5. The term *ray* (*first ray, second ray,* etc.) may be used.

Terminal Transverse

acheiria: absence of the hand (carpals, metacarpals, phalanges).
acheiropodia: an extremely rare congenital absence of forearms, hands, and feet.
adactylia: absence of all five rays (metacarpals and phalanges).
amelia: complete absence of a limb.
apodia: absence of the foot.
complete aphalangia: absence of one or more phalanges from all five digits.
ectromelia: severe form of hypoplasia or actual absence of one or more long bones involving one or more limbs. This term generally includes amelia, hemimelia, and phocomelia.
hemimelia: absence of the forearm and hand or leg and foot portion of a limb.
partial hemimelia: absence of part of the forearm or leg.

Terminal Longitudinal

complete paraxial hemimelia: lengthwise loss of one side or the other of the forearm and hand or leg and foot.
incomplete paraxial hemimelia: similar to hemimelia, but a portion of affected bone remains, for example, complete absence of the ulna with a portion of the diameter of the radius intact.
partial adactylia: absence of one to four rays (phalanges and metacarpals).
partial aphalangia: absence of one or more of the three phalanges from one to four digits.

Intercalary Transverse

complete phocomelia: presence of only a hand or foot.
distal phocomelia: hand directly attached to upper arm; or foot directly attached to thigh.
proximal phocomelia: presence of hand and forearm or leg and foot.

Intercalary Longitudinal

complete paraxial hemimelia: absence of radius or ulna with intact hand or absence of tibia or fibula with intact foot.
incomplete paraxial hemimelia: similar to complete hemimelia, except a portion of affected bone remains intact.
partial adactylia: absence of all or part of the first through fifth rays.
partial aphalangia: absence of the proximal or middle phalanx from one or more digits, one through five. A common deformity is a complete loss of the radius with the rest of the arm and hand being intact—intercalary complete paraxial hemimelia. Proximal focal femoral deficiency is an absence of a portion of the hip and/or proximal femur.

Miscellaneous Congenital Deficiencies

amniotic band syndrome: congenital presence of constricting bands that may affect trunk, limbs, and cranium; partial amputations may result.
arachnodactyly: unusually long spidery fingers and toes characteristically seen in patients with Marfan syndrome.
dolichostenomelia: increased length of the limb compared with that of the trunk.
fragile-X syndrome: familial form of mental retardation associated with flat feet and excessive joint laxity.
Larsen syndrome: associated skeletal abnormalities seen in infancy: dislocation of the elbows and hips, equinovarus deformities of the feet, long cylindrical fingers and shortened metacarpals, wide-spaced eyes, prominent forehead, and depressed nasal bridge.
Prader-Willi syndrome: spontaneous genetic mutation resulting in uncommon infantile disorder characterized by hypotonia, hypogonadism, obesity caused by overeating, diabetes mellitus, delayed psychomotor development, mental deficiency, short stature, small hands and feet, hypermobile joints, and kyphosis.

rhizomelic: short proximal end of a limb, such as seen in achondroplastic dwarfism.

tibial dysplasia: rare congenital deformity. Must be distinguished from more common fibular dysplasia.
  Three types: Type I—total absence of tibia; Type II—distal tibial aplasia; Type III—distal dysplasia with tibiofibular diastasis.

ulnar dimelia: a rare congenital disorder, characterized by duplication of the ulna, absence of the radius and polydactyly.

Specific Regional Classification Systems for Congenital Limb Absences

Achterman and Kalamchi Classification for Fibular Hemimelia
Type I: fibula present.
Type Ia: absence of proximal fibula. Distal fibular physis proximal to dome of talus.
Type Ib: only partial fibula present.
Type II: fibula absent.

Aitken Classification for Longitudinal Deficiency of the Femur, Partial
A: portion of the femoral neck distal to the femoral head is deficient but the hip is reasonably well developed.
B: a larger portion is deficient or absent.
C: the femoral head is absent, the femur is short, and the acetabulum is dysplastic.
D: the femoral head is absent, the femur is very short, and the acetabulum is very dysplastic.

Bayne Classification for Radial Bone Deficiencies
Type 0: hypoplasia of the radial carpus (scaphoid); radius of normal length.
Type I: radius slightly shorter than normal; physis evident both proximal and distal.
Type II: radius in miniature: normally shaped, but smaller radius with both proximal and distal physis.
Type III: partial aplasia of the radius; absence of the distal part of the radius, including the distal epiphysis.
Type IV: absence of radius.

Bayne Classification for Longitudinal Ulnar Deficiencies
Type I: hypoplasia, distal epiphysis intact.
Type II: partial hypoplasia distal epiphysis absent.
Type III: total aplasia.
Type IV: radiohumeral synostosis with total ulna hypoplasia.

Birch Classification for Fibular Deficiencies
Type I: functional foot.
  A: 0%–5% predicted leg-length inequality at maturity.
  B: 6%–10% predicted leg-length inequality.
  C: 11%–30% predicted leg-length inequality.
  D: > 30% predicted leg-length inequality.

Type II: nonfunctional foot.
  A: functional upper extremity.
  B: nonfunctional upper extremity.

Cole and Manske Classification for the First Distal Ray Absence with Ulnar Deficiency
Type A: normal thumb and first web space.
Type B: mild first web and thumb deficiency.
Type C: moderate to severe first web and thumb deficiency (loss of opposition, malrotation, thumb index syndactyly, absent extrinsic tendon function).
Type D: thumb absent.

Gillespie Classification for Longitudinal Deficiency of the Femur, Partial
Group I: the femur is 40%–60% shorter than normal and the hip and knee can be made functional.
Group II: the femur is shorter and the hip and knee cannot be made functional.

Jones, Barnes, and Lloyd-Roberts Classification for Tibial Deficiency
1a: tibia not seen, hypoplastic lower femoral epiphysis.
1b: tibia not seen, normal lower femoral epiphysis.
2: distal tibia not seen.
3: proximal tibia not seen.
4: diastasis.

Kalamchi and Dawe Classification for Tibial Deficiency
Type I: complete absence of the tibia.
Type II: presence of proximal tibia.
Type III: severe diastasis at ankle.

Kummel Classification for Longitudinal Ulnar Deficiency at Elbow Joint
Type A: normal radiohumeral joint.
Type B: radiohumeral synostosis.
Type C: dislocation of the radiohumeral joint.

Specific Regional Classification Systems for Congenital Limb Absences—cont'd

Letts Classification for Fibular Deficiencies

Type A: affected side less than 10% shorter than opposite side, discrepancy projected to be less than 6 cm at maturity, foot nearly normal, minimal femoral shortening.

Type B: affected side 10%–20% shorter than opposite side, discrepancy projected to be 6 to 10 cm at maturity, minimal foot deformities, minimal femoral shortening.

Type C: affected side greater than 30% shorter than opposite side, discrepancy projected to be greater than 10 cm at maturity, severe foot deformity, severe femoral shortening.

Type D: bilateral fibular deficiency or partial longitudinal deficiency of the femur.

Ogden Classification for Ulnar Longitudinal Deficiency

Type I: hypoplasia of otherwise normal ulna with a distal epiphysis.

Type II: partial aplasia (absence of distal part of ulna, including the distal epiphysis).

Type III: total, aplasia.

Pappas Classification: a complex classification for congenital abnormalities of femur

See Pappas AM, 1983.

Stanitski and Stanitski Classification for Fibular Hemimelia

Type I: fibula nearly normal.

Type II: small or miniature fibula, regardless of its portion in the limb.

Type III: total absence of fibula.

Tibiotalar Joint and Distal Tibial Morphology Classification System

H: horizontal

V: valgus (triangular distal tibial epiphysis.

S: spherical (ball and socket ankle)

Presence of a tarsal coalition denoted with lower case.

Number of foot rays medial to lateral (denoted 1–5).

Venn-Watson classification system: foot polydactyly based on preaxial and postaxial duplication.

Wassel Classification for Thumb Polydactyly

Type I: split distal tuft.

Type II: split distal phalanx.

Type III: split distal middle phalanx and distal phalanx.

Type IV: split middle and distal phalanx.

Type V: split distal metacarpal and distal phalanges.

Type VI: split distal metacarpal and distal phalanges.

Type VII: split distal phalanx with ulnar ray having three phalanges.

Symbols

The following symbols are used for congenital limb absences:

-: transverse.

/: longitudinal.

I: intercalary.

T: terminal.

1, 2, 3, 4, 5: denotes ray involved.

-: when line is used above a letter, indicates the lower extremity.

-: when line is used below a letter, indicates the upper extremity.

TI: tibia, complete.

ti: tibia, incomplete.

FI: fibula, complete.

fi: fibula, incomplete.

R: radius, complete.

r: radius, incomplete.

U: ulna, complete.

u: ulna, incomplete.

Associated Disease Terminology

Diseases of the musculoskeletal system are often described by other terms relating to the disease process or some qualitative nature of the disease. These associated defined terms are given in alphabetic order.

abrasion: any superficial scraping of skin tissue or mucous membrane mechanically or through injury.

abscess: localized collection of pus in a cavity, which may form in any tissue.

acute: describes symptoms, conditions, or diseases of recent onset or recurrence that are severe or of short duration. *Acute* refers to the initial stage, short stage, or most severe stage of disease (e.g., acute low-back strain may take a protracted course, becoming chronic, or may occur a number of times as part of a long-term chronic low-back syndrome).

adenopathy: glandular swelling of the lymph nodes with morbid pathologic condition.

adhesions: tissue structures normally separated that adhere together because of inflammation or injury.

adventitious: acquired, not congenital; found out of normal place.
afebrile: without fever.
aggravated: made worse, more serious, or severe.
-agra (suffix): violent pain or seizure of acute pain.
-algia (suffix): painful.
allergy: hypersensitive state manifested by specific tissue changes after repeated exposure to particular allergens; an antibody-antigen reaction.
analgesia: loss of sensitivity to pain.
analgia: absence of pain.
anastomosis: connection of two distinct parts of cavities forming a passageway; the results of trauma or surgery. For example, the reattachment of a ruptured blood vessel after the injured portion has been removed.
anesthesia: loss of feeling or sensation of pain with or without loss of consciousness.
anomaly: malformation; a deviation from normal, usually referring to a congenital or hereditary defect.
anteflexion: the abnormal forward bending of an organ or part, not commonly used for skeletal disorders.
anteversion: forward rotation, as commonly seen in the femoral neck.
aphasia: either partial or complete, transient or permanent inability to understand or speak the spoken word as a result of a central neurologic occurrence such as stroke or injury.
apoplexy: old term describing a stroke, a bleeding into or loss of blood supply to the brain.
aseptic: free of bacterial or fungal contamination.
asphyxia: lack of oxygen.
aspiration: withdrawal of fluids from a joint cavity, such as a bloody effusion in the knee. Also, the inhalation of a liquid or solid such as the aspiration of vomit in an unconscious patient.
asthenia: lack of strength and energy.
asymmetry: dissimilarity between two corresponding parts of the body.
asymptomatic: absence of symptoms.
asynergia: disturbance of coordination.
ataxia: lack of muscle coordination with voluntary movement; numerous types.
athetosis: involuntary writhing motions of the body (usually upper extremities).
atonia: lack of normal muscle tone; also called **atony**.
atrophy: wasting away of tissue, usually refers to muscle tissue.

atypical: irregular; appearing abnormal.
avascular: absence of adequate blood supply.
avulsion: tearing away of a part or structure from its attachment.
Beighton hyperlaxity score: a nine points scoring system of multiple joints. See Beighton Hypermobility Score, 2014.
benign: not causing destruction of life or limb; when used in reference to tumors, denotes the absence of metastasis (noncancerous).
bifurcation: site at which any given structure divides in two.
bipartite: having two parts where only one is expected, for example, a bipartite patella.
bossing: rounded prominence of bone that is abnormally visible under the skin.
bruit (pronounced *bru-ee*): abnormal sound heard on auscultation of a blood vessel or the heart.
cachexia: systemic symptoms of malnutrition, malfunction, or debility that accompanies ill health or tissue breakdown.
café-au-lait: brown spots on surface of skin, often symptomatic of a systemic disease. Smooth borders ("Coast of California") are associated with neurofibromatosis, and irregular borders ("Coast of Maine") are associated with McCune-Albright syndrome.
calcification: deposition of calcium salts, either in normal bone or abnormally in soft tissue.
callosity: hardening of the epidermis because of persistent pressure.
callus: formation of new bone around a fracture site.
campomelia: a syndrome associated with angulation of the long bones, classified into long- and short-limb varieties. One genetic mutation is Sox9.
caries: decay and death of bone from bacterial action.
caries sicca: dry form of infection (i.e., less fluid associated with purulent material), characteristic of tuberculosis.
cellulitis: swelling and inflammation of soft tissues; may be caused by bacteria or chemical irritation.
chronic: describes symptoms, conditions, or diseases of long duration, as opposed to acute.
chylothorax: chyle (lymph duct fluid) that accumulates in the chest cavity that may occur after thoracic spine surgery with inadvertent transsection of lymph duct.
cicatrix: scar, may be formed by healing of any wound or tissue injury.

clonus: the uncontrolled spasmodic muscle jerking seen in conditions such as epilepsy or cerebral palsy. This term can refer to the spasmodic contraction of a reflex such as the ankle reflex that once elicited, continues indefinitely. When there are only several "jerks" in the muscle reflex, the term **unsustained clonus** is used.

-coele (suffix): indicates a sac or cavity; *-cele.*

comatose: semiconscious state; in a coma.

congenital: present at birth.

contagious: refers to a disease or condition that can be transmitted from one person to another; communicable.

contractions: forceful shortening of muscle.

contracture: permanent shortening of muscle tissue caused by paralysis or spasm; loss of motion of a joint caused by fibrosis of tissue around the joint.

contrecoup: a blow to one side of the body that causes damage on the other, as often seen in head injuries.

contusion: bruise of any tissue but without disruption.

convalescence: any given period of recovery.

conversion disorder: a response to psychologic conflict or need, manifested by unintentionally produced signs of a physical disorder, in which there is no known identifiable cause.

convulsion: violent involuntary contractions of voluntary muscles; paroxysm, seizure.

cramp: painful muscle spasm affecting the nerve supply to that muscle caused by overexertion. Recumbency cramps are often felt in the legs and feet and occur at rest. Tonic muscle contractions can be anywhere and are associated with job-related activity. A true cramp is a motor unit hyperactivity that occurs at rest in the lower limbs. It is associated with motor neuron disease, fluid and electrolyte disorders, drug therapy, alcohol ingestion, or heat exposure.

crepitus: any crackling or grating sound with sensation on movement of surfaces at the joint; may indicate wearing away of cartilage.

cyanosis (*adj.* cyanotic): bluish discoloration of skin resulting from abnormally low levels of oxygen in blood; the actual cause is an excessive concentration of reduced hemoglobin.

cyst: any sac, normal or abnormal, containing liquid or semisolid material.

debridement: removal of foreign material or devitalized tissue from a wound.

decalcification: loss of calcium salts from bone or soft tissue.

defervescence: period of abatement of fever.

degenerative: deterioration of quality of tissue; rarely refers to dead tissue; usually describes a state of abnormal remodeling or replacement of tissue, sometimes making it less functional.

degloving: closed soft tissue injuries to subcutaneous tissue with separation of fascia.

dehiscence: splitting or separation of a part or all of a closed wound.

deossification: loss or removal of bone of osseous tissue.

derangement: displacement of position of any given anatomic part; commonly used in reference to joints.

diagnosis: identifying a disease process or the agent responsible by means of cultures, tests, surgery, or intuition (recognizing patterns of disease).

diffuse: widely distributed; used in association with symptoms or disease terms.

diverticulum: in orthopaedics, usually refers to outpouching of a joint or tendon sheath.

dowager's hump: round upper back deformity.

-dynia (suffix): denotes pain.

dys- (prefix): denotes defective, difficult, or painful.

dysesthesia: pinprick or other abnormal sensations; painful touch perception.

dysfunction: impairment of function.

dysplasia: abnormal development or replacement of tissue.

dystonia: simultaneous contraction of agonist and antagonist muscles.

dystrophy: failure of normal replacement of tissue; see osteo-, chondro-, and muscular dystrophies.

eburnation: in degenerative joint disease, changes in subchondral bone render its substance dense, smooth, and ivory-like. The bone surface becomes exposed as a result of complete loss of cartilage surface.

ecchymosis: extravasation of blood under the skin, as seen in a bruise.

edema: excessive accumulations of fluid in soft tissues causing swelling; may be the result of heart failure, venous insufficiency, kidney failure, or malnutrition. More specifically, in inflammation, an increase in postcapillary intraluminal pressure causes a shift in equilibrium so that fluid return is impeded and accumulates in tissues, which results in edema.

effusion: collection of fluid in a cavity such as the joint space.

emaciation: wasted condition of the body; malnutrition.

enucleation: removal, either surgically or traumatically, of a tissue, organ, or foreign body.

erosion: uneven wearing away of a surface, as seen on radiographs of diseased bones.

erythema: redness of skin, as seen in sunburn; caused by an increased blood supply (capillary congestion).

eschar: term usually restricted to skin; refers to full-thickness skin injury with the formation of a hard, black, leathery, contracted material that, if removed, would reveal living tissue underneath.

esthesia: perception, feeling, sensation.

etiologic factors: causes of a condition or disease, separated or related, based on what is presently known about that disease process.

exacerbation: aggravation of symptoms or increased severity of disease.

exudate: escape of fluid, cells, or cellular debris that escapes from blood vessels and deposits into soft tissues, cavities, or wounds as a result of inflammation. An exudate, in contrast to a transudate, is characterized by a high content of protein cells or solid materials derived from cells.

factitious injury: unconscious production of symptoms or actual physical injury for purposes of secondary gain, that is, attention or preferential treatment.

Fanconi anemia: radial clubhand deformity associated with dwarfism, brownish pigmentation of the skin, anomalies of the thumb, and then at 5 to 10 years of age a diminished number of all blood cells develops; also called **congenital pancytopenia** and **idiopathic refractory anemia.**

febrile: with fever.

fibrillation: involuntary contraction of small groups of muscle fibers as occurs with nerve root irritation; the fraying of a tissue such as seen in degenerative cartilage.

fissures: groove or natural division in tissue; also, ulcer-like sore.

flaccid: lacking muscle tone, whether voluntary or involuntary muscle.

flail: absence of motor control, as seen in a flail joint, may connote an abnormal mobility associated with loss of normal control such as flail chest, which is a chest crush injury.

foreign body: anything within a tissue that may lead to infection, inflammation, or scarring, requiring removal.

fretting: mechanical abrasion from relative micromotion between two surfaces. For orthopaedic appliances, this is between metal and bone or metal and cement. Microscopic particles are produced, initiating an inflammatory process that produces more loosening.

friable: tissue that is easily crumbled or separated.

fusiform: spindle-shaped, tapered at ends.

gangrene: death of tissue caused by loss of blood supply (ischemia), bacterial infection, or both.

glycocalyx: extracellular polysaccharide elaborated by some bacteria that provides a binding material to internal prosthetic and fixation devices resulting in resistance to antibiotics.

granulation: reddish, moist, new tissue along edges of a healing wound.

hair tourniquet syndrome: in infants, one or more appendages are strangulated by circumferential hair fibers that may be buried under the skin and not visible.

hemorrhage: abnormal bleeding into soft tissues or a cavity. Should this process form a discrete pocket of blood, it is called a **hematoma;** if the blood is evenly distributed in the tissue, it may appear as petechiae (very small), purpura (up to 1 cm), or ecchymosis (larger than 1 cm).

hereditary: familial or genetic transmission of a quality or trait from parent to offspring by a gene. When the gene is inherited from the chromosome associated with the sex of the offspring, it is said to be **sex-linked inheritance.** When the characteristic is inherited from the other chromosomes, it is called **autosomal inheritance.** If both chromosomes need the same gene to have the characteristic expressed, the condition is said to be **recessive inheritance.** If only one chromosome must carry the affected gene, the condition is called **dominant inheritance.**

herniation: abnormal protrusion of a body structure beyond its normal limits, such as disk herniation.

hibernoma: a rare, benign soft tissue tumor originating from brown fat and named for the brown appearance of fat seen in hibernating animals.

Holt-Oram syndrome: atrial septal defect or other cardiac abnormality associated with a radial clubhand deformity.

hypalgesia: diminished sensitivity to pain; hypoesthesia.

hyperalgesia: increased sensitivity to pain; hyperesthesia.

hyperextension: excessive extension of joint.

hyperglycemia: abnormally high blood glucose level increasing risk of infection.

hyperplasia: excessive increase in the number of normal cells in tissue, producing an increase in size.

hypertension: high blood pressure.

hypertonia: excessive tension of muscle or arteries.

hypertrophy: increase in size of a structure resulting from a functional activity such as in muscle hypertrophy.

hypoglycemia: abnormally low blood glucose level.

hypoplasia: defective or incomplete development of tissue or an organ (e.g., hypoplastic labrum; an abnormally small rim of cartilage in the shoulder joint can lead to a laxity of that joint).

hypotension: low blood pressure.

iatrogenic: adverse effects of medical or surgical treatment.

idiopathic: disease process with an unknown cause.

impingement: pressure transmitted from one tissue to the next, such as nerve impingement.

induration: firmness of soft tissue caused by extravasation of fluids or cells from blood vessels.

infarct: local area tissue death resulting from reduced or completely obliterated blood supply.

infection: an imbalance of pathogenic and normal microorganisms with an immune response by the host to the viable irritant. The terms *infection* and *inflammation* are not interchangeable. The distinction is important in that inflammation is a vascular response that may not specifically or necessarily be due to infection.

inflammation: localized increase in blood supply, resulting in small vessel dilatation or migration of white blood cells into the tissue. Inflammation is the normal response of living tissue to an injury with tissue alteration. The inflammatory process mobilizes the body's defense mechanism to initiate the healing process and react against any microbes that may be introduced at the site of injury with resultant heat, pain, swelling, and loss of function. Inflammation involves two basic sequences that develop separately: vascular alteration and cellular phenomena. Examples are bursitis and arthritis.

insidious: undetectable development of symptoms or disease, usually gradual in onset.

intractable: resistant to therapy, relief, cure, or control.

ischemia: insufficient blood supply to a tissue or organ.

laceration: a cut; any wound made by a sharp or blunt object.

lesion: circumscribed area of tissue altered by structural or functional disease. The word *lesion* describes a wound, injury, or pathologic change in tissue. A gross lesion is visible to the naked eye.

line of demarcation: zone of inflammatory reaction separating a gangrenous area from healthy tissue.

lipping: development of excess bone at the margins of a joint, as seen in arthritis.

loxoscelism: condition caused by a bite from a brown recluse spider. A local rash progresses to full-thickness skin death. Small hemorrhage or blister may form, surrounded by blanched skin caused by ischemia. A classic description is a nonhealing ulcer with red, white, and blue phenomenon.

lytic: denoting dissolution of tissue; used to refer to radiographic appearance of bone that has been displaced by some pathologic process.

maceration: softening or loss of surface tissue caused by constant exposure to moisture.

malaise: subjective feeling of being ill.

malignant: applied to neoplasms and implies the properties of anaplasia, invasion, and metastasis. A disease resistant to treatment, resulting in eventual destruction of tissue; in tumors, implies that the tumor spreads by seeding itself in distant regions of the body or by local uncontrolled invasion.

malingering: act of pretending to be ill only when being observed. This differs from *secondary gain,* in which the person derives an emotional gain from believing that he or she is ill.

melioidosis: an infectious disease caused by *Burkholderia pseudomallei,* which, when it affects the skeleton, may mimic tuberculosis or tumors.

mesenchymoma: neoplastic tumors in which there are at least two cells of mesenchymal derivation other than fibrous tissue; for example, chondrolipoangioma (cartilage, fat, and blood vessel).

metastasis: spread of malignant cells to other organs or tissues—a malignant tumor is said to **metastasize.**

microgeodic d.: transient phalangeal osteolysis that presents with pain and swelling and is followed by spontaneous resolution.

morbid: the disease state; however, the term may denote ready visibility, such as morbid anatomy.

morbidity: condition of being diseased with untoward results; could be congenital, acquired, or iatrogenic.

mucopurulent: denotes an exudate containing mucus and pus.

mucosanguineous: denotes an exudate containing mucus and blood.

myxedema: dry, waxy type of swelling associated with abnormal deposits of mucin in the skin; also called **nonpitting edema.**

necrosis: death of tissue or group of cells in tissue from trauma or disease.

neoplasm: abnormal new growth of tissue, either benign or malignant.

nevus: mole or birthmark.

nidus: place or source of infection or reaction.

node: confined tissue swelling or mass that can be readily seen or palpated, for example, lymph node.

nodule: small node, usually hard.

nutritional index: minimum metabolic condition required for wound healing that includes a total serum protein of at least 6.2 g/dl, serum albumin of at least 3.5 g/dl, and a total lymphocyte count of $1500/mm^3$.

obesity: abnormal accumulation of body fat.

occlusion: obstruction.

occult: hidden, not observable unless closely examined.

-odynia (suffix): pain.

onco- (prefix): combining form denoting relationship to swelling, mass, or tumor.

-orrhagia (suffix): hemorrhage.

-orrhea (suffix): discharge.

-orrhexis (suffix): rupture.

-osis (suffix): abnormal condition.

panniculitis: inflammation in subcutaneous tissue.

paresthesia: sensation of numbness or tingling and heightened sensitivity experienced in the central and peripheral nervous systems.

pectus carinatum: pigeon chest.

pectus excavatum: central depression of breast bone.

petechiae: tiny hemorrhages into the tissue; when seen in the skin, they appear as little violet dots.

phantom limb syndrome: sensations of an amputated part still being present. The perception of the phantom limb gradually shrinks to localization of sensation appropriate to the level of the stump.

-phyma (suffix): swelling produced by exudate to subcutaneous tissue.

pleomorphic: taking on a shape that lacks description such as round, square, angular, and so forth. The term is often used to describe the shape of cells.

plexiform: taking on a tortuous or multiple-form shape. Often used to describe the shape of a tumor.

polyps: protruding growths from mucous membranes.

procurvatum: angulation of a bone or joint that is convexed anteriorly.

prognosis: prediction of the outcome of disease or surgery.

prophylaxis: prevention of disease.

proprioception: sensibility to position, whether conscious or unconscious.

purpura: hemorrhage into the skin or other area with extravasation of blood into a congested area that is eventually resorbed.

purulent: pus-forming.

pyoderma gangrenosum: rare, destructive cutaneous lesion that starts as a painful, rapidly enlarging ulcer leading to a chronic, draining wound; often associated with other diseases.

pyogenic: having the ability to produce pus.

pyrexia: fever.

quiescence: discontinuation of symptoms or a disease, the connotation being an expectation of the return of symptoms or disease.

rarefaction: decrease in density, usually used to refer to appearance of bone on radiograph.

recrudescence: relapse or recurrence of symptoms.

recurvatum: angulation of bone or joint that is convexed posteriorly.

regressive remodeling: removal and replacement of bone such that the replacement occurs progressively away from the original maximal border of bone, for example, codfish vertebrae.

rigidus: stiffness.

rubor: redness of the skin.

rudimentary: insufficient development of a part or the development of an extra part such that no function is served by its presence; a rudimentary limb is so deficient that it serves no function, and a thirteenth rib similarly serves no function and is rudimentary.

rupture: discontinuity of tissue, usually referring to muscles and tendons.

sanguineous: bloody, as in a wound. This is in contrast to serosanguineous fluid, which is serous fluid containing some red cells.

saponification: calcification that occurs with the breakdown of fatty acids in the avascular area of aseptic necrosis.

sarcoidosis: granulomatous disorder of unknown cause affecting mostly the skin, lungs, and eyes. The condition usually is seen in the third and fourth decade of life. When bone is involved, the disorder usually affects the hands and feet.

sebaceous: secreting a greasy substance, as in oily skin or sebaceous cyst.

sepsis: denotes the presence of infection caused by bacteria.

septicemia: bacteria in the blood. It should be noted that blood poisoning often refers to the red streaks seen in a limb that has an infection; however, this condition is more accurately a lymphangitis.

sequela (*pl.* sequelae): sequel that follows, that is, a morbid condition that follows the consequence of disease, meaning one pathologic condition leads to another discrete pathologic condition; for example, muscle spasticity is a sequela of cerebral palsy.

seropurulent: denotes an exudate containing both pus and serous material.

serosanguineous: denotes an exudate containing both blood and serous material.

serous: denotes an exudate that is usually yellow, fairly fluid, and possibly blood-tinged.

slough: spontaneous separation of devitalized tissue from living tissue.

somatization disorder: in some patients with chronic pain, there are recurrent somatic complaints without an apparent significant physical disorder. Physical symptoms are related to anxiety, and the patient may seek medical attention over a period of years.

spasm: sudden or violent involuntary contractions of muscle.

splaying: to spread out, as in flatfoot deformity.

spurs: abnormal projection of bone at the margin or joints or strong ligamentous or tendinous attachments.

stenosis: stricture or narrowing of a canal or opening.

stigma: physical mark that aids in the identification of an abnormal process.

subliminal: below the threshold of sensation; weak; no muscle contractions.

supernumerary: excess number of anatomic parts, for example, six fingers on one hand.

suppurative: producing pus.

syncope: fainting caused by lack of oxygen or blood flow to the brain.

TAR syndrome: *t*hrombocytopenia *a*genesis *r*adius; the coincidental findings of bilateral failure of formation of the radius associated with petechiae, black stools, and other signs of thrombocytopenia resulting from a failure of normal formation of platelets. This autosomal recessive disorder improves with proper support, leaving the skeletal deformity as the primary problem.

tardy: denotes delayed onset or appearance of a disease process (e.g., tardy ulnar nerve palsy, which may occur years after an elbow fracture).

tetany: symptom of a biochemical disturbance or imbalance in the body characterized by hyperactivity of sensory and motor units and marked by spasms and twitching of muscles of the hands and feet and possibly spinal muscles. Most common causes are hypocalcemia, hypokalemia, hypoparathyroidism (rare), hyperventilation, or lack of vitamin D. (Not to be confused with tetanus, an infection.)

tonus: involuntary continued contraction of a muscle after the patient has attempted voluntary relaxation.

torticollis: postural neck deformity associated with a turning or bending of the head and neck. It may be due to congenital muscle tightness or disorders such as birth injury, psychogenic spasm, or spasm resulting from trauma. The term **wry neck** is sometimes used to describe this condition.

toxic: poisonous.

transudate: fluid passage through a normal membrane caused by imbalance in osmotic and hydrostatic forces.

trauma: any injury to tissue or psyche; can result from chemical, physical, or temporal events.

tumefaction: swelling, puffiness, edema.

tumor: a swelling, in the most generalized sense. However, the term connotes a neoplasm, that is, a new uncontrolled growth of tissue.

turgid: swollen or congested, describing a physical finding on palpation.

ulcer: penetrating disruption of mucous membrane of skin.

VATER association: acronym for a nonrandom group of occurrences that include *v*ertebral segmentation disorders and fusion, *a*nal atresia, *t*racheoesophageal fistula, *e*sophageal atresia, and *r*adial ray defects. Other defects may occur.

vertigo: loss of equilibrium caused by disease of the central nervous system, ear infection, or from unknown causes.

vestigial: remnants of a structure that functioned in a previous stage of species or individual development.

wear debris disease: absorption of bone seen around a joint prosthesis. This is due to macrophage response to numerous microscopic particles generated by the prosthesis.

wound: any disruption of normal tissue. A break in the skin is usually implied, but the term can be applied to a traumatic injury in which deep tissue is injured but the skin has not been broken.

wry neck: torticollis; stiff condition of the neck caused by spastic muscle contractions.

Imaging Techniques

Computerized diagnostic imaging techniques applied to the field of radiology has contributed more to medicine than any other method in diagnosing diseases, injuries, and other conditions. The computer is an indispensable tool for managing information and recording programs from various scanning devices that are retrieved and read out by a central computer bank. This technology has provided computer graphics and anatomic color images, has changed diagnostic procedures, and given medical specialists a more accurate diagnostic picture that saves considerable time. In addition, the most important contribution of imaging technology is that it enables physicians to see detailed images of the body without surgery.

The standard radiographic technique depicts a body part as a simple two-dimensional shadow portrayed on a negative film. Today, imaging technology creates two- and three-dimensional views from any angle. The types of diagnostic imaging are as follows:

- **Nuclear medicine studies**—Invasive (requiring an injection) tests that use radioisotopes; examples are positron emission tomography (PET) and bone scan (scintigraphy) (Fig. 3-1).
- **Magnetic resonance imaging (MRI)**—Noninvasive technology that combines radio waves and a strong magnetic field with the hydrogen atoms in the body to produce images of soft tissue structures.
- **Ultrasound (sonography, ultrasonography), digital color Doppler, pulsed Doppler, or power Doppler**—Noninvasive forms of imaging that use a small transducer (transmitter/receiver) that is in contact with the area being examined to produce high-frequency sound waves that penetrate the area involved and reflect back to the receiver.
- **Computed axial tomography (CAT scan, CT) and radioisotope imaging (RII)**—This may be an invasive (requiring intravenous injection of a radiopaque solution) or a noninvasive technique. Scans can now be obtained in a continuous helical motion and not just by a single slice at a time. These and other radiographic techniques have been updated and defined in this edition.

Radiography has been an integral part of the orthopaedic examination, and the new diagnostic imaging techniques enable the orthopaedic surgeon to not only identify the anatomic site, but to evaluate the physiologic conditions within and surrounding this site. Specifically, bone density, pathologic changes (necrosis of bone tissue, tumors, infections), spur formation, joint space narrowing, synovial inflammation, nerve impingements, and soft tissue changes can be evaluated. A computer compiles vast amounts of digital data during an examination, and these data are turned into picture form. Physicians compare the many views, which can ultimately be made into a single video image.

The radiologist, a board-certified physician and specialist in radiology, is often consulted by the orthopaedist and other physicians to give interpretations of

FIG 3-1 Bone scan image with areas of more active bone formation brighter at knee joint with arthritis.

imaging technology and of more complicated pathologic conditions. Using image guidance and minimally invasive techniques to gain access to bone, organs, vessels, and other soft tissues, interventional radiologists can diagnose and treat certain conditions that may otherwise require surgery. The radiologist is assisted by qualified technologists who have learned the fundamentals of working with the radiographic and imaging equipment, developing film, and positioning patients. These specialists are challenged to meet the ever-changing technologic demands in their field to capably assist all branches of medicine.

This chapter presents the specialized terminology of radiology, new imaging technology, and its application to orthopaedics.

General Radiologic Terms

baseline radiograph: radiograph taken at time of first examination and compared with those taken later.
catheter: a thin plastic tube inserted through the skin and into an artery or vein for the injection of contrast material in a vascular arteriography procedure. An example is femoral arteriography.
cathode ray tube: vacuum tube that, with a high enough voltage, will produce x-rays.
contrast: a radiopaque medium that appears white on x-ray and can be given intravenously, intraarterially, intrathecally, orally, rectally, or into a joint to aid visualization of internal structures; also called **contrast radiography, contrast study.** New **nonionic contrast agents** have been developed. Advantages over standard ionic agents are that there are fewer serious allergic reactions in patients at risk for allergic reactions; nonionic agents should be used.
echogenic: tissue or structure that reflects sound waves and give rise to ultrasound echoes. Examples are bone, metal, and air; produce white (hyperintense) areas on ultrasound images. Also called **hyperechoic.**
Hounsfield unit: a measure of radiodensity relative to water, with air being −1000, water 0, and bone between 700 and 3000.
hypoechoic: Tissue or structure that reflects few ultrasound waves. Examples are fluid, muscle, and cartilage; produce dark (hypointense) areas on ultrasound images.
oscilloscope: instrument that displays computer data of electrical variations on the fluorescent screen of a cathode-ray tube.
Pantopaque: trade name for an iodinated oil (radiopaque contrast medium) used in a contrast radiographic procedure (i.e., myelography). It is no longer used due to its lack of resorption, which required complete removal through aspiration at the end of the procedure. This was usually not possible, and the residual material occasionally resulted in chronic irritation and arachnoiditis. Also called **iodophenylundecylic acid.**
rad: measure of *r*adiation *a*bsorbed *d*ose, 100 erg/g (energy per gram).
radiograph: image produced on a film by means of ionizing radiation. **X-ray**, as in a *chest x-ray*, is a commonly used synonym.
radiology: the specialized branch of medicine concerned with the diagnosis of disease utilizing ionizing (e.g., x-rays) and nonionizing (e.g., ultrasound and MRI) radiation; also called **roentgenology.** A **radiologist** is a physician specialist who interprets the radiology studies.
radiolucent: permitting free passage of ionizing energy (x-ray) through an area, with dark appearance on exposed film.

radiopaque: preventing passage of ionizing energy (x-ray), thus allowing the representative area to appear light or white on exposed film.

roentgen (R): unit of x- or gamma-radiation exposure; 1 **gray** = 100 roentgen; 1 **centigray** = 1 roentgen.

roentgenography: the use of x-irradiation to produce either positive or negative film images or fluoroscopic images of objects; also called **radiography.**

scout film: general term for a radiograph prior to the injection of contrast. The purpose is to check the radiographic technique and to look for abnormalities that may be obscured once contrast is given; also called **scout radiograph.**

translucent: allowing some light to pass through but not clearly transparent; for example, soft tissue appears as a light shadow on a radiograph when compared with bone.

wet reading: as implied. Today, films are dried automatically and are read dry. In the past, if an immediate interpretation of the film was required, it was read while still wet. Thus a request for an immediate interpretation is still called *wet reading.*

x-ray: electromagnetic radiation generally greater than 10 Kev in energy and less than 1 nanometer in wavelength, capable of penetrating tissue; also called **roentgen ray.**

Orthopaedic Radiographic Techniques and Procedures

arthrography: procedure showing interior outline of a joint after contrast (dye) medium or air has been injected intraarticularly; tendon, ligament, or meniscal tears and articular cartilage injuries can be detected in this manner; also called **arthrogram.** Imaging modalities include MRI, CT, and conventional radiographs.

bone densitometry: procedure for determining the relative density of bone by using several different radiographic techniques. A density gradient plate can be placed on the film at the same time radiography of the part is being performed. From this plate, a comparative density of the bone can be made, usually of the spine. Photons from a single emitting source can be used to directly measure the density of bone, such as that of the distal radius and lumbar spine. These studies can then be compared with age-matched normal values. This procedure is called **photon densitometry.**

dual photon densitometry (DPD), dual photon absorptiometry (DPA): the use of two different emitting sources to help correct for soft tissue density.

dual x-ray absorptiometry (DEXA): the use of two different x-ray voltages to correct for soft tissue density.

quantitative computed tomography (QCT): another method of measuring bone density by using computerized tomographic images through lumbar vertebral bodies and comparing the measured density with age-matched normal values.

bone marrow pressure: measurement taken to detect bone necrosis. The pressure is taken while *intraosseous venography* and *core decompression* are performed to aid in diagnosis of ischemic necrosis of the femoral head, forming an early basis for treatment.

bursography: injection of radiopaque dye to show a bursa such as a retrocalcaneal bursa.

diskography: visualization of the cervical and lumbar intervertebral disks after direct injection of a radiopaque contrast medium into the disk; also called **diskogram.**

femoral arteriography: radiographic examination in which the femoral artery of the groin is catheterized. Through the femoral artery, the catheter can be directed to arteries throughout the body, including the brain, chest, abdomen, and legs. Contrast is injected through the catheter to identify abnormalities in the arterial system or can be useful in outlining extent of a tumor; also called **arteriogram.** In some cases, a vascular abnormality can be treated through the catheter (e.g., by angioplasty).

fluoroscopy: direct visual radiographic procedure with the use of x-ray tube, fluoroscopic screen, and television monitor for intensification, that is, continuous monitoring showing organ function that can be videotaped; used in gastrointestinal studies, arthrography, and angiography.

kidneys, ureters, bladder (KUB): plain frontal supine radiograph of the abdomen, generally not an orthopaedic radiographic procedure, but taken occasionally to study the abdominal wall or suspected masses.

Iopamidol (Isovue) myelography: this and iohexol (Omnipaque) are water-soluble contrast agents used for myelography after injection of an iodine-based water-soluble contrast medium. The material does not have to be withdrawn after completion of the study, giving some advantages over the oil-based material that must be withdrawn.

lymphangiography: radiographic examination after introduction of radiopaque contrast medium into peripheral lymphatic vessels to determine presence of blockage or tumor in proximal lymphatic vessels.

myelography: radiographic examination with contrast medium injected into the subarachnoid space under fluoroscopy to examine the spinal cord and canal for possible disk protrusions or lesions; also called **myelogram**.

orthoroentgenography: for measuring limb-length disparity; three separate exposures are taken of the hip, knee, and ankle (or shoulder, elbow, and wrist) to produce an image of the entire limb; also called **orthoroentgenogram**.

pneumoarthrography: injection of air into a joint before radiographic examination to determine internal outline, as in meniscal tear or other injuries and abnormalities; also called **pneumoarthrogram**.

roentgen stereophotogrammetry: simultaneous anterior-posterior and lateral radiographic examination performed with the examined part in a calibration cage. Radiographs can be obtained serially over time to study the progression of bony changes. Computer-driven calculations allow for the identification of three-dimensional changes as small as 2 mm. The technique is particularly useful in the study of prosthetic wear and migration over time.

scanography: for measuring leg-length discrepancy, a film is moved beneath the patient for three successive exposures of the three pairs of joints, and a radiopaque scale is placed beneath the limbs so that measurements may be made from the scale of the film. A film 43 cm in length may be used rather than a film two to three times longer; also called **scanogram**.

sinography: radiographic examination for sinus tract infection in bone, performed after injection of water-soluble contrast medium, after saline cleanser, to determine the course of a deep draining wound; also called **sinogram**.

teleroentgenography: for measuring limb-length disparity; radiographic examination performed with the x-ray tube 2 to 3 m (6 to 7.5 feet) from the plate to obtain a more parallel roentgenogram. The entire bone is visualized, but the degree of magnification (approximately 10%) is difficult to assess; also called **teleroentgenogram**.

tomography: used to show detailed images of structures lying in a predetermined plane of tissue, while blurring or eliminating details of images of structures in other planes as in polytomography, planography, or zonography. It is used with radiographic magnification to detect abnormalities of the spine (laminography) or joints and in malunion fractures; also called **tomogram**.

Routine Radiographic Views

The number of views varies and is determined by the history and physical examination. For instance, an anteroposterior (AP) view may be unremarkable, but a lateral view may reveal a fracture or dislocation, depending on the angle of view taken. A complaint of knee pain often arises from a hip disorder, making radiographic (x-ray) views of the knee or hip important in diagnostic evaluation. Asymmetry of two identical bones (comparing femur to femur) can also exhibit an underlying abnormality. More than one view is usually required to diagnose the chief complaint. The terms are defined first and then given in abbreviated form by anatomic region.

Alexander v.: lateral view of scapula with shoulders protracted forward.

AP v.: anteroposterior view (x-ray beam passes from front to back).

apical v.: apex, tip, or point of subject radiographed.

apical lordotic v.: usually of the chest for the apices of the lungs, but for the clavicle if a patient's symptoms suggest an orthopaedic problem.

axillary lateral v.: for the shoulder, lateral view through axilla.

Breuerton v.: special view of the hand to search for early joint changes in rheumatoid arthritis.

Broden v.: for injuries affecting subtalar joint; lateral view of foot with a 45-degree rotation and various tilts.

Bura v.: for ulnar side of wrist; a supinated oblique view taken as an AP with 35 degrees supination.

Burnham v.: AP hyperextended view of thumb with dorsum on cassette and 15-degree cephalic tilt.

Canale v.: for the talus; an AP view with 75-degree cephalic tilt and 15-degree pronation.

carpal tunnel v.: for hook-of-hamate fracture; tangential view of volar wrist taken with wrist in dorsiflexion.

Carter-Rowe v.: view of the hip taken at a 45-degree oblique angle to determine size of bone fragment in a posterior acetabular hip fracture or other abnormality of the pelvis.

clenched fist v.: to demonstrate scapholunate instability; an AP view is taken with the fist clenched.

coned-down v.: close-up of a particular area, with radiation shielded from the rest of the patient's body.

cross-table lateral v.: for hip fracture; lateral view obtained with opposite hip in flexion.

Dunn v.: for hip dysplasia, an AP of the pelvis centered at the pubic symphysis with hips flexed 90 degrees and abducted 20 degrees.

false profile view: standing lateral x-ray of pelvis with person turned with the hip furthest from the cassette slightly posterior.

frog-leg lateral v.: AP view of hip in abduction and external rotation.

Garth v.: for acromioclavicular joint injury; apical oblique with 45-degree caudal and AP tilt.

Grashey v.: for shoulder impingement by acromion; scapular lateral with a 10-degree caudal tilt; also called **supraspinatus outlet v.**

Harris v.: for calcaneus; AP standing with 45-degree tilt.

Hobb v.: for sternoclavicular joint; while standing, the patient bends over end of x-ray table and cassette with hands on head, neck parallel to table, and chest approximately 45 degrees to table. The x-ray beam is vertical to the cassette.

Holmberg v.: for femoral notch architecture, two views with patient on hands and knees. A PA radiograph is obtained with beam perpendicular to knee and leg, and knee flexed at 45 degrees and 70 degrees.

Hughston v.: knee is flexed to 60 degrees, and view is obtained at a 55-degree angle to show a cartilage-osseous fracture of the femoral condyle or subluxing patella.

inlet v.: for pelvic injury; 45- to 50-degree caudad; an AP view.

inversion ankle stress v.: AP view of the ankle, which is stressed in inversion to test the integrity of the lateral collateral ankle ligaments.

lateral v.: view taken side to side, left or right.

lateral monopodal stance v.: for anterior cruciate deficiency; lateral x-ray to detect posterior shift of femur on tibia.

Lowenstein v.: a frog-leg lateral.

lumbosacral series: multiple views of the lumbosacral spine to include AP, lateral, and oblique views.

Merchant v.: tangential superior to inferior patellar view taken with the knee flexed at 45 degrees; also called **Knuttson v.**

mortise v.: view of the ankle rotated internally until medial and lateral malleoli are parallel to film; demonstrates the talus, tibia, and fibula without superimposition; used for comparison with normal AP view and to detect joint abnormalities.

Neer transscapular v.: posterior oblique scapular projection to help obtain a lateral view of the shoulder in trauma; also called **Neer lateral v.**

notch v.: prone view of knee with 45-degree caudal from vertical.

oblique v.: any view that is off angle from AP, PA, or lateral.

odontoid v.: specific for the odontoid process of C2 vertebra; AP view obtained with mouth open; also called **open-mouth v.**

outlet v.: for pelvic injury; 45-degree cephalad AP view.

PA: posteroanterior view (from back to front).

plantar axial v. of foot: offers visualization of the plantar aspect of the metatarsal heads.

prayer v.: for wrist instabilities; lateral view of both wrists at same time with palms pressed together to bring about maximum wrist extension.

push-pull ankle stress v.: lateral view of the ankle, which is stressed in an attempt to evaluate the anterior talofibular ligament.

Robert v.: AP hyperextended view of thumb with dorsum on cassette.

Rosenberg v.: for osteoarthrosis knee; weight-bearing PA with knee at 45-degree flexion and x-ray tube positioned 10 degrees above the horizontal.

serendipity v.: for sternoclavicular dislocation or proximal-third fracture of the clavicle; AP view taken with patient supine and tube angled upward 40 degrees from the vertical position.

Slomann v.: for tarsal coalition; a 45-degree oblique view of the foot.

Stryker notch v.: for scapular notch; view taken with patient supine, hand on head, and camera with 10-degree cephalic tilt.

sunset v.: view of patella with knee bent at 120 degrees to permit a profile view; used for examination of patella and adjacent femoral surfaces; also called **sunrise v.** and **tangential v.**

swimmer's v.: for lower cervical spine injuries; lateral view obtained with one arm held overhead while other arm is pulled down.

transthoracic lateral v.: for proximal humeral fracture or dislocation; view obtained with one arm held overhead and x-ray beam directed through chest.

trauma v.: for shoulder injuries; true AP, 45-degree oblique, and Y scapular (tangential) views.

true lateral v.: perfectly positioned lateral projection without rotation.

tunnel v.: view of tibia, fibula, and femur only with patella out of the way; a knee notch or intercondylar view; the radiographic examination is done with the tibia and fibula straight and the femur at a 45-degree angle.

von Rosen v.: view of the hips in 45 degrees abduction and internal rotation for determining dislocation of the hip(s) in developmental dysplasia.

West Point v.: for shoulder (glenoid) injuries; prone axillary lateral view with 25-degree lateral and posterior tilt to camera.

Y scapular v.: lateral view of scapula taken at an angle to view scapular blade such that it appears as the stem of a Y with coracoid and spine as the branches of the Y.

Zanca v.: for distal-third clavicle fractures or acromioclavicular joint, a 10-degree cephalad view.

Radiographic Views by Anatomic Region

Thoracic Region

chest: PA, lateral
clavicle: AP, apical lordotic, tangential
ribs:
  anterior: PA, obliques
  posterior: AP, obliques

scapula: AP, oblique, lateral
shoulder: AP, internal rotation; AP, external rotation; axillary lateral; transthoracic lateral
sternum: right anterior oblique, lateral

Upper Limbs

elbow: AP, lateral, oblique
hands/fingers: AP, lateral, oblique
humerus: AP, lateral, transthoracic lateral
radius/ulna: AP, lateral
wrist: AP, lateral, oblique, AP with ulnar and radial deviation (for scaphoid fracture), carpal tunnel

Spinal Region

C-spine: AP, lateral, both obliques, open-mouth odontoid
coccyx: AP, lateral
L-spine: AP, lateral, both obliques, coned-down L-5 to S-1 lateral
pelvis: AP, inlet, outlet
SI joints: AP, both obliques
sacrum: AP, lateral
T-spine: AP, lateral

Lower Limbs

ankle: AP, lateral, and mortise oblique
femur: AP, lateral
foot/toes: AP, lateral, oblique
hip: AP, frog-leg, and/or cross-table lateral
knee: AP, lateral, tunnel, Hughston
patella: tunnel, sunset, lateral, PA, merchant
tibia/fibula: AP, lateral
calcaneus: lateral, plantodorsal, axial

Additional views requested may be views in flexion and extension, special views of the skull, push-pull films of hips for piston sign, and cine (movies) of x-ray images.

Radiographic Angles, Lines, Signs, and Methods

Angles

The anatomic description is taken directly from points using the intersection of two straight lines to form the angle.

FIG 3-2 Radiographic measurements for hip dysplasia. **1,** horizontal Y line (Hilgenreiner line); **2,** vertical line (Perkins line); **3,** quadrants (formed by lines 1 and 2); **4,** acetabular index (Kleinberg and Lieberman); **5,** Shenton line; **6,** upward displacement of femoral head; **7,** lateral displacement of femoral head; **8,** U figure of teardrop shadow (Kohler); **9,** Y coordinate (Ponseti); **10,** capital epiphyseal dysplasia (**a,** delayed appearance of center of ossification of femoral head; **b,** irregular maturation of center of ossification); **11,** bifurcation (furrowing of acetabular roof in late infancy [Ponseti]); **12,** hypoplasia of pelvis (ilium); **13,** delayed fusion (ischiopubic juncture); **14,** adduction attitude of extremity. *(Modified from Kelly DM: Congenital and developmental anomalies of the hip and pelvis. In Canale ST and Beaty JH, editors: Campbell's operative orthopaedics, ed 12, Philadelphia, 2013, Elsevier, Fig. 30-4B.)*

acetabular a.: angle created by the intersection of a line from the inferior margin to the superior margin of the acetabulum and a line horizontal to the pelvis (connecting two inferior acetabuli; Fig. 3-2).

acetabular index: angle formed between lateral margin of acetabular roof and inferior aspect of the pelvic "teardrop" and horizontal line between the inferior aspect of both pelvic "teardrops."

acromial a.: measured in patients with shoulder impingement by drawing a line along the inferior acromial cortex on either side of the apex, resulting in anterior and posterior lines that cross to form an angle.

alpha a (α angle): a measure for femoral acetabular impingement; angle made by the intersection of a line from the center line of the femoral neck to the central part of the femoral head, to a line from the center of the femoral head to the anterior superior edge of the femoral neck.

anatomic femorotibial a. (FTA): angle created by the intersection of lines through the shaft of the tibia and the shaft of the femur.

Baumann a.: angle created by intersection of two lines drawn on an AP view of a child; one line is drawn from the medial margin of the distal humeral physeal line to the lateral margin of the lateral condylar epiphysis, and the other line is drawn in the line of the lateral condylar epiphysis. This angle is usually 11 degrees.

bimalleolar a.: angle drawn by bisection of line horizontal to ankle joint with line crossing medial and lateral malleolar tips. This angle is typically 23 degrees.

Böhler a.: angle formed by intersection of a line drawn from the cephalic aspect of the anterior calcaneal tuberosity to the superior point of the posterior facet with a line drawn from the superior point of the posterior facet to the superior posterior calcaneus, normally 20 to 40 degrees.

carrying a.: for the AP angle of the extended elbow, that is, the angle of the forearm when arm is extended.

center edge (CE) a.: created by two lines drawn from the center of the femoral capital epiphysis, one line being vertical and the other extending to the acetabular edge. Also called **Wiberg a.**

Codman a.: discrete angle at edge of the bone cortex produced by periosteal elevation and reactive bone in the area of a tumor; also called **Codman triangle.**

condylar-plateau a. (CPA): angle created by the intersection of a line parallel to the tibial plateau surfaces and the distal femoral condyles.

congruence a.: bisecting angle of the patella intersecting with vertical angle from trochlea (Fig. 3-3).

coronal femoral component a.: for knee replacement positioning, the angle of distal femoral cut to the anatomic line through the femur seen on AP projection.

coronal tibial component a.: for knee replacement positioning, the angle of proximal tibial cut to the anatomic line through the tibia seen on AP projection.

FIG 3-3 Radiographic measurements to evaluate patellar instability. **A,** Insall-Salveti ratio, LT–LP, normally 0.8 to 1.2. **B,** Measurements of patellofemoral congruence described by Merchant et al. *F,* facet; *L,* lateral condyle; *M,* medial condyle; *P,* patellar ridge; *S,* sulcus. Angle *MSL* is sulcus angle (average, 137 degrees; standard deviation, 6 degrees). Line *SO* is zero reference line bisecting sulcus angle. Angle *PSO* is congruence angle (average, −8 degrees; standard deviation, 6 degrees). Line *PF* (lateral facet) and line *ML* form patellofemoral angle that should diverge laterally. Ratio of lateral height at L to medial height at M is normally 1.65. *(Modified from Phillips BB: Recurrent dislocations. In Canale ST and Beaty JH, editors:* Campbell's operative orthopaedics, *ed 12, Philadelphia, 2013, Elsevier, Figs. 47-4 and 47-10.)*

costophrenic a.: angle formed at the junction of the costal and diaphragmatic parietal pleura.

costovertebral a.: angle made between the twelfth thoracic rib and the T12 vertebra at the posterior inferior margin of the thoracic cage on each side.

crucial angle of Gissane: seen on lateral radiograph of foot; angle created by posterior facet of calcaneus and the superior anterolateral surface of the calcaneus.

femoral tibial a.: angle created by anatomic axis of the femur and tibia (line drawn from midpoint of proximal and distal shaft). Average is 6 degrees of valgus.

Ferguson's a.: represents the angle of the lumbosacral junction as measured by the inclination of the superior surface of the first sacral vertebra to another line parallel to the ground (usually measured from a standing lateral film); also called **sacral base a.**

Fick a.: standing foot angle or Fick's angle represents the amount of toeing in (**decreased foot a.**) or toeing out (**increased foot a.**) observed during stance.

Fowler-Phillip a.: to measure degree of pump bump; angle created by intersection of a line from the posterior surface and the plantar surface of the calcaneus.

hallux valgus a.: angle created by intersection of a longitudinal line through shaft of first metatarsal and the shaft of the proximal first phalanx.

head-shaft a.: for slipped capital femoral epiphysis; angle between the femoral head physis and a vertical line drawn through the femoral shaft seen on frog-leg projection; also called **Southwick a.**

Hibbs a.: two angles created by intersection of a longitudinal line of first metatarsal and the line of the plantar surface of the calcaneus.

Hilgenreiner a.: angle of the acetabular slope to the Y-line (horizontal line drawn through both acetabular centers); also called **acetabular index a.**

Hilgenreiner epiphyseal a.: for coxa vara or slipped epiphysis angle of intersection of Y-line with line drawn through femoral physis.

Kager triangle: triangular space anterior to the Achilles tendon normally visible on radiographs as a radiolucent area.

Konstram a.: for gibbus deformity; the obtuse angle created by the intersection of the two lines drawn parallel to the surface of the superior vertebral body above and inferior surface of vertebral body below the deformed segment.

lateral distal femoral a.: angle of a line from the femoral head to the tibial spine to a horizontal line across the two femoral condylar surfaces; measured in the superolateral of the four quadrants obtained.

Laquena and Deseze a.: for acetabular coverage of femoral head in developmental hip dysplasia; using a lateral x-ray view, the angle between a line seen in the shaft of the femur and from the center of the femoral head to the anterior acetabular rim; also called **ventral inclination a. (VCA).**

Laurin a. (lateral patellofemoral a.): acute angle created by intersection of line drawn from medial to lateral condylar points and a line parallel to the lateral undersurface of the patella. The angle is positive when it opens laterally.

Levine Drennan a.: angle that lies between a line drawn through the most distal points of the medial and lateral beaks of the metaphysis and a line perpendicular to the lateral cortex of the tibia; also called **metaphyseal-diaphyseal a.**

lumbosacral a.: angle between the inferior plate of L5 to line of superior plate of sacrum. Typically the sacrum is inclined such that the sacral line opens anteriorly in reference to the lumbar line.

Meary a.: angle formed between the long axis of the talus and the first metatarsal on a lateral weight-bearing view. This line is used as a measurement collapse of the longitudinal arch. An angle that is greater than 4 degrees convex downward is considered pes planus.

mechanical axis: line created between the center of the femoral head and the center of the talus. In a normal knee, this axis passes close to the center of the joint; also called **Maquet line.**

medial proximal tibial a.: for tibial plateau slope; the angle created by a vertical tibial shaft line and a line across the tibial plateaus; measured in the inferomedial of the four quadrants drawn.

Merchant a.: created on a Merchant view by intersection of two lines, one drawn from the intracondylar apex of patella to center and a line perpendicular to plane of condyles.

Mikulicz a.: angle of declination of the proximal femur formed by the neck of the femoral epiphysis and diaphysis center lines. It is the same as the neck shaft angle.

neck shaft a.: created by intersection of a line drawn through the femoral shaft and a line through the femoral head and neck.

Pauwels a.: of a femoral neck fracture in reference to the horizontal line of a standing patient.

pelvic femoral a.: of inclination formed by a line parallel to the tilt of the pelvis with line of femoral shaft.

physeal a.: for Legg-Calvé-Perthes disease; the angle created by intersection of a line drawn vertically though the femoral shaft and the line of femoral head physis; also called **physeal slope.**

pitch a.: a line is drawn from the plantar-most surface of the calcaneus to the inferior border of the distal articular surface. The angle made between this line and the transverse plane of the floor is the calcaneal pitch angle. A decreased pitch is consistent with pes planus. Also called **calcaneal inclination a.**

Q angle: made by intersection of lines drawn from anterosuperior iliac spine to midpatella and from midpatella to anterior tibial tuberosity.

radial inclination a.: measured by drawing a perpendicular line to the radial axis through the distal sigmoid notch and by drawing another line joining the tip of the radial styloid and the distal sigmoid notch. These two lines form the radial inclination angle (normal angle 21–25 degrees).

sacrovertebral a.: obtained by junction of lines through lateral projection of sacrum and lumbar spine.

sagittal femoral component a.: for knee replacement positioning, the angle of distal femoral cut to the anatomic line through the femur seen on lateral projection

sagittal tibial component a.: for knee replacement positioning, the angle of proximal tibial cut to the anatomic line through the tibia seen on lateral projection

Sharp a.: defined by intersection of lines from inferior acetabulum (bottom of teardrop) to superolateral acetabulum and a horizontal line.

slip a.: angle of the line of the inferior body of L5 to the line of the superior body of S1. As L5 slips forward on S1, this angle reverses.

Southwick a.: for slipped capital femoral epiphysis, on lateral radiograph of the hip the angle created by a line through the center of the shaft of the femur to a perpendicular line to a line through the base of the epiphysis. The angle is compared to the normal side. If both sides affected at an angle greater that 12 degrees is considered abnormal, less than 30 degrees is mild, 30 to 50 degrees is moderate, and more than 50 degrees is severe; also called **posterior slip a. and epiphyseal shaft a.**

sternal a: angle formed by the junction of the manubrium and the body of the sternum; also called **angle of Louis.**

sulcus a.: on Merchant view, lines drawn from apex of medial and lateral condyles to lowest point in groove to create this obtuse angle.

talocrural a.: angle created by intersection of lines, one drawn parallel to the tibial plafond, the other across the tips of the medial and lateral malleoli; normally 8 to 15 degrees.

Tönnis a.: on an AP projection of the pelvis, the angle created by the intersection of a line parallel to the ischial tuberosities and the slope of the sourcil, which is the dense subchondral bone of the roof of the acetabulum.

Ward triangle: relatively radiolucent area of bone in the intertrochanteric area of the femur.

Lines, Indices, and Ratios

A *line* is defined as that seen or drawn directly on the film to help in the interpretation of the radiograph or an anatomic line of reference.

acetabular coverage: may be expressed as distance from lateral lip of acetabulum to lateral edge of the femoral head, or as a ratio of the width of the femoral head divided into distance from the lateral lip of acetabulum to the lateral edge of the femoral head.

acetabular depth: depth of the longest possible vertical line drawn perpendicular to a line crossing the superior and inferior acetabular margins.

acetabular head quotient: for hip dysplasia; the ratio of the radius of the femoral head divided by the distance from the femoral head center to a vertical line drawn from the acetabular lip.

acetabular l.: line drawn from superolateral tip of both acetabuli for measuring femoral head or prosthetic migration.

anteversion: descriptive of axial rotation. For example, the normal relationship of femoral head is 20 degrees anterior to axis of femur.

Blackburne-Peel ratio: for a patella alta, the distance from the inferior articular margin of the patella to the line parallel to the tibial surface is divided by the length of the articular surface. Normal range is 0.54 to 1.06.

Blumensaat l.: line parallel to superior part of intercondylar notch as seen on lateral radiographs; used to judge the relative height of the patella.

canal-to-calcar isthmus ratio: for proximal femoral canal cylindrical configuration; two vertical lines are drawn from points on the inner cortex, one 10 cm from the mid-lesser trochanter and the other 3 cm from the mid-lesser trochanter. The ratio is the width of the space between these two lines at the mid-lesser trochanter divided by the width of the canal 10 cm distal to that point.

carpal height ratio: for capitate instability in the wrist; the ratio of the length of the third metacarpal to the length of the wrist from the base of the third metacarpal to the distal radius. The **revised carpal height ratio** is the width of the wrist from the base of the third metacarpal divided by the length of the capitate.

Caton-Deschamps ratio: for patella baja or alta, from a lateral projection of the knee. The ratio of a line drawn from the anterior corner of the tibial surface to the lower articular margin of the patella divided by the length of the patellar articular surface. Normal range is 0.6 to 1.2.

central sacral l.: the vertical line on a frontal radiograph that passes through the center of the sacrum.

cervico-obturator l.: a curve that can be drawn on an AP view of the pelvis. This line continues from the inferior border of the femoral neck to the inferior border of the pubic ramus. An interruption in the line is suggestive of an abnormal position of the femoral head. Also called **Shenton l.**

Chamberlain l.: for developmental basilar skull impression onto cervical spine; a line drawn from the posterior edge of the foramen magnum to the posterior edge of the hard palate, on a lateral projection.

demarcation l.: zone between normal and abnormal tissue, most commonly used to denote area or line of normal-appearing tissue next to gangrenous tissue in a devitalized limb. This term is also used in describing radiographic evidence of disease that shows a clear line or zone of activity.

Dorr ratio: for proximal femoral canal cylindrical configuration; width of the canal at the mid-lesser trochanter divided by the width of the canal 10 cm distal to that point.

epiphyseal l.: line of fusion of the physeal growth plate.

Feiss l.: a line drawn on a standing lateral radiograph between the tip of the medial malleolus and the base of the first metatarsophalangeal joint. The position of the navicular tuberosity is noted, and it should not lie below the line. The Feiss line is used in evaluation of pes planus.

femoral cortical index: ratio of the femoral diameter of the outer cortex to the inner cortex 10 cm distal to the mid-lesser trochanter.

femoral head neck offset: not to be confused with femoral offset, this measures the ratio of the distance from the outermost margin of the femoral head to the femoral neck to the radius of the femoral head

femoral offset: perpendicular distance from the center line of the femoral shaft to the center of the femoral head.

femoral shaft l.: line drawn from midpoint of proximal and distal shaft; also called the **anatomic femoral axis.**

fracture l.: any line thought to be the result of a fracture.

Frankel l.: a white line around the outer margins of the bony epiphysis, which can be seen on a bone radiograph in a patient with scurvy.

growth-arrest l.: line of bony density seen on radiograph of a long bone. This may represent a growth-arrest scar from the growth plate as a result of stress (fracture or an illness) during a period of growth; also called **Harris l.** and **Harris-Park l.**

herniation pit: not a true herniation, but a point of wear in the femoral neck caused by misshaped femoral head or acetabulum leading to impingement on the anterior acetabulum.

Hilgenreiner l.: a horizontal line drawn between the two triradiate cartilage centers of the hips defines a horizontal plane and an approximation to the flexion axis of the hips.

Hueter l.: line drawn horizontal to the medial epicondyle of the humerus, passing tip of olecranon when elbow is extended.

Insall ratio: for patella alta; with the knee flexed at 30 degrees, the ratio is the length of the patella tendon to the height of the patella. A number greater than 1.3 indicates patella alta; also called **Insall-Salvati ratio.**

Klein l.: a line tangential to the superior femoral neck on an AP view of the pelvis. Normally, a portion of the femoral head is above this line. In patients with a slipped capital femoral epiphysis, the femoral head is below this line or a smaller portion of the femoral head is above this line when compared with the contralateral view.

Kohler l.: slanted line drawn from the acetabular teardrop to the most lateral tangent of the pelvic ring (commonly the sciatic notch).

lead l.: radiopaque (white) thin line in the metaphysis (end region) of bones in a patient with lead poisoning.

Maquet l.: line drawn from center of femoral head to midtalus; normally passes through middle of the knee.

McGregor l.: for developmental basilar skull impression onto cervical spine; line drawn from base of occiput to posterior edge of hard palate.

McRae l.: for developmental basilar skull impression onto cervical spine; a line drawn from anterior to posterior edge of the foramen magnum.

medialization ratio: percentage of the horizontal radius of the cartilaginous femoral head medial to vertical line drawn from lateral tip of acetabulum, as seen on an arthrogram with the hip in the position of reduction.

Nélaton l.: drawn from the anterosuperior iliac spine to the ischial tuberosity; normally goes through the greater trochanter forming one side of Bryant triangle.

obturator/brim l.: drawn from inner pelvic brim to midobturator foramen. It is used in determining the degree of femoral head or prosthetic migration.

Ogston l.: drawn from adduction tubercle to intercondylar notch; used as a guide for transection of condyle in osteotomy for knock-knee deformity.

patella subluxation ratio: for patellar subluxation; ratio created by the distance of medial femoral condylar margin to apex of patella divided by the depth of the patella groove.

Pavlov ratio: for spinal cord space in cervical spine; ratio of vertebral body width to spinal canal diameter (Fig. 3-4).

Perkin l.: a line drawn perpendicular to the horizontal Hilgenreiner line through the most lateral edge of the ossified acetabular cartilage. In normal newborns and infants, the medial aspect of the femoral neck or the ossified capital femoral epiphysis falls in the lower inner quadrant. The appearance of either of these structures in the lower outer or upper outer quadrants indicates subluxation or dislocation of the hip; also called **Ombrédanne l.**

retroversion: descriptive of axial rotation. For example, in hip dysplasia, the femoral head is posterior to the axis of the femur.

sacroiliac l.: line drawn from both inferior sacroiliac joints, used in measuring proximal migration of femoral head or prosthesis.

sacroiliac/symphysis l.: horizontal line drawn from midpoint between superior symphysis pubis and sacroiliac line, used in measuring proximal migration of femoral head or prosthesis.

Shenton l.: curved line seen on radiographs of a normal hip joint, drawn from the top of the obturator foramen to medial femoral neck and lesser trochanter.

FIG 3-4 Pavlov ratio used to determine relative narrowness of cervical spinal canal, a:b, where a value 1 is normal and less than 0.8 indicates a developmentally narrow canal. *(From Pavlov H, Porter IS: Criteria for cervical instability and stenosis, Op Tech Sports Med 1:170, 1993.)*

sourcil: eyebrow-shaped area of dense bone on the superior acetabulum seen on AP radiograph of hip.

Spontorno index: for proximal femoral canal cylindrical configuration; outer cortical diameter at the mid-lesser trochanter divided by the width of the canal 7 cm distal to that point.

teardrop: the appearance of a teardrop found on the AP radiograph of the acetabular joint. The outer border of the teardrop is the inner border of the acetabulum. The inner border of the drop is the outer wall of the pelvis next to the inferior acetabulum. In grading acetabular dysplasia, the position of the teardrop is graded as *A,* open, when the medial line is lateral to the ilioischial line; *B* when it overlaps that line; *C* when it is medial to that line; and *D* when the lateral border of the teardrop is medial to the ilioischial line.

trough l.: a vertical or archlike line of cortical bone projecting parallel and lateral to the articular cortical surface of the humeral head. It is seen on a conventional AP radiograph of the shoulder. The trough line represents an anteromedial impaction fracture of the humeral head secondary to posterior dislocation of the shoulder.

Ullmann l.: line of displacement in spondylolisthesis.

Winberger l.: infraction (appearing as a radiolucent line) in the metaphysis, as seen in syphilis. (Not to be confused with Wimberger sign seen in scurvy.)

Y-line: line drawn through both triradiate cartilages at the acetabular center; also called **Hilgenreiner l.**

Radiographic Signs

anteater nose s.: seen in tarsal coalition; caused by the elongation of the anterior process of the calcaneus that approaches or overlaps the navicular bone, assuming the appearance of anteater nose, seen on lateral radiograph.

anterior hiatal s.: seen in posterior ligament ankle instability; a lateral radiograph shows a wedge-shaped opening at the anterior dome of the talus when the foot is flexed and pushed backward.

Ashhurst s.: seen in ankle diastasis; a widening of the normal overlap of the distal anterior tubercle and fibula at the ankle joint.

bamboo spine: bamboo appearance of spine seen in ankylosing spondylitis.

celery stalk s.: Thickened hyperintense appearance of the anterior cruciate ligament on sagittal T2-weighted MRI scan, with otherwise normal course of collagen fibers, reflecting mucoid degeneration without tear.[*]

cement-wedge s.: wedge-shaped area of radiographic lucency seen under tibial prosthetic component, implying motion of the component.

chalk-stick fracture: appearance on a radiograph of a fracture through bone in a patient with Paget disease of bone.

choppy sea s.: an apparent but not real tear of a meniscus seen on arthrogram.

codfish vertebrae: radiographic appearance of vertebrae severely involved with osteoporosis, in which the central portion is depressed secondary to collapse.

crescent s.: radiographic finding in avascular necrosis in which there is a space between the subchondral plate and impacted bone of the femoral head, leaving a crescent-shaped area that is radiolucent (relatively black) on a radiograph.

crossing s.: for femoral trochlear dysplasia. On a lateral radiograph with the posterior condyles parallel there are three image types at the point of crossing of the line drawn following the anterior margin of the condyles and the line of the trochlear groove.

cross-over s: in acetabular retroversion, the margin of the anterior acetabulum crosses over the posterior margin when seen on an AP radiograph of the pelvis.

dripping candle wax s.: Irregular cortical hyperostosis, typically along one side of the involved bone, which has the appearance of thickened melted wax flowing down one side of a candle; indicates melorheostosis.[†]

double density s.: for os acromiale, overlap of two transversely elongated radiographic cortical densities seen in the AP projection of the shoulder, one representing the cortex of the os acromiale and the second the cortical margin of the residual acromial base.

double posterior cruciate ligament s.: seen on midline sagittal MRI scan of the knee as a low-signal-intensity band that is parallel and anteroinferior to the posterior cruciate ligament, and is indicative of bucket-handle tears of the medial or lateral menisci.[*]

double popliteus tendon s.: seen on sagittal MRI scan of the knee as a low-signal-intensity band parallel to the popliteus tendon at the level of the popliteus hiatus. It is the result of a displaced complex flap tear of the lateral meniscus.[†]

Fat pad s.: Elevated anterior lucency and visible posterior lucency along the articular surface of the distal humerus on a lateral radiograph of the elbow held in 90 degrees of flexion, which is indicative of joint capsule distention, classically seen in hemarthrosis from acute fracture.[‡]

four-tendon s.: presence of four, rather than the usual three, separate tendons in the medial margin of the ankle on axial MRI scan, reflecting longitudinal splitting and separation of the posterior tibial tendon.[§]

Gage s.: seen in Legg-Calvé-Perthes disease; a small osteoporotic segment forms a translucent V on the lateral side of the femoral head epiphysis; seen on AP view.

geyser s.: seen on shoulder arthrogram, shoulder ultrasound, or MRI. Characterized by leakage of contrast material from the glenohumeral joint into the subdeltoid bursa, and then through the AC joint. It normally indicates a large full-thickness tear of the rotator cuff.

gull wing s.: appearance of a finger anterior posterior radiograph looks like a gull wing because of cartilage loss. Seen in erosive osteoarthritis.

hair-on-end s.: long, thin, vertical striations within a widened diploic space and thin outer table of the skull, seen on radiographs, MRI and CT scan, caused by red marrow hyperplasia in response to chronic severe anemia (i.e., thalassemia major, iron deficiency anemia, sickle cell disease, and spherocytosis).[**]

Hawkins s.: zone of radiographic translucency beneath the subchondral plate of the dome of the

---

[*] Papadopoulou P, 2007.
[†] Bansal A, 2008.

[*] Camacho MA, 2004.
[†] Lesniak B, et al, 2011
[‡] Goswami GK, 2002.
[§] Ly JQ, 2008.
[**] Hollar M, 2001.

talus on frontal radiographs of the ankle, usually seen after 6–8 weeks of disuse or immobilization. It results from increased bone resorption relative to bone formation with active hyperemia. It indicates a preserved blood supply to the talar dome, and therefore that avascular necrosis is not likely to occur.*

ivory vertebra s.: radiographic appearance of a dense vertebral body that looks like ivory compared with other vertebral bodies. It can be a sign of metastatic carcinoma, lymphoma, postradiation necrosis, primary sarcoma, and condensing osteoses such as mastocytosis or osteopetrosis.

inverted Napoleon's hat s.: seen in spondylolisthesis on frontal radiographs of the spine when a severely anteriorly subluxed L5 vertebral body (dome of the hat) projects end-on and overlaps the sacrum, with the transverse processes forming the hat's tapered brim.†

J s.: Refers to J-shaped appearance of the anterior band of the inferior glenohumeral ligament on coronal MRI scan of the shoulder and indicates humeral avulsion of the anterior band of the inferior glenohumeral ligament.‡

Matev s.: seen in median nerve entrapment; a gap in the fracture callus of the medial epicondyle of the humerus.

Pelkan spur: seen in vitamin C deficiency; an elevation of distal metaphyseal periosteum resulting in the development of a spur of bone.

pencil-in-cup deformity: radiographs of the hand of a person with psoriatic arthritis that has a characteristic area of narrowing of the distal part of the proximal phalanx, and a widening of the proximal base of the middle phalanx, to give the appearance of a pencil in a cup; third through fifth ray most commonly affected.

polka-dot s.: numerous high attenuation dots from thickened trabeculae within the medullary cavity of a vertebral body, seen on transverse CT images, simulating the polka-dot pattern on clothing and reflecting vertebral body hemangioma.§

---
* Donnelly E, 1999.
† Talangbayan LE, 2007.
‡ Carlson CL, 2004.
§ Persaud T, 2008.

posterior hiatal s.: anterior ligament ankle instability; a lateral radiograph with the foot pulled forward shows a wedge-shaped opening at the posterior dome of the talus.

posterior wall s.: seen on AP radiograph the posterior wall of the acetabulum is medial to the center of the femoral head. This reflects that the posterior coverage is deficient, and may be seen in femoroacetabular impingement.

posterior vertebral scalloping s: Exaggeration of the normal concavity of the posterior margin of vertebral bodies on a lateral radiograph of the spine, and on the sagittal planes on CT and MRI scans, which results from increased intraspinal pressure (intraspinal tumor), dural ectasia (Marfan syndrome, Ehlers-Danlos syndrome, neurofibromatosis, ankylosing spondylitis), small spinal canal (achondroplasia), congenital skeletal disorders (Morquio and Hurler syndromes), and soft tissue hypertrophy (acromegaly).*

Reimers index (migration index): for lateral acetabular deficiency; the lateral border of the femoral head to Perkin line (vertical line from lateral tip of acetabulum) divided by the width of the femoral head parallel to Hilgenreiner line (line drawn through the inferior points of both acetabuli) and multiplied by 100.

ring s.: secondary to scaphoid ligament disruption, which causes rotation of the scaphoid, giving it a ring appearance on a radiograph.

Risser s.: for skeletal maturity, the degree of capping of the iliac apophysis.

Risser I: iliac apophysis ossification of 25%; anterior superior iliac spine (anterolateral). Seen in prepuberty or early puberty.

Risser II: iliac apophysis ossification of 50%. Ossification extends halfway across iliac wing. Seen immediately before or during growth spurt.

Risser III: iliac apophysis ossification of 75%. Indicates slowing of growth.

Risser IV: one-hundred percent ossification with no fusion to iliac crest. Indicates slowing of growth.

Risser V: Iliac apophysis fuses to iliac crest. Indicates cessation of growth.

rugger jersey spine: the appearance of alternate white and black zones seen on spine radiographs, frequently

---
* Wakely SL, 2006.

in patients with hyperparathyroidism or renal osteodystrophy.

Scotty dog s.: seen in spondylolysis; the oblique radiograph reveals what looks like a Scotty dog. The eye is a pedicle seen end on; the nose, the transverse process; the collar, the lysis (fracture of the pars interarticularis); the body, the lamina; the tail, the posterior spinous process; the ears, the superior facet; and the forefoot, the inferior facet. Also called **Scotch terrier s.**

spur: a bony protrusion or lip at the edge of a joint, usually related to degenerative disease or osteoarthritis; also called **lipping** and **osteophyte.**

spur s.: Seen on transverse CT images or obturator oblique radiographs of the pelvis. Inferiorly directed apex of triangular fracture fragment from iliac bone that remains attached to the sacroiliac joint, but separated from a fractured acetabulum. It is indicative of a fracture involving the anterior and posterior acetabular columns (both-column fracture).*

Terry-Thomas s.: in scapholunate dissociation, there is an apparent gap between the scaphoid and lunate seen on a neutral anteroposterior wrist radiograph.

Thurston-Holland s.: small fragment of bone seen at margin of metaphysis just proximal to epiphysis that indicates a type II Salter fracture; also called **corner s.**

trough line s.: Seen on frontal radiographs of the shoulder as a vertical line of cortical bone projecting parallel and lateral to the articular surface of the humeral head; indicates a posterior dislocation of the glenohumeral joint.†

Waldenström s.: apparent lateral displacement of femoral head seen in early Legg-Calvé-Perthes disease.

Wimberger s.: relatively dense margin representing the provisional zone of calcification surrounding an osteopenic epiphysis seen in scurvy; not to be confused with Winberger line seen in syphilis.

windshield wiper s.: radiographic view outlines the shadow of a prosthesis with the appearance of a windshield wiper; with a loose internal prosthesis, there is bone absorption and formation secondary to a to-and-fro motion of the stem of the prosthesis in the shaft of the bone.

Methods

acromial profile: for impingement in the shoulder caused by an anterolateral hook that develops in adults on the inferior surface of the acromion.
  type I: flat acromial profile
  type II: curved acromial profile
  type III: hooked acromial profile

Ahlback changes: grading system for degenerative arthritic changes seen on anteroposterior knee radiographs.
  grade 0: normal joint space
  grade I: joint space narrowing
  grade II: joint space obliteration
  grade III: minor bone attrition
  grade IV: moderate bone attrition
  grade V: severe bone attrition
  grade VI: subluxation

Anderson Orthopaedic Research Institute Periprosthetic Bone Loss (AORI): periprosthetic bone loss, scoring femur and tibia separately.
  type 1: intact metaphyseal bone with minor defect that will not compromise the stability of a revision component.
  type 2: damaged metaphyseal bone. Loss of cancellous bone in the metaphyseal segment that will need to be filled with cement, augments, or a bone graft at revision to restore the joint line. Defects can occur in one femoral condyle or tibial plateau (2A), or in both condyles and plateaus (2B).
  type 3: deficient metaphyseal bone. Bone loss that compromises a major portion of either condyle or plateau. The defects are occasionally associated with detachment of the collateral or patellar ligaments and usually require long-stemmed revision implants with bone grafts or a custom-made hinged prosthesis.

Association Research Circulation Osseous Classification for Osteonecrosis (ARCO)

An international classification for femoral head avascular necrosis:

Stage 0: All present diagnostic techniques are normal or nondiagnostic.

---
* Johnson TS, 2005.
† Gor DM, 2002.

Stage 1: Plain x-ray and CT scan are normal. At least one of the following techniques is positive: scintigraphy and MRI.
  By location: medial, central, and lateral
  By size: by area of femoral head involvement: minimal (< 15%), moderate (15–30%), and extensive (> 30%)

Stage 2: There is no subchondral fracture; areas of abnormalities such as mottled aspect, sclerosis, osteolysis and focal porosis seen on radiograph; the femoral head remains spherical on AP and lateral views on x-ray and CT-scan; and scintigraphy and MRI remain positive with stage 1 subclassification.

Stage 3: subchondral crescent sign visible on the x-ray. The femoral head fails mechanically by size or joint surface depression. Minimal = < 15% involvement or a depression of < 2 mm; moderate = 15–30% involvement or a depression of 2–4 mm; extensive = > 30% involvement or a depression of more than 4 mm.

Stage 4: Progression to osteoarthritis.

Bertol method: for dysplastic hips in newborn infants; the ratio of two lines, one being the distance from the top of the femoral physis to central acetabular horizontal line and the other being the distance from the medial acetabular wall and superior medial femoral shaft. A ratio of 2 or greater is normal, and progressive instability produces a line ratio that progresses to 1.

bone age: in pediatric orthopaedics and radiology, refers to the predictable skeletal changes of bone that take place from infancy to adulthood. Bone age studies observe the size of bone, development of ossification centers, and outline of bones in the hand and wrist. Comparison with radiographs of normal patients at specific ages allows determination if a patient's bones are growing too rapidly or too slowly. Standard sets of radiographs are found in Greulich and Pyle (1959).

Bucholz and Ogden's Classification for Osteonecrosis

For evaluation of osteonecrosis that occurs after hip dysplasia treatment:

Type I: Complete fragmentation of the capital femoral ossific nucleus. Physis shows no irregularities and no propensity to premature closure. Minimal to mild residual deformity.

Type II: The physis became irregular in its lateral aspect soon after fragmentation of the ossification center. Localized premature fusion of the superolateral portion of the plate. This premature fusion is not evident until the patients are 7 to 12½ years of age, with the mean age of roentgenographically evident partial premature fusion being 9 years.

Type III: The entire physis is irregular, and premature fusion of the entire plate occurred at an average age of 7½ years. Marked coxa vara with a variably deformed femoral head, an extremely short femoral neck, and severe overgrowth of the greater trochanter.

Type IV: Variable abnormalities that seem to affect the medial epiphyseal ossification center and to a lesser degree, the medial metaphysis. Severe coxa magna with shortening of the femoral neck.

Campanacci Radiographic Classification for Benign Bone Tumors

For benign bone tumors adapted from the Enneking clinical system:

Grade 1: tumors are surrounded by a reactive rind.

Grade 2: tumors are contained within at least a neocortex, if not the original cortex.

Grade 3: tumors, including soft-tissue masses, extend beyond the cortex.

Canadian C-spine rule: to determine if additional imaging is required after initial normal radiographs following trauma of the neck.
  Any high-risk factor, including age 65 or older, a dangerous mechanism of trauma (such a high-speed crash or fall from more than a 3-foot elevation), or paresthesias in extremities
  Absence of a low-risk factor that allows for safe assessment of range of motion (such as being ambulatory at any point, delayed onset of neck pain, or a simple rear-end car crash)
  Inability to rotate the neck 45 degrees to the left and right

Catterall hip score: for pediatric avascular necrosis of the femoral head or Legg-Calvé-Perthes disease (Fig. 3-5).
  I: no finding on AP, compression on frog-leg lateral
  II: central compression on both AP and frog-leg lateral
  III: lateral femoral head compression seen on AP, not covered by acetabulum, and intact medial femoral head
  IV: entire femoral head involvement

Cierny-Mader Staging System: for osteomyelitis anatomic location.
  stage 1: medullary osteomyelitis
  stage 2: superficial osteomyelitis
  stage 3: localized osteomyelitis
  stage 4: diffuse osteomyelitis

Cobb method: for measuring degree of curvature in scoliosis; a line is drawn across the superior vertebral plate of the superior vertebra with the greatest tilt and the inferior plate of the inferior vertebra with the greatest tilt. The intersection of these two lines creates the angle.

Dejour Classification for Trochlear Dysplasia

Type I: normal, and the outline of the condyles is symmetric, crossing the floor line at its apex.

Type II: the crossing of the two condylar outlines with the outline of the trochlear floor is asymmetrical.

Type III: the crossing of the two condylar outlines with the trochlear floor is distal and asymmetrical.

Edinburgh method: for dysplastic hip; radiograph obtained with a newborn's legs held parallel with slight traction and no rotation. Proximal migration is measured by distance from superior femoral shaft to a line through the central acetabulum (inferior ilium). The gap from the lateral ischium to the most medial part of the femoral metaphysis is the index of dislocation. This gap is normally 4 mm, suspicious if more than 5 mm, and diagnostic if 6 mm or more.

Fairbanks changes: a grading scale for the changes seen on the AP radiographs of osteoarthritic knees, originally used in postmeniscectomy patients seen in long-term follow-up.

grade 0: normal

grade I: ridge from margin of femoral condyles

Group I

Group II

Group III

Group IV

FIG 3-5 Catterall classification of Legg-Calvé-Perthes disease. I: anterior head only involved, no collapse; II: only anterior head with sequestrum; III: only a small part of epiphysis not involved; IV: total head involvement. *(© 1996 American Academy of Orthopaedic Surgeons. Reprinted from the Journal of the American Academy of Orthopaedic Surgeons, Volume 4(1), pp. 9-16 with permission.)*

grade II: joint-space narrowing on side of meniscectomy

grade III: flattening of femoral condyle

Fergusson method: for measuring angle of degree of curvature in scoliosis, using vertical lines through spinous processes.

Arlet Ficat Marcus Classification for Femoral Head Osteonecrosis

I: Mottled densities, may be obscure, anterosuperior weight-bearing area of femoral head

II: Well-demarcated infarction, rim of increased density of bone at base of area of infarction

III: Subtle flattening of femoral head or subchondral radiolucent crescent

IV: Pronounced collapse of avascular segment

V: Degenerative arthritis with loss of cartilage space

VI: Marked degenerative changes

Ficat Classification for Avascular Necrosis Femoral Head

Stage 0: x-rays and MRI normal, no symptoms present.

Stage 1: x-rays show normal or minor osteopenia; bone scan shows increased uptake below lesion; clinical symptoms present.

Stage 2: x-ray shows mixed osteopenia or sclerosis; MRI shows geographic defect; bone scans show increased uptake; pain and stiffness present.

Stage 3: x-ray and MRI show crescent sign and eventual cortical collapse, pain and stiffness present with or without radiation to knee.

Stage 4: x-ray and MRI show end stage with degenerative disease, pain and limp present.

Gruen zones: for topographic description of loosening in patients with femoral prosthetic component; on the lateral margin of the prosthesis three zones are numbered from proximal to distal 1 to 3, zone 4 is at prosthetic tip, and zones 5 to 7 are from distal to proximal on the medial side, with zone 7 at the medial femoral neck.

Herring Lateral Pillar Classification

For prognosis in Legg-Calvé-Perthes disease (Fig. 3-6):

Group A: height of pillar (lateral head above physis) normal.

Group B: height of pillar 50% to 100% of original height.

Group C: height of pillar less than 50% of original height.

Ishihara cervical spine curve index: for spondylolytic changes in the neck; a vertical line is drawn from the base of C2 to the base of C7. The sum of the distance of the posterior vertebral bodies of C3–C6 to that vertical line is divided by that vertical line and multiplied by 100 to get the percent value.

Kalamchi and MacEwen Classification

For osteonecrosis that occurs after hip dysplasia treatment*:

Group I: Changes affecting the ossific nucleus, either delay in the appearance of the ossific nucleus or mottling of the ossific nucleus. With revascularization, there is flattening and fragmentation of the shadow of the ossific nucleus, but the head will usually regain its spherical shape. Some femoral heads will show the head-within-head appearance. This is the most common with the best prognosis.

FIG 3-6 Herring classification of Legg-Calvé-Perthes disease. **A,** Lateral pillar retains its height, no collapse. **B,** Lateral pillar shows density changes with height loss. **C,** Lateral pillar loses more than 50% of its height. (© 1996 American Academy of Orthopaedic Surgeons. Reprinted from the Journal of the American Academy of Orthopaedic Surgeons, Volume 4(1), pp. 9-16 with permission.)

Group A   Group B   Group C

> **Group II:** Lateral Physeal Damage
>
> The initial changes in the ossific center may follow exactly those seen in Group I, but in addition there is damage to the lateral part of the physis. The early roentgenographic signs indicating lateral physeal damage are:
>
> 1. lateral ossification
> 2. lateral physeal irregularity and bridging
> 3. lateral notching of the epiphysis
> 4. a lateral metaphyseal defect
>
> The damage to the physis may remain dormant. By the age of 10 years, however, valgus deformity of the head on the neck develops. (This type occurred in 35% of total [avascular necrosis] at [the Alfred I. DuPont Hospital for Children].)
>
> **Group III:** Central Physeal Damage
>
> The early changes in the ossific nucleus are similar to those observed in Group I and II. The damage to the growth plate is more centrally located. Commonly, patients develop a short femoral neck without varus or valgus. Relative overgrowth of the greater trochanter and limb length discrepancy are the principal problems.
>
> **Group IV:** Total Damage to the Head and the Physis

*Homma M and Kumar J, 1996.

Kellgren osteoarthritis grade:
- **grade 1:** one or more osteophytes without joint-space narrowing.
- **grade 2:** sclerosis of the acetabulum and joint-space narrowing; may be accompanied by small osteophytes.
- **grade 3:** clear formation of osteophytes and narrowing of the joint space.
- **grade 4:** deformation of the femoral head with distinctive joint-space narrowing; cyst formation in femoral head and acetabulum; both bones sclerosed. This scoring method is also used for degenerative disk in the spine.

Knee Society total-knee arthroplasty roentgenographic evaluation and scoring system: a system of angles and absorption at specific numerical points of prosthetic fixation to bone.*

Lamparski method: for skeletal maturity using cervical vertebral bodies C2-C6.
- **stage I:** initiation
- **stage II:** development of concavities on the lower borders of the vertebral bodies
- **stage III:** increase of the anterior portion and of the total height of these vertical bodies causing changes in their shape

---
* Ewald FC, 1989.

- **stage IV:** changing from a wedge shape to a rectangular shape
- **stage V:** change from rectangular shape to a square shape
- **stage VI:** a predominance of height over width

Larsen index: for knee osteoarthritis
- **grade 0:** Normal
- **grade 1:** Slight abnormality; one or more minor lesions (periarticular soft tissue swelling, periarticular osteoporosis, and slight joint space narrowing)
- **grade 2:** Definite early abnormality; erosion (not obligatory) and joint space narrowing
- **grade 3:** Medium destructive abnormality (erosion obligatory)
- **grade 4:** Severe destructive abnormality (bone deformation present)
- **grade 5:** Mutilating abnormality (gross bone deformation)

> **Lenke Scoliosis Classification**
>
> Thoraco-lumbar scoliosis classification uses central sacral vertical line (CSVL):
>
> Lumbar modifiers are:
>
> **A:** CSVL between lumbar pedicles
> **B:** CSVL touches apical bodies
> **C:** CSVL medial to body
>
> Thoracic modifiers are:
>
> hypokyphosis less than 10 degrees
> normal 10–40 degrees
> hyperkyphosis more than 40 degrees

Modic intervertebral disk changes on MRI:
- **Type I:** Decreased signal on T1 and increased signal T2
- **Type II:** Increased signal intensity T1 and an isointense or slightly hyperintense signal intensity T2
- **Type III:** Decreased signal intensity on both T1 and T2 images

Mose concentric rings: for avascular necrosis of femoral head in children; a system using concentric rings with 2-mm separations.
- **Good:** both hips perfect circles.
- **Fair:** deviation is less than 2 mm.
- **Poor:** deviation more than 2 mm.

NEXUS cervical spine criteria: to determine if additional imaging is required after initial normal radiographs following trauma of the neck.
No tenderness in the posterior midline cervical spine
No evidence of intoxication
No focal neurologic deficit
No painful distracting injuries
Normal alertness with a score of 15 or better on the Glasgow Coma Scale

Perdriolle torsiometer: for measuring spinal rotation in scoliosis; a transparent celluloid overlay is placed on radiographs to help estimate the rotation.

Salter-Thompson Classification for Legg-Calvé-Perthes Disease

For dividing Legg-Calvé-Perthes d. into two groups of expected outcome:

Group A: bone underlying fracture presumed to be necrotic and any bone lateral presumed to be viable; involves approximately one half of the femoral head; similar to Catterall groups I and II.

Group B: no evidence of an intact, visible lateral margin seen on AP radiograph; subchondral fracture extends to most lateral extent of epiphysis; similar to Catterall groups III and IV.

Sauvegrain skeletal age: method of assessment of age base on elbow radiographs.

Severin hip dysplasia scale: for staging severity of hip deformity that may lead to dysplastic dislocation.
  Group I: normal hips
    A: Center Edge (CE) angle of more than 19 degrees for ages 6 to 13 years; CE angle of more than 25 degrees for ages 14 years and older.
    B: CE angle of 15 to 19 degrees for ages 3 to 13 years; CE angle 20 to 25 degrees for ages 14 years and older.
  Group II: moderate deformity of femoral head, neck, or acetabulum; otherwise normal joint. A and B same as group I.
  Group III: dysplastic hip without subluxation; CE angles less than 15 degrees for ages 6 to 13 years and less than 20 degrees for ages 14 years and older.
  Group IV: subluxation.
    A: moderate, CE angle positive or equal to 0 degrees.
    B: severe, CE angle negative.
  Group V: head articulating with secondary acetabulum in the upper part of original acetabulum.
  Group VI: redislocation.

Singh index: an index of osteoporosis accomplished by a grading system using the three major trabecular patterns in the femoral intertrochanteric and head region; Grades I through VI, with lowest grade being the most osteoporotic.

Stahl index: for staging lunate necrosis in wrist, uses ratio of height to width.
  stage I: index more than 45%.
  stage II: index 30% to 44%.
  stage III: index less than 30%.

Steinberg Classification Hip Osteonecrosis

For aseptic necrosis of the femoral head, Steinberg's stage II and IV are equivalent to Ficat stage III; and stage V and VI are equivalent to Ficat stage IV:

Stage 0: normal radiograph and bone scan

Stage I: normal radiograph and abnormal bone scan

Stage II: sclerosis and/or cyst in femoral head
  A: mild (< **B:** moderate (20–40%)
  C: severe (> 40%)

Stage III: subchondral collapse (crescent sign) with collapse.
  A: mild (< 15%)
  B: moderate (15–30%)
  C: severe (> 30%)

Stage IV: head flattening with joint narrowing or acetabular change
  A: mild (< 15% surface and 2-mm depression)
  B: moderate (15–30% surface or 2- to 4-mm depression)
  C: severe (> 30% surface or > 4-mm depression)

Stage V: flattening of head with joint narrowing and/or acetabular changes
  A: mild
  B: moderate
  C: severe

Stulberg method: system for measuring concentricity of femoral heads in Legg-Calvé-Perthes disease

Tönnis osteoarthritis grade: for degree of severity of degenerative changes:
  grade 0: No signs of OA
  grade 1: Increased sclerosis, slight joint space narrowing, no or slight loss of head sphericity

grade 2: Small cysts, moderate joint space narrowing, moderate loss of head sphericity

grade 3: Large cysts, severe joint space narrowing, severe deformity of the head

Tönnis system for hip dysplasia: for hip dysplasia as seen on radiograph:

grade 1: dysplasia of the hip and mild subluxation

grade 2: center of ossification of femoral head displaced laterally, inferior to superolateral corner of the true acetabulum

grade 3: center of ossification at level of superolateral corner of acetabulum

grade 4: center of ossification proximal to the superolateral corner of acetabulum

Waldenström stage: stage of healing in Legg-Calvé-Perthes disease

stage A: formation stage:

1: initial stage; epiphysis is denser, patchy, more distal, and uneven at the margins.

2: fragmentation stage; epiphysis in pieces, can be further divided into a mass of small granules.

stage B: healing period; the epiphysis becomes homogeneous, evidence of diffuse and extensive revascularization.

stage C: period of growth; normal growth and ossification of deformed femoral head.

Invasive and Noninvasive Techniques

bone scan: a commonly employed nuclear medicine study in orthopaedics. A radioactive material (radioisotope) is attached chemically to a substance that is taken up by active bone cells, and specifically by osteoblasts. The radioisotope is then injected into a vein, and the radioactivity emitted can be detected by a gamma camera. Usefulness of the study includes detection of infection, fractures, and metastatic lesions. A bone scan demonstrates where bone is actively being produced, whereas a radiograph shows only where bone is present; also called **bone scintigraphy.**

three-phase bone scan: a modification of the routine bone scan applied when osteomyelitis is suspected. This scan examines the perfusion, immediate soft tissue blood pool, and delayed bone uptake, whereas a routine bone scan examines only the delayed bone uptake phase. The advantages of a three-phase bone scan is that it improves the specificity of the examination for osteomyelitis. A normal perfusion phase excludes an active inflammatory process.

calcium 47: for bone formation; an in vivo total body accretion test.

cinefluoroscopy: recorded fluoroscopic study for relative motion of bones in a joint, for example, to detect carpal instability; also called **videofluoroscopy, cineroentgenogram,** and **cineradiography.**

computed tomography (CT) scan: a computer generates a two-dimensional, cross-sectional image from a series of x-ray beams that rotate in a circular and forward motion around the patient. CT images show detailed anatomy and allow detection of differences in tissue density and shape. In orthopaedics, CT is especially useful for analyzing complicated fractures and may be performed after arthrography to aid visualization of pathologic conditions of the joint. With CT, bone structures are clearly defined without the need of intravenous contrast medium, tumors are located with precision, tissue is recognized as normal or abnormal, and blockages in blood vessels can be sought invasively. The advantages of this technique are that it can be invasive or noninvasive, and it provides a sharp, detailed image. This method is best for patients who cannot tolerate rigorous radiographic examinations. The terms **CT scan** and **computed axial tomography (CAT) scan** are the same (Fig. 3-7).

spiral CT (helical CT): the latest development in CT, it allows scanning of a volume of tissue during a single breathhold by continuous scanning as the patient is moved through the gantry. Advantages over the conventional CT are that it eliminates motion artifacts and shortens examination time. The trade-off is some loss of resolution. It is not used in cases in which high resolution is important, for example, bone detail.

dual photon densitometry: to estimate bone density, the part being measured is exposed to two beams of photons of different intensity. A two-dimensional picture of bone density is obtained with calculated subtraction of soft tissue density. The results are

FIG 3-7 Computed tomography scan slice showing arthritis in left anterior sacroiliac joint.

expressed in grams of bone mineral per square centimeter.

fat saturation: a technique used in MRI to suppress the signal from fat, causing it to appear black on the MRI scan. This technique allows pathologic conditions to be more easily identified. Also called **fat sat** and **fat suppression.**

gadolinium (Gd)–enhanced MRI: the element Gd has paramagnetic properties and is used to enhance magnetic resonance imaging. Gd is especially useful in distinguishing scar tissue from disk herniation in cases of prior spine surgery. It is also useful in tumor imaging and in evaluating the blood supply to bone to exclude avascular necrosis. **Gadopentetate dimeglumine** is a Gd preparation used in Gd-enhanced MRI.

gallium-67 (^{67}Ga) scan: radioactive ^{67}Ga is introduced intravenously and localizes in areas of concentrated granulocytes; used to detect hidden infections, such as osteomyelitis.

gamma camera: instrument used for nuclear medicine studies. The camera contains many radiation detectors, which detect the radiation emitted from a radioisotope inside the patient's body. The gamma camera generates an image of the whole body or of a specific area of interest (e.g., see **bone scan**).

indium scan: radioactive indium-111 is incubated with white blood cells (WBCs) taken from the patient. The indium-111 is taken up inside the WBCs, which are then injected back into the bloodstream and localized in areas of acute osteomyelitis (infection). Also called **indium leukocyte scan.**

integrated-shape imaging system (ISIS): for scoliosis; computer analysis of spinal and rib contours, may replace need for repeated radiographic evaluations.

LeukoScan: commercial term used for the method to localize infection in bone or soft tissue. Technetium-99m is attached to a monoclonal antibody that attaches to a specific cell surface protein seen only on neutrophils, the type of white cells that localize to areas of infection. It is then injected into the bloodstream.

magnetic resonance imaging (MRI): A radiographic technique in which the patient is exposed to a magnetic field. The movement of photons (water molecules) is usually random and is aligned by the magnetic field. Radiowaves are then used to change the alignment of the protons. When the radiowaves are turned off, the protons emit a weak signal. The signals are detected and transformed into cross-sectional images. The signal decay curves of the protons as they return to their relaxed state depend on two factors: **T1** (spin-lattice) longitudinal relaxation depends on the relationship between protons and their surrounding environment, and **T2** (spin-spin) transverse relaxation is the effect of spinning protons on each other. By adjusting certain imaging parameters, images can be more influenced by T1 or T2. Referred to as *T1-weighted images* or *T2-weighted images* (Figs. 3-8 and 3-9). In orthopaedics, MRI is especially useful for diagnosing injuries to ligaments, meniscal tears, muscle injury, tumors, avascular necrosis, and infection. It is also useful for diagnosing fractures that are difficult to see on radiographs, such as nondisplaced fractures of the hip in older adults. An MRI is also helpful in diagnosing growth-plate injuries; characterizing neuropathic changes in diabetic feet; characterizing metabolic bone diseases; and detecting radiographically occult articular cartilage lesions, which can be seen in osteoarthritis, inflammatory arthropathy, and trauma. MRI techniques have been designed to highlight the vasculature and are referred to as **magnetic resonance angiography (MRA).** This technology has a terminology unique to the system (Fig. 3-10).

Imaging Techniques | 127

FIG 3-8 T1-weighted image of knee highlights fat in the bone marrow and subcutaneous tissue; cortical bone appears black.

FIG 3-9 Matched fat suppressed T2-weighted image of the knee highlights water; cortical bone appears black as does the suppressed subcutaneous fat and bone marrow.

magnetic resonance spectroscopy: technique using magnetic resonance to determine the relative amounts of specific chemicals in an anatomic part. One such study is the evaluation of chemical reactions involving phosphate in the muscle. This type of evaluation helps to determine the metabolic adequacy of the muscle.

neutron radiography: technique helpful in visualizing bony tissue. A narrow beam of neutrons is passed through tissue from a nuclear reactor.

perfusion imaging: technique using dynamic magnetic resonance or computed tomography to determine blood flow through tissues (perfusion). It facilitates various hemodynamic measurements including blood volume, blood flow, and mean transit time, and therefore helps characterize tissue ischemia and necrosis. It also aids in the histologic evaluation of tumors, and assesses tumor response to chemotherapy or radiation therapy.

proton density: an MRI study in which the image is strongly affected by the differences in the density of protons in the tissue. Such images are usually produced with a spin-echo pulse sequence having repetition time of more than 600 msec and an echo time of less than 80 msec.

short tau inversion recovery (STIR): imaging signal acquisition that helps enhance image to detect fractures that are difficult to see on x-ray; particularly useful in occult hip fractures.

single photon emission computerized tomography (SPECT): use of a single-beam emission source to make two-dimensional images revealing relative areas of bone abnormality. It may be used to diagnose avascular necrosis, fractures, and infection.

spoiled grass (SPGR): image obtained with lower flip angle, giving a fat-suppressed image that makes articular cartilage appear white on a MRI.

strontium-85 resorption rate: a nuclear medicine in vivo study to determine bone absorption rate.

T1-weighted image: an MRI study in which the image is strongly affected by the longitudinal magnetic relaxation time, T1. Such images are usually produced with a spin-echo pulse sequence generally having repetition time less than 600 msec and an echo time less than 20 msec.

T2-weighted image: an MRI study in which the image is strongly affected by the transverse magnetic relaxation time, T2. Such images are usually produced with a spin-echo pulse sequence having repetition time of 2000 msec or more and echo time of 80 msec or more.

FIG 3-10 Cervical spinal cord as would be seen on magnetic resonance imaging or computed tomography scan with myelography. The ratio of the transverse diameter to the sagittal diameter greater than 0.4 is a sign of good recovery prognosis after surgical decompression. *(From J Bone Joint Surg 76A:1422, 1994.)*

technetium-99m (Tc^{99}m): a radioactive substance that can be chemically attached to a variety of substances for nuclear medicine imaging studies. For example, Tc^{99}m can be attached to diphosphonate for imaging of bones, attached to white blood cells for imaging of infection, or attached to red blood cells for detection of a pulmonary embolus (blood clot to the lung); also called **technetium scan.**

thermography: to differentiate nerve irritation, vascular disorders, and increased muscle tone; a temperature-sensitive plate displaying color gradients reveals differences in skin surface temperature.

tomosynthesis: computer-driven radiographic techniques that allow for a 5-second radiation exposure, equivalent to a standard radiograph, and less than CT.

ultrasound: the use of mechanical radiant energy having a 1 to 10 million MHz (megahertz = 1 million cycles per second) frequency to obtain images. The ultrahigh frequency sound (well beyond the upper limits of human hearing, which is 20,000 Hertz) is emitted, reflects off tissue surfaces, and is received and processed by a computer to form an image. In orthopaedics, this imaging technique is used to evaluate fluid collections, tendon and tissue abnormalities, tumors, cysts, and hemorrhages and infant hip disorders. Also called **ultrasound study, ultrasonography,** and **sonography.**

Vascular Diagnostic Studies

After the history and physical examination are complete, other tests may be required to diagnose abnormalities in the peripheral circulation to the limbs. These specific tests are often made in conjunction with an orthopaedic problem. These studies fall into two categories: invasive and noninvasive tests. The invasive tests are performed at the direction of vascular surgeons by radiologists.

Invasive Tests

To perform an invasive test, radiographic contrast is injected through a catheter placed into an artery or vein, and a computer-guided radiographic machine obtains an image as the iodinated contrast material courses through the vessel network. This contrast material enables visualization of any degree of narrowing (blockage) and the extent of blood flow around a blockage. Other abnormalities of vessels can also be detected. New computer technology allows vessel procedures to be performed in a short time.

angioplasty: can be performed following arteriography in which an area of narrowing has been identified. A special catheter with an inflatable balloon is placed at the area of narrowing. The balloon is inflated to open the narrowing. This procedure can treat areas of arterial narrowing that otherwise would require surgery.

angioscopy: tiny cameras are used to visualize the inside of blood vessels and bypass grafts, and assess the lining and, in some cases, facilitate repair from within the vessel.

arteriography: a radiographic examination in which an artery is catheterized and contrast injected to study the blood supply to an area or detect blockages of arteries. May be performed following an ultrasound study that indicates the presence of vascular compromise or in a patient with symptoms of blockage of blood vessels in the extremities. In some cases, a blockage or narrowing of an artery can be treated through the catheter (e.g., angioplasty); also called **arteriogram, angiogram,** and **angiography.** Arteriography may be enhanced with the use of CT and is referred to as **CT angiography.**

digital subtraction angiography (DSA): two-step imaging technique in which a radiograph is obtained of the area of interest before adding contrast medium. This first image is stored in the computer. Contrast medium that is opaque to x-ray is injected, and a second image is obtained. The opacity creates a shadow that allows visualization of blood flow. The computer subtracts the first image from the second image to produce a clear view of flowing blood and its blockages by narrowed vessels, ruptured vessels, or abnormal tissue.

phlebography: invasive radiographic procedure in which radiopaque material is injected into a vein to visualize possible blockage or other abnormalities; also called **phlebogram, venography,** and **venogram.**

sclerotherapy: a procedure whereby a chemical (sclerosing agent) is injected into a blood vessel to scar the vessel shut. Usually done electively for veins but can also be used for small bleeding arteries.

venogram: a diagnostic procedure in which a contrast medium is injected into a vein and an x-ray is used to visualize venous anatomy and pathologic conditions, for example, a blockage, clots, or chronic changes; also called **venography, phlebography,** and **phlebogram.**

Noninvasive Tests

These tests apply external techniques, and the body is not entered. These methods frequently provide dynamic information.

ankle-brachial index (ABI): comparison of pressure measured by blood pressure cuff or B-mode Doppler signal between arms and legs (e.g., normal –1, moderate decrease –0.75, severe decrease –0.35). Test principle relies on compressibility of blood vessels and results are often affected by diabetes. Also called **ankle-arm index.**

Doppler ultrasound (duplex Doppler or pulsed Doppler): Low-intensity sound waves are reflected off blood vessels or other organs or moving blood and passed through a computer to produce sound (B-mode) or pictures. Provides detailed information of anatomy and pathologic conditions (clots, narrowing, dilatations, obstructions). Combining with duplex techniques provides physiologic information as well.

color Doppler: assigns colors (usually red and blue) to blood flowing in specific directions, and can be used to analyze blood flow. A **power Doppler** is an ultrasound technique that is more sensitive in detecting the presence of blood flow; however, it does not assess the direction of blood flow. Doppler studies are commonly used to detect narrowing of the carotid arteries and blood clots in the veins of the legs.

duplex ultrasound: provides both a two-dimensional image of the vessel and the velocity of flow. There are many uses, including carotid artery stenosis and venous blood flow to test blood clots. Duplex imaging for clots in leg veins is less invasive than venography and is the first imaging test of choice for this common clinical problem.

electrocardiogram: graphic recording of electrical activity of the heart.

plethysmography: noninvasive procedure that measures volume changes in an organ or extremity. Principle is applied in various forms to include volume displacement (air or water), strain gauge, mechanical, photoelectric, or impedance.

impedance plethysmography: instrument to measure changes in electrical impedance in a limb, which indicates changes in blood content and limb volume.

oculoplethysmography (OPG): noninvasive diagnostic procedure measuring carotid artery pressure indirectly by measuring blood pressure in the eyes. The medium of measurement may either be air (oculopneumoplethysmography) or water (oculohydroplethysmography).

photoplethysmography (PPG): noninvasive procedure with an instrument that uses light to measure blood flow to skin and thereby measure blood in larger vessels that may be occluded by arteriosclerosis.

pulse volume recorder (PVR): segmental air plethysmograph to determine change in limb blood flow by change in cuff pressure.

transcutaneous oximetry (TcPO$_2$): produces local measurement of skin oxygen tension and can give measures of capillary perfusion and predict wound healing.

Radiation Therapy

Ionizing radiation causes molecules to split when the radiation particle or wave hits the molecule. This event can cause injury to cells, particularly those that are dividing rapidly such as in tumors, blood cells, and normal gastrointestinal lining.

As a result, ionizing radiation for diagnostic purposes is kept to a minimum, and treatment is made focal by a variety of techniques. The terminology listed here is restricted to techniques commonly applied to orthopaedic conditions and to some dosimetry terms.

roentgen: measure of the change resulting from the exposure of air to radiation.

roentgen absorbed dose (rad): the actual energy absorbed by the local tissue, measured in ergs per gram. This is not a whole-body count of absorbed dose, but a number that looks at each tissue system or organ.

roentgen-equivalent-man (rem): biologic effectiveness of radiation in a human subject. For diagnostic purposes, *rad* is equal to *rem*.

strontium-89: treatment for metastatic bone pain. A beta-emitting radioactive material is injected intravenously. The isotope is taken up in bone and delivers the radiation to the affected areas. The effect lasts for several months. Also called **Metastron.**

Orthopaedic Tests, Signs, and Maneuvers

This chapter identifies the many names used in orthopaedics to describe tests, signs, and maneuvers that are synonymous with other names having the same definition and meaning. This occurs as a reflection of the influence of educational institutions around the country in that the names of prominent physicians are named for these examinations, along with generic names given to describe a test, sign, or maneuver. Eponyms are routinely used in the physical evaluation process. Familiarity with the names and techniques enables physicians and assistants to accurately record an orthopaedic examination. When more than one name is given for a single definition, the synonym follows at the end of the definition.

The physical examination is performed by direct visual observation, noting the way a patient walks (gait) or the manner in which the upper and lower limbs are used; by auditory findings such as auscultation of pulses; or by palpation, which is the use of hands in determining firmness, shape, and motion of a part. All of these can stand alone or be combined to aid in diagnosis.

A **test** may be part of the physical examination in which direct contact with the patient is made, or it may be a chemical test, radiographic examination, or other study. All tests described in this chapter relate to the physical examination only.

A **sign** may be elucidated by a test, maneuver, or simply a visual observation, for example, a list. It is an indication of the existence of a problem as perceived by the examiner. The terms *sign* and *test* are often interchanged.

A **maneuver** is a complex motion or series of movements used as either a test or treatment. It is also referred to as a *method* or *technique*.

A **phenomenon** is any sign or objective symptom; it is any observable occurrence or fact.

This chapter presents the many categories of tests, signs, and maneuvers. An alphabetized list is presented first to guide the reader to the appropriate section. The categories are neck, back, shoulder, upper limbs, hands, hips, lower limbs, knees, feet and ankles, neurologic, metabolic, general, gait, scales and rating, and other examinations. A table of knee examinations is included. Scales and ratings, as pertains to outcomes assessment as well as degree of impairment, are listed along with a grading system for spinal cord injury.

In addition to many new terms, a table has been included on knee instability tests, an area that receives much attention. Scales and ratings, as pertains to preoperative and postoperative assessment of joints and degree of functional impairment, have been expanded to include a neurologic assessment grading system for spinal cord injury.

Tests, Signs, and Maneuvers

Abbott method (back)
abduction sign (shoulder)
abduction external rotation test (shoulder)
Achilles bulge sign (feet, ankles)

Achilles squeeze test (lower limb)
active compression test (shoulder)
active glide test (knee)
Addis test (lower limbs)
adduction sign (shoulder)
Adson maneuver or test (neck)
Allen maneuver (neck)
Allen test (hands)
Allis maneuver (hips)
Allis sign (hips)
ambling (gaits)
American Shoulder and Elbow Surgeons (scales and ratings)
American Spinal Injury Association (ASIA) scale (scales and ratings)
Amoss sign (back)
André Thomas sign (hands)
Anghelescu sign (back)
ankle clonus test (neurologic)
Anstrom suspension test (back)
antalgic (gait)
antecedent sign (general)
anterior cruciate ligament instability (knee)
anterior drawer sign (feet, ankles)
anterior slide test (shoulder)
anterior tibial sign (lower limb)
anvil test (neck; hips)
Apley test (knees)
Apley scratch test (shoulder)
apprehension test (shoulder)
arthrometer test (knees)
artifact (general)
ataxic (gaits)
axial compression test (hand)
Babinski reflex (back)
Babinski sign (neurologic)
ballotment test (hands)
ballotable patella sign (knee)
Barlow test (hips)
bayonet sign (knees)
Beevor sign (neurologic)
Beighton laxity score (scales and ratings)
Bekhterev test (back)
belly press test (shoulder)
bench test (back)
benediction attitude sign (hands)

benediction sign (hands)
Bigelow reduction maneuver (hips)
Booth test (shoulder)
bounce home test (knees)
Bouvier maneuver (hands)
bowstring sign (back)
Boyes test (hands)
Bozan maneuver (hips)
bracelet test (hands)
Bragard sign (back)
British test (knees)
Brudzinski sign (neck, neurologic)
Bryant sign (shoulders)
bulge sign (knee)
café-au-lait (general)
Callaway test (shoulders)
camelback sign (knees)
Carducci test (hands)
carpal compression test (hands)
Chaddock sign (neurologic)
Chapple test (hips)
Charnley hip scale (scales and ratings)
Chicago test (back)
Chiene test (hips)
Childress test (knee)
Chvostek sign (metabolic)
circumduction (gaits)
circumduction maneuver (hands)
circumduction test (shoulder)
claw hand sign (hands)
Cleeman sign (lower limb)
Codman sign (shoulders)
cogwheel phenomenon (general)
Coleman lateral standing block test (feet, ankles)
commemorative sign (general)
Comolli sign (shoulders)
confrontational test (hands)
contralateral straight leg raising test (back)
Coopernail sign (back)
costoclavicular maneuver (neck)
Cotton test (feet, ankles)
Cozen test (back)
cram test (back)
crank test (shoulder)
cross-body abduction maneuver (shoulder)
cross-chest test (shoulder)

cross-over test (knee)
Dawbarn sign (shoulders)
Dejerine sign (back)
Demianoff sign (back)
Desault sign (hips)
Destot sign (hips)
Deyerle maneuver (hip)
Deyerle sign (back)
Dial test (knee)
dimple sign (feet, ankle)
dimple sign (neurologic)
doll's eye sign (neurologic)
drop-arm test (shoulder)
drop-back phenomenon (knee)
double camelback sign (knee)
double PCL sign (knee)
drawer sign (knee; feet, ankles)
drawer test (shoulder)
Dugas test (shoulders)
Duchenne sign (hands)
Dupuytren sign (general)
Durkan test (hands)
Earle sign (hips)
East Baltimore maneuver (hips)
elbow flexion test (elbow)
Elson middle slip test (hands)
Ely test (hips, neurologic)
Erichsen sign (back)
extension lag (knee)
external rotation drawer test (knee)
external rotation recurvatum test (knee)
extrinsic tightness test (hands)
FABERE test (back)
FADIRE test (back)
Fairbank sign (knee)
fan sign (neurologic)
Fellar patellar score (scales and ratings)
femoral nerve traction test (back)
Fick angle (gaits)
figure 4 test (knee)
Finacetto sign (knee)
finger to nose test (neurologic)
Finkelstein sign (hands)
flexion rotation drawer test (knees)
foot slap (gait)
forced adduction test (shoulder)

Forestier (back)
Fouchet sign (knee)
Fournier test (neurologic)
Fowler maneuver (hands)
Fowler test (shoulder)
Frankel scale (scales and ratings)
Fränkel sign (neurologic)
Froment sign (hands)
fulcrum test (shoulder)
Gaenslen sign (back)
Galeazzi sign (hips)
gear-stick sign (hips)
Gerber test (shoulder)
Gilliat tourniquet test (hand)
Glasgow coma score (scales and ratings)
gluteus maximus (gait)
gluteus medius (gait)
Godfrey test (knee)
Goldthwait sign (back)
Gordon reflex sign (neurologic)
Gower sign (general)
grand piano sign (knees)
gravity stress test (elbow)
Green-Anderson growth chart (scales and ratings)
grimace test (knees)
grip-strength test (hands)
Guilland sign (neurologic)
Halstead test (neck)
Hamilton test (shoulder)
Harris-Beath footprinting mat (feet)
Harris hip scale (scales and ratings)
Hawkins impingement sign (shoulder)
head tilt sign (neck)
heel-bisector method (neurologic)
heel height difference (knee)
heel-to-buttocks difference (knee)
Helbing sign (feet, ankles)
Helft test (knee)
hemodynamic test (general)
Hirschberg sign (neurologic)
Hoffmann sign (neurologic)
Homan sign (lower limbs)
hook test (elbow; feet, ankles)
Hoover test (back)
hop test (knee)
hornblower sign (shoulder)

Hueter sign (general)
Hughston jerk test (knee)
Huntington sign (neurologic)
Hutchinson sign (hands)
hyperabduction test (neck)
hyperextension test (neck)
impingement sign (shoulder)
impingement test (shoulder)
internal-rotation drawer test (knees)
International Classification for Surgery of the
    Hand in Tetraplegia (hands)
intrinsic tightness test (hands)
inverted radial reflex (back)
J sign (knee)
Jansen test (hips)
Jeanne test (hands)
Jendrassik maneuver (back; neurologic)
jerk test (shoulder)
Jobe test (shoulder)
Kanavel sign (hands)
Kapandji thumb opposition score (hand)
Keen sign (feet, ankles)
Kernig sign (neurologic)
Kerr sign (neurologic)
Kim test (shoulder)
Kleinman shear test (hands)
Klippel-Feil sign (neurologic)
knee instability tests (knees)
Knee Society clinical rating system (scales and ratings)
King maneuver (hips)
Kocher maneuver (shoulders)
Kujala score (scales and ratings)
Lachman test (knees)
lack of extension sign (knees)
Langer line (general)
Langoria sign (hips)
Lasègue sign (back)
Laugier sign (upper limbs)
lead line (metabolic)
Leadbetter maneuver (hips)
Lefkowitz maneuver (hips)
Leichtenstern sign (neurologic)
Léri sign (neurologic)
Lhermitte sign (neurologic)
Lichtman test (hands)
lift-off test (shoulder)

Linder sign (back)
list (back)
load-and-shift test (shoulder)
long finger extension test
long tract sign (neurologic)
Lorenz sign (back)
loss of extension test (knee)
Losse test (knee)
Lovett test (hands)
Ludington sign (shoulder)
Ludloff sign (hips)
Lynholm knee-scoring scale (scales and ratings)
Magnuson test (back)
Maisonneuve sign (hands)
Marie-Foix sign (feet, ankles)
Marshall knee-scoring scale (scales and ratings)
Marvel test (shoulder)
masses sign (hands)
Matles test (feet, ankles)
Mazur ankle rating (scales and ratings)
McBride test (foot)
McCarthy sign (hips)
McElvenny maneuver (hips)
McMurray test (knees)
Mendel-Bekhterev sign (neurologic)
medial subluxation test (knees)
Mennell sign (back)
Merke sign (knee)
Merle d'Aubigne and Postel hip scale
    (scales and ratings)
Meryon sign (metabolic)
Meyn and Quigley maneuver (upper limbs)
Michele buckling sign (back)
Michele flip sign (back)
Milch maneuver (shoulder)
Milgram test (back)
military brace maneuver (back)
Mills test (upper limbs)
Mimori test (shoulder)
Minor sign (back)
modified lift-off test (shoulder)
Moro reflex sign (neurologic)
Morquio sign (neurologic)
Morton test (feet, ankles)
Medical Research Council sensory grade (neurologic)
Mulder sign (feet)

Murphy sign (feet, ankles; hand)
Nachlas (back)
Naffziger sign (back)
Napoleon test (shoulder)
Neer impingement sign (shoulder)
Neer impingement test (shoulder)
Nélaton line (hips)
Neri bowing sign (back)
Neviaser test (shoulder)
Norton scoring system (scales and ratings)
no touch test (knees)
nuchocephalic reflex (neurologic)
O'Brien test (shoulder)
O'Connell test (back)
O'Driscoll SLAP test (shoulder)
Ober test (hips)
objective sign (general)
obturator sign (hips)
Oppenheim sign (neurologic)
Ortolani test (hips)
Oshsner clasping test (hand)
overhead exercise test (neck)
paratonia (neurologic)
Parvin maneuver (upper limbs)
patellar apprehension test (knees)
patellar glide test (knee)
patellar grind test (knee)
patellar retraction test (knee)
patellar tilt test (knees)
Patrick test (hips)
Payr sign (lower limbs)
pelvic rock test (back)
Phalen test and maneuver (hands)
piano key sign (hands)
Piotrowski sign (neurologic)
piston sign (hips)
pivot-jerk test (knees)
pivot-shift test (knees)
Pitres-Testut sign (hand)
Pollock sign (hands)
Popeye deformity (upper limbs)
posterior drawer test (knees)
post-total hip internal rotation (hip)
posterior lift-off test (shoulder)
posterolateral instability (elbow)
postural fixation (back)

pronation sign (neurologic)
prone external rotation test (knees)
prone hanging test (knees)
pseudo-Babinski sign (neurologic)
pseudostability test (hand)
push-pull test (shoulder)
quadriceps test (general)
quadriceps active test (knees)
Queckenstedt sign (neurologic)
radialis sign (neurologic)
Raimiste sign (neurologic)
Raynaud phenomenon (general)
release test (shoulder)
relocation test (shoulder)
reverse Bigelow maneuver (hips)
reverse pivot-shift test (knees)
Romberg test (neurologic)
Roos test (neck)
Roux sign (hip)
rubber band sign (shoulder)
Rust sign (neck)
sag sign (knee)
sagittal stress test (feet, ankles)
Sarbo sign (neurologic)
scaphoid test (hands)
scapular assistance test (shoulder)
scapular dyskinesis sign (shoulder)
scapular sign of Putti (shoulder)
scapular winging sign (shoulder)
Schlesinger sign (lower limbs)
Schreiber maneuver (neurologic)
scissors (gaits)
screw-home mechanism (knee)
Seimon sign (neck)
Semmes and Weinstein monofilament test
    (scales and ratings)
Sharp-Purser test (neck)
shuffling (gait)
Silfreskiöld test (feet, ankles)
Slocum test (knees)
Smith maneuver (hips)
Smith and Ross test (hand)
Smith-Peterson test (back)
somatic sign (general)
Soto-Hall sign (back)
Speed test (shoulder)

spilled teacup sign (hands)
spine sign (back)
sponge test (back)
Spurling test (neck)
stairs sign (neurologic)
standing apprehension test (knees)
station test (neurologic)
Steinmann test (knee)
Stimson maneuver (hips)
stoop test (back)
straight leg raising (SLR) test (back)
Strümpell confusion test (neurologic)
Strunsky sign (feet, ankles)
succinylcholine test (neurologic)
sulcus sign (shoulder)
swallow-tail sign (shoulder)
symmetrical extension test (knee)
table top test (hand)
talar tilt test (feet, ankles)
tendon reflexes (neurologic)
tenodesis test (hands)
Tensilon test (metabolic)
Terry-Thomas sign (hand)
Thessaly test (knee)
Thomas sign (hips, neurologic)
Thomas squeeze test (feet, ankles)
thumbnail test (knees)
thumb-to-forearm test (neurologic)
tibial sag sign (knees)
tibialis sign (neurologic)
tilt test (knees)
Tinel sign (neurologic)
toe spread sign (feet, ankles)
too many toes sign (feet, ankles)
total hip arthroplasty outcome evaluation (scales and ratings)
tourniquet test (lower limbs)
towel clip test (knees)
Trendelenburg gait (hips)
Trendelenburg test (hips)
Trotter bulge test (knee)
tuck sign (hands)
Turyn sign (back)
two-point discrimination test (hands)
ulna fovea sign (hands)
valgus stress test (elbow, knee)

valgus thrust (knee)
Valsalva maneuver (back)
Vanzetti sign (back)
varus recurvatum test (knee)
varus stress test (knee)
vertical patella test (knees)
Waddell sign (back)
Walker-Mureloch wrist sign (metabolic)
Wartenberg sign (hands)
Watson test (hands)
Wellmerling maneuver (hips)
wet leather sign (hands)
Whitman maneuver (hips)
Wilson sign (knees)
WOMAC (scales and ratings)
Wright maneuver or test (shoulder, neck/test)
wrinkle test (neurologic)
Wu sole opposition test (feet, ankles)
Yergason test (shoulders)

Neck (Fig. 4-1)

Adson m. (test): for scalenus anticus (thoracic outlet) syndrome, noted on obliteration of radial pulse; upper limb to be tested is held in dependent position while head is rotated to the ipsilateral shoulder while inhaling.

Allen m.: for same diagnosis as *Adson m.*, except the forearm is flexed at right angle with the arm extended horizontally and rotated externally at the shoulder, with the head rotated to the contralateral shoulder.

anvil t.: for vertebral disorders; a closed fist striking blow on top of the head elicits pain in the vertebra(e).

costoclavicular m.: for thoracic outlet syndrome; pulling shoulders and chin back at the same time reduces the radial pulse when arm is by side; also called **military brace m.**

Halstead t.: for thoracic outlet; the standing patient keeps arm by side while pulse is taken; extending neck and turning head to opposite side obliterates pulse.

head tilt s.: seen in a complete brachial plexus injury, the head tilts to the side opposite the injury.

hyperabduction t.: for thoracic outlet syndrome, after obtaining the patient's radial pulse the shoulder

FIG 4-1 Cervical radiculopathy. **A,** Herniated disk compressing nerve root. **B,** Spurling maneuver. Hyperextension of neck and rotation and tilt toward the side of lesion cause radicular pain in neck and down arm. *(Netter illustration from www.netterimages.com. © Elsevier Inc. All rights reserved.)*

is abducted to greater than 90 degrees with extension. The patient is instructed to take a deep breath and hold. A positive test is a decrease in radial pulse intensity.

hyperextension t.: for thoracic outlet; both arms are fully abducted after confirming radial pulse with arms at side. The pulse is obliterated on the affected side.

overhead exercise t.: for thoracic outlet syndrome; the hand is held overhead and making repeated fists results in immediate soreness in the forearm muscles; also called **Roos t.**

Rust s.: for osteomyelitis or malignant disease of the spine; the patient supports head with hands while moving body.

Seimon s.: for fractured odontoid in small child; child cries if sat upright without support to head and neck.

Sharp-Purser t.: for chronic subluxation of the first on second cervical vertebra; with the patient sitting, the head is tilted forward and then backward with the examining finger on the first cervical spinous process to detect slippage.

Spurling t.: for cervical spine and foraminal nerve encroachment; compression on the head with extension and rotation of the neck causes radicular pain into the upper extremities. Often helpful in distinguishing pathologic conditions of the neck from shoulder conditions when symptoms are found in the shoulder.

Wright m.: in thoracic outlet syndrome, downward pressure on shoulder with shoulder being pulled back obstructs the radial pulse; also called **costoclavicular m.**

Back

Abbott method: for scoliosis of the spine; traction is applied to produce overcorrection, followed by casting.

Amoss s.: for painful flexure of the spine; pain is produced when the patient places hands far behind body in bed and tries rising from supine position to sitting position.

Anghelescu s.: for testing tuberculosis of the vertebrae or other destructive processes of the spine; in the supine position the patient places weight on head and heels while lifting body upward; inability to bend the spine indicates an ongoing disease process.

Anstrom suspension t.: for sciatica; while tapping on the affected area of the lumbar spine the patient will have pain while standing, but not if suspending weight using arms to hold the spine in suspension.

Bekhterev t.: for nerve root irritability in sciatica; while sitting up in bed, the patient is asked to stretch out both legs; with sciatica, patient cannot sit up in bed this way but can only stretch out each leg in turn.

bench t.: for nonorganic back pain; in normal hip motion, the patient should be able to bend over and touch the floor kneeling on a 12-inch high bench; not being able to do so implies a nonorganic (or psychologic) back pain; also called **Burns t.**

bowstring s.: with leg raised with knee bent in same position, pain is felt in the back of the limb pressing on the central popliteal fossa. Increased pain is a sign of nerve irritability depending on position of the patient. Also called **cram t., Forestier t.,** and **Deyerle t.**

Bragard s.: for nerve or muscular involvement; with the knee stiff, the lower extremity is flexed at the hip until the patient experiences pain; the foot is then dorsiflexed. Increased pain points to nerve involvement; no increase in pain indicates muscular involvement.

Chicago t.: to distinguish between back strain with muscle spasm and disk disease without spasm, the patient kneels on a chair and attempts to touch the floor. With muscle spasm the patient has difficulty; also called **Bench Burn disease.** Note: this same test is also used to study the way the patient returns to a more erect position. Slow movement implies an emotional component.

contralateral straight leg raising t.: for sciatica; when the leg is flexed, the hip can also be flexed, but not when the leg is held straight. Flexing the sound thigh with the leg held straight causes pain on the affected side. Also called **Fajersztajn crossed sciatic s.**

Coopernail s.: for fracture of pelvis; ecchymosis of the perineum, scrotum, or labia indicates a pelvic fracture.

Cozen t.: to distinguish sciatica from muscle spasm, the supine patient is assisted in sitting up with the knees out straight. An inability to do this without flexing the knee implies nerve irritation or muscle spasm in the lower limb.

cram t. (bowstring t.): for radiculopathy, with the patient supine the examiner does a passive straight leg raise on involved side and if the patient has radiating pain the examiner then flexes the knee to approximately 20 degrees to reduce the pain. Pressure then applied to popliteal area to reproduces radicular pain.

Dejerine s.: for herniated intervertebral disk causing radiating limb symptoms; a Valsalva maneuver, such as coughing, sneezing, or straining at stool, accentuates the symptoms.

Demianoff s.: for differentiation of pain originating in the lumbosacral muscle from lumbar pain of any other origin; the pain is caused by stretching of the lumbosacral muscle.

Erichsen s.: in sacroiliac disease, when the iliac bones are sharply pressed toward each other, pain is felt in the sacroiliac area.

FABERE t.: for testing lower back or sacroiliac joint disorder by using a forced position of the hip; the patient crosses the leg with the foot of the affected side resting on the opposite knee, then in extension by pressing down on the knee. *FABERE* is an acronym for *f*lexion *ab*duction *e*xternal *r*otation in *e*xtension; also called **Patrick t.**, **figure of 4 t.**, and **LaGuerre t.**

FADIRE t.: forced position of the hip causing pain. An acronym for *f*lexion *ad*duction *i*nternal *r*otation in *e*xtension; also called **Patrick t.** and **FADIRE s.**

femoral nerve traction t.: for radiculopathy of the second through fourth lumbar nerves; with patient prone, the knee is flexed, causing back or thigh pain; also called **Ely t.**

Forestier t.: for early ankylosing spondylitis, in free lateral bending, the early ankylosing spondylitis (AS) patient has palpably firm, due to contracted dorsolumbar muscles on the concave side.

Gaenslen s.: for sacroiliac disease; pressure on hyperextended thigh with the opposite hip held in flexion elicits pain on the affected side over edge of bed, indicating a sacroiliac problem.

Goldthwait s.: for distinguishing lumbosacral from sacroiliac pain; with the patient supine, the leg is raised with one hand, while the examiner's other hand is placed under the patient's lower back. Leverage is then applied to the side of the pelvis. If pain is felt by the patient before the lumbar spine is moved, the lesion is a sprain of the SI joint; if pain is not felt until after the lumbar spine is moved, the lesion is in the SI or lumbosacral articulation.

Hoover t.: for a supposed malingering back disorder; while lying supine, the patient is asked to raise one leg with the knee straight and with the examiner holding the opposite heel. Any active effort to do this will result in pressure of the opposite heel against the examiner's hand. The lack of such effort implies malingering. Excessive pressure of the heel against the examiner's hand implies abdominal muscle weakness.

inverted radial reflex: for cervical spondylotic myelopathy (cord compression); there is spontaneous flexion of the digits when the brachialis reflex is being tested.

Jendrassik m.: to help distract the patient or to help determine presence or absence of a weak reflex, patient is asked to push hands together or lock fingers and pull hands apart while reflex is tested; also called **reinforcement m.**

Lasègue s.: for sciatica; flexion of thigh on hips is painless, and when the knee is bent, such flexion is easily made. If painless, there is no hip joint disease. If test produces pain when the knee is straightened, nerve root irritation or lower back disorder may be present; also called **straight leg raising t.**

Linder s.: for sciatica; with the patient sitting or recumbent with outstretched legs, passive flexion of the head will cause pain in the leg or lumbar region.

list: said of a patient who leans to one side or another when standing or walking; most commonly seen in lumbar disk disease.

Lorenz s.: for ankylosing spondylitis and Marie-Strumpell disease; ankylotic rigidity of the spinal column, especially thoracic and lumbar segments.

Magnuson t.: for malingering; put an x mark on spot where patient reports pain. At a later time in the examination, test for tender points by palpation. The patient indicating pain not including that mark implies malingering.

Mennell s.: for spinal problems; examiner's thumb is taken over the posterosuperior spine of sacrum outward and inward for noting tenderness, which may be caused by sensitive deposits in gluteal aspect of posterosuperior spine; ligamentous strain and sensitivity.

Michele buckling s.: for sciatica; the continued straight-leg raising past the point of nerve irritation will cause the patient to flex the knee if he or she has true sciatica.

Michele flip s.: for sciatica; the sitting patient who has the flexed knees passively extended will lean backward if true sciatica exists.

Milgram t.: for a lesion within the dural sac; while lying supine, the patient flexes both hips so that the knees are straight and both feet are lifted by only several inches. If the patient is able to hold this position without pain for 30 seconds, there is no problem within the dural sac. However, a positive test may occur for both intrathecal and extrathecal disorders.

military brace maneuver: for thoracic outlet syndrome, the person first stands in a relaxed posture, with the head looking forward. They then depress and retract the shoulders as if standing at attention in a military brace. Production of symptoms is a positive sign.

Minor s.: for sciatica; patient rises from sitting position supporting body on healthy side, placing hand on back, and bending affected leg, revealing pain.

Nachlas t.: sacroiliac disorder, the prone patient has the knee flexed to a right angle with pressure against the anterior surface of the ankle and the heel is slowly directed straight toward the ipsilateral buttock. The contralateral ilium should be stabilized by the examiner's other hand. If a sharp pain is elicited in the ipsilateral buttock or sacral area, a sacroiliac disorder should be suspected.

Naffziger t.: for sciatica or herniated nucleus pulposus; nerve root irritation is produced by external jugular venous compression by examiner.

Neri bowing s.: for sciatica; the standing patient with knees extended is asked to bend forward. Knee flexion implies sciatica.

O'Connell t.: for lumbar nerve irritability. With knee extended, both lower limbs are raised to maximum hip flexion to the point of pain; lowering the unaffected limb will exacerbate pain in sciatica.

pelvic rock t.: for sacroiliac joint disorder; forcible compression of the iliac crest toward the midline will produce pain.

postural fixation: a sign noted on range of motion of the back; any postural deformity (stiffness) noted does not reverse with range of motion.

Smith-Peterson t.: for sacroiliac joint origin of pain; with one hand under the spine the opposite hand raises the leg. If the hamstrings are tight, apply posterior leverage to the pelvis. Pain prior to lumbar movement can be present in both lumbar and sacroiliac joint disorders. If this occurs at the same level for both legs, sacroiliac disease is implied.

Soto-Hall s.: for lesions in back abnormalities; with the patient supine, flexion of the spine beginning at the neck and going downward will elicit pain in the area of the lesion.

spine s.: for poliomyelitis; the patient is unable to flex the spine anteriorly because of pain.

sponge t.: for detecting lesions of the spine; the examiner passes a hot sponge up and down the spine, and the patient feels pain over the lesion.

stoop t.: for spinal stenosis; with persistent walking the patient will begin to stoop forward to reverse lumbar lordosis and improve spinal space. Likewise, in a sitting position the patient will lean forward.

straight leg raising (SLR) t.: for determining nerve root irritation; the supine patient elevates the leg straight until there is back or ipsilateral extremity pain or until the pain is increased with dorsiflexion of the foot; also called **Lasègue s.**

Turyn s.: for sciatica; when examiner bends the patient's great toe dorsally, pain is felt in the gluteal region.

Valsalva m.: for determining nerve root irritability within the spinal canal. This maneuver is also used for many other unrelated reasons. Taking a deep breath and bearing down, such when lifting a heavy object, elicits pain.

Vanzetti s.: for sciatica; the pelvis is horizontal in the presence of scoliosis. In other scoliotic conditions, the pelvis is inclined as part of the deformity.

Waddell s.: for nonphysical-origin back pain; pressure on tender area results in jump-away pain in excess of that expected for level of disease, implying a strong emotional component. The term *Waddell* has commonly been used on other areas to reflect the same implications.

Shoulder

abduction external rotation t.: abduct shoulder to 90 degrees with elbow at 90 degrees. On external rotation, pain without apprehension implies rotator cuff disorder. Apprehension implies anterior instability.

abduction s.: for subacromial impingement or pathologic conditions of the rotator cuff; the examiner places the shoulder in 90 degrees abduction and 30 degrees flexion and then internally rotates arm, producing pain.

active compression t.: with the arm at 10 degrees adduction, 90 degrees forward flexion, and maximal forearm pronation, pain with resistance to downward force is correlative with a superior labrum anterior to posterior lesion; also called **O'Brien t.**

adduction s.: for acromioclavicular joint disease; the shoulder is abducted 90 degrees, brought horizontally forward 90 degrees, and then flexed maximally forward, producing pain at the acromioclavicular joint. Also called **cross-body adduction t.**

anterior slide t.: while patient is sitting, humeral head is pressed anteriorly with examiner's hand, resulting in increased pressure if anterior capsular laxity exits.

Apley scratch t.: the patient is asked to put hand behind the back and elevate the hand as far as possible as when trying to scratch the midback. A measurement of shoulder extension combined with internal rotation is measured by the thoracic level at which the finger can reach, typically T7. A reasonable measure of internal rotatory shoulder strength as well.

apprehension t.: for anterior subluxing or dislocating shoulder; the arm is held abducted and extended while in external rotation, best completed in a supine position. The patient is apprehensive in a positive examination. Placing a posterior directed force at the proximal humerus may relieve the feeling of shoulder instability experienced by the patient, further confirming the instability.

belly press t.: for ruptured or neurologically impaired subscapularis; patient is unable to hold hand on abdomen when hand is forcibly being pulled away or unable to compress belly and actively forward push the elbow against resistance. Also called **anterior lift-off t.** and **Napoleon t.**

Booth t.: for transverse humeral ligament rupture; with pressure on biceps groove, the arm is abducted and externally rotated. A snap indicates subluxation of the biceps tendon caused by ligament insufficiency. Also called **Marvel t.**

Bryant s.: for dislocation of the shoulder with lowering of the axillary folds, as noted on visual examination.

Callaway t.: for dislocation of the humerus; the circumference of the affected shoulder measured over the acromion and through the axilla is greater than that on the opposite, unaffected side.

circumduction t.: for posterior shoulder instability; to bring the shoulder passively from an abducted and extended position to anterior adduction position results in subluxation in the provocative anterior position. Not to be confused with circumduction maneuver for the knee to determine torn meniscus.

Codman s.: for rupture of the supraspinatus tendon; the arm can be passively abducted without pain, but when support of the arm is removed and the deltoid muscle contracts suddenly, pain occurs again.

Comolli s.: for scapular fracture; shortly after injury, there is triangular swelling, reproducing the shape of the body of the scapula.

crank t.: for anterior shoulder instability; the supine patient has the shoulder abducted and externally rotated. On full external rotation, there is apprehension and resistance, similar to apprehension test.

cross-chest t.: for acromioclavicular joint arthritis; passively or actively bringing the affected arm across the chest causes pain in the acromioclavicular joint region. Also called **cross-body abduction m., forced adduction t.,** and **cross-body adduction t.**

Dawbarn s.: for acute subacromial bursitis; with arm hanging by side, palpation over the bursa causes pain; when the arm is abducted, pain disappears.

drawer t.: for shoulder instability; the patient may be sitting or lying. The scapula and clavicle are held securely in one hand and the head of the humerus in the other; the humeral head is pushed forward and backward to compare the two sides for crepitus and ligamentous stability. Also called **load and shift t.**

drop-arm t.: for rotator cuff tear; the patient is unable to actively control bringing the arm down from a full abducted position past 90 degrees. The arm drops at 90 degrees. This test is best performed with a local anesthetic injected into the subacromial space.

Dugas t.: for dislocation of the shoulder; placing hand of affected side on opposite shoulder and bringing elbow to side of chest, a dislocation may be present if the patient's elbow will not touch side of the chest; also called **Dugas s.**

Fowler t.: for anterior shoulder instability; patient lies supine and the shoulder is held in an abducted and externally rotated position using the edge of the examining surface as a fulcrum. Posterior force is then applied to the humerus. Relief of apprehension is a sign of anterior instability; also called **push-pull t.**

fulcrum t.: for anterior-inferior shoulder instability; patient lies supine and the shoulder is held in an abducted and externally rotated position. The arm is then further abducted and extended using the edge of the examining surface as a fulcrum (support).

Gerber t.: for subacromial impingement; forward elevation of the arm while adducted and internally rotated causes anterior shoulder pain.

Hamilton t.: for luxated shoulder; a rod applied to the humerus can be made to touch the lateral condyle and acromion at the same time to determine a dislocation.

Hawkins impingement s.: for rotator cuff disorder; forward flexion of humerus to 90 degrees followed by horizontal adduction and internal rotation produces pain.

hornblower s.: a patient with a rotator-cuff tear of the infraspinatus or teres minor is unable to bring both hands to the mouth without abducting the affected arm, indicating a weakness of external rotation. Also seen as weakness of external rotation at 90 degrees of abduction; also called **trumpet s.**

impingement s.: the examiner forces the shoulder into flexion and internal rotation with downward pressure on the acromion produced by the other hand. Pain is a positive sign of impingement.

impingement t.: after a subacromial injection of an anesthetic such as lidocaine, the shoulder becomes pain free or significantly less painful when taken through the motion to produce the impingement sign. A positive result may indicate bursitis, impingement, or rotator cuff disease.

jerk t.: for posterior shoulder instability; when the supine patient has the shoulder flexed to 90 degrees with the elbow at 90 degrees, pressure in a posterior direction causes a jerk or jump with subluxation. By bringing the humerus out of flexion and back midline at 90 degrees of abduction, the humeral head will noticeably "clunk" back to its reduced position within the glenoid.

Jobe t.: for supraspinatus pathologic conditions; standing patient is asked to actively abduct the shoulder to 90 degrees and forward flex 30 degrees with thumbs down. Pain occurs if patient is asked to push arm toward the ceiling; also called **supraspinatus isolation t.**

Kim t.: for posteroinferior labral pathologic conditions. Pain is elicited through an arc of motion with the examiner placing an axial force on a forward-flexed shoulder.

Kocher m.: for reducing anterior dislocations of the shoulder; done by abducting the arm, externally rotating, adducting, and then internally rotating.

lift off t.: for rupture of the subscapularis in the shoulder, when placing the back of their hand on the middle of their back the patient in unable to lift their hand from their back.

load-and-shift t.: with the patient supine and the shoulder slightly abducted on the edge of the examining table, the humeral head is shifted anteriorly and posteriorly while the forearm or scapula is stabilized by the examiner's opposite hand. This is a method of determining shoulder joint laxity or instability when compared side to side.

Ludington s.: for integrity of the long head of the biceps tendon; patient interlocks hands overhead and then presses hands together. Failure of biceps contraction implies long head rupture.

Milch m: for anterior shoulder dislocation reduction; with one hand on the acromion to support thumb pressure on humeral head, the arm is abducted and externally rotated followed by pressure on humeral head to reduce over glenoid rim.

Mimori t.: for superior labral tears; the sitting patient has the shoulder abducted to 90 to 100 degrees, externally rotated with the elbow at 90 degrees, and the forearm supinated. If there is an increase in pain with forearm pronation, the test is positive for a tear.

modified lift-off t.: inability to keep the arm in a position posterior to or not touching the back when placed there by the examiner and released, indicating weakness or a pathologic condition of the subscapularis.

Napolean t.: for subscapularis rupture, with the patient's hand placed on their abdomen, they cannot resist the examiner pulling the hand away from the abdomen.

Neer impingement s.: for rotator cuff disorder; examiner passively flexes humerus to maximal forward flexion with one hand while depressing the scapula with the other to produce pain.

Neer impingement t: injection of the subacromial bursa eliminates pain elicited with Neer s. The terms *Neer test* and *Neer sign* are often used without discrimination.

Neviaser t.: for proximal triceps tendonitis; with shoulder fully adducted, tenderness over origin of triceps is increased with subsequent active elbow extension against force.

O'Brien t.: for superior labral tear the patient points the thumb down with the shoulder flexed to 90 degrees and adduct across midline. Resistance against further shoulder flexion causes pain with the thumb pointing down. If pain was present with the thumb down but relieved with the thumb up, it is considered a positive test.

O'Driscoll superior labrum anterior to posterior (SLAP) t.: for SLAP tear. With the patient supine, the examiner abducts the shoulder to 90 degrees and allows external rotation of the shoulder to its natural limit. The shoulder is then elevated. A click may be palpated, or pain may be produced. The shoulder is then returned following full overhead elevation, again looking for pain or a click.

posterior lift-off t.: for rupture of subscapularis muscle; weakness of internal rotation is demonstrated by inability of patient to lift hand from back. Also called **modified lift off t.**

push-pull t.: for anterior shoulder instability. Also called **Fowler t.**

release t.: for anterior instability of the shoulder; supine patient with arm abducted at 90 degrees and maximally externally rotated with posterior direct pressure on humeral head is comfortable. Release of humeral head pressure causes apprehension or subluxation; also called **apprehension t.**

relocation t.: for occult anterior shoulder subluxation in throwers; patient lies supine, the shoulder is held in abducted and externally rotated position using the edge of the examining surface. Posterior force is then applied to the humerus with relief of pain apprehension or symptoms of shoulder instability. Less specific when pain is the only symptom.

rubber band s.: weakness and pain with resisted external rotation with the humerus slightly abducted and hands facing forward indicating infraspinatus tendon pathologic condition.

scapular assistance t.: for shoulder impingement syndrome. The examiner elicits pain with forward flexion of the humerus to 90 degrees with internal rotation. A positive test occurs when there is relief of pain when this maneuver is repeated while holding the scapula against the posterior chest wall.

scapular dyskinesis s.: with active forward elevation of the arm comparing to the opposite side the side with rotator cuff impingement, instability, or neurologic injury will often show a noticeable asymmetry of scapular function manifested most often by a medial border of the scapula winging or protruding. Although sensitive, this sign is not particularly specific for any pathologic condition.

scapular sign of Putti: for contractures about the scapula; when the arm is forcibly drawn into the chest and externally rotated, the superior lateral side of the scapula wings out; also called **Putti s.**

Speed t.: for proximal long head of biceps tendonitis; anterior proximal humeral pain created with humerus forward flexed against force while elbow is in full extension.

sulcus s.: for inferior shoulder instability; a downward longitudinal force is applied to the humerus of a resting arm with relaxed shoulder girdle, creating a noticeable sulcus between the acromion and the humeral head. The thumb of the opposite hand can press into the lateral subacromial area, indicating a developing sulcus.

swallow-tail s.: for deltoid muscle function; extension of both arms posteriorly results in a lag on the side that has axillary nerve palsy.

Yergason t.: for pathologic conditions of the proximal long head of biceps or subluxation of the long head of the biceps tendon; while pulling distally on the elbow, the patient holds it flexed at 90 degrees with supination and forced external rotation of the shoulder against resistance by the examiner. Painful subluxation of the tendon can be palpated.

Upper Limbs and Elbow

elbow flexion t.: for cubital tunnel syndrome (ulnar nerve compression at elbow); the examiner holds the elbow in passive maximal flexion. Tingling in the ring and little finger is positive for ulnar nerve irritation.

gravity stress t.: for medial instability; the supine patient has the externally rotated arm out over the edged of the table. With elbow at 20 degrees, the weight of the forearm reveals the laxity.

hook t.: While the patient actively supinates with the elbow flexed 90 degrees, an intact hook test permits the examiner to hook his or her index finger over and behind the intact distal biceps tendon in the antecubital fossa. Inability to "hook" the tendon indicates a distal biceps rupture.

Laugier s.: for a displaced distal radial fracture; condition in which the styloid process of radius and ulna are on same level.

lateral key pinch s.: for ulnar nerve palsy wherein the patient must compensate for index finger adductor tendon flexor loss by pressing the thumb on the radial side of the index finger.

Meyn and Quigley m.: for dislocation of the elbow; the patient lies prone with the arm resting on the examining table and the elbow flexed at 90 degrees. The forearm is pulled distally while the opposite hand guides the olecranon.

Mills t.: for tennis elbow; with wrist and fingers fully flexed and the forearm pronated, complete extension of the elbow is painful.

Parvin m.: for dislocated elbow; the patient lies prone with the arms and forearm over the edge of the examining table. Traction is applied on the wrist in a distal direction while the opposite hand pushes on the anterior distal arm in a posterior direction.

Popeye deformity: loss of continuity of either the proximal or distal attachments of the biceps brachii resulting in a balled-up appearance of the biceps in the front of the upper arm similar to the depicted flexed biceps muscle of the cartoon caricature after which it is named.

posterolateral instability of elbow: for lateral ulnar collateral ligament laxity; with patient supine, shoulder flexed to 90 degrees, elbow extended, the forearm is supinated with a concurrent valgus stress. The instability will increase at 40 degrees of elbow flexion. Also called **pivot shift of elbow.**

Hands

Allen t.: for occlusion of radial or ulnar artery; a method of determining if radial and ulnar arteries communicate through the two palmar arches. Both arteries are occluded digitally. First one artery is released, then the other, to observe pattern of capillary refill in the hand. This can be performed with a Doppler placed on the digits during test. The test is valuable prior to an invasive procedure on the arteries at the wrist.

André Thomas s.: in low ulnar nerve palsy; in an effort to extend the fingers, flexing the wrist using the tenodesis effect will increase the claw.

axial compression t.: for thumb carpometacarpal joint arthritis; thumb is compressed with rotation causing pain in that joint.

ballottement t.: assesses triquetrolunate dissociation; stabilize the lunate with one hand, the triquetrum with the other. Displace one from the other dorsally and volarly. If there is crepitus, pain, and extreme laxity, the test is positive.

benediction attitude s.: for paralysis of the anterior interosseous branch of the median nerve; in the resting hand the index finger and thumb are held in full extension.

benediction s.: in low ulnar nerve palsy; there is metacarpophalangeal hyperextension, proximal and distal interphalangeal joint flexion in the fourth and fifth digits, and the index and middle fingers are relatively spared.

Bouvier m.: in low ulnar nerve palsy; passively preventing metacarpophalangeal hyperextension will allow proximal and distal interphalangeal extension.

Boyes t.: for boutonnière deformity; with full extension of the proximal interphalangeal joint of the finger, there is decreased distal interphalangeal flexion compared with the contralateral finger.

bracelet t.: for early rheumatoid arthritis involving the distal radioulnar joint; compression of the lower ends of the ulna and radius elicits moderate lateral pain.

Carducci t.: for boutonnière deformity; with full metaphalangeal and wrist flexion there is 15- to 20-degree loss of proximal interphalangeal extension compared with the contralateral finger.

carpal compression t.: compression of the carpal tunnel for as long as 30 seconds will produce or exacerbate symptoms of carpal tunnel syndrome. A sphygmomanometer bulb can gauge the proper pressure of approximately 150 mm Hg.

circumduction m.: for the thumb; any general test or motion involving a rotation action of a group of joints; a range-of-motion examination.

claw hand s.: in lower ulnar nerve palsy, there is metacarpophalangeal hyperextension with proximal and distal interphalangeal flexion, and intrinsic minus posture in all palmar digits. These may be static or dynamic.

confrontational t.: for intrinsic muscle weakness of the hand; the strength of specific muscle or muscle groups is compared by pressing the thumb or finger against opposite thumb or finger in a fashion to produce resistance against those muscles. Weakness is indicated by an inability to oppose the compared digits with equal strength (i.e., one side gives out).

Duchenne s.: in low ulnar nerve palsy with extrinsic muscles intact; the ring and little fingers will claw with metacarpophalangeal hyperextension and flexion of the middle and distal phalanges.

Durkan t.: median nerve compression at the wrist exacerbates symptoms in carpal tunnel syndrome.

Elson middle slip t.: for ruptured central extensor tendon slip of the proximal interphalangeal (PIP) joint; the finger is flexed to 90 degrees. If the central slip is intact, the patient can extend the PIP joint, but the distal interphalangeal (DIP) joint is flail. Otherwise, the PIP joint will not have extension power, and the DIP joint will extend while in that position.

extrinsic tightness t.: to assess extrinsic extensor tendon adherence or foreshortening; passive metacarpophalangeal (MCP) joint flexion will cause MCP joint hyperextension. MCP flexion will force the PIP joint into extension.

Finkelstein s.: bending the thumb into the palm to determine synovitis of the abductor pollicis longus tendon to wrist. Passively flexing and ulnar deviating the wrist with the thumb in full opposition will elicit pain over the first dorsal extensor compartment in de Quervain disease.

Fowler m.: for testing rheumatoid arthritis; tight intrinsic muscles in ulnar deviation of the digits and a heavy, taut ulnar band are demonstrated when the digit is held in its normal axial relationship.

Froment s.: for ulnar nerve loss; there is paralysis of the adductor pollicis and first dorsal interosseous and second palmar interosseous. The flexor pollicis longus flexes the interphalangeal joint up to 90 degrees to effect power pinch.

Guilliatt tourniquet t.: to diagnose carpal tunnel syndrome; a tourniquet is placed on the upper arm of affected limb. Inflate cuff to a point above the systolic pressure to 220 mm Hg. Arm pain normally occurs within 2 to 3 minutes. Tingling in the median nerve distribution of thumb, index, and long finger will occur in 30 to 60 seconds in carpal tunnel syndrome.

grip-strength t.: to measure the strength of coordination of intrinsic and extrinsic finger and thumb flexors; a grip dynamometer is used.

Hutchinson s.: seen in malignant melanoma; lesion under a fingernail or toenail in which the pigment extends into the proximal nail fold.

International Classification for Surgery of the Hand in Tetraplegia
To determine extent of muscle capacity for intrinsic and extrinsic muscle and tendon transfers that improve hand function:
Motor Group
0: no muscle below elbow available
1: BR > 4+
2: BR and ECRL > 4+
3: BR, ECRL, and ECRB > 4+
4: BR, ECRL, ECRB, and PT > 4+
5: BR, ECRL, ECRB, PT, and FCR > 4+
6: BR, ECRL, ECRB, PT, FCR, and finger extensors > 4+
7: BR, ECRL, ECRB, PT, FCR, finger extensors, and thumb extensors > 4+
8: BR, ECRL, ECRB, PT, FCR, finger and thumb extensors, and partial digital flexors > 4+
9: lacks only intrinsic muscle function
X: exceptions
Sensation
0: two-point discrimination in the thumb > 10 mm
Ocu: two-point discrimination in the thumb < 10 mm

BR, *Brachioradialis*; ECRB, *extensor carpi radialis brevis*; ECRL, *extensor carpi radialis longus*; FCR, *flexor carpi radialis*; PT, *pronator teres*.

intrinsic tightness t: to assess adherence or contracture of intrinsic muscles with metacarpophalangeal joint passively extended. Active or passive proximal interphalangeal flexion is limited.

Jeanne t.: in ulnar nerve palsy; with adduction, pollicis dysfunction with metacarpophalangeal hyperextension will result with key pinch or gross grip.

Kanavel s.: for infection of a tendon sheath; there is a point of maximum tenderness in the palm 1 inch proximal to the base of the little finger. In pyogenic tenosynovitis, the four signs are a flexed position of the finger, symmetric fusiform enlargement of the fingers, marked tendon sheath tenderness, and pain on passive digital extension.

Kapandji thumb opposition score: for ability to oppose thumb; with fingers extended, increasing ability to oppose from base of index to the finger tip, graded 1 to 3; 4, opposition to long finger tip; 5, opposition to ring finger tip; 6 to 8, opposition from tip of little finger to base; 9, opposition to palm distal to flexion crease; 10, opposition to palm proximal to flexion crease.

key pinch: the strength in the ability to grasp, as in holding a key; see also **pulp pinch**.

Kleinman shear t.: to assess triquetrolunate disability. Stabilize the lunate with a thumb placed on the dorsum of the lunate. If the test is positive, the pisotriquetral joint is pushed dorsally from the volar side with pain, crepitus, and increased motion.

Lichtman t.: in nondissociative midcarpal instability; a painful clunk is elicited with passive (and sometimes active) ulnar deviation of the wrist. The clunk occurs as the hamate reduces on the triquetrum and the entire proximal row rotates rapidly from its flexed to an extended position.

long finger extension t.: for radial (supinator) tunnel compression; the patient holds wrist at 30 degrees extension while extending all fingers. The examiner attempts to press on the dorsum of the long finger to produce the dorsal forearm symptoms.

Lovett t.: for boutonnière deformity; with full metaphalangeal and wrist flexion there is decrease in proximal interphalangeal extension strength compared with the contralateral finger.

Maisonneuve s.: for Colles fracture; there is marked hyperextensibility of the hand.

masses s.: in ulnar nerve palsy; there is flattening of the metacarpal arch and hypothenar atrophy caused by intrinsic dysfunction with loss of metacarpophalangeal flexion of the fifth digit.

Murphy s.: for scaphoid fracture or lunate dislocation; tapping on the index metacarpal head causes pain with navicular fracture and tapping long finger metacarpal head causes pain with lunate dislocation.

Oshsner clasping t.: for high median nerve paralysis; the index finger will not flex when clasped hands are brought together.

Phalen t. or Phalen m.: for carpal tunnel syndrome; irritation of the median nerve is determined by holding the wrist flexed or extended for 30 to 60 seconds, reproducing symptoms.

piano key s.: test for distal radioulnar joint instability; the wrist is pronated, the radius and ulna are grasped in examiner's hands, and moving each bone up and down relative to the other, a painful movement indicates instability.

Pitres-Testut s.: for ulnar nerve paralysis; the patient is unable to make a cone shape with the hand and fingers because of intrinsic muscle weakness.

Pollock s.: in high ulnar nerve palsy; inability to flex the distal interphalangeal joints of the fourth and fifth digits with paralysis of the flexor digitorum profundus to fourth and fifth digits.

Prehension t.: the ability to grasp with the fingers and thumb in opposition.

pseudostability t.: for carpal bone stability; in the normal wrist, if the hand is held in one hand and the distal forearm in the other, there is a normal anterior posterior translation. This translation is lost in carpal bone instability.

pulp pinch: the strength in the position one would use to pick up a piece of paper. See also **key pinch**.

scaphoid t.: for dynamic scapholunate instability; the examiner places his or her thumb under the scaphoid tubercle, moving wrist from ulnar to radial deviation. The scaphoid flexes against the thumbs in an upward push causing a painful clunk at the scapholunate articulation; also called a **Watson t.**

Smith and Ross t.: for boutonnière deformity; with passive metaphalangeal joint and wrist flexion, there is passive posterior interphalangeal extension if the central slip is intact, and a greater than 20-degree lag if there is central slip rupture.

spilled teacup s.: in perilunate dislocation; the lunate will assume a volar flexed posture as seen on lateral radiographs. A spectrum exists from normal lunate position to complete volar dislocation of the lunate.

table top t.: for timing of surgery in Dupuytren contracture; the patient has limitation putting hand flat on table top.

tenodesis t.: to check structure integrity of the extrinsic extensors; extreme wrist flexion will passively extend the metacarpophalangeal joints, whereas wrist extension will allow passive digital proximal and distal interphalangeal flexion. This is due to resting tension of extrinsic extensor and flexor groups, respectively.

Terry Thomas sign: for scapholunate ligament disruption, separation of the lunate from the scaphoid seen on AP radiograph.

tuck s.: the puckering seen just proximal to a mass of chronically inflamed dorsal tenosynovium. This is accentuated by digital extension and commonly seen in rheumatoid arthritis.

two-point discrimination t.: measures innervation density under the skin. Static two-point discrimination t. is for *slowly* adapting fibers; moving two-point discrimination t. is for *rapidly* adapting fibers. It is the ability to distinguish one point and two points with eyes closed. (Normal range is 1–5 mm.)

ulnar fovea s.: for split tear of the ulnar triquetral ligament or foveal disruption of the radial ulnar ligament; direct pressure between the flexor carpi ulnaris and the distal ulnar styloid (fovea) produces exquisite pain.

Wartenberg s.: for intrinsic muscle weakness of the hand; while the fingers are extended there is an inability to bring together the ring and little finger. In ulnar nerve palsy with interosseous paralysis, there is an inability to adduct the extended fifth digit to fourth digit; also called **oriental prayer s.**

Watson t.: for scapholunate instability; the examiner can elicit a painful wrist click by compressing the scaphoid while the patient moves the wrist; also called **rotary click t.**

wet leather s.: subcutaneous palpable crepitus or squeaking with movement of tendons affected by tenosynovitis.

Hips

Allis m.: for reduction of anterior hip dislocation; the supine patient has the knee flexed, hip slightly flexed with longitudinal traction, and an assistant stabilizes the pelvis while applying a lateral traction force to the medial thigh. The surgeon then adducts and internally rotates the femur.

Allis s.: for femoral neck fracture or congenital dislocation hip; there is relaxation of the fascia between the crest of the ilium and the greater trochanter.

anvil t.: for early hip joint disease or diseased vertebrae; a closed fist striking a blow to the sole of the foot with leg extended produces pain in the hip or vertebrae.

Barlow t.: for dysplastic hip in infants; holding the symphysis pubis to sacrum with one hand, the opposite hip is flexed and an attempt is made to dislocate the hip. Pulling the hip back up or abducting the hip should produce a perceptible reduction.

Bigelow reduction m.: for posterior dislocation of the hip. The hip is flexed and adducted. While traction is maintained, the femoral head is levered into the acetabulum by abduction, external rotation, and extension of the hip.

Bozan m.: for reducing femoral neck fractures; a large swathe is placed around the crest of the ilium of the affected limb and a small swathe in the inguinal fold; traction, abduction, and internal rotation forces are then applied.

Chapple t.: for infant congenital hip dislocation; the hips cannot be abducted past 45 degrees while in flexion.

Chiene t.: for determining fracture of the neck of the femur by use of a tape measure.

Desault s.: for intracapsular fracture of the hip; alternation of the arc described by rotation of the greater trochanter, which normally describes the segment of a circle, but in this fracture, rotates only as the apex of the femur rotates about its own axis.

Destot s.: in a pelvic fracture; there is the formation of a large superficial hematoma beneath the inguinal ligament and in the scrotum.

Deyerle m.: for femoral neck fracture reduction; patient placed in traction with over-distraction and external rotation. The leg is then internally rotated with some traction release and inward pressure on the greater trochanter to reduce and impact fracture site.

Earle s.: for pelvic fracture; bony prominence or hematoma associated with tenderness on rectal examination.

East Baltimore m.: for posterior hip dislocation; two-person reduction maneuver with patient supine and hip in 90 degrees flexion.

Ely t.: for determining tightness of the rectus femoris, contracture of the lateral fascia of the thigh, or femoral nerve irritation; with patient in prone position, flexion of the leg on the thigh causes buttocks to arch away and leg to abduct at the hip joint; also called **Nachlas knee flexion t.**

Galeazzi s.: for congenital dislocation of the hip; the dislocated side is shorter when both thighs are flexed to 90 degrees, as demonstrated in infants; in an older patient, a curvature of the spine is produced by shortened leg.

gear-stick s.: for femoral head deformity of dysplastic hip or Legg-Calvé-Perthes disease; thigh abduction is full in flexion, but as the hip is extended with the hip abducted, there is impingement between the greater trochanter and ilium.

Jansen t.: for osteoarthritic deformity of the hip; the patient is asked to cross the legs with a point just above the ankle resting on the opposite knee. If significant disease exists, this motion is impossible.

King m.: for femoral neck fracture reduction; on fracture table, the affected leg is in traction with pressure placed on the posterior thigh with internal rotation. Lateral traction with a groin sling may be added.

Langoria s.: for symptoms of intracapsular fracture of the femur; relaxation of the extensor muscles of the thigh is present.

Leadbetter m.: for slipped capital femoral epiphysis or femoral head fracture; injured hip is flexed to 90 degrees and manual traction applied to axis of the flexed thigh with adduction. The leg is then circumducted slowly to abduction maintaining internal rotation, and then the thigh and leg are brought down to the horizontal level.

Lefkowitz m.: for posterior dislocation of the hip. The patient's hip and knee are flexed, with the patient's leg over the provider's flexed knee. A downward force is applied to the patient's foot while the provider raises the knee, reducing the hip.

Ludloff s.: for traumatic separation of the epiphysis of the lesser trochanter; swelling and ecchymosis are present at the base of Scarpa triangle, together with inability to raise the thigh when in a sitting position.

McCarthy s.: for labral tears; with both hips flexed the patient's pain is reproduced by extending the hip in external rotation first, followed by extending the hip in internal rotation. Also, there is inguinal pain with flexion, adduction, and internal rotation.

McElvenny m.: for femoral neck fracture reduction; with 36- to 45-kg traction, the hip is abducted and internally rotated. Medial to inferior force is produced over the greater trochanter, and then the hip is adducted.

Nélaton l.: for detecting dislocation of the hip; there is a line from the anterosuperior iliac spine to the ischial tuberosity, which normally passes through the greater trochanter. Term is also used in radiology.

Ober t.: for tight tensor fascia lata; with patient lying on side with hip and knee flexed, the opposite hip is extended while the knee is flexed. Inability to place the knee being tested on the table surface indicates a tight fascia lata.

obturator s.: inward rotation of the hip so that the obturator internus muscle is stretched. Results may be positive in acute appendicitis.

Ortolani t.: for congenitally dislocated hip; an audible click is heard when the hip goes into the socket as noted in infancy. If the sign is elicited, the dislocation should be corrected at that time to avoid hip dysfunction later; also called **Ortolani click.**

Patrick t.: for pathologic conditions of the sacroiliac joint; the patient's hip is placed into abduction, flexion, and external rotation, and pain is elicited with further forced abduction. Also called **FABERE t.**

piston s.: for congenital dislocation of the head of the femur; if positive, there is up-and-down movement of the head of the femur; also called **Dupuytren s.**

post-total hip internal rotation t.: for assessing hip dislocation risk after capsular healing; hip is flexed to 90 degrees and then internal rotation to end point. Internal rotation of 15 degrees or less indicate that hip dislocation precautions can be discontinued.

reverse Bigelow m.: for anterior dislocation of the hip; two maneuvers are done, both starting in hip flexion and abduction. In the first maneuver, while lifting the lower leg of the supine patient, there is a quick jerk on the flexed thigh; the second maneuver involves traction in the line of deformity with the hip then being adducted, sharply internally rotated, and extended.

Roux s.: in a pelvic lateral compression fracture, there is a distance between the greater trochanter and pubic spine on the affected side.

Smith m.: for reduction of femoral neck fractures; thigh is externally rotated and placed in traction, then fully abducted, internally rotated, and subsequently adducted.

Stimson m.: for posterior hip dislocation; the patient is placed prone on a table with the involved hip flexed and the opposite hip extended. With the involved knee flexed downward, pressure is applied to the calf, resulting in reduction of the dislocation.

Thomas s.: for hip joint flexion contracture; when the patient is walking, the fixed flexion of the hip can be compensated by lumbar lordosis. With the patient supine and flexing the opposite hip, the affected thigh raises off the table; also called **Strümpell s.** and **Thomas t.**

Trendelenburg t.: for muscular weakness in poliomyelitis, ununited fracture of the femoral neck, rheumatoid arthritis, coxa vara, and congenital dislocations. With the patient standing, weight is removed from one extremity. If gluteal fold drops on that side, it signifies muscular weakness of the opposite weight-bearing hip; also called **Trendelenburg s.**

Wellmerling m.: for femoral neck fracture reduction; the affected hip is overdistracted by 0.64 cm (¼ inch) in external rotation, and the foot is then internally rotated and traction released.

Whitman m.: for femoral neck fracture reduction; the hip is flexed and then extended with traction being applied and the normal hip abducted. The affected side is then abducted and a spica cast applied.

Lower Limbs

Achilles squeeze t.: for Achilles tendon rupture; with patient prone and knees flexed, squeezing the calf muscle fails to produce plantar flexion of the ankle joint; also called **Thompson t.** and **Simmons t.**

Addis t.: for determination of leg-length discrepancy; with patient in prone position, flexing the knees to 90 degrees reveals the potential discrepancies of both tibial and femoral lengths.

anterior tibial s.: for spastic paraplegia; involuntary extension of the tibialis anterior muscle when thigh is actively flexed on the abdomen.

Cleeman s.: for distal fracture of femur with overriding of the fragments; shows creasing of the skin just above the patella.

Homan s.: pain in calf on dorsiflexion of foot (active or passive). Once considered a reliable test in diagnosing deep vein thrombophlebitis but no longer considered valid.

Payr s.: early sign of impending postoperative thrombosis, indicated by tenderness when pressure is placed over the inner side of the foot.

Schlesinger s.: for extensor spasm at the knee joint; with patient's leg held at the knee joint and flexed strongly at the hip joint, there will follow an extensor spasm at the knee joint with extreme supination of the foot.

tourniquet t.: for phlebitis of the leg; tourniquet is applied to the thigh and pressure gradually increased until the patient complains of pain in the calf; result is compared with the effect on the opposite leg.

Knees (Table 4-1)

active glide t.: the appearance of lateral excursion of the patella greater than proximal excursion, with quadriceps contraction, indicates an increased functional Q angle.

anterior cruciate instability t.: with the knee flexed, a supine patient extends the knee slowly with the foot against the table surface; there is a sudden anterior shift of the tibia. This test might be confused with a quadriceps active test for posterior cruciate ligament

TABLE 4-1 Knee Instability Tests

Instability	Positive Test	Deficient Structure
Medial	Valgus stress at 30 degrees	Medial collateral ligament
Lateral	Varus stress at 30 degrees	Minor lateral complex tear
Anterior	Anterior drawer at 90 degrees, neutral rotation	Anterior cruciate and partial medial and lateral collateral ligaments
Posterior	Posterior drawer at 90 degrees	Posterior cruciate, arcuate complex, posterior oblique ligaments
Anteromedial	Slocum at 30 degrees external rotation accented	Medial capsular, tibial collateral, posterior oblique, anterior cruciate ligaments
Anterolateral	Slocum at 15 degrees internal rotation accented	Lateral capsular ligament
	Jerk test	Arcuate complex
	Lateral pivot shift	Anterior cruciate ligament
Posterolateral	Reverse pivot shift	Arcuate complex, lateral capsular ligament, popliteus tendon, some posterior cruciate ligament
Posteromedial (controversial)	Medial tibial plateau shifts posterior on stress	Tibial collateral, medial capsular, posterior oblique, semimembranosus, anterior cruciate ligaments

injury, which gives the same forward motion of the tibia on the femoral condyles, but from a posterior subluxed position to a reduced position. In the case of the anterior cruciate instability test, the forward motion of the tibia begins from a position of a reduced joint and subluxes anteriorly.

Apley t.: for differentiating ligament from meniscal injury; with a prone patient and the knee flexed 90 degrees, tibial rotation while applying compression results in pain caused by meniscal pathologic findings and is generally specific to the side of the meniscal injury. Articular injury or chondromalacia may result in a positive Apley t.; also called **Apley grind t.**

arthrometer t.: mechanical testing device for measuring anteroposterior ligament stability of the knee. The arthrometer is most often used in a physician's office to document the outcome of anterior cruciate ligament replacement surgery.

ballotable patella t.: for knee effusion; with knee extension, pushing patella onto distal femoral surface results in rebound caused by swelling.

bayonet s.: lateral placement of infrapatellar tendon with a valgus knee produces a bayonet appearance in the quadriceps-patellar-tendon complex.

bounce home t.: for bucket-handle tear of meniscus; passive pressure past maximum active extension results in a bounce back to more flexion.

British t.: for knee pain or injury; compression of patella during active quadriceps contraction as knee is extended elicits pain. Generally specific for patellofemoral chondromalacia or pathologic condition.

bulge s.: for knee effusion; fluid is pressed into the superior pouch and then medially or laterally, resulting in a fluid bulge.

camelback s.: an unusually prominent infrapatellar fat pad of the knee and hypertrophy of the vastus lateralis.

Childress t.: for torn meniscus; when duck walking, the supporting leg will have pain on the side of the torn meniscus.

cross-over t.: for anterior cruciate ligament laxity; with patient's permission, the examiner stands on the foot of the affected side of standing patient. When the patient attempts to cross the opposite leg over the knee there is a sense of the knee feeling unstable.

dial t.: for posterolateral corner and posterior cruciate instability; isolated posterior cruciate instability will allow 15 degree plus increased passive external rotation of the foot and ankle when the knee is flexed at 90 degrees. Posterolateral corner instability will have 15 degree or greater increased external rotation of the foot and ankle at 30 degrees; also called **Cooper t.**

double camelback s.: prominence of a high-riding patella and infrapatellar fat pad, producing the appearance of a camelback.

double PCL sign: on magnetic resonance imaging there appears to be two posterior cruciate ligaments due to a displaced bucket handle meniscal tear seen on midline sagittal images of the knee. There is a low-signal-intensity band that is parallel and antero-inferior to the ligament.

drawer s.: may be anterior or posterior for ligamentous instability or ruptured cruciate ligaments; with the patient supine and knee flexed to 90 degrees and the foot plantigrade on the table, the sign is positive if the tibia can be delivered either anteriorly or posteriorly beyond normal when compared with the uninjured knee. Excessive anterior drawer indicates an incompetent anterior cruciate ligament whereas excessive posterior drawer is a sign of posterior cruciate ligament injury.

drop-back phenomenon: for posterior cruciate rupture; posterior sag of tibia in relationship to distal femur when knee is flexed and patient is at rest; also called **sag s.**

extension lag: a sign of patella or quadriceps tendon rupture; there is an injury-related change in the ability of the patient to actively extend the knee.

external rotation drawer t.: with the foot held in external rotation, an anterior drawer test is completed. A slight increase in anterior drawer is found in normal knees, whereas a larger amount of anterior laxity is indicative of anterior cruciate ligament and medial collateral ligament injury.

external rotation recurvatum t: with the patient supine, lifting the entire leg off the table by the great toe results in a posterior sag and external rotation of the tibia in reference to the normal alignment of the leg, indicating a posterior cruciate ligament tear with or without a posterior lateral ligamentous injury as well.

Fairbank s.: for subluxating patella; with the affected knee in extension the examiner pushes the patella in a lateral direction, causing apprehension.

figure 4 t.: placing the knee in a figure four position, the lateral collateral ligament (LCL) can often be palpated coursing from the fibular head to the lateral epicondyle and checked for integrity. When injured, this position puts stress on the LCL and can result in pain in the presence of an injury to the lateral and posterolateral ligamentous structures.

Finacetto s.: Lachman test with tibial subluxation beyond the posterior horns of the meniscus indicates a severe anterior cruciate ligament deficiency and instability.

flexion rotation drawer t.: with the knee extended and the thigh relaxed, there is anterolateral tibial subluxation. The knee is gradually flexed with reduction of the subluxation occurring at approximately 30 degrees of flexion. Roughly synonymous with pivot shift test as it relates to evidence of anterior cruciate ligament insufficiency and is less painful to most patients. Also called **Noyes t.**

Fouchet s. (Allis t.): for tibial or femoral insufficiency, with the patient supine and knees flexed with equal rotation of the tibia, a short tibia can be distinguished for a short femur.

Godfrey t.: for posterior cruciate ligament laxity; with patient supine and the knee and hip flexed at 90 degrees and the examiner supporting heel, the proximal tibia is more posterior on the affected side. Best seen on a side-to-side comparison; also called **sag t.**

grand piano s.: the appearance of the trochlear surface after the anterior femoral cut has been made in preparation for the femoral prosthetic component. If the rotation of the femoral guide is correct, that cut surface should have two times greater exposed bone on the lateral than on the medial side, appearing like a grand piano seen from above.

grimace t.: for knee pain or crepitus; if compression of the patella elicits pain or crepitus is noted, the patient will grimace.

heel height difference: for knee flexion contracture; prone patient in knee extension has different level of heels; also called **prone hanging t.**

heel-to-buttocks difference: for swelling or obstruction of flexion; the heel is further from the buttocks in flexion compared with the unaffected side; also called **symmetrical extension t.**

Helft t.: for proximal tibiofibular instability; the standing patient is asked to gradually flex the involved knee. If laxity exists the person will cross the opposite leg and foot behind the affected knee to stabilize it.

hop t.: for anterior cruciate examination; patient hops forward on affected knee. Ability to do this is one sign of adequate anterior cruciate stability. Also called **one-legged hop t.**

Hughston jerk t.: for anterolateral instability of the knee; noted by starting at 90 degrees flexion with tibia internally rotated and applying valgus force while rotating fibula medially. There is a jerk at approximately 20 degrees from full extension.

internal-rotation drawer t.: with the foot internally rotated, an anterior drawer test should in a normal knee result in less anterior displacement, whereas a looser drawer is found in anterior cruciate ligament–deficient knees. Also called **anterior drawer s.**

J s.: bringing the knee into extension results in a lateral deviation of the patella thought to reproduce the track of an inverted J, which may indicate patellar instability or maltracking.

Lachman t.: with the patient supine and the knee flexed to 20 degrees, the tibia is pulled anteriorly. A lack of a solid endpoint to when the anterior cruciate ligament (ACL) reaches its limit of length indicates a probable ACL tear. It is important to always compare the injured knee to the normal knee to determine the extent and feel for a normal end-point. Also called **Noulis t.**

lack of extension s.: a perceptible lack of passive full extension in the early postinjury period following an anterior cruciate ligament (ACL) tear; the possible result of soft tissue impingement in the intercondylar notch from the tibial sided remnant of the torn ACL.

loss of extension t.: for anterior cruciate injury, in the absence of extensor mechanism injury, when compared to the uninjured knee the patient is unable to fully extend the knee when in a supine position.

Losse t.: for posterolateral laxity; the supine patient has the affected knee held at 30 degrees flexion with the distal leg on the examiner's chest and the examiner's opposite thumb behind the head of the fibula and fingers on the patella. As the thumb pulls the fibular head forward, the knee is gradually extended and a shift should occur as the plateau subluxes anteriorly.

McMurray t.: internal and external tibial rotation while moving from a starting point of maximal flexion into extension results in pain isolated to the side of meniscal pathologic condition. In general, internal rotation of the tibia results in lateral meniscus tear symptoms whereas external rotation results in medial meniscus pathologic symptoms; also called **McMurray s.**

medial subluxation t.: for tight lateral patellar retinaculum; the patella is pressed in a medial direction with the knee at full extension and then at 30 degrees of flexion. More that 15 mm of medial displacement in flexion implies that the patella tracks laterally because of a tight retinaculum.

Merke s.: for meniscal tear; the standing patient will have a meniscal tear on the medial side if there is pain on internal rotation, and a tear on the lateral side if there is pain on external rotation.

no touch t.: for checking patellar stability after total knee joint replacement and for anterior cruciate instability; with the patient supine and the knee flexed, there is a sudden anterior shift of the tibia when the patient extends the knee slowly with the foot on the surface; also called **quadriceps active t.**

patellar apprehension t.: pushing patella laterally, the most common direction of instability, results in patient apprehension for symptoms of patellar instability.

patellar glide t.: for maltracking of the patella; the sitting patient is asked to extend the knee and the tracking of the patella is observed. Maltracking is typically in a lateral direction.

patellar grind t.: described as being for chondromalacia patella; this is a nonspecific test in which the patella is pressed into the trochlea on active or passive knee extension from flexion. Pain may be from the patella or from regional synovium; also called **Fouchet s.**

patellar retraction t.: for synovitis; compression of patella causes pain when the patient attempts to set the quadriceps muscles with the knee in full extension.

patellar tilt t.: for lateral retinacular tightness; examiner tries to lift up the outside edge of the patella (kneecap) using his thumb. The patella should not be pushed to the inside or the outside. Inability to lift implies tight retinaculum.

pivot-jerk t.: a lesser utilized test for anterior cruciate ligament insufficiency wherein the knee goes from a position of anterolateral femoral tibial reduction to an anterolateral shift when taking the knee from flexion to extension while applying a valgus movement with internal tibial rotation. Also called **pivot shift t.**

pivot-shift t.: with the knee extended, the examiner internally rotates the leg and with a valgus stress gradually flexes the knee. There is a shift at 30 to 40 degrees of flexion, from anterolateral subluxation to a reduced knee, which is the result of the mechanical advantage of the hamstrings in pulling the tibia posteriorly behind a flexed knee. Patient relaxation is key for optimal results, and, although it can be achieved outside the operating room, results are best noted under anesthesia. Also called **MacIntosh t.**

posterior drawer t.: with the hips at 45 degrees and the knees flexed at 90 degrees the examiner sits on the foot and pushes the tibia backward; also with the hips and knees flexed at 90 degrees the heels are held together and the two knees observed for comparison of relative posterior sag of the tibia.

prone external rotation t.: for posterior cruciate knee rupture; with the patient prone and knees flexed at 30 degrees, the test is considered positive for rupture if the foot externally rotates more than 15 degrees compared with the normal side. Increasing the flexion to 90 degrees with an accompanying further increase of external rotation difference, when compared side to side, indicates the presence of a posterior cruciate ligament injury as well; also called **dial t.**

prone hanging (prone hang) t.: for knee flexion tightness, with patient prone, knee resting on the end of the examination table, the height of the heels is measured.

quadriceps active t.: with the patient supine, the involved knee is flexed at 90 degrees and the foot rests on the table. With one hand, the examiner supports the thigh and palpates the relaxed quadriceps muscle; the other hand stabilizes the foot. When the patient is asked to slide the foot down the table, the proximal leg is pulled forward to its posteriorly subluxed resting point by the patellar tendon, indicating a posterior cruciate tear with resulting posterior sagging of the leg.

reverse pivot-shift t.: with the patient supine, the lateral tibial plateau shifts from posterior subluxation to reduction as the knee is brought from flexion to extension. Also called **Jacob t.** and **jerk t.**

sag sign: for posterior cruciate rupture, with the patient supine and the knee flexed to 90 degrees, the tibial appears more posteriorly displaced compared to the unaffected knee.

screw-home mechanism: the small degree of external rotation that occurs as the knee is brought to the last few degrees of extension.

Slocum t.: for rotary instability of the knee; the examiner pulls on the upper calf of a supine patient with the knees flexed 90 degrees. Then, while sitting on the patient's foot, the examiner pulls anteriorly, comparing the amount of give with the foot turned in 15 degrees neutral and turned out 30 degrees.

standing apprehension t.: for anterior cruciate laxity; with patient standing and knee slightly flexed, examiner's hand holds the knee firmly with the thumb pushing the lateral femoral condyle medially, resulting in motion.

Steinmann t.: for medial meniscal tear; on the supine patient the knee is held flexed at 90 degrees, the calf held firmly, and the tibia rotated internally and externally. Sharp medial pain implies a meniscal tear.

symmetrical extension t.: a noticeable difference in the back of the knee to examination table with the patient in the supine position or in prone heel height indicates an extension deficit that can be the result of contractures, bucket-handle meniscal tears, mechanical block, or ligamentous injury. Also called **lack of extension test for ACL injury.**

Thessaly t: for meniscal injury; with support, the patient stands and rotates the knee and body internally and externally three times, keeping the knee flexed at 20 degrees. Joint-line discomfort medial or lateral is a positive test.

thumbnail t.: for patellar fracture; fracture is felt as a sharp crevice when the examiner's thumbnail is passed over the subcutaneous surface of the patella.

tibial sag s.: a noticeable posterior sag of the tibia in reference to the femoral condyles with the knee flexed 90 degrees and the foot plantigrade on the examination table. This test and sign is best noted when both limbs are symmetrically placed and a side-to-side difference is visualized. This may be thought of as a passive posterior drawer.

tilt t.: for lateral retinacular tightness; examiner tries to lift up the outside edge of the patella (kneecap) using his thumb. The patella should not be pushed to the inside or the outside. Inability to lift implies tight retinaculum.

towel clip t.: for patellar subluxability in joint replacement surgery; the vastus medialis and medial retinaculum is approximated to the medial border of the patella using a towel clip or a stitch. The knee is taken through a range of motion. Any elevation of the medial edge of the patella is considered a positive test for a tight lateral retinaculum.

Trotter bulge t.: for knee swelling; massaging pressure on medial side of knee may make swelling move superiorly so that pressure from above may make fluid more apparent on return to medial side.

varus recurvatum t.: for posterior lateral instability, with the patient supine, the examiner presses down on the distal femur while hyperextending the knee and applying a varus stress.

valgus stress t.: although this term is commonly applied to the knee, the test may also be done on the elbow. The upper part of the limb is supported while a laterally directed force is produced on the distal limb. If knee laxity is found in full extension, both the anterior cruciate and medial collateral ligaments are compromised. If there is laxity at only 30 degrees, there is an isolated medial collateral ligament tear.

valgus thrust t.: for isolated medial collateral ligament rupture, the knee is flexed at 30 degrees and with the examiners hand on the lateral knee there is sudden lateral pressure applied to the ankle.

varus stress t.: although this term is commonly applied to the knee, the test may also be done on the elbow. The upper part of the limb is supported while a medially directed force is produced on the distal limb. If knee laxity is found in full extension, both the anterior cruciate and lateral collateral ligaments are compromised. If there is laxity at only 30 degrees, an isolated medial collateral ligament tear or posterolateral corner injury is likely.

vertical patella t.: during knee joint replacement surgery the patella is initially everted to 90 degrees in relation to the femoral component and then translated medially so that its lateral border is past the middle of the intercondylar groove of the femoral component while still everted. The inability to translate it past the midpoint of the intercondylar groove of the femoral component suggests a tight lateral retinaculum.

Wilson s.: with knee extended from 90 degrees to 30 degrees with valgus stress and internal rotation of the foot, a click is heard in cases of osteochondritis dissecans. The pain is relieved by externally rotating the tibia. Loss of the sign is an index of healing.

Feet and Ankles

Achilles bulge s.: seen in ankle instability; a bulging Achilles tendon occurs when the foot is pulled forward while the leg is pushed backward with the knee flexed; also called **heel-cord s.**

anterior drawer s.: for ankle instability; the heel is pulled forward with the leg being restrained by the opposite hand. A precise lateral radiograph is obtained with the patient supine and both the popliteal area and heel supported and 5 kg applied to the ankle.

Coleman lateral standing block t.: to detect flexibility of cavovarus deformity of foot; lateral side of foot and full heel are placed on a 1-inch block, and loss of varus deformity implies flexibility.

Cotton t.: for distal tibial-fibular diastasis; direct pressure on the heel pressing in a lateral direction widens the medial joint space and tibial-fibular space.

dimple s.: for ruptured lateral collateral ligament of ankle; an anterior force is directed on the heel while a posterior force is directed on the distal leg. In the case of a ruptured ligament, a dimple will appear.

drawer s.: for lateral collateral ligament injury in the ankle; with the foot and ankle at rest and the knee flexed and the ankle flexed at 10- to 15-degree plantar flexion, the heel is pulled forward. The center of rotation is the deltoid ligament.

Harris-Beath footprinting mat: a pressure sensitive mat used to reflect the various pressure points under the foot.

Helbing s.: for hyperpronation of foot; medialward curving of the Achilles tendon as viewed from behind.

hook t.: for lateral ankle instability with fixed medial malleolus; the tibia is grasped with one hand and a hook is placed on the distal fibula. The test is considered positive if there is greater than 2 mm fibular distraction.

Keen s.: for Pott fracture of the fibula; if fracture exists, there is increased diameter around the malleoli area of the ankle.

Marie-Foix s.: for central nervous system disorder; there is withdrawal of the lower leg on transverse pressure of the tarsus or forced flexion of toes, even when the leg is incapable of voluntary movement.

Matles t.: for Achilles tendon rupture; patient lies prone and with knee to 90 degrees. Any dorsiflexion of the foot indicates a ruptured tendon.

McBride t.: for contracture of lateral capsule metatarsal phalangeal joint of the big toe or tight adductor; the patient has an ability to passively put toe in neutral position.

Morton t.: for metatarsalgia or neuroma; transverse pressure across heads of the metatarsals causes sharp pain in the forefoot.

Mulder s.: for interdigital neuroma in the foot; a palpable click can be heard on motion of the metatarsal heads.

Murphy s.: for Achilles tendon bursitis at the heel; dorsiflexion of the foot produces pain.

sagittal stress t.: for ankle instability; with the knee flexed to at least 45 degrees, the foot is pulled forward while the leg is pushed backward. If the usual concavity of the Achilles tendon is flattened or reversed, the sign is positive for an instability of the anterior fibular collateral ligament.

Silfverskiöld t.: for ankle equinus contracture; test passive restriction of ankle dorsiflexion with knee in flexion and extension. Contracture that is due to soleus alone will not change with knee flexion. That caused by gastrocnemius that will have better ankle dorsiflexion when knee is flexed.

Strunsky s.: for detecting lesions of the anterior arch of the foot; sudden flexing of the toes is painless in a normal foot, but painful if inflammation exists in the anterior arch.

talar tilt t.: with the ankle in neutral position, the heel is grasped in one hand and the ankle in the other. The ankle is then supinated with maximum force. An anteroposterior radiograph may be obtained to define the talar tilt.

Thomas squeeze (Simmonds) t.: for Achilles tendon rupture; the prone patient with knee flexed at 90 degrees has calf squeezed. Failure of foot flexion indicated Achilles rupture.

toe spread s.: for Morton neuroma; disproportional spreading of the toes, comparing one foot with the other.

too many toes s.: increased hindfoot, valgus, pronation, and abduction of forefoot. On clinical observation, refers to the excessive number of toes that appear laterally when foot is viewed from behind. Often indicates collapse of the medial arch and flatfoot deformity.

Wu sole opposition t.: for posterior tendon rupture; a visual test that shows a defect as both feet are opposed to each other.

Neurologic Examination

ankle clonus t.: implies a central nervous system condition of cord or brain; sudden forced dorsiflexion of the ankles results in repeated flexion. **Sustained clonus** does not stop as long as dorsiflexion pressure is applied to the foot.

Babinski reflex: for loss of brain control over lower extremities; scraping the soles causes toes to pull up.

Babinski s.: for testing of pathologic conditions of the first sacral nerve root; an absent Achilles tendon reflex or diminished reflex as compared with the other side.

Beevor s: for segmental nerve disease involving T5–T12 or L1 nerve roots; the patient does an active sit-up with the arms held behind the head. In a positive examination, the umbilicus moves toward the segment that is weak.

Brudzinski s.: for meningitis; flexion of the neck forward results in flexion of the hip and knee; when passive flexion of the lower limb on one side is made, a similar movement will be seen in the opposite limb; also called **neck s.** and **contralateral s.**

Chaddock s.: for upper motor neuron loss (brain); the big toe extends when irritating the skin in the external malleolar region; indicates lesions of the corticospinal paths; also called **external malleolus s.** and **Chaddock reflex.**

doll's eye s.: for testing normal or abnormal brain function; the normal coordinated eye motions seen when passively turning the head of an unconscious patient; also called **Cantelli s.**

Ely t.: for L3 and L4 nerve root irritation; flexing thigh with patient prone causes back or thigh pain; also called **femoral nerve stretch t.** and **Ely s.**

fan s.: for central nerve problems; stroking the sole of the foot with a needle causes toes to spread; part of Babinski reflex examination.

finger to nose t.: for cerebellar disease; patient attempts to put a finger on nose and then on the examiner's finger, back and forth rapidly; any incoordination indicates positive test. Also called **coordination extremity t.**

Fournier t.: for determining ataxic gait; it is noted with the patient moving about abruptly in walking, starting, and stopping.

Fränkel s.: for tabes dorsalis; noted by diminished tonicity of muscles about the hip joint.

Gordon reflex: for loss of brain control; percussion on lateral thigh causes toes to go up rather than the normal downward motion.

Guilland s.: for meningeal irritation; when the contralateral quadriceps muscle group is pinched, there is brisk flexion at the hip and knee joint.

heel-bisector method: used for assessing metatarsus adductus. The heel-bisector line passes through the longitudinal axis of the heel. When the foot is held in the simulated weight-bearing position, the line should pass through the second toe. Metatarsus adductus is mild if the line passes through the third toe, moderate if through the fourth toe, and severe if through the fifth toe.

Hirschberg s.: for pyramidal tract disease; internal rotation and adduction of foot on rubbing inner lateral side.

Hoffmann s.: for testing digital reflex; nipping of three fingernails (index, middle, ring) produces flexion of terminal phalanx of thumb and second and third phalanx of some other finger; digital reflex.

Huntington s.: for lesions of the pyramidal tract; patient is supine, with legs hanging over the examining table, and is asked to cough; if coughing produces flexion of the thigh and extension of the leg in the paralyzed limb, a lesion is indicated.

Jendrassik m.: to enhance a patellar reflex; the reflex is tested when the patient hooks hands together with flexed fingers and pulls apart as hard as possible.

Kernig s.: for meningitis; in dorsal decubitus, the patient can easily and completely extend the leg; when sitting or lying down with thigh flexed on the abdomen, the leg cannot be completely extended.

Kerr s.: for spinal cord lesions; alteration of the texture of the skin below the somatic level is used to locate level of lesions.

Klippel-Feil s.: for pyramidal track disorders; passive flexion and extension of index finger causes thumb flexion and adduction.

Leichtenstern s.: for cerebrospinal meningitis; tapping lightly on any bone of the extremities causes patient to wince suddenly.

Léri s.: for hemiplegia; passive flexion of the hand and wrist of the affected side shows no normal flexion at the elbow.

Lhermitte s.: for cervical cord injuries or unstable cervical spine; transient dysesthesia and weakness are noted in all four limbs when the patient flexes the head forward.

long tract s.: any sign that one would see in affection of either sensory or motor tracts in the spinal cord. Examples are the Babinski reflex and the Romberg test.

Mendel-Bekhterev reflex: for organic hemiplegia; using a percussion hammer, the examiner notes flexion of the small toes if the dorsal surface of the cuboid bone is struck.

Moro reflex s.: for testing normal early neurologic development or the failure to progress neurologically; the infant is placed on a table, then the table is forcibly struck from either side, causing the infant's arms to be thrown out as in an embrace; should disappear as infancy progresses.

Morquio s.: for epidemic poliomyelitis; the supine patient resists attempts to raise trunk to a sitting position until the legs are passively flexed.

Medical Research Council (MRC) sensory grade: for assessment of sensation of peripheral nerve after injury or repair. Also called **Zachary sensory grade.**

  S 0: absence of any sensory recovery
  S 1: recovery of deep cutaneous pain sensibility
  S 2: return of some superficial pain and tactile sensibility

- **S 2+:** recovery of touch and pain sensibility throughout the autonomous zone, but with persistent overreaction
- **S 3:** return of superficial pain and tactile sensibility throughout the autonomous zone with disappearance of overreaction
- **S 3+:** as S 3 but with good localization and some return of two-point discrimination
- **S 4:** return of sensibility as in S 3, with recovery of two-point discrimination

nuchocephalic reflex: for diffuse cerebral dysfunction as in senility; when the shoulders are turned to the left or right, there is a failure of the head to turn in that direction within 0.5 second.

Oppenheim s.: for pyramidal tract disease; dorsal extension of the big toe is present when the medial side of the tibia is stroked in a downward direction.

paratonia: for diffuse cerebral dysfunction as in senility; the patient is asked to relax with the elbow passively flexed and extended. Intermittent opposition is abnormal.

Piotrowski s.: for organic disease of the central nervous system; percussion of tibialis muscle produces dorsiflexion and supination; also called **anticus reflex** or **s.**

pronation s.: for central nervous disorders; there is a strong tendency for the forearm to pronate; also called **Strümpell s.**

pseudo-Babinski s.: in poliomyelitis; the Babinski reflex is modified so only the big toe is extended, because all foot muscles except dorsiflexors of the big toe are paralyzed.

Queckenstedt s.: for detecting a block in the vertebral canal; compression of veins in the neck on one or both sides produces rapid rise in pressure of cerebrospinal fluid of a healthy person and quickly disappears. In a patient with blockage in vertebral canal, pressure of cerebrospinal fluid is little or not at all affected.

radialis s.: for nerve impairment; inability to close the fist without marked dorsal extension of the wrist; also called **Strümpell s.**

Raimiste s.: for paretic condition; patient's hand and arm are held upright by examiner; a sound hand remains upright on being released, but a paretic hand flexes abruptly at the wrist.

Romberg t.: for differentiation between peripheral and cerebellar ataxia; increase in clumsiness in movements and in width and uncertainty of gait when patient's eyes are closed indicate peripheral ataxia; no change indicates cerebellar type. (Note: Romberg sign is similar in testing but used for noting tabes dorsalis.)

Sarbó s.: for locomotor ataxia; analgesia of peroneal nerve is noted.

Schreiber m.: for patellar reflex testing; rubbing the inner side of the upper part of thigh enhances the reflex.

stairs s.: in locomotor ataxia; there is difficulty or failure of ability to descend stairs.

station t.: for coordination disturbance; feet are planted firmly together; if the body sways, lack of coordination is indicated.

Strümpell confusion t.: for dyskinesia as seen in cerebral palsy; the sitting patient is asked to flex hips while knee is bent. Ankle dorsiflexion will occur with dyskinesia.

tendon reflexes: for testing continuity of normal muscle to spinal cord to muscle reflex arc. Any tendon may be so tested, but the most common are the deep tendon reflexes:
- **Achilles r.:** ankle jerk
- **biceps r.:** elbow jerk
- **mental r.:** jaw jerk or reflex
- **quadriceps r.:** patellar tendon or knee jerk
- **triceps r.:** elbow jerk

Thomas s.: for cord lesions; pinching of the trapezius muscle causes goose bumps above the level of the cord lesion.

tibialis s.: for spastic paralysis of the lower limb; there is dorsiflexion of the foot when the thigh is drawn toward the body; also called **tibial phenomenon.**

Tinel s: for noting a partial lesion or beginning regeneration of a nerve; tingling sensation of the distal end of a limb when percussion is made over the site of divided nerve as in carpal tunnel impingement on the median nerve of the hand; also called **formication s.** and **distal tingling on percussion (DTP) s.**

Metabolic Tests

Chvostek s.: for determining low serum calcium leading to tetany; tapping the cheek near the facial nerves causes the muscles to twitch or go into spasm; also called **Chvostek t., Chvostek-Weiss s., Weiss s.,** and **Schultze-Chvostek s.**

lead line: a blue line seen in the gums of a patient with lead poisoning; also called **Burton s.**

Tensilon t.: for myasthenia gravis; a chemical test for denoting muscle strength or weakness; injection of edrophonium chloride (Tensilon) will reverse the symptoms in patients whose muscle weakness is caused by myasthenia gravis.

Walker-Mureloch wrist s.: for Marfan syndrome; ability of patient to grasp opposite wrist with fingers and thumb such that the little finger overlaps with thumb caused by narrow wrists and long digits characteristic of that condition.

wrinkle t.: for sensory nerve loss; skin of part that is denervated will not wrinkle like normal skin on prolonged immersion.

General Observations

antecedent s.: any precursory indication of a malady.

artifact: a feature of a *test* that stimulates pathologic condition or interference with the correct results of the test.

café-au-lait: flat, hyperpigmented areas of skin with rugged coast of Maine borders or smooth borders. The presence of four or more café-au-lait spots with coast of Maine borders is seen often in von Recklinghausen disease.

cogwheel phenomenon: jerky motions produced on testing a muscle's strength; the jerks are neither rhythmic nor equal and represent malingering or protection from pain; also called **cogwheel s.**

commemorative s: any sign of a previous disease.

dimple s.: for a variety of joint dislocations; in the shoulder, when there is an anterior dislocation, there is a dimple in the deltoid below the acromion; in a posterolateral dislocation of the knee where the medial femoral condyle buttonholes the anteromedial capsule, the skin is furrowed.

Dupuytren s.: for determining sarcomatous bone; a crackling sensation on compression of that area is noted.

Gower s.: for progressive muscular dystrophy or congenital myopathy; the patient must use hands to press on leg and then thighs to stand up.

hemodynamic t.: to determine the relationship of blood flow in normal as compared with diseased anatomic structures.

Hueter s.: for indication of fracture; absence of the transmission of osseous vibration in fractures as heard by a stethoscope, where the fibrous material is interposed between the fragments.

Langer l.: the normal tension lines of skin commonly used to define direction of scar, as to how the scar runs with or across those lines.

Meryon s.: for muscular dystrophy; when a child is lifted by the underarms, the child will slide through because of shoulder muscle weakness.

objective s.: one that can be seen, heard, measured, or felt by the diagnostician to confirm or deny an ongoing symptom; also called **physical s.**

quadriceps t.: for hyperthyroidism or debilitating condition; while standing, the patient is asked to hold leg up and straight out; a disease is present if patient cannot maintain this position for 1 minute.

Raynaud phenomenon: pallor or blueness of fingers, toes, or nose brought about by exposure to cold and less commonly by other stresses.

somatic s.: any sign presented by trunk or limbs rather than sensory apparatus.

succinylcholine t.: for differentiation of muscle power loss caused by nerve injury or tendon rupture; injection of succinylcholine will produce contractions lasting several minutes when there is denervation.

thumb-to-forearm t.: an index of generalized joint laxity; the examiner places the tip of the thumb on the forearm while flexing the wrist.

Gaits

A patient's walking pattern (gait) is very important in the evaluation of disorders, particularly those affecting the lower limbs. A limp is more apparent in the stance phase of walking. Of the various gait patterns, some have very specific characteristics.

ambling g.: for observing a patient's gait; both upper and lower limbs on the same side advance at the same time.

antalgic g.: because of pain in the stance phase (while walking through on the foot), the time spent on the affected side is shortened compared with that on the normal side.

ataxic g.: usually caused by cerebellar or cord disease; uncoordinated gait with legs lifted high; whole sole of foot strikes at once. Also called **cerebellar g.**

circumduction g.: typically with spastic hemiplegia or cerebral palsy, lower limb is swung forward in a circumduction manner.

Fick angle g.: a measure of toe in and toe out during normal gait; the angle formed by the axis of the foot and the direction of the gait.

foot slap g.: seen in peroneal nerve palsy and other source of ankle dorsiflexor weakness; forefoot comes down hard on the ground after heel strike; also called **drop foot g., equinus g.,** and **slap foot g.**

gluteus maximus g.: because of weak or nonfunctioning hip extensor muscles, the patient thrusts the thorax posteriorly to maintain hip extension; also called **gluteal gait.**

gluteus medius g.: because of weak or nonfunctioning hip abductor muscles, the patient lurches toward the weak side to place the center of gravity over the hip; also called **abductor lurch** and **gluteal lurch.**

scissors g.: in paraplegia or spastic diplegia, thighs cross on ambulation because of overpowering hip adductors. Often the hips are internally rotated with knees and ankles flexed.

shuffling g.: seen in Parkinson disease; walking with feet barely leaving the ground and with short steps.

Trendelenburg g.: lateral bending of trunk when in stance. This can reflect hip disease with pain, muscle weakness of abductors, or lumbar nerve insufficiency.

Scales and Ratings

To have a reproducible presentation of the preoperative and postoperative condition of certain joints, various scales and rating systems have been developed. The scales and ratings are usually based on pain and the degree of functional impairment.

American Shoulder and Elbow Surgeons system: a five-point grading system for level of pain and four-point system for lowest to highest level of function in activities of daily living, work, and sports.

American Spinal Injury Association (ASIA) scale: for spinal cord injury and deficit below injury:
  Grade A: Complete with no motor or sensory function
  Grade B: Incomplete with intact sensory function but no motor function
  Grade C: Incomplete motor function with most muscles Grade < 3
  Grade D: Incomplete motor function with most muscles Grade > or = 3
  Grade E: Normal motor or sensory function

Beighton laxity score: for evaluating generalized laxity; maximum of nine points. One point each (on each side) for hyperextension of the metaphalangeal joints of the hand, ability to touch the volar forearm with the thumb, hyperextension of the elbow, hyperextension of the knee, ability to place hands flat on the floor during toe-touch.

Charnley hip scale: for evaluating hip disease and postoperative results; scale uses pain, range of motion, and function for scoring.

Feller patellar score: for patellar disorders or postsurgical evaluation
  Anterior knee pain
    None: 15
    Mild: 10
    Moderate: 5
    Severe: 0
  Quadriceps strength
    Good (5/5): 5
    Fair (4/5): 3
    Poor (</5): 1
  Ability to rise from chair
    Able with ease (no arms): 5
    Able with ease (with arms): 3
    Able with difficulty: 1
    Unable: 0
  Stair-climbing
    1 foot/stair no support: 5
    1 foot/stair with support: 4

2 feet/stair no support: 3
2 feet/stair with support: 2

Frankel neurologic assessment: for spinal cord injury.
  complete (A): no motor power below the level of the lesion
  sensory (B): no motor power but some sensation below the level of the lesion
  motor useless (C): some motor power below the level of the lesion, but of no functional use to the patient
  motor useful (D): motor power of functional use below the level of the lesion; the patient is able to walk with or without aids
  recovery (E): full motor power, normal sensation, and no sphincter disturbance, although reflexes may be abnormal

Frankel scale: for spinal cord injury and deficit below injury
  Grade A: complete motor and sensory loss
  Grade B: incomplete sensory loss, complete motor loss
  Grade C: sensory function useless, some motor function; no functional strength
  Grade D: sensory function useless; weak but useful motor function.
  Grade E: normal motor or sensory function

Glasgow Coma Score (GCS): for brain injury, score based on eye, verbal and motor. The three values can be used separately or for a sum total score (3–15). The lowest possible sum score is 3, which indicates deep coma or death. The highest is 15, which is a fully awake person. The score is expressed in the form such as GCS 9 = E2 V4 M3. The severity of brain injury is classified as severe (GCS ≤ 8), moderate (GCS 9–12), and minor (GCS ≥ 13).

Best eye response (E)
1. No eye opening
2. Eye opening in response to pain.
3. Eye opening to speech
4. Eyes opening spontaneously

Best verbal response (V)
1. No verbal response
2. Incomprehensible sounds (moaning but no words)
3. Inappropriate words (random or exclamatory articulated speech, but no conversational exchange)
4. Confused (the patient responds to questions coherently but there is some disorientation and confusion)
5. Oriented (patient responds coherently and appropriately to questions such as the patient's name and age, where the patient is and why, the year, month, etc.)

Best motor response (M)
1. No motor response
2. Extension to pain with abduction of arm, internal rotation of shoulder, and pronation of forearm, extension of wrist; decerebrate response
3. Abnormal flexion to pain with adduction of arm, internal rotation of shoulder, pronation of forearm, flexion of wrist; decorticate response
4. Flexion or withdrawal to pain: flexion of elbow, supination of forearm, flexion of wrist when supraorbital pressure applied; pulls part of body away when nail bed is pinched
5. Localizes to pain with purposeful movements toward painful stimuli
6. Obeys commands and does simple things as asked

Green-Anderson growth chart: chart used for measuring height and weight development with comparison to norms.

Harris hip scale: 100-point scale with 40 points for function and 60 points for pain in the hip.

Iowa hip scale: for evaluating hip disease and postoperative results; scale uses pain, range of motion, and function for scoring.

Knee Society clinical rating system: the Knee Society presented this rating system as a uniform system for research. It uses pain and physical examination for a maximum of 100 points. Function is scored by walking and use of stairs for a maximum total of 100 points.

Kujala score: A new questionnaire used to evaluate subjective symptoms and functional limitations in patellofemoral disorders.

Lynholm knee-scoring scale: knee scale incorporating pain, swelling, function, and stability.

Marshall knee-scoring scale: knee scale including symptoms, function, and examination references.

Mazur ankle rating: grading system for the ankle using pain and function as a basis for the rating.

Merle d'Aubigne and Postel hip scale: for evaluating hip disease and postoperative result; scale uses pain, range of motion, and function for scoring.

Norton scoring system: to evaluate pressure ulcer risk. The system is a global scale used by nurses to evaluate pressure ulcer risk. It includes five domains: physical condition, mental condition, activity, mobility, and incontinence.

Semmes Weinstein monofilament t.: for sensory testing. The filament is applied perpendicular to the surface to be tested. The filament will bend at a specific force defined by the diameter of the filament. If the blinded patient can properly locate the area of the sensation over different areas, the test is normal. In diabetic feet a 5.07 filament will bend with 10 gm of force and is used for the test.

total hip arthroplasty outcome evaluation: designed by the American Academy of Orthopaedic Surgeons for universal definition of outcome of total hip arthroplasty. Includes function, satisfaction, physical examination, complications, and radiographic examination. This form also takes into account preoperative factors.*

WOMAC: specific scales designed at the Western Ontario and MacMasters Universities for hip, knee, and other disorders.

Other Physical Examinations

The portions of a physical examination that are not described as a test, sign, or maneuver include tests for ranges of motion, muscle strength and sensation, and sensory examinations. These tests are found in Chapter 12 and Appendix B.

---

*Liang MH et al., 1991.

Laboratory Evaluations

Laboratory medicine, or *clinical pathology* as it is also called, is the field of science and medicine that tests and examines tissue samples from the human body relevant to the diagnosis, treatment, and prognosis of diseases. The studies and tests, performed in the areas of biochemistry, bacteriology, hematology, histology, cytology, and serology, are ordered by physicians and other health care providers.

This chapter discusses the examination of blood and its components, synovial fluid, and urine specimens. The first section deals with those tests commonly performed as part of the routine evaluation of outpatients or preoperative patients. The next section discusses the laboratory findings of specific diseases as relates to orthopaedic physicians, taking into account that some generalized diseases result in orthopaedic problems. The definitions are designed to be comprehensive. According to accreditation and regulation, reference ranges of laboratory values must be reported with each laboratory result.

Because reference values depend on the geographic area, patient population, test methodology, and laboratory standardization, such values are not considered useful when published in textbooks because they are likely to be misleading. Therefore reference values have been deleted and the initial statement or sentence in either section should be an adequate overview for those not concerned with the complete nature of the study.

Care should be exercised when using laboratory terminology, decimal points, significant figures in laboratory data, and other specific information. Forms are provided for most tests requested. Laboratory results should never be given over the telephone except in emergency situations. Laboratory requests may be emergency (stat), urgent, or routine.

A blood test may examine the quantity and type of cells, the concentration of chemicals in the serum, and (rarely) the chemical composition of the blood cell. For each laboratory test, the definition states what component of the blood is tested. Note that is a test is on both cells and fluid of the blood, the phrase *whole blood* is used. The preferred unit of volume is the liter (L).

The last two sections give a list of laboratory abbreviations and annotation of units.

Routine Evaluations

Complete Blood Count

The complete blood count (CBC) is a series of whole-blood tests to determine the quantity and other characteristics of blood cells. Some physicians prefer only a hemoglobin, hematocrit, and white count. Most laboratories use automated instruments to provide all the parameters as a part of a standard report, and a limited study such as a hematocrit and hemoglobin (H&H) test is not cost-effective. The comprehensive CBC may include the following tests.

bone marrow biopsy: laboratory test performed on bone marrow from a medullary cavity, such as the posterior iliac crest, to determine by microscopic examination the adequacy and morphologic characteristics of hematopoietic cells.

hematocrit (HCV), packed cell volume (PCV): the proportion of the red cells in whole blood expressed as a percentage.

hemoglobin (Hb, Hgb): the iron-carrying protein in the blood. Normal values depend on age and gender (g/dl).

hematocrit and hemoglobin (H&H): determination of hematocrit and hemoglobin levels only.

mean corpuscular hemoglobin (MCH): the average amount of hemoglobin in each red cell (pg).

mean corpuscular hemoglobin concentration (MCHC): the average concentration of hemoglobin in the red cells (g Hb/dl red cells).

mean corpuscular volume (MCV): average volume of a red cell. May not be reliable if red cells are abnormal (i.e., sickle cell disease) (fl).

platelets (Plt): a blood test measuring the number of platelets (thrombocytes) per volume of whole blood. Platelet counts are routinely done by automated instruments. Platelets play an important role in hemostasis ($\times 10^9$/L).

red blood count (RBC): the number of red cells per unit volume of whole blood (million cells/μl) (# cells $\times 10^{12}$/L).

white blood count (WBC): number of white blood cells per unit volume of whole blood (thousand cells/μl) ($\times 10^9$/L).

> **differential WBC (diff):** percentage of different white cell types: neutrophils (segmented [mature] and precursors [immature]), lymphocytes, monocytes, eosinophils, basophils, and occasionally other forms. With present laboratory technology, the differential count is usually performed automatically and may not indicate the maturity of the neutrophils. In the unusual cases in which segmented neutrophils must be distinguished from more immature forms, the test may be performed by microscopic examination of the stained blood smear ($\times 10^9$/L).

Basic Chemistry Profiles

Many hospitals offer groups of chemistry tests (called *profiles* or *panels*) because these tests are frequently ordered together (e.g., serum electrolytes, hepatitis panel, renal panel). The basic components of these panels are listed here.

albumin: serum concentration of the major osmotically active component of the blood. May be decreased in acute or chronic inflammation, liver disease, severe burns, or fever (mg/dl).

alanine aminotransferase (ALT): enzyme present in several organs but generally used to assess liver disease (U/L); also called **SGPT**.

alkaline phosphatase (ALP), serum: enzyme present in bone, liver, and other organs. Marked elevations over adult normal values may be seen in healthy adolescents (U/dl, U/L).

aspartate aminotransferase (AST): enzyme present in many organs, particularly muscle and liver. Increased values may indicate damage to the organ (U/L); also called **SGOT**.

blood urea nitrogen (BUN): a metabolic waste product usually cleared by the kidney. When increased, may indicate kidney disease (mg/dl).

calcium (Ca) and phosphorus (P): in general constitute the two main bone mineral ions. The blood levels of these two ions do not necessarily denote bone problems (mg/dl). *Phosphorus* is also called **phosphate**.

cholesterol: a steroid-based compound that has been associated with predisposition to coronary artery disease. The level of cholesterol depends on both genetic and dietary factors. Cholesterol is usually bound to a carrier lipoprotein, which comes in two primary densities: high and low. High-density lipoprotein (HDL) cholesterol appears to vary inversely with coronary artery disease—the higher the level, the lower the disease frequency. On the other hand, low-density lipoprotein (LDL) cholesterol appears to vary directly with coronary artery disease (mg/dl).

creatinine (Cr): a metabolic byproduct usually cleared by the kidney. Increased levels may indicate kidney disease (mg/dl).

gamma-glutamyltransferase (gamma-GGT), gamma-glutamyltranspeptidase (GGTP): serum enzyme that is frequently increased in liver disease caused by obstruction of the bile duct(s) (U/L).

lactate dehydrogenase (LDH): enzyme present in many organs. Increased values may indicate liver disease, red blood cell destruction within blood vessels, or recent heart attack (within 24 to 36 hours) (U/L).

total bilirubin: metabolic byproduct of liver metabolism of hemoglobin. Usually an indicator of liver function (mg/dl).

total serum protein: concentration of all proteins in the serum (g/dl).

uric acid (UA): metabolic byproduct usually elevated in cases of chronic gout. Elevated levels of uric acid are not necessarily correlated with acute attacks of gout (mg/dl).

Urinalysis (UA; Routine and Microscopic [R&M])

The routine urinalysis includes a notation of the color turbidity (appearance); specific gravity (density with respect to that of water, which tells how concentrated the urine is); pH (acidity or alkalinity); and the presence or absence of glucose, protein, bilirubin, ketone bodies, urobilinogen, and occult blood. A microscopic examination may be done on the urinary sediment, and the material seen may be described as white cells, red cells, epithelial cells, and a variety of crystals and casts (microscopic debris usually from diseased kidneys). The quantity of cells and crystals is expressed in the number of observed objects per high-power field (HPF) of the microscope, whereas the quantity of casts is expressed in the number of observed objects per low-power field (LPF).

General Blood and Serum Tests

The general orthopaedic and related laboratory examinations and results found in this section are grouped according to similar disease processes, such as arthritis, infection, metabolic disturbances, and hematologic disorders, and also for assessment of spinal fluid and liver function.

However, these categories are not used as unit headings because the tests are often used to study a variety of problems, depending on the clinical circumstance. The orthopaedic laboratory work-up may include any or all of the following.

acid phosphatase (AcP): a serum assay for acid phosphatase activity. Elevations are usually associated with disease of the prostate, particularly cancer. *Prostate-specific antigen (PSA)* may be increased in prostatic disease, particularly in prostatic cancer. High PSA values (> 20 ng/ml) have been shown to correlate with metastatic disease. The % free PSA also correlates with disease. In general, lower percentage free PSA correlates with higher risk of disease. Greater than 30% free PSA has a lower probability of prostate cancer. Serial PSA levels are of value in following patients with prostate cancer after surgery or radiation (ng/ml).

activated partial thromboplastin time (APTT, PTT): a test that measures the clotting factors in the *in*trinsic coagulation system. It is the test of choice in monitoring patients receiving heparin to retard blood clotting.

alanine aminotransferase (ALT): an enzyme present in several organs but generally used to assess liver disease (U/L).

alkaline phosphatase (ALP, alk PO^4 tase): test to determine the level of this enzyme. The most common sources of high values are rapid growth or fracture healing. In any growth spurt the value may be as high as three times normal. Other bone disorders causing an increase in alkaline phosphatase include Paget disease, primary bone tumors, some metastatic diseases, and osteomalacia. Because elevations in alkaline phosphatase can result from liver disorders, two additional tests may be performed: (1) heating the enzyme will destroy it if it comes from the liver and (2) abnormally high values of serum gamma-glutamyl transpeptidase (gamma GT) and alanine aminotransferase (ALT) indicate liver disease. Isoenzymes of alkaline phosphatase can be measured by indicating the organ of origin (U/L).

anti–double-stranded (native) DNA: test for antibodies against the genetic chemical information in the cell. High values are highly suggestive of systemic lupus erythematosus (IU/ml).

antinuclear antibody (ANA): an immunologic screening test that reveals the presence of serum antibodies against cellular nuclear material (DNA); usually reported as positive or negative. Elevations of ANA, especially when accompanied by the peripheral rim pattern of fluorescence, are associated with lupus erythematosus.

antistreptolysin O titer (ASO): this test is done mostly on children with joint complaints who are suspected of having rheumatic fever. The most meaningful finding for this test is an increase in the values during the course of 1 week. Values greater than 100 IU/ml in children and greater than 200 IU/ml in adults are associated with strep throat infection.

blood gases: a measurement of the amount of oxygen (O_2) and carbon dioxide (CO_2) in the blood. The oxygen is usually presented with a percent saturation value, which is normally more than 90%. The pH (acidity) of the blood is simultaneously determined.

C-reactive protein (CRP): a plasma protein not affected by the presence of circulating hormones or antiinflammatory drugs. Good indicator of inflammation or trauma. Correlates well with ESR (see later), but elevations appear and disappear before changes in ESR (mg/L or µg/L).

creatinine: byproduct of metabolism that is cleared by the kidney. A 2-hour *creatinine clearance (Ccr)* indicates how effectively the kidney is functioning as a blood filter (mg/dl).

creatine kinase (CK; creatine phosphokinase [CPK]): an enzyme contained in many organs, principally skeletal muscle, heart muscle, and brain. In muscle disorders, particularly muscular dystrophy, it is elevated. In cases of suspected acute myocardial infarction, isoenzyme determinations help distinguish the organ of origin of the elevated enzyme level (U/L).

erythrocyte sedimentation rate (sed. rate, sedimentation rate, ESR):
- *modified Westergren method:* test performed on anticoagulated whole blood to determine the speed of settling of cells in 1 hour. Three stages of sedimentation occur: initial aggregation and rouleaux formation, quick settling, and packing. The test is nonspecific, similar to determination of temperature or pulse, and a normal value is perfectly consistent with many disease states. An increased sedimentation rate may indicate certain conditions, particularly inflammation. Therefore this test is often used in evaluating bone and joint infections and other inflammatory diseases (mm/hr).

fasting blood sugar (FBS): test done to detect diabetes. Blood sample must be obtained at least 12 hours after the last meal. In the past, a *glucose tolerance test (GTT)* was a 2- to 5-hour study of both the blood and urine obtained from a patient who had taken 75 g of sugar after fasting. The most efficient GTT is a fasting and 2-hour postprandial (after eating) blood glucose. If these values are sufficiently abnormal according to the expected values for that particular laboratory, diabetes mellitus can be diagnosed. Three different sets of criteria are available for interpreting the plasma glucose levels in the GTT. These include the National Diabetes Data Group (NDDG), the World Health Organization (WHO) criteria, and age-related expected values for glucose criteria. Those values are available on request from your laboratory. There is usually little value in performing a 3- to 5-hour GTT (mg/dl).

hemoglobin electrophoresis: a test to determine types of red cell hemoglobin. Abnormalities are present in sickle cell disease, thalassemia, and other red cell disorders. The results of this test are reported as normal or described by the specific abnormality.

human leukocyte antigen–B27 (HLA-B27): an antigen on the surface of cells frequently present in patients with ankylosing spondylitis.

international normalized ratio (INR): ratio of value of patient's prothrombin time to the mean of normal raised to the power of the international standard index.

prothrombin time (pro time, PT): a test that measures the clotting factors in the *ex*trinsic coagulation system, commonly done to monitor patients taking blood thinners such as warfarin sodium (Coumadin).

reticulocyte count: a blood cell test to determine the erythropoietic activity, thereby helping in the classification of anemia. When observed under the microscope, only 1 of 100 red cells will normally take up a stain, indicating it is less than 24 hours old. Finding an increased number of reticulocytes means probable increased red blood cell production, usually in response to anemia. However, the percentage of reticulocytes is relative to the total red cell count, so that mathematical correction of the percent reticulocytes is necessary for proper interpretation. Some centers have moved to reporting *absolute* reticulocyte counts (reference range: 25,000 to 75,000 cells/μl or 25 to 75 × 10^9/L).

rheumatoid factor (RF): a serologic test to determine the presence of certain antibodies frequently seen in autoimmune diseases. The antibodies may be detected by several methods; some are more sensitive than others. The individual laboratory will interpret the importance of positive, negative, or numeric results.

salicylates: a test can be done on the blood to determine the specific levels of salicylates or on the urine as a screening test for the presence of aspirin. This can be done to follow the treatment of arthritis or in the event of an accidental overdose. Salicylate is also present in oil of wintergreen, which some people use topically for relief of muscle pain, so elevated levels do not always indicate aspirin therapy or overdose (μg/ml).

serum lead: in cases of lead poisoning, the serum can be tested for that element specifically. Because lead is a heavy metal, a heavy metal screening test is frequently used to determine the presence of lead poisoning. Elevated lead levels can also be indirectly tested for by measuring the free red cell protoporphyrin or zinc protoporphyrin levels (μg/dl).

serum protein electrophoresis (SPE, SPEP): a test to determine the presence and amount of particular types of serum proteins; used to detect multiple myeloma—a malignancy of the cells that produces immunoglobulin (Ig). A report of a high immunoglobulin or monoclonal pattern may indicate myeloma. An *immunoelectrophoresis* is a similar test reporting the concentrations of various immunoglobulins (IgG, IgA, and IgM) in the serum.

triiodothyronine (T^3), thyroxine (T^4), and thyroid-stimulating hormone (TSH): measures of the levels of thyroid-active hormones and the pituitary hormone controlling thyroid function. There are various methods for determining these levels to help recognize hyperthyroidism and hypothyroidism. A caution in interpreting such values should be made in chronically ill patients (ng/dl, μg/dl, μU/ml).

troponin: screen for evidence of myocardial infarction.

Serum and Urine Tests for Metabolic Disease

The following tests, as well as some urine excretion tests, are done to assess bone metabolism (i.e., bone formation and resorption). These tests are used most often for diagnosing and following therapeutic response in patients with osteoporosis, Paget disease, hyperparathyroidism, and other metabolic bone diseases. In Paget disease, patients can have either evidence of decreased bone formation or increased bone resorption. These studies are often ordered by an endocrinologist but are of interest to the orthopaedist.

Serum Tests for General Bone Turnover Markers

25-hydroxyvitamin D, 25-hydroxycholecalciferol (25[OH]D): measurement of 25(OH)D, a liver metabolite of vitamin D, in the serum is a good index for determining vitamin D deficiency and intoxication and aids in diagnosis of patients with metabolic bone diseases. It is measured by radioimmunoassay or competition binding protein assay (ng/ml).

1,25-dihydroxyvitamin D, 1,25-hydroxycholecalciferol 1,25(OH)2D: measurement of 1,25(OH)2D is used in the management of hypocalcemic and hypercalcemic disorders, specifically the bone diseases parathyroid gland disorders, renal failure, and sarcoidosis, and for therapeutic management of treatment. It is measured by radioreceptor assay (pg/ml).

calcitonin: serum calcitonin is most frequently used for the diagnosis and management of medullary thyroid carcinoma. It is measured by either radioimmunoassay or the concentration technique (pg/ml).

parathyroid hormone (PTH): measured in serum for evaluation and differentiation of disorders of calcium metabolism. Intact PTH is measured by either immunoradiometric or immunochemiluminescent assay (pg/dl, pmol/L).

serum calcium (Ca): measures serum calcium concentration. Serum calcium levels are increased in hyperparathyroidism, while there is a concurrent decrease in serum phosphorus (PO_4). The phosphorus determination in parathyroid disease depends on renal function. Calcium and phosphorus levels are commonly measured as a screening measure. Many diseases affect the blood levels of these two chemicals (mg/dl).

Serum Tests for Bone Formation

bone specific alkaline phosphatase (BAP, BSAP): determined by alkaline phosphatase isoenzyme electrophoresis or enzyme-linked immunosorbent assay (ELISA); can be a useful marker for the rate of bone formation (or bone turnover). It is usually elevated in Paget disease, after menopause, in hyperparathyroidism, and in other conditions, and its determination can help monitor patients with these conditions who are treated with antiresorptive therapy (U/L, IU/L).

osteocalcin or bone Gla protein (OC, ON, BGP): a serum marker for assessment of bone formation; most abundant noncollagenous protein in bone, measured by radioimmunoassay or immunoradiometric assay (ng/ml).

procollagen propeptide: serum marker of osteoblast activity measured in two chemical forms: the **carboxyterminal propeptide (c-PCP, PICP)** and the **aminoterminal propeptide (N-PCP).**

Serum Tests for Bone Resorption

C-telopeptide (cross-links, CTx or CTX): enzyme-linked immunosorbent assay is used to measure Type I collagen degradation products in urine as a bone resorption marker. It is reported as cross-links nmol/mmol creatinine. It is used for research and approved for clinical applications such as to monitor effectiveness of different antiresorptive therapies. CTX can also be measured in the serum, and must be evaluated in the fasting state.

free pyridinium cross-links: for bone resorption; these are the cross-links of Type I collagen, which constitutes 90% of the organic bone matrix. **Pyridinoline (PYD) and deoxypyridinoline (Dpd, DPYD)** are excreted in the urine and not affected by diet. Dpd is more specific for bone metabolism. It is a useful marker to monitor therapies for metabolic bone diseases.

N-telopeptide (NTx or NTX): quantitative measure of excretion of cross-linked N-telopeptides of Type I collagen (NTx) is done by ELISA as a resorption marker. NTx is reported as bone collagen equivalents or creatinine. Measurement of NTx is intended for use in predicting skeletal response to hormonal antiresorptive therapy in postmenopausal women and therapeutic monitoring of other antiresorptive therapies (ng/ml). NTX can also be measured in the serum, and must be evaluated in the fasting state.

tartrate-resistant acid phosphatase (TRAP): a serum test to measure bone resorption and to determine the metabolic activity of osteoclasts; specific acid phosphatase seen from active metabolic osteoclastic activity.

Urine Chemical Tests

Some minerals and other chemicals measured in blood are also measured in urine. These include calcium, phosphorus, creatinine, and uric acid. The following are indicators of bone resorption, with the exception of the mucopolysaccharides, which are an index of proteoglycan metabolic abnormalities.

hydroxyproline (HYP): urine test that measures the degradation products of bone matrix; total fasting urinary hydroxyproline-creatinine ratio is used traditionally as a marker of bone resorption. It is markedly increased in Paget disease. It is used to monitor treatment with antiresorptive drugs.

mucopolysaccharides: test done on the urine to determine the excretion of abnormal amounts of specific mucopolysaccharides that are seen in diseases causing dwarfism, Hurler syndrome, mental retardation, and other congenital problems.

pyridinoline collagen cross-links (PYD) and pyridinium collagen cross-links (PYD): these two names refer to the same urine tests used to measure cross-linked fragments of collagen that result from bone degradation.

Bacteriologic Studies

acid-fast bacillus (AFB): refers to the bright red appearance of mycobacteria when stained by a special technique and observed under a microscope. A more efficient method involving fluorescence microscopy is presently used.

anaerobic culture: bacterial culture grown in the absence of oxygen (obligate anaerobes) or minimal free oxygen (facultative anaerobes). Certain organisms require this environment for growth in contrast to the standard aerobic cultures grown in the presence of normal oxygen. Anaerobic bacteria, like their aerobic counterparts, can be pathogenic or nonpathogenic.

colony count (CC): the placement of a known amount of urine on culture media; the report is usually given in number of bacterial colonies per milliliter of urine.

culture and sensitivity (C&S): bacteria from a wound, urine, blood, joint fluid, throat, or any other source are grown in tubes or on plates. The bacteria are identified by combinations of biochemical reactions that they can or cannot carry out. The results of bacterial cultures are usually listed by individual organism along with its antimicrobial sensitivity.

typical bacterial species reports: the following bacterial species are frequently encountered in laboratory studies; they are listed for spelling purposes, without definitions. The terms *common flora* and *normal flora* denote the presence of normal, nonpathogenic bacteria.

Acinetobacter baumannii
Escherichia coli (E. coli)
Klebsiella pneumoniae
Mycobacterium avium
Mycobacterium marinum
Mycobacterium tuberculosis
Neisseria gonorrhoeae (cause of gonorrhea)
Pseudomonas aeruginosa
Salmonella organisms
Staphylococcus aureus (Staph. aureus)
Streptococcus organisms

Common fungal organisms are:

Actinomyces
Aspergillus
Blastomyces
Candida
Coccidioides
Cryptococcus
Histoplasma

fluorescent treponemal antibody (FTA): a highly specific treponemal serologic test for syphilis; usually interpreted as positive or negative. Nontreponemal screening tests commonly used are the Venereal Disease Research Laboratory (**VDRL**) and rapid plasma reagin (RPR). These are essentially the same test, with VDRL used on cerebrospinal fluid (CSF) and RPR used on serum.

Gram stain: a general stain used on microscopic slide specimens to aid in seeing various organisms and estimating their numbers. Depending on their color after processing, they are described as *gram-positive* or *gram-negative*. This aids in the initial selection of antibiotics likely to be useful. Also, white blood cells should be noted in sputum and wound specimens to indicate whether one is dealing with colonization (if white cells are not present) or actual infection (if they are).

polymerase chain reaction (PCR): used as a rapid identification for microorganisms of DNA, bacteria, human virus, anthrax, and in bioterrorism.

Other Special Studies

cerebrospinal fluid (CSF): a study that includes the following:

protein: normally 45 mg/dl.

glucose: normally two thirds that of the serum glucose; decreased in bacterial infections.

white blood cells: normally 0 to $3/mm^3$; when an increased number of cells are present, they are divided into polys and lymphs.

culture: some fluid is placed on a growth medium to see if any organisms are present; occasionally, a slide is made from a smear of the fluid and a Gram stain done directly to determine the presence of bacteria.

bacterial antigen assay: used predominantly on pediatric population for rapid screening of bacterial surface antigens.

Cryptococcus latex antigen test: a rapid latex agglutination test for the qualitative and semiquantitative detection of the capsular polysaccharide antigens of *Cryptococcus neoformans*.

TABLE 5-1 Classification of Synovial Effusions

		Routine Laboratory Examination				
Gross Examination	Normal	Noninflammatory (Group I)	Inflammatory (Group II)	Septic (Group III)	Crystal (Group IV)	Hemorrhagic (Group IV)
WBC (mm³)	<200	200–2000	2000–75,000	Often > 100,000	2000–75,000	50–10,000
PMN leukocytes (%)	<25	<25	>50 often	>75	>50 often	>50
Crystals present	No	No	No	No	Yes	No
Glucose (AM fasting)	Nearly equal to blood	Nearly equal to blood	<50 mg% lower than blood	<50 mg% lower than blood	<50 mg% lower than blood	Nearly equal to blood

PMN, Polymorphonuclear; WBC, white blood cell.
In septic arthritis, the leukocyte count is almost always greater than 50,000 cells/μl. Occasionally, however, a patient with gout, pseudogout, or rheumatoid arthritis may have counts in this range. Noninflammatory synovial findings reveal a white count of up to 5000 with less than 30% PMN leukocytes. In inflammatory synovitis, a 2000 to 200,000 white count can be anticipated with greater than 50% polys. In infectious or septic arthritis, greater than 90% PMN leukocytes can be expected. In crystal-induced arthritis, the synovial cell count can be 500 to 200,000 with less than 90% PMN leukocytes. In hemorrhagic arthritis, 50 to 10,000 white cells may be present, but fewer than 50% are PMN leukocytes.
Adapted from Schumacher HR: Synovial fluid analysis and synovial biopsy. In Kelley WN, Harris ED, Ruddy S, Sledge CB, editors: Textbook of rheumatology, ed 3, Philadelphia, 1989, WB Saunders.

flow cytometry: for evaluation of tumors. A stream of single-file tumor cells is passed by the path of a laser that is able to measure the relative amounts of DNA. This may help in the relative grading of the tumor cells. Also, after staining with certain antibodies that have been linked to fluorescent chemicals, lymphocytes from patients with acquired immunodeficiency syndrome (AIDS) can be counted by flow cytometry to determine the concentration of helper T lymphocytes—an indication of response to therapy.

synovial fluid evaluation (Table 5-1): evaluation of synovial fluid for the type and quantity of cells in the fluid. The normal white count of synovial fluid is considered to be less than 200 cells/μl or mm³. The leukocyte count is performed in a standard hemocytometer.

Gram stains are routinely performed for the detection of infectious arthritis, and, under certain circumstances, bacterial, fungal, and mycobacterial cultures are done. Viscosity may be useful; inflammation is associated with decreased viscosity. If crystals are seen, **polarized light microscopy** may be used to distinguish the two types of crystal-induced arthritis, gout and pseudogout, allowing the distinction between uric acid crystals seen in gout and calcium pyrophosphate crystals in pseudogout.

Histologic and Pathologic Techniques

Using special stains, tissue samples can be examined for normal or abnormal architecture. Abnormal changes are described as *pathologic*. Special staining techniques may also be used to detect alterations in normal musculoskeletal growth and repair.

desmin stain: useful for detecting the presence of muscle-related process in pathologic tissue sections.

Factor VIII stain: the stain is actually for von Willebrand factor (vWF), also known as *factor VIII–related antigen*. It is seen in both normal and pathologic vascular endothelium and is useful in distinguishing the origin of some tumors.

hematoxylin and eosin staining (H&E): for standard tissue histology. This is a double stain designed to distinguish areas of tissue with a greater propensity for these two stains. The result is a light orange and purple appearance.

keratins stain: stain for a specific molecule that can be an indication for a variety of pathologic conditions, including sarcoid and adamantinoma.

Masson trichrome: for both histologic and pathologic examination. Three dyes are employed on the same tissue sample, resulting in selective staining for muscle, collagen fibers, fibrin, and erythrocytes.

neurofilament stains: a stain useful to detect neurofilament material in some tumors as well as some cancers such as Merkel cell carcinoma.

safranin O fast green staining: particularly useful in cartilage samples, safranin O stains for proteoglycans and fast green for collagen.

tetracycline labeling: to determine the rate of bone formation, tetracycline is given orally 11 to 14 days prior to obtaining a tissue sample for bone. This helps determine the rate of bone formation as well as abnormal bone matrix resulting in widened osteoid seams.

vimentin stain: for a specific molecule wherein its presence will help distinguish the mesenchymal origin of some tumors.

Laboratory Evaluations in Musculoskeletal Tumors

Using special stains, chromosomes can be seen under the microscope. The 46 human chromosomes are paired and numbered 1 through 23. The first 22 pairs are called *autosomes*. The twenty-third pair, the *sex chromosome*, is either an XX or XY pair. The arms of these chromosomes can exchange a portion of one of the arms with another chromosome. This is called a *translocation*. With translocations, specific gene products result in specific proteins that may be associated with specific tumors. The short arm of the chromosome is indicated by *p* and the long arm is indicated by *q*. Table 5-2 shows currently used studies for musculoskeletal tumors.

TABLE 5-2 Current Studies for Musculoskeletal Tumors

Tumor	Translocation	Gene product
Alveolar rhabdomyosarcoma	t(2;13)(q35;q14)	PAX3-FKHR
	t(1;13)(p36;q14)	PAX7-FKHR
Myxoid/round cell liposarcoma	t(12;16)(q13;p11)	EWS-CHOP
	t(12;22)(q13;q12)	TLS-CHOP (Type 1)
		TLS-CHOP (Type 2)
Synovial sarcoma	t(X;18) (p11;q11)	SYT-SSX1
		SYT-SSX2
		SYT-SSX4
Ewing sarcoma	t(11;22) (q24;q12)	EWS-FLI-1
	21;22 and 7;22 also reported	
Alveolar soft part sarcoma	t(X;17) (p11;q25)	N/A
Clear cell sarcoma	t(12;22)(q13;q12)	EWS-ATF1

Blood Bank Procedures and Products*

Procedures and Terms

autologous donor: a patient who donates his or her own blood that is labeled and tagged specifically for use by the same patient. Donations typically occur once a week during the weeks prior to surgery; however, the final unit must be collected more than 72 hours prior to the anticipated surgery or transfusion. There is controversy regarding the use of autologous blood. Many feel it is a safer product because the donor and patient are one and the same. However, risks associated with patient misidentification and bacterial contamination of the blood products still exist. Patients who provide their own blood may also be more likely to require a blood transfusion because of lower presurgical hemoglobin and hematocrit levels caused by the autologous donations.

directed donor: blood from a certain donor targeted specifically for use by a particular patient. Blood products supplied are subject to the same testing requirements as allogeneic donors. Controversy exists as to the use of directed donors because these donors often feel peer pressure to provide blood for a friend or family member when in reality these donors may not be the best choice for blood donation.

intraoperative autologous transfusion (IAT): the intraoperative recovery of red cells for reinfusion during the course of surgery. The efficiency of this system has been improved with a *hemodilution* technique.

irradiation: American Association of Blood Bank Standards state that cellular blood products should be

---

*Prepared by Corey Jenkins, MS, MT (ASCP) SBB, Blood Bank Officer, National Naval Medical Center, Bethesda, MD.

irradiated prior to issue when the patient is at risk for developing transfusion associated graft versus host disease, when the donor is a blood relative of the recipient, or when the donor is selected for HLA compatibility. Irradiation is accomplished by delivering at least 25 Gy of irradiation to the center plane of the blood product. Radiation sources are usually cesium-137, cobalt-60, or x-ray.

leukocyte reduction: a process that removes a majority of the leukocytes in cellular blood products (< 5.0 × 10^6 leukocytes/unit for random and single donor platelets). The process usually involves filtration either at the bedside, in the laboratory prior to issue, or shortly after collection (prestorage). Leukocyte-reduced products are indicated for patients who experience repeated febrile reactions from blood transfusions and to prevent alloimmunization to HLA antigens. Leukocyte-reduced products have been shown to be as effective as cytomegalovirus (CMV)–negative products in preventing transmission of CMV.

maximum surgical blood order schedule (MSBOS): a preoperative blood ordering guideline established by many institutions based on past surgical blood use. The MSBOS provides a list of common surgical procedures along with the recommended blood use for each procedure (e.g., hip arthroplasty = type and cross-match [T&C] two units red blood cells [RBCs]; open reduction and internal fixation [ORIF] ankle = type and screen [T&S]).

type and cross-match (T&C): the potential blood recipient's ABO and Rh type is determined through antigen/antibody testing. In addition, the recipient's serum/plasma is screened for unexpected antibodies. Compatible donor units are then selected based on the results of the recipient's blood type and antibody screen. Cells from segments attached to these units are then cross-matched against the recipient's serum to determine true compatibility. Some facilities perform a computer cross-match provided certain regulatory agency requirements are met.

type and screen (T&S): the potential blood recipient's ABO and Rh type is determined through antigen/antibody testing. In addition, the recipients' serum/plasma is screened for unexpected antibodies. Antibodies detected in the antibody screen are identified through additional testing. For patients with a positive antibody screen, many facilities will antigen type ABO/Rh compatible donor units to find products that are antigen negative for the corresponding antibody(s) in case red cell transfusions are needed.

Blood Products

cryoprecipitate (Cryo): cryo is the cold-insoluble portion of FFP that has been prepared by thawing FFP at 1°–6° C, removing the plasma, and then refreezing the precipitated portion of the FFP, along with a small volume of plasma, for up to 1 year at less than –18° C. Cryo contains fibrinogen, factor VIII (VIII:C and VIII:vWF) and factor XIII. Each unit of Cryo contains at least 80 units of factor VIII and 150 mg of fibrinogen.

fresh frozen plasma (FFP): the plasma portion of whole blood is separated within 8 hours of collection, frozen, and stored at less than –18° C for up to 1 year. Once thawed, FFP is good for 24 hours and contains one unit of coagulation factor per ml of FFP.

platelets: platelets can be prepared from whole blood via centrifugation and then pooled or collected from a single donor via apheresis. One single donor platelet is equivalent to approximately five or six random pooled platelets. Platelet transfusions are indicated in cases of thrombocytopenia or abnormal functioning platelets. One unit of apheresis platelets is expected to increase the platelet count by 30,000 to 60,000/μl in an average adult. Platelets are stored at room temperature with gentle agitation and expire 5 days after collection. Platelets can be leukoreduced, irradiated, or both.

red blood cells (RBCs): RBCs are made by removing most of the plasma from whole blood. RBCs contain the same oxygen-carrying capacity as whole blood with less risk of volume overload. Depending on the anticoagulant solution used, RBCs can be stored at 1°–6° C for up to 42 days. One unit of RBCs is expected to increase the average adult hemoglobin by 1 g/dl or the hematocrit by 3%. RBCs can be leukocyte reduced, irradiated, and washed.

thawed plasma: thawed plasma is FFP that has been thawed for more than 24 hours. This product is good for 4 additional days but has decreased amounts of the labile clotting factors (V and VIII).

whole blood: approximately 500 ml of blood. After 24 hours, platelets and granulocytes are not viable. The labile clotting factors (V and VIII) also decrease with prolonged storage. Whole blood is seldom used. Instead, component therapy is usually indicated, providing the patient with the specific component needed. Whole blood may be useful when oxygen carrying capacity and volume replacement are both required.

Blood Bank Immunologic Tests

alloantibodies: circulating atypical antibodies that are the result of prior antigenic stimulation from previous transfusion of blood products, pregnancy, or some other event. The presence of these antibodies may cause a delay in locating compatible blood products.

anti-hepatitis C virus (anti-HCV): test performed on donor blood to detect the presence of the antibody to hepatitis C antigen. This is also necessary in preventing transmission of hepatitis to a blood recipient. Its presence is detectable in certain patients who currently have, or have previously had, clinical or subclinical hepatitis C. This test may be negative in patients with hepatitis A, hepatitis B, or hepatitis E. Positive results are confirmed with a recombinant immunoblot assay (RIBA) test. HCV genotyping is done to identify genotypes responsive to medication.

anti-human immunodeficiency virus antibodies (anti-HIV): test for antibodies to the viruses causing autoimmune deficiency syndrome (AIDS)—human immunodeficiency virus 1 and 2 (HIV-1 and HIV-2). It is performed routinely on every donated unit of blood to prevent the transmission of this disease to blood recipients. In patients, it is used to detect those who are suspected of having AIDS, although a positive test (i.e., having the antibody) is not necessarily the same as having AIDS. The screening methodology for this antibody can give falsely positive results, so each positive must be confirmed by the Western blot technique.

direct Coombs test, direct anti–human globulin test (DAT): performed on patient's red blood cells to detect the presence of antibodies or complement components attached to the red cells. The red cells with attached antibodies or complement components usually have a shortened life.

factor VIII and factor IX: blood coagulation factors that may be absent or substantially reduced in hemophilia A (factor VIII) or hemophilia B (factor IX). These factors and certain specially prepared blood products are available for replacement in acquired disorders of the labile coagulant system.

HB$_s$Ag: test performed on donor blood to detect the hepatitis B surface antigen. This is also necessary in preventing transmission of hepatitis to a blood recipient. Its presence is detectable in certain patients who currently have, or have previously had, clinical or subclinical hepatitis B. This test may be negative in patients with hepatitis A, hepatitis C, or hepatitis E.

human immunodeficiency virus-1 antigen (HIV-1 antigen): test for the actual HIV-1 virus itself. This test measures a specific molecular portion (antigen) of the virus and is used in addition to anti-HIV-1 for screening blood and blood products. Reported as positive or negative.

human immunodeficiency virus, viral load test (HIV, viral load): quantitative test for determining the actual number of HIV particles within a patient's blood. The test uses polymerase chain reactive methodology to detect and measure levels of HIV RNA. The test is used to determine when to initiate drug therapy and to monitor response to therapy.

immune serum globulins: various immunoglobulins produced from sensitized individuals whose serum contains these antibodies; used for disease prophylaxis or attenuation, for example, Rh$_o$(D). Immune globulin is given to RH$_o$(D)-negative women to prevent the sensitization to the Rh antigen and the resulting potential for Rh hemolytic disease of the newborn.

indirect Coombs test (indirect anti–human globulin test): performed on patient's serum to detect abnormal circulating antibodies. Presence of these atypical antibodies may cause a transfusion reaction. If present in women of childbearing age, these antibodies may cause hemolytic disease of the newborn (erythroblastosis fetalis).

isoantibodies: circulating, naturally occurring antibodies, which are usually of the IgM classification of immunoglobulins. Group O individuals usually have isoantibodies A and B in their plasma, group

AB usually have neither, group A usually have anti-B, and group B usually have anti-A.

Routine Physiologic Parameters

electrocardiogram (ECG): recorded measurement of the spontaneous electrical activity of the heart, using multiple leads to assess the heart from a variety of directions. This study is commonly obtained before surgery to give a baseline in the event of operative or postoperative complications, such as pulmonary embolus or cardiac arrest.

electroencephalogram (EEG): recorded measurement of the spontaneous electrical activity of the brain using multiple leads placed on the head and ears. This study is obtained to detect certain seizures and brain disorders and the lack of activity when there has been severe damage leading to brain death.

height and weight: taken into consideration in an orthopaedic work-up because many back problems are related to being overweight and the stress that is placed on the vertebrae. A formula for relative obesity uses height and weight to determine body mass index.

vital signs: the easily measurable sustaining functions include temperature, pulse, respiration rate, and blood pressure. A fifth vital sign, pain, has been added and is graded on a scale from 0 (no pain) to 10 (most severe pain imaginable). These vital signs have been and will continue to be the major index of a patient's general progress.

Laboratory Abbreviations

Blood Components and Clotting

ABO: blood group system comprising A, B, AB, and O blood
CBC: complete blood count
diff: differential white blood cell count
  basos: basophils, basophilic granulocytes
  blasts: extremely immature blood cells
  eos: eosinophils, eosinophilic granulocytes
  lymphs: lymphocytes
  monos: monocytes
  nonsegs: bands, stabs, metamyelocytes, myelocytes, promyelocytes, myeloblasts
  polys: polymorphonuclear leukocytes
  segs: segmented neutrophils
ESR: erythrocyte sedimentation rate
FFP: fresh frozen plasma
H&H: hemoglobin and hematocrit
Hct: hematocrit
Hgb, Hb: hemoglobin
IAT: intraoperative autologous transfusion
INR: international normalized ratio
MCH: mean corpuscular hemoglobin
MCHC: mean corpuscular hemoglobin concentration
MCV: mean corpuscular volume
MSBOS: maximum surgical blood order schedule
Plt: platelet (thrombocyte)
PT: prothrombin time
PTT: partial thromboplastin time; (activated) **APTT**
RBC: red blood cell count
rbc: red blood cell
Rh: rhesus factor ($Rh_o[D]$)
T&C: type and crossmatch
T&S: type and screen
WBC: white blood cell count
wbc: white blood cell

Serum Chemistries

25(OH)D: calcidiol, 25OH vitamin D
1,25(OH)2D: calcitriol, 1,25OH vitamin D
AcP: acid phosphatase
Alk P: alkaline phosphatase
Alb: albumin
ALP: alkaline phosphatase
ALT: alanine aminotransferase (SGPT)
AST: aspartate aminotransferase (SGOT)
BAP, BSAP: bone specific alkaline phosphatase
BUN: blood urea nitrogen
Ca: calcium, serum calcium
Chol: cholesterol
CK: creatine kinase
Cl: chloride
CO_2: carbon dioxide (bicarbonate)
CPK: creatine phosphokinase (same as CK)
Cr: creatinine
CRP: c-reactive protein
FBS: fasting blood sugar

GGTP: gamma-glutamyl transpeptidase
GTT: glucose tolerance test
HDL: high-density lipoprotein
Ig: immunoglobulin. There are five classes: IgA, IgD, IgE, IgG, and IgM
K: potassium
LDH: lactate dehydrogenase
LDL: low-density lipoprotein
Na: sodium
OC, BGP: osteocalcin or bone Gla protein
PAP: prostatic acid phosphatase
PO$_4$: phosphorus, phosphate
PSA: prostate-specific antigen
PTH: parathyroid hormone
SGOT: serum glutamic oxaloacetic transaminase (obsolete)
SGPT: serum glutamic pyruvic transaminase (obsolete)
SPE, SPEP: serum protein electrophoresis
T. Bili: total bilirubin
TRAP: tartrate-resistant acid phosphatase
UA: urinalysis, uric acid
VLDL: very low-density lipoprotein

Serology

ANA: antinuclear antibody
anti-DNA: anti–double-stranded (native) DNA antibody
anti-HIV-1: anti–human immunodeficiency virus 1 antibody
anti-HIV-2: anti–human immunodeficiency virus 2 antibody
ASO: antistreptolysin O titer
DAT: direct anti–human globulin test
ELISA: enzyme-linked immunosorbent assay
EMIT: enzyme-multiplied immunoassay technique
FTA (ABS): fluorescent treponemal antibody (absorbed)
HbC: hepatitis C antigen
HB$_c$Ab: hepatitis B core antibody
HB$_e$Ab: hepatitis B e antibody
HB$_s$Ab: hepatitis B surface antibody
HB$_e$Ag: hepatitis B e antigen
HB$_s$Ag: hepatitis B surface antigen
HIV: human immunodeficiency virus
HLF: human leukocyte antigen
RF: rheumatoid factor assay
STS: serologic test for syphilis
VDRL: Venereal Disease Research Laboratory

Urine

Ace: acetone
BHB: beta-hydroxybutyrate
Ccr: creatinine clearance
c-PCP, PICP: carboxyterminal propeptide
C-Tx: cross-links: C-telopeptide
DPYD, Dpd: deoxypyridinoline
Glu: glucose
HPF: high-power field
HYP: hydroxyproline
KB: ketone bodies
LPF: low-power field
NTx: N-telopeptide
pH: concentration of hydrogen ions; solution to measure acidity and alkalinity
Prot: protein
PYD: pyridinoline and pyridinium collagen cross-links
R&M: routine and microscopic examinations
s.g.: specific gravity
spec grav: specific gravity
spgr: specific gravity
UA: urinalysis

Other

AFB: acid-fast bacteria
C&S: culture and sensitivity
CC: colony count
CSF: cerebrospinal fluid
ECG: electrocardiogram
EKG: electrocardiogram
PPD: purified protein derivative (tuberculosis skin test)
spec: specimen
T$_3$: L-triiodothyronine
T$_4$: L-tetraiodothyronine (thyroxine)
TSH: thyroid-stimulating hormone (also called **thyrotropin**)

Annotation of Units

Weight

g: gram (454 gram = 1 pound)
kg: kilogram (1000 gram = 2.2 pounds)

µg: microgram = 1/1,000,000 gram
mg: milligram = 1/1000 gram
ng: nanogram = 1/1,000,000,000 gram
pg: picogram = 1/1,000,000,000,000 gram

Volume

dl: deciliter = 1/10 liter
fl: femtoliter = 1/1,000,000,000,000,000 liter
L: liter (0.943 quarts; 1.06 liter = 1 quart)
µl: microliter = 1/1,000,000 liter
ml: milliliter = 1/1000 liter

Length

cm: centimeter = 1/100 meter (0.39 inch; 2.54 cm = 1 inch)
m: meter (39.37 inch)
µm: micrometer = 1/1,000,000 meter
µ: micron = micrometer (obsolete)
mm: millimeter = 1/1000 meter

Other

Eq: equivalent; 6.023×10^{23} ionic charges
mEq: milliequivalent; 1/1000 equivalent weight

Important Laboratory Notes

In an attempt to standardize the way medical (and other scientific) units are reported, Le Système Internationale d'Unités was developed. Among others, it makes the following specifications:

Omit periods in abbreviations (kg, mm, ml, mg).
Omit plurals (70 kg, not 70 kgs).
Avoid commas as a spacer in expressing large numbers. (In some countries, the comma is used as a decimal point.)
Compound prefixes should not be used (10^{-9} meter = nanometer, not millimicrometer [mµm]).
Omit the degree sign for the Kelvin temperature scale (310 K, not 310° K).
Multiples and submultiples are used in steps of 10^3 or 10^{-3} as follows:

Multiplier	Prefix	Abbreviation
10^3	kilo-	k
10^6	mega-	M
10^9	giga-	G
10^{12}	tera-	T
10^{-1}	deci-	d
10^{-2}	centi-	c
10^{-3}	milli-	m
10^{-6}	micro-	µ
10^{-9}	nano-	n
10^{-12}	pico-	p
10^{-15}	femto-	f
10^{-18}	atto-	a

Only one solidus (/) may be used when indicated per or a denominator: acceleration = velocity per second = m/s^2, not m/s/s.
When the compound unit is derived from the multiplication of two base units, a point (·) is used to so indicate. A unit of torque is the Newton-meter, written N·m not Nm.
Preferred spellings are *meter*, not *metre*; *liter*, not *litre*; and *kilogram*, not *kilogramme*.

Casts, Splints, Dressings, and Traction

This chapter defines the materials applied and prescribed by an orthopaedist or assigned individual in the direct care of patients with fractures, dislocations, and conditions of the musculoskeletal system. The types of cast immobilization materials are described, as are the traction devices and weights designed for hospital or home care. Some emergency stabilization devices are included at the end of the chapter.

The techniques of cast immobilization, splints, dressings, and traction devices are designed to provide an external means of support or protective covering while healing proceeds under optimal conditions. Casts are generally applied in fracture reduction and immobilization, but they are also helpful in the correction of pediatric deformities, dysplastic hip disease, scoliosis, and foot deformities such as club foot, with the goal being to maintain or obtain a correction of deformity, promote alignment following surgery, and give support to damaged soft tissues in the healing process of fractures, dislocations, and sprains.

Because the care of the orthopaedic patient is a team approach, orthopaedists in private or group practice and in hospital settings are assisted by qualified orthopaedic nurses and technologists who are also involved in patient care. The orthopaedic nurse may choose to work in a doctor's office or an outpatient clinic of a hospital or become directly involved with inpatient management by assuming diverse responsibilities for a plan of quality care from admission to discharge. This requires specialized knowledge of orthopaedic nursing, to include skills in the use of traction equipment and appliances, and the ability to manage patients with this armamentarium. Depending on educational background, training, and hospital policies, qualified nurses and technologists scrub in on orthopaedic surgical procedures in the operating room, clinic, or physician's office.

The National Association of Orthopaedic Nurses (NAON), founded in 1980, is the professional organization that offers a certification program to orthopaedic nurses who wish to further develop their skills in the management and care of orthopaedic patients. The NAON provides support and educational opportunities through its sponsored activities to promote continued professional development.

There are numerous organizations that support orthopaedic technicians in professional growth. One is the National Board for Certification of Orthopaedic Technologists, founded in 1982, that offers a certifying examination and an ongoing program of education and training to promote skills in the practice of orthopaedic technology. In 1999, the American Society of Orthopaedic Professionals, an Internet organization, was formed to include all allied professionals working within orthopaedics, such as the orthopaedic, radiologic, and surgical technicians; physician assistants; paramedics; emergency room technicians; and orthopaedic product representatives. Under this organization is the certified Orthopaedic Allied Professionals and the Registered Orthopaedic Technologists, a designation that will become recognized as the standard of orthopaedic knowledge required by allied professionals who are actively upgrading their skills.

With appropriate orders the technologist assists in setting up traction appliances, Circ-O-Lectric beds, and similar devices of care, and has the shared responsibility of proper application of traction, weights, and equipment required for patient rehabilitation. Administrative tasks involve ordering supplies and equipment for the plaster rooms, examining rooms, wings, and clinics and conferring with medical suppliers on catalogue items and supplies.

The orthopaedic technologist, with training and practice, becomes skilled in the art and science of cast application and the many types needed for specific injuries and conditions. Under a physician's directions, technologists instruct patients on cast care and prevention of complications. In addition, they may assist patients in gait training (crutch-walking, ascending and descending stairs) and various home exercises after immobilization. Technologists also maintain and prepare the plaster room for specific procedures, as well as assume the clean-up duties that follow. In some orthopaedic offices, the technologist is skilled in basic orthopaedic radiographic techniques—skills that clearly enhance the team approach.

The orthopaedic specialty is so diversified that opportunities for continuing medical education for nurses and technologists are offered through the American Academy of Orthopaedic Surgeons instructional courses across the country and within the specialty organizations of orthopaedics. Corporate-sponsored activities have also been instrumental in updating product designs and state-of-the-art equipment. Together, these groups seek to promote the highest standards of quality care in cooperation with orthopaedic surgeons and other members of the health care team.

The basic tools of the trade are as follows.

A **cast** is a circumferentially wrapped plaster of Paris–impregnated bandage or encasement applied to a portion of the body. Additional materials, such as fiberglass and plastics, are also used instead of plaster of Paris.

A **splint** is a rigid or semirigid, noncircumferential material used to reinforce a soft dressing or to provide additional support for or immobilization of the body part being treated. The splint may be made of plaster of Paris, metal, wood, plastic, or, in an emergency, newspapers or magazines.

A **dressing** involves those materials used to cover a wound or surgical incision, a fabric with or without accessory medications or self-adhesive properties.

A **bandage** is a nonrigid, usually cotton material that holds a dressing in place or acts as the dressing by itself. It may be applied to provide padding over a body prominence under a cast. An elastic bandage provides support for a joint or soft tissue to control swelling.

Traction devices are any adjustable external appliances used in early treatment of fractures that suspend or deliver pull to any given part of the body. Traction is also used for temporary treatment of specific spinal conditions.

Cast Materials

Casting materials have improved considerably over the years; however, plaster of Paris casts are still widely used and familiar to all practitioners. These rolled crinoline bandages are impregnated with gypsum powder (calcium salt) that, when exposed to water, crystallizes. The reaction then slows to a maturation process (hardening) that takes approximately 24 hours to dry. The heat felt by the patient is the crystallization process that takes place within the cast material. To fabricate and mold plaster of Paris bandages is considered an art, and the technician soon learns the numerous techniques of application.

Fiberglass and thermoplast casts have become a popular form of treatment. They are lightweight, are radiolucent, are easier to apply, can tolerate moisture, and harden within 5 minutes, allowing for immediate weight-bearing. This rolled type consists of fiberglass and resin, fiberglass and plastic polymer, and polyurethane that also crystallize on exposure to water. Most fiberglass casts are long-wearing.

cast cutter: electrical circular oscillating saw for splitting or removing a cast. Long-handled cast-cutting instruments are also designed to remove small plaster casts from children.

cast padding: soft cotton wrap or synthetic wraparound material used with a plaster or fiberglass cast.

cotton roll: material made from cotton that can be rolled as a bandage and acts as a buffer between the skin and plaster material; also called **Webril.**

felt padding: thick felt or feltlike material added to the undersurface of a cast to relieve pressure on local areas of bony prominences or pressure areas; also called **Reston.**

fiberglass cast: lightweight fiberglass wrap material that is impregnated with resin or another substance that polymerizes when exposed to water.

moleskin: adhesive, thin, velvetlike material used to smooth edges of casts or to buffer areas of excessive skin wear.

plaster rolls: gauze roll impregnated with plaster of Paris, which, when dipped in warm water, can be applied, rolled smoothly, and molded, becoming hard within minutes.

sheet wadding: strong, cotton material that clings to part being applied and molded to contour of that part.

stockinettte: cloth stocking roll used initially in cast applications; comes in many sizes; can be covered by padding followed by firm cast material. Bias-cut and tubular are two different varieties.

Cast Immobilization

Cast immobilization involves the following anatomic areas: upper and lower limbs, cervical to chest region, and chest to lower spine. The various types are described later.

Body Casts

A body cast is a circumferential cast enclosing the trunk of the body and may extend from the head or upper chest to the groin or thigh. This type of cast immobilization is used in treating disorders of the cervical, thoracic, and lumbar spine such as fractures and scoliosis, or it may be applied following some types of surgery on the spine. There are several types of body casts.

extension body c.: chest-pubis cast in which the patient is positioned so that the trunk is extended backward; applied for specific fractures.

flexion body c.: chest-pubis cast in which the patient is positioned so that the trunk is flexed forward; for treatment of painful lower back conditions.

halo c.: for high-level cervical fractures; a thoracic-to-pelvic level cast incorporating the necessary extensions used to support the posts that are attached to a metal halo skeletally affixed to the head.

Minerva c.: cast immobilization extending along the side and in back of the head and neck, chest to hip area, incorporating a plaster-of-Paris headband; for fractures of the neck and in certain scoliosis problems.

scoliosis c.: special modification of the body cast for preoperative and postoperative treatment of scoliosis (curvature of the spine). These casts have in large part been replaced by operative fixation and custom fabricated orthoses. Modifications of this type are as follows:

    Cotrel c.: modified scoliosis cast applied following Cotrel traction.

    turnbuckle c.: special modification to allow changes in angle by use of turnbuckles on either side of the cast.

    Risser localizer: specialized body cast with localizer pressing over convex side of curve.

Spica Casts

A spica cast immobilizes an appendage by incorporating a part of the body proximal to that appendage. The most common spica casts are hip, thumb, and shoulder spicas. They are listed by anatomic region in the following sections.

Limb Casts

Upper Limb Casts

arm cylinder c.: long-arm cast with the elbow set in flexion and free motion at the wrist.

Dehne c.: cast incorporating the thumb with a separate extension incorporating the index and middle fingers; for fractures of the navicular. Also called **three-finger spica.**

drop out c.: for elbow contracture, a modification of the long-arm cast with posterior portion above elbow, cut out to allow arms extension resulting from gravity on forearm. By allowing elbow extension, the patient is also able to operate a manual wheelchair for independence.

gauntlet c.: short cast extending from slightly above or proximal to the wrist to some point in the palm; usually has an outrigger to control one or more fingers; indicated for metacarpal fractures, phalangeal fractures, or dislocations.

hanging arm c.: long-arm cast that, through suspension from a sling around the neck, brings about traction of fracture fragments of the distal humerus.

long-arm c. (LAC): extends from the palm and wrist to the axilla, with the elbow at 90 degrees and the wrist at neutral, preventing movement at the elbow; for treatment of fractures of the forearm, elbow, and humerus.

   cotton-loader position c.: rarely used long-arm cast applied with the wrist in full pronation, flexion, and ulnar deviation; for distal radial fractures.

Munster c.: cast that comes above the humeral epicondyles to prevent pronation and supination but allows some flexion and extension of the elbow; also called **supracondylar c.**

short-arm c. (SAC): any of a number of casts extending from the elbow to the palm or fingers; commonly used for distal forearm and wrist fractures.

shoulder spica c.: cast that incorporates the upper torso and envelops a part or all of the limb in a position of abduction; for proximal humeral fractures. Also called **airplane c.** and **statue of liberty c.**

thumb spica c.: short- or long-arm cast that incorporates the thumb; for treatment of navicular fractures. Also called **navicula c.** and **scaphoid c.**

Lower Limb Casts

cylinder c.: cast from proximal thigh to just above the ankle with the knee in extention; for injuries of the knee.

Delbert c.: a short-leg cast that is trimmed away from the anterior and posterior portions of the ankle and from the heel. This allows dorsiflexion and plantar flexion while maintaining lateral stability.

gel c.: semirigid cast, usually applied to the lower leg and foot for ankle injuries, lymphedema, or venous ulcers; also called **Unna boot.**

hip spica c.: cast incorporating the lower torso and extending to one or both lower limbs.

   Batchelor plaster: hip spica cast that holds the hip in internal rotation but allows motion in other planes; for dysplastic hip in an infant.

   bilateral hip spica c.: cast incorporating both the lower torso and lower limbs, usually because of bilateral fractures of the hips, femur, or tibia. If only the thighs are incorporated leaving the knees and leg free, called a **panty c.** Also called **double c.**

   1½ hip spica: cast that incorporates the lower torso, the entire affected limb, and the opposite limb to just above the knee; for proximal femoral fractures and some pelvic fractures.

   Petrie spica c.: specially applied cast for abduction to assist in ambulation for Legg-Calvé-Perthes disease; also called **broom-stick c.**

   unilateral hip spica c.: cast incorporating the lower torso and entire position of only one leg; for femoral fractures. Also called **single-hip spica c.**

long-leg c. (LLC): non–weight-bearing cast extending from the upper thigh to the toes; for fractures of the tibia and fibula or ligament injuries of the knee.

   long-leg walking c. (LLWC): a cast from the upper thigh to the toes, with a cast shoe or with an attached rubber sole device called a *walker*.

Quengle c.: for flexion contracture of the knee, a two-part cast hinged at the knee level, with the distal portion of the cast terminating at the ankle or foot, and the proximal portion terminating at the upper thigh.

short-leg c. (SLC): non–weight-bearing cast extending from just below the knee to the toes; for injuries of the lower limb, ankle, and foot.

   short-leg walking c. (SLWC): reinforced to accept a cast shoe or with an attached rubber walker; for ankle and foot injuries.

   patellar tendon bearing (PTB) c.: indicated for fractures in the distal third of the tibia. A short-leg walking cast with special molding at the patellar tendon, condyles, and calf to reduce rotation and reduce the axial force on the tibia during ambulation. Also called a **Sarmiento cast.**

slipper c.: incorporating the foot up to the ankle; a rigid postoperative dressing following forefoot procedures.

toe spica c.: cast specifically designed to incorporate all of the great toe and a portion or all of the foot; usually after bunion surgery.

well-leg c.: casts applied to both lower limbs and then attached together; used in some rare instances for treatment of femoral fractures.

Other Cast-Related Terms

air cast c.: term use for a wide variety of items. Most commonly used for ankle stirrups, which have air bags on both sides. However, the term is often used for larger devices such as a walking boot with air bladders.

ankle stirrup: for ankle sprains and some fractures; a hard plastic that covers the lateral and medial ankle and lower part of the leg, held in place with Velcro straps. May contain air bladder for increased stabilization.

bivalve c.: cast that is split in half (shelled) by cuts made on opposite sides of the cast to release pressure or allow removal and reapplication of the cast such as would be needed for wound care and physical therapy treatments.

Boston bivalve c.: cast split in half with a step cut rather than a straight line; most often done when the cast is going to be removed, often for physical therapy, and then reapplied.

univalve c.: cast split on one side to relieve pressure.

cast boot: any of a variety of commercially available walking boots that can often serve the function of a short-leg cast. These devices can have adjustable ankle motion and are called **controlled ankle motion (CAM) walkers**. Some of these commercially available boots have adjustable air-filled bags and are referred to as an **air cast walker**. Also called **high-tide walker, low-tide walker, short CAM walker or boot,** and **tibial gaiter.**

collar and cuff: sling with a soft portion wrapped around the neck and a cufflike device wrapped around to support the distal forearm, sometimes with the additional support of a waist band; for humeral fractures.

corrective c.: made to correct a deformity by nonsurgical technique; commonly applied to clubfeet.

fenestrate: to cut an opening (window) in a dressing or cast to allow inspection of a part.

petaling edges: to eliminate abrasion from the edge of a cast, small vertical slits are made at the edges of the cast, and then the edges (petals) are folded out and held in place by adhesive tape, moleskin, or other material.

serial c.: any sequence of casts applied in the progressive correction of deformity.

wedge c.: circumferential cutting of the cast and reapplication of plaster over the same cast after a manipulation has been performed to change bone position.

closing wedge c.: removal of a segment of plaster, with closing of that wedge by manipulation and reapplication of plaster.

opening wedge c.: circular cut cast that is opened by manipulation and then covered with a new layer of plaster.

window: removal of a piece of cast, usually square or rectangular, to allow inspection of a wound or relieve pressure at a specific point. Also said to fenestrate.

Devices Applied to Casts

abduction bar: to help maintain hip abduction; any bar placed between two long-leg casts.

cast orthosis: modifications of standard casts often applied to facilitate early motion. The cast orthosis (brace) is designed with normal physiologic characteristics in mind while still protecting the fracture site; it is molded in the manner of orthotic-type devices. In addition, it is usually hinged at the joints to allow some free motion of joints and to improve muscle recovery. Also called **cast brace.**

cast protectors: waterproof covers for a limb cast, allowing patient to shower or bathe.

cast shoe: for the most part replaces walking heels, a hook-and-loop strap-on shoe to protect the bottom of the cast from weight bearing.

walker (walking heel): hard rubber wedge directly incorporated into the sole of a cast to allow walking or resting the leg.

Cast Complications

Generally, a neurovascular and neuromuscular examination is made before, during, and after cast immobilization. However, even with close attention to treatment, the following complications can occur.

cast burns: applying cast material with water temperature too warm, which, when added to the crystallization process that produces heat, can produce skin burns.

constrictive edema: disruption of normal venous drainage with resulting fluid accumulation in soft tissue and swelling distal to the point of constriction caused by circulatory impairment. Severe swelling may lead to neurovascular involvement to include compartment syndrome.

decubitus ulcer: an area of breakdown of skin or subcutaneous tissue as a result of unrelieved pressure on a bony prominence or portion of the body resting on a firm surface for a long time. The lesions are staged as follows:
  Stage I: only the dermis is involved.
  Stage II: dermis and subcutaneous fat are involved.
  Stage III: ulcer involves some deep fascia or muscle; bone not uncovered.
  Stage IV: bone is exposed.

dropfoot: when referring to a complication of cast treatment, applies to paralysis of the peroneal nerve resulting from pressure over the fibular head leading to inability to dorsiflex the ankle.

muscle atrophy: loss of muscle tissue resulting from protracted disuse secondary to joint immobilization.

pin tract infection: direct bacterial contamination of area where pins have been used for external traction or skeletal fixation; could potentially lead to osteomyelitis.

pressure sore: breakdown of skin or subcutaneous tissue because of direct pressure of displaced or bunched cotton padding under cast, creating pressure lasting usually in excess of 4 hours; often caused by patient inserting object in cast to reach an area that is itching from plaster dust in cast; also called **decubitus ulcer.**

superior mesenteric artery syndrome: disruption of circulation to the bowel; occurs after application of body cast and results in abdominal pain, diarrhea, and, if unrecognized, severe problems; also called **cast syndrome.**

Splints and Accessories

This section is restricted to descriptions of those splints applied in the early treatment of injury or management of postoperative conditions and their accessories.

Splints

airplane s.: removable cast or prefabricated device used to hold the arm in abduction and limit shoulder flexion.

aluminum foam s.: straight, metallic foam, padded splint of various widths from ½ to 2 inches; can be used separately or in association with casts for hand and finger injuries.

baseball s.: prefabricated metallic splint applied to the volar forearm and hand; the palm portion of the splint positions the hand as if it were holding a baseball.

Bohler s.: for spiral phalangeal fractures of the fingers; a device designed to maintain proper position and continuous traction.

coaptation s.: for limb injuries; two slabs of plaster are placed on either side of the limb and held together by some outer dressing.

dynamic s.: any splint device that incorporates springs, elastic bands, and other materials that produce a constant active force to help reduce a deformity or counteract deforming forces.

frog s.: aluminum foam splint for finger injuries; before application the splint has a frog-shaped appearance.

gutter s.: semicircular or U-shaped splint fashioned around the injured part, usually in metacarpal and phalangeal fractures of the ulnar side of the hand.

hairpin s.: spring-assisted splint to help gain extension in a finger injury affecting the joint.

half shell: usually refers to spica casts; the section of cast that remains after it has been bivalved and a portion removed.

laced splint: for ankle sprains, a laced canvas ankle and proximal foot wrap that is held in place by laces; some have side pockets for insertion of more rigid plastic inserts. Also called **Swede-o.**

long-arm s.: splint applied from the axilla to wrist or distal palm posteriorly; holds the elbow and wrist in any given position.

long-leg s.: splint extending from the thigh to the lower calf or distally to the toes.

night s.: any splint or similar device used only at night. Commonly refers to a volar splint for treatment of carpal tunnel syndrome and leg splints in ankle dorsiflexion for treatment of plantar fasciitis.

pneumatic compression boot or sleeve: provides periodic compression to a limb to help prevent venous thrombosis and is often used on an uninjured limb. This is in contrast to the sequential type of pump used in lymphedema. The pneumatic sequential compression boot is another type used after knee replacement and is effective against deep vein thrombosis after lower limb surgery.

short-arm s.: splint extending from distal elbow to palm; used for nondisplaced fractures or after advanced fracture healing.

short-leg s.: splint extending from the upper calf to toes for initial immobilization.

sugar tong s.: long slab of plaster applied to the affected limb in the fashion of a sugar tong and held together with outer dressing; for wrist fractures and injuries to the shoulder, arm, and forearm; sugar tong cast.

universal gutter s.: wire mesh splint for lower extremity fractures.

Velcro s.: commercial name becoming generic referring to splints that have straps or surfaces that adhere to each other; these surfaces may be approximated and separated as many times as needed, and there is no loss of the original strength of the adhesion of the two surfaces; can be used for any part of the body.

Velpeau s.: for shoulder dislocation, humeral fracture, and other condition of the upper limb; soft dressing that surrounds the shoulder and arm with arm held close to chest and typically elbow flexed more that 90 degrees. Commercially available devices have an adjustable waist belt and shoulder immobilizer. Also called **sling and swathe,** and **Velpeau dressing.**

volar s.: specifies a splint applied to the anterior forearm.

wraparound s.: various commercially available splints that can be wrapped around a limb but are easily removable for physical therapy or wound care.

Accessories

In the area of casts, splints, and dressings, the following important aids to patient management are provided.

canes: for a painful hip; the patient is instructed to hold cane in the hand opposite the affected hip to transmit load through cane at the same moment that weight-bearing takes place on affected extremity.

crutches: when a three-point gait is needed to relieve weight-bearing on affected side; used in fractures, sprains, and after surgery. A three-point gait is when both crutches are placed on the ground simultaneously with the affected limb, decreasing body weight from three to one.

spring-loaded crutches: crutch design that absorbs peak stress, reduces shock, and reduces fatigue in upper limbs. The down-directed weight is borne by the crutches that have energy-storing ability on weight bearing.

walkers: assistive lightweight metallic devices (usually with four legs) that allow patient to apply weight bearing bilaterally when there is instability in walking. New variations in these devices include the option for a pair or quartet of wheels, hand brakes, and baskets for carrying items.

Dressings

The term *dressing* may apply to any material used to cover a wound; however, when there is considerable swelling without a wound, a dressing is used to apply pressure.

General Types of Dressings

Adaptic d.: nonadhesive mesh dressing for the direct covering of wounds.

Betadine d.: any dressing that has been impregnated with povidone-iodine (Betadine) and then applied directly to the wound.

compression d.: any dressing intended to apply pressure to reduce or prevent swelling or bleeding.

dry d.: dressing that has not been impregnated with any solution.

figure 8 d.: dressing applied in the shape of an 8, as is often done for clavicular fractures; commercially prefabricated dressings, referred to as **clavicle straps,** are available.

gauze d.: any dressing made of cheesecloth-type material, for example, Kling, Kerlix, 4 × 4.

iodoform d.: narrow gauze strip impregnated with an iodine compound; for the treatment of open wounds.

Kerlix d.: broad elastic gauze dressing often a part of a compression dressing.

Kling d.: narrow gauze elastic bandage for compression.

Koch-Mason d.: warm occlusive saline dressing placed over a limb with cellulitis.

occlusive d.: any dressing that protects a wound from outside contamination.

packing: describes that portion of a dressing that is placed inside an open wound.

pressure d.: dressing designed to apply pressure to a specific location.

protective d.: any dressing that protects a wound from trauma.

saline d.: any dressing impregnated with normal saline; for treatment of open wounds.

Telfa d.: sterile nonadherent dressing, often applied on fresh wounds or incisions.

transparent d.: a class of transparent, occlusive dressings that are weatherproof and allow direct observation of the wound. Brand name terms include **Op Site** and **Tegaderm.**

vacuum assisted closure (VAC) dressing: commercially available dressing that is applied directly to an open wound. Vacuum pressure is believed to help speed wound healing.

wet-to-dry d.: dressing that is impregnated with normal saline and allowed to dry; used as a part of open-wound treatment.

Xeroform d.: nonadherent mesh dressing applied to fresh wounds or incisions.

Other Dressing Materials

Ace bandage: nonadhesive, elastic material that is a direct compressive wrap or holds other dressings or splints in place. The trade name is now used generically.

adhesive tape: sticky nonpermeable tape used to secure local dressing.

bandage adhesive: sticky material applied to the skin to help in the application of various forms of tape; commonly used adhesive is *tincture of benzoin*.

pads: variety of bulky materials (rectangular or square) that cover large wounds; often referred to as *abdominal pads*.

Specialized Dressings

Esmarch bandage: special rubber, rolled bandages used to expel blood from a limb before surgery; also called **Martin bandage.**

Gibney bandage: strips of adhesive tape applied in alternate directions about the ankle; for ligament and other injuries.

high Dye dressing: method of noncircumferential ankle taping designed to support the ankle after an inversion injury.

Kenny-Howard splint (A/C harness): for acromioclavicular separations, a sling that supports wrist and elbow with a counterforce strap to push the clavicle down and a chest strap to hold the device in place.

low Dye dressing: taping technique for plantar fasciitis.

Robert Jones bandage: layered bulk dressing applied to the lower limbs for a variety of injuries but specifically following knee surgery or injury; also called **Shands dressing.**

Shands d.: composed of two layers of cast padding and two layers of elastic bandage applied to the leg and foot; for ankle sprains and nondisplaced fractures of the metatarsals.

universal hand d.: for compression or extensive injuries involving the hand and fingers; a bulky, even-pressured hand dressing composed of cotton or gauze fluffs and wrapped with gauze or other circular dressing material, leaving the fingertips exposed. Over this dressing, a cock-up splint is applied to hold the wrist in 15-degree extension. Some of these dressings are incorporated into a stockinet sling for elevation.

Velpeau d.: bandage applied to the arm and torso such that the elbow is at the side in flexion and the hand is pressed against the upper chest.

Suspensions, Tractions, and Frames

Suspension, traction, and frames are adjustable appliances used with pulleys, bars, weights, and other supports in the treatment of fractures with casts or splints, for scoliosis, and in the care of patients before and after surgery. This method of treatment is offered to ensure proper alignment in healing and to provide suspension or deliver pull, directly or indirectly, to bone, muscle, skin, and fascia.

Many of the parts of various suspensions and traction devices are known by the originator's name. Devices are listed by placement, each with its component.

New techniques and methods of traction can be found in suppliers' catalogs, but the user should find this section helpful in deciphering why such devices are used in the care of patients. The various types of traction equipment are defined, followed by some emergency stabilization equipment.

Suspension

Suspension is the means by which a limb or part is held suspended by some external device. Traction often accompanies the suspension.

balanced suspension (Fig. 6-1): suspension device that allows the patient to move the affected limb without changing the fracture position of that limb; preferred for treatment of long-bone injuries. There are two components:

Arizona universal leg support: for lower limb fracture; a balanced suspension device with adjustable anterior thigh pad and suspension support by two parallel lines from the knee and foot.

Thomas splint: originally designed to help splint fresh fractures; composed of a full ring around the thigh and two metal rods that extend down either side of the limb and are joined distally to the foot. The **half-ring Thomas splint** is the most commonly used. Most are adjustable for length and are thus called **adjustable Thomas splints.**

Pearson attachment: attached to a Thomas splint; consists of two metal rods joined distally, allowing flexion of the knee.

overhead suspension: the forearm is suspended overhead with the elbow bent; used in treatment of forearm and elbow fractures.

Traction (Fig. 6-2)

In general, traction is the pull on a limb or a part thereof. Skin traction (indirect traction) is applied by using a bandage to pull on the skin and fascia when light traction is required. Skeletal traction (direct traction), however, uses pins or wires inserted through bone and is attached to weights, pulleys, and ropes. This is applied when a longer period is needed in traction. External fixators can be attached to the traction apparatus to help in the healing process. Internal and external fixation techniques have mostly replaced the devices. The following devices are applied:

Barton tongs: skull tongs for cervical skeletal traction.
Böhler-Braun frame: metallic adjustable frame for support of the thigh and leg; for leg elevation and often in severe ankle fractures in which os calcis traction is applied.

FIG 6-1 Balanced suspension. *(Modified from Smith RM: Femoral shaft fractures. In Browner BD et al, editors: Skeletal trauma, ed 4, Philadelphia, 2009, Elsevier, Fig. 52-10.)*

FIG 6-2 **A,** Skin traction. **B,** Skeletal traction. (**A** *modified from Herring JA, editor: Tachdjian's pediatric orthopaedics, ed 4, Philadelphia, 2008, Elsevier, Fig. 43-74.* **B** *modified from Thompson SR: Handbook of splinting and casting, Philadelphia, 2012, Elsevier, Fig. 15-9.)*

Bryant t. (Fig. 6-3): for infants only; an overhead suspension of leg and thigh such that the knees are extended and the thighs flexed to 90 degrees.

Buck t.: originally designed as skin traction incorporating the entire lower limb but now describes skin traction of the leg only; generally used in knee injuries but also a temporary measure applied in hip fractures.

cervical halter t.: a cloth, halterlike sling for traction of the neck; applied when patient is sitting or lying down, continuously or intermittently; also called **head halter traction.**

Charnley t.: for femoral fractures; wire or pin through proximal tibia, incorporated into a short-leg cast that has a flanged extension at heel to prevent leg rotation.

continuous passive motion (CPM): for early knee or hip motion following injury or surgery; frames that support calf and thigh. The electric motor-driven device allows passive continuous flexion and extension of knee.

Cotrel t.: combination of a cervical sling and pelvic traction used in scoliosis before surgery or casting to help straighten the back.

Crutchfield tongs: type of cranial skeletal tongs used for traction of the cervical spine.

Dunlop t.: commonly used for elbow fractures; the arm is held suspended by skin or a combination of skin and skeletal traction, with a weight applied to the lower arm.

Gardner-Wells tongs: device for immobilization of cervical spine injuries in which two sharp metal pins are screwed into the superficial layer of the skull. They are then connected to hanging weights or other traction devices for stabilization of the spine. They may also be used for definitive treatment of spine injuries.

halo-femoral t.: bed-type traction using a ring-shaped device directly affixed to the bone of the skull in conjunction with femoral skeletal traction; used in scoliosis or injury distraction.

halo-pelvic t.: ambulatory-type traction for cervical spine injuries that uses a ring-shaped device directly affixed to the bone of the skull in conjunction with pelvic skeletal pins. These are interconnected to hold the spine rigid when the patient is ambulatory.

Kirschner wire (K-wire): skeletal t. in which small wires are placed across bone(s) so that a traction device can be placed externally; applied to some pediatric and hand fractures. May be threaded or nonthreaded.

FIG 6-3 Various traction devices. *(From the American Orthopaedic Association: Manual of orthopaedic surgery,* ed 5, *Chicago, 1979, American Orthopaedic Association.)*

Bryant's traction

Buck's extension

Thomas splint

Pearson attachment

Suspended or floating traction

Lyman-Smith t.: use of olecranon pin and overhead traction for supracondylar (elbow) fractures.

Neufeld roller t.: for fractured femur; a cast for the calf and thigh is hinged at the knee and suspended by a line to the anterior midthigh looped around a pulley and to a spring attached to the anterior midleg. The pulley for this loop is then supported by an overhead suspension with weight and a second pulley.

pelvic sling: sling encircling the hip and pelvic region in treatment of pelvic injuries; sling is suspended overhead.

pelvic t.: cloth, girdle-type device with traction directed at the foot of the bed; for lower-back disorders such as herniated disks.

Quigley t.: for lateral malleolar and trimalleolar fractures; a stockinet is placed around the leg and ankle, with the ankle being suspended by the stockinet attached to an overhead frame.

Russell t.: skin traction on the lower limb from thigh to ankle or knee to ankle, attached to a sling that suspends the distal thigh. This may be done with a continuous rope and a number of pulleys (simple) or with two different weights, one for the leg and the other for thigh suspension portion (split). Russell traction is often used with older adults as a temporizing treatment for fractured hips or in the very young in treatment of femoral fractures. Also called **Hamilton-Russell.**

semi-Fowler position: semisitting position with knees flexed; used in lower back and lumbar disk disorders.

skeletal t.: any traction using a pin through the bone to deliver traction; for the tibia, femur, olecranon, os calcis, and metacarpal.

Steinmann pin: wide-diameter pin for heavy skeletal traction such as in the tibia or femur. May be threaded or nonthreaded.

traction bow: U-shaped piece of metal for placement into a K-wire or Steinmann pin in skeletal traction.

Vinke tongs: special set of skeletal traction tongs used for skull traction in neck injuries.

well-leg t.: bilateral casting of lower limbs with an interconnecting metal bar that allows traction on one leg to be supported by the other; for femoral fractures, it has the advantage that a patient can be moved out of bed.

90–90 t.: for some femur fractures and low-back disorders; the patient is placed supine, with hips and knees flexed to 90 degrees such that the calf is suspended; for femoral fractures.

Frames

Frames are specialty units for an entire bed or additions to a bed.

Balkan f.: upright metal bars based at the corners of a bed and connected by overhead metal bars that hold suspension and traction pulleys.

Bradford f.: canvas bed suspended from rectangular poles with opening for the buttocks; split Bradford.

claw-type basic f.: traction frame that is attached to the bed by a clawlike clamp device.

Foster f.: special bed composed of two stretcherlike parts that, when connected, hold the patient sandwiched firmly between them, allowing the patient to be completely turned without injury to the spine; used for tuberculosis and spinal fractures or for patients with scoliosis following a Harrington instrumentation and fusion. A **Stryker frame** is a similarly constructed device.

Heffington f.: device that attaches to a standard operating table to allow prone position of a patient for lumbar spine surgery. The table end is dropped 90 degrees with patient's hips flexed over the edge and the patient further flexed to reverse the lumbar lordosis.

intravenous (IV)-type basic f.: traction frame that is attached to the bed by a device similar to that used for holding IV poles.

Jones abduction f.: a special frame used on standard beds to assist in gaining hip abduction in tuberculosis, acute arthritis, and other diseases of the hip.

Watson-Jones f.: for holding tibial fractures in surgery; a semicircular posterior-inferior thigh cuff with an attached adjustable extension that runs posterior to the leg with the knee in 90-degrees flexion. Tibial traction is maintained with a Steinmann pin.

Whitman f.: specially constructed frame to assist in gaining spine extension; may be used when cast application is necessary.

Emergency Stabilization

The use of emergency measures in trauma situations has saved many lives and limbs. There are many new types of equipment made for stabilization of the injured. These temporary measures of tamponade, fracture immobilization, and tissue protection are generally performed by trained emergency medical technicians and paramedics acting under the guidance of emergency room physicians. The various types of air splints should be used only by those trained in their use. The following emergency equipment may be used before the patient reaches the hospital.

air pressure splints: double-walled plastic tubes that, in the deflated state, are placed around the injured limb and are then inflated (either by mouth or inflation device) to bring about even pressure and immobilization.

Hare traction: metallic splint with multiple straps and a special distal traction device for use in transporting unstable lower-limb-injured patients.

inflatable splint: sometimes referred to as an **air splint,** it is a first-aid device used at the onset of injury; when blown up, this balloonlike splint provides good immobilization with even pressure. It is usually applied to the lower leg and foot, but other inflatable splints incorporate the entire arm or entire lower limb.

medical antishock trousers (MAST): pneumatic sleeve for immediate stabilization of lower limbs in cases of trauma. MAST encompasses lower limbs and abdomen to provide sufficient pressure to force blood to the central portion of the body. This provides some stabilization of shock and provides stability for pelvic, hip, and femoral fractures and aids in preventing further tissue damage. In addition to tamponading sites of bleeding, this device sometimes acts by increasing pulse and blood pressure. Its use is controversial, and it should be used carefully and briefly (if at all) to avoid prolonged muscle ischemia and MAST-associated compartment syndrome. MAST is inflated by a foot-operated pump.

Neal-Robertson litter: modified spine board for transporting trauma patients with spinal injuries to the emergency room.

posterior splint: for emergency immobilization; rigid devices used for initial stabilization of upper and lower limb fractures.

Sager traction splint: for femoral fractures; emergency traction splint with a unit that measures the force of traction at the ankle. For children and adults, this device maintains fracture position and alignment without excessive pressure around the ankle or sciatic nerve injury.

spinal board: rigid board with multiple slots for straps used for head and thoracolumbar restraints; designed to transport patients in a relatively immobile state.

For further information on emergency stabilization measures, refer to Crosby LA, et al.

Prosthetics and Orthotics

Prosthetists and orthotists are allied health professionals who measure, design, fabricate, and fit prostheses (artificial limbs) and orthoses (braces).

Prosthetics is the science that specializes with functional and cosmetic restoration of all or part of a missing limb, following the directive of a physician's prescription.

Orthotics is the science that focuses on orthoses designed to provide external control, correction, and support for the patient in need for nonoperative management of musculoskeletal disorders. Service in this area is also provided on a prescription basis.

The words *prosthetics* and *orthotics* may be used as nouns to describe the body of knowledge each pertains to, as in the preceding two paragraphs. The devices are referred to as *prostheses* and *orthoses*. When referring to a specific device, the words *prosthetic* and *orthotic* are adjectives needing an appropriate noun.

Specialists in these areas are certified by the American Board for Certification and titled **certified prosthetist (CP)** and **certified orthotist (CO). A certified prosthetist-orthotist (CPO)** has demonstrated proficiency in both fields during examinations by the national board. Supportive personnel are orthotic and prosthetic assistants, orthotic fitters, and technicians, with varying responsibilities and duties.

Many major institutions have ongoing prosthetic and orthotic clinics or conferences that meet as often as patient need requires. Members of the clinic team consist of a chief physician, physical and occupational therapists, a prosthetist, an orthotist, a rehabilitation nurse, and a social worker. The clinic team approach is oriented toward management of the total patient, so although the rationale for prescription of an appropriate prosthetic or orthotic system is a prerequisite, the complete rehabilitation program is the long-range goal and responsibility of the team. Factors such as vocational retraining, if necessary, financial considerations of various phases of management, the necessity and duration of physical or occupational therapy, and a possible need for psychologic counseling are all taken into account. Perhaps most important, the patient must feel comfortable in the clinical setting and be assured that the result will be as satisfactory as is realistic and attainable.

The prosthetist or orthotist is responsible for assisting with the prescription regarding components, elements of design, definitive and proper fitting of the system, and follow-up and adjustments as indicated at future visits to the clinic.

If prosthetic and orthotic practitioners are to serve patients at the highest professional level, they must maintain a program of further education to remain informed of new techniques, components, and concepts. Such programs are available through the American Academy of Orthotists and Prosthetists. Other groups are the American Orthotics and Prosthetics Association (AOPA) and the Children's Amputee Prosthetic Program (CAPP).

Prosthetics

Prosthetics, or artificial limbs, are designed to replace function and sometimes cosmesis of a missing body part. Internal prostheses are surgically implanted devices, such as the artificial hip, and are described in Chapter 8.

Upper Limb Prosthetics

An upper limb prosthesis is an external system designed for the partial hand level amputation distally to the interscapulothoracic (forequarter) level proximally. This terminology is different from that that used by surgeons in describing the amputation levels.

elbow disarticulation (ED): amputation through the elbow joint. Correct with elbow disarticulation prosthesis with socket encompassing the residual limb and trimmed at the proximal humerus to allow good range of motion. This socket design is used with cable and figure-eight harness control, external elbow hinges with lock, wrist unit, and terminal device. The cable design can be either a Bowden, fair-lead or triple control cabling system.

interscapulothoracic (forequarter amputation): this level of amputation includes the resection of the scapula. Correct with cosmetic shoulder cap to restore normal appearance for clothing, but differing in that an extension usually goes around and over the sound shoulder to provide additional suspension. The weight of the prosthesis assists in balance during sitting, standing, and walking. This system will be used with cable (Bowden, fair-lead or triple control), modified chest strap, and waist belt-type harnessing, excursion amplifier, shoulder joint similar to that used in shoulder disarticulations, internal locking elbow, forearm lift assist, wrist unit, and terminal device.

partial hand amputation: distal to or through one or more of the phalanges, metacarpals or resection at any level of the thumb. Restore function with cosmetic individual finger replacements with fillers and/or opposition-type posts. More proximal amputation sites necessitate cosmetic gloves and wired finger fillers or more intricately designed opposition posts to restore function. Proximal partial hand amputations for more active individuals or individuals with careers that require more hand dexterity can benefit from myoelectric partial hand prosthetic components.

shoulder disarticulation (SD): amputation through the glenohumeral joint. Correct with shoulder disarticulation prosthesis with larger socket extending from the spine posteriorly to near the xiphoid process anteriorly and fitted closely at the neck; used with a fair-lead cable, modified chest strap–type harness, shoulder joint or bulkhead (spacer) to allow passive positioning in abduction and adduction, passive positioning, and flexion and extension, internal locking elbow, forearm lift assist, wrist unit, and terminal device.

transhumeral amputation (TH): Previously referred to as an *above elbow amputation*; proximal to elbow joint but distal to shoulder. Prosthetic socket will extend over the acromion to support axial loading and carefully fitted at axilla. This design is used with a fair-lead cable and figure-eight harness, elbow unit, forearm lift assist, wrist unit, and terminal device. Depending on the length of the transhumeral amputation, the component will change. For example, a class I transhumeral amputation level will use outside locking hinges, whereas a class III amputation level will incorporate an internal locking elbow unit

transradial amputation (TR): Previously referred to as a *below elbow amputation*. Level of involvement is proximal to wrist but distal to elbow. TR prostheses are designed to fit the residual limb, retaining pronation and supination in the longer levels, while allowing flexion. Several cable options are available based on length of residual limb, including a Bowden cable and fair-lead cable, additional components include a figure-eight harness control, flexible or rigid elbow hinges, wrist unit, and terminal device. **Münster** prosthetic socket design makes the system applicable for short to very short transradial amputations. This socket design must be carefully fitted proximal to the epicondyles at the elbow to provide adequate suspension without the aid of additional devices.

wrist disarticulation (WD): amputation through the wrist joint. The prosthetic socket is designed to be donned over the bulbous ("screwdriver" shape) distal end of the residual limb, retaining as much pronation and supination as possible. The prosthetist will trim the anterior, medial, lateral, and posterior trim of the socket to allow functional motion. This socket design is used with a Bowden cable system, a figure-nine or figure-eight harness, flexible elbow hinges, wrist unit, and terminal device.

Upper Limb Prosthetic Components

The components of an upper limb prosthesis include any device that is a supportive or integral part of the prosthesis, including terminal devices.

control cables: steel cable traveling inside housing to move and lock mechanical joints, for example, flexion and locking of the elbow joint; also provide prehension to the terminal device. The housing is sometimes lined with Teflon to reduce friction and thereby increase efficiency. Cable systems are generally lightweight, as for small children, with standard 1/8-inch or heavy-duty cable (e.g., Bowden single, Fair-Lead dual, and triple control cables). Fig. 7-1 illustrates single control only.

elbow hinges: mechanical types of hinges to provide specific strength or allow controlled mobility. The following types are commonly used: single pivot providing mediolateral control, suspension polycentric, multiple action, sliding action step-up, and residual limb activated locking. These are all designed to provide additional forearm flexion for very short below-elbow amputations or the patient with flexion contracture.

electrical switch control: prosthesis for the patient with shoulder disarticulation or transhumeral or forequarter amputation; uses switches to control current from a battery that operates an electrical elbow or hand. The switches are placed in strategic positions within the harness system, and by opening these switches the patient is able to operate the electrical elbow or hand. This type of system is most feasible for patients with limited excursion from causes such as contractures, higher levels of amputation, or bilateral limbs, because each position in the switch is 1/16-inch excursion—considerably less than that required to operate the standard system.

excursion amplifier sleeve: pulley and cable system used to increase efficiency in patients with limited excursion; generally used in shoulder disarticulation and forequarter systems.

flexible hinges: hinges made of Dacron tape or metal spirals to provide suspension while allowing retention of available pronation and supination for long transradial and wrist disarticulation residual limb length. Supination and pronation are not available in very short, short, and some standard levels of amputation

forearm lift assist: adjustable spring-loaded device attached to the elbow to provide initial forearm flexion; especially applicable for those with higher level amputations such as shorter above-elbow amputation and shoulder disarticulation.

Griefer prosthesis: electrically enhanced, strong-gripping hand component.

myoelectric control: sophisticated prosthesis available for the patient with wrist disarticulation, below-elbow or above-elbow amputation: uses electrodes placed over the flexor and extensor muscle groups to pick up the milliamperes of electricity emitted by a muscle during contraction. This electrical stimulus is then used to operate a switch that controls a motor in a mechanical hand or other component. Prosthetic sockets are generally self-suspended, thereby eliminating the need for any harness.

FIG 7-1 Control cable housing. *(From* Below and Above Harness and Control System, *Evanston, IL, 1966, Northwestern University Prosthetic-Orthotic Center.)*

nudge control: mechanical unit that can be pressed by the chin to lock or unlock one or more joints of the prosthesis; seen in forequarter systems.

outside locking hinge: used on the elbow disarticulation system because of length of residual limb. Outside locking elbow and internal positive locking elbow hinges with multiple locking positions are used for above-elbow, shoulder disarticulation, and forequarter systems.

shoulder harness, chest straps, and waist belts: an infinite variety of Dacron, cloth, and leather materials is used to fabricate these components, which provide suspension as well as control through their attachment to cables that operate locks for various joints and provide function for the terminal device. The figure-eight ring harness is one of the most common and provides suspension and control of prosthesis. The figure-nine harness supplies only control, as the Müenster socket provides suspension (Fig. 7-2).

terminal devices: hooks or hands affixed to the wrist unit, affording function and cosmesis.

   hands: a number of functional and passive hands are available. The mechanically functional hand provides prehension through several options. Options include a voluntary opening hand, voluntary closing hand, or myoelectrically controlled hand. A cosmetic glove matched to the patient's skin color is applied externally. Passive hands, although nonfunctional, generally provide increased cosmesis. Some specific hands are **Dorrance voluntary-opening hand, Sierra voluntary-opening hand, APRL voluntary-closing hand, soft voluntary-closing hand, Becker locking grip hand,** and **CAPP terminal device.**

hooks: Prosthetic hooks have lyre or canted fingers, rubber bands, and a ball terminal attachment for the cable system. Lyre-shaped hooks provide a "straight approach" to pick up different objects. The lyre shaped hook allows for fine point prehension (such as picking up a needle), but the individuals line of sight is slightly obstructed. Canted shape hooks allow for a "side approach" for prehensile activities, such as using a pencil, and allows for better line of sight for the individual. Hooks are available in numerous sizes, generally in aluminum with Plastisol covering for children, aluminum or stainless steel with neoprene or nitrile lining, stainless steel with serrated inner finger surface such as the model 5X, and for heavy-duty tasks the 7 or 7LO (large opening) types **(farmer's hook),** designed to hold devices such as shovels or rakes. Although certain hooks differ, such as the Army Prosthetics Research Laboratory (APRL) types, most use rubber bands or springs to close (voluntary opening), and prehension is directly proportional to the strength and number used. Other devices are model 8x small adult, model 10 children, model 12P infants, mitts, and **N-Alber II** for task-specific tool interchange. Hooks may also be classified as voluntary closing, where the individual controls the force of grip during prehensile activities. Voluntary closing hooks involve more complexity of use compared to a voluntary opening terminal device.

wrist flexion unit: allows prepositioning of terminal device closer to the midline of the body; generally used for the bilateral patient.

FIG 7-2 Cross-point of harness connected by stainless steel ring. *(From Below and Above Elbow Harness and Control System, Evanston, IL, 1966, Northwestern University Prosthetic-Orthotic Center.)*

wrist units: integral components at the distal end of the prosthesis that allow attachment, interchangeability, and pronation and supination of the terminal devices. Types are standard, constant friction, and quick change; units are oval or round to match the distal anatomic aspect of the residual limb.

Lower Limb Prostheses and Components (Fig. 7-3)

Lower limb prostheses are any external system designed for the amputation levels from the partial foot level distally to the hemipelvectomy level proximally. They are categorized as *exoskeletal* or *endoskeletal*. The exoskeletal prosthesis has a rigid outer shell that provides structural strength and cosmetic shape. The endoskeletal prosthesis has a tubular structure connecting the components and is covered by cosmetic foam. The primary components of the prosthesis are the socket, suspension system, foot, and knee unit. This terminology is different from that used by surgeons in describing the amputation levels.

Chopart: distal to the ankle joint. Correct with distal weight-bearing socket with partial foot replacement.

FIG 7-3 A patellar tendon-bearing exoskeletal prosthesis with supracondylar cuff and solid ankle cushioned heel foot.

hemipelvectomy: amputation at hip level with ablation of the ischial tuberosity. Correct with plastic socket designed to distribute weight using remaining musculature, rib margin, cosmetic socket build-up, mechanical hip and knee joints, and prosthetic foot.

hip disarticulation (HD): amputation at the hip level but with the ischial tuberosity intact. Correct with plastic socket designed to transpose weight through the ischial tuberosity and related gluteal musculature, mechanical hip and knee joints, and prosthetic foot.

Jaipur foot: foot device using readily available materials attached to end of prosthesis for barefoot individuals. The prosthesis is cheap and can be made in 1 hour. It enables individuals to work in rural conditions and muddy, wet fields, and to climb trees. It has been widely used in India, southeast Asia, and Africa, where local variations to the design have now been made.

knee disarticulation: amputation through the knee joint. The socket is self-suspending with either a medial opening or a soft liner to facilitate donning. A Silesian belt can be worn as an auxiliary suspension. There is also a polycentric (four-bar linkage) knee unit and prosthetic foot. End-bearing leather or plastic sockets with external hinges, fork straps, and waist belts are still in use. Also called **knee bearing (K/B).**

Lisfranc: a disarticulation through the medial metatarsophalangeal joint or metatarsal-tarsal joints. Correct with extended steel shank in shoe to provide a place to push off and toe filler or foot plate with toe filler.

stubbies: short lower-limb prosthesis, typically for bilateral above-knee amputations that do not include knee units. Designed to increase stability during initial ambulation by lowering the individual's center of gravity.

Syme: through the ankle joint; results in a bulbous distal weight-bearing residual limb. Correct with a medial-opening or expandable-wall prosthesis, which facilitates application and removal. Weight-bearing is distributed between the distal end and the patellar tendon. The socket is self-suspending because of the reduced circumference above the distal limb.

transfemoral: formerly called *above knee*, it is proximal to the knee joint but distal to the hip joint. Correct with quadrilateral or narrow medial-lateral ischial containment socket prosthesis.

computer-assisted design/computer-assisted manufacturing (CAD-CAM): refers to the contour of the socket and how it is modified. It is a handmade, computer-assisted method of providing a cosmetically accurate fit that can use any of the ischial containment sockets.

ischial containment sockets: an transfemoral amputation socket design incorporates a narrow M/L shape, high lateral wall, and a slanted pocket to encompass the ischium. Provides greater control of lateral forces during gait and a more even distribution of proximal weight-bearing areas. Also called **narrow medial-lateral** and **contour adducted trochanteric controlled alignment method (CAT-CAM).**

quadrilateral ischial weight-bearing socket: wooden or plastic socket designed with a shelf to transpose weight through the ischial tuberosity; suspension may be achieved by a hip joint with a pelvic band and control belt or with a suction socket.

transtibial: formerly called *below knee,* it is proximal to the ankle but distal to the knee. Correct with patellar tendon–bearing (PTB) prosthesis, designed to bear weight through the patellar tendon, medial tibial flare, and other pressure-tolerant areas; socket may be hard or have a soft liner. Suspension is with supracondylar cuff strap or with waist belt, sleeve, or suction. Self-suspending variations of the PTB prosthesis include the following:

side joint and thigh laser (joint and corset): for the patient with mediolateral instability of the knee, for a very short below-knee amputation, or for residual limb incapable of supporting total body weight because of conditions such as burns and skin-adherent tissue. A typical prescription is as follows: PTB type of socket, external mechanical knee joints, thigh corset, fork strap, waist belt, and prosthetic foot.

suction socket suspension: for transtibial prosthesis, a design of suspension that incorporates a valve, silicone and other materials for a liner, and suspension sleeve to stabilize the residual limb in the socket without volume fluctuation. The silicone liner may incorporate a liner with silicone ring to achieve socket suction without having to apply the suspension sleeve. Differs from PTB type.

supracondylar (PTB-SC): PTB with supracondylar stability incorporates higher medial and lateral walls that encompass the femoral condyles. A medial wedge, either movable or built into a soft liner, is placed firmly over the medial epicondyle.

supracondylar-suprapatellar (SC-SP): similar to supracondylar but also includes a high anterior wall that encompasses the patella. This provides increased suspension and increased surface area to decrease pressure on the residual limb, and limits hyperextension of the knee.

Lower Limb Prosthetic Components

below-knee suspension: used to support below-knee prostheses.

billet: connects supracondylar cuff to waist belt.

condylar cuff: mediolateral attachment to a transtibial prosthesis with strap proximal to femoral condyles.

fork strap: anterolateral attachment to prosthesis connecting to waist belt.

suction socket: cushion liners are used for suction prosthetics and are worn directly over residual limb. Can assist in achieving suction by adding a vacuum to the socket, or by adding a suspension liner over the cushion liner and socket to achieve suction suspension.

supracondylar cuff: tabs that attach mediolaterally to prosthesis with cuff strap going around knee proximally to femoral condyles.

waist belt: webbing wrapped circumferentially at pelvis with connection to billet or fork strap.

foot and ankle components: allow normal gait patterns. There are five clinical categories of prosthetic feet designed according to the level of activity of the wearer:

dynamic response foot: curved metal strip that brings about spring action to assist in toe-off.

energy storing feet: incorporates a cushioned heel with a resilient toe lever that stores energy in stance phase and releases it at toe-off. Typically lighter than a solid ankle cushioned heel (SACH) foot.

multiaxial ankle: allows plantar flexion and dorsiflexion, and inversion and eversion. It is the traditional SACH foot with sides to flex.

SACH foot: solid ankle cushioned heel (wedge).

single-axis ankle: allows anteroposterior motion and controlled plantar flexion with dorsiflexion stop.

hip disarticulation or hemipelvectomy suspension: webbing over shoulder on sound side with anteroposterior socket attachments.

knee disarticulation suspension: the most common type of suspension for a knee disarticulation patient is self-suspension over the femoral condyles or suction, then a total elastic suspension belt, not a waist belt.

knee prosthetic components: designed to provide stability during early and middle stance phases and bend in late stance and swing phase, as well as in kneeling and sitting.

  external: most common application in knee bearing; no controlled friction.

  fluid-controlled knee (hydraulic or pneumatic): provides swing phase control for a variable rate of gait, eliminating excessive heel rise and terminal impact. Varieties include Dupaco, Dynaplex, Daw, Otto Bock, and Mauch.

  four-bar linkage: a polycentric system that is inherently stable, this unit can be adjusted to change the instantaneous center of rotation during dynamic alignment.

  hybrid knee: combined polycentric knee with pneumatic fluid-control cylinder component.

  manual locking knee: knee automatically locks at full extension. Patient-controlled lock disengages for sitting.

  safety knee: weight-activated stance control. When knee is extended and weight-bearing, an adjustable braking mechanism is activated to resist flexion.

  single axis knee: single point of rotation with constant friction to control swing phase.

  swing and stance knee (S n' S): a hydraulic knee unit that can be adjusted to control resistance during swing and stance phases of gait.

transfemoral suspension: used to suspend above-knee prostheses.

control belt: leather wrapped circumferentially at pelvis and attached to pelvic band.

pelvic band: mechanical free-motion joint positioned anatomically on lateral wall of socket with metal band contoured to pelvis and attached to upright of hip joint. Also called **hip joint.**

shoulder harness or suspenders: webbing straps traversing shoulders with roller and cord or various attachments to socket.

Silesian bandage or belt: webbing over hip on sound side with one lateral and two anterior socket attachments. Used in conjunction with a looser-fitting suction socket.

Other Components, Materials, and Techniques

cast sock: used to take negative plaster impressions; sometimes used with or in place of residual limb socks; especially applicable for the new transtibial amputations during volume reduction of the residual limb.

check socket: an adjustable, clear plastic socket used to ensure proper fit before definitive fabrication; also called **test sock.**

distal end pad: injection of Silastic or an equivalent foam into end of socket of below- or above-knee systems; provides total contact distally and reduces possibility of edema.

donning sleeve: for transfemoral amputation a tubular cotton or nylon material allowing the patient to don suction socket of the prosthesis during volume reduction of the residual limb.

extension aid: to assist knee extension in the above-knee prosthesis.

pylon: height-adjustable tubular component that connects the socket and prosthetic foot (endoskeletal construction).

residual limb-compression garment: compression sleeve worn on residual limb to reduce volume.

rigid dressing: device worn on residual limb to reduce volume, protect the residual limb during transfers, and desensitize the limb. A rigid dressing can be fabricated using plaster, fiberglass, or a plastic.

rotator unit: component in the prosthesis designed to compensate for shear forces, thereby reducing torque and friction between the residual limb and interface of the socket; also called **torsion unit.**

sheath: nylon interface worn between residual limb and stump socks to reduce shear forces.

silicone gel socket insert: inner liner made of silicone gel designed to absorb shear forces. Often used for problem-fitting transtibial patients.

suspension sleeve: neoprene, gel, or latex sleeve worn over proximal portion of the prosthesis and extending onto the patient's thigh. Provides suction suspension.

socket: custom-fabricated component into which the residual limb fits.

soft cosmetic cover: foam material covering endoskeletal components; shaped cosmetically.

soft socket insert: soft inner liner for a patellar tendon–bearing socket. Petite or silicone gel most common.

sock: wool or cotton sock worn over residual limb to provide a cushion for friction between skin and socket interface. Available in various plies (thicknesses) from the thinnest (1 ply) to the thickest (6 ply).

total contact: for transtibial amputation intimacy between socket and residual limb, particularly at distal end, to control edema.

Specialized Systems

immediate operative prosthesis (IPOP): procedure performed immediately after surgery; patient is fitted with plaster type of socket, adjustable pylon, and prosthetic foot. Advantages include early ambulation, protection of the residual limb, and psychologic benefits.

intermediate prosthesis: thermoplastic type of socket with adjustable pylon and prosthetic foot; intermediate phase of management used to expedite fitting, establish early ambulation, and reduce volume of residual limb prior to definitive fitting. Also called **temporary prosthesis.**

modular prosthesis: selectively applicable for below-knee or any level of proximal amputations; use socket according to prescription with adjustable pylon and foot and socket attachment plates; exterior surface is made of custom-shaped foam and covered with cosmetic material. Also called **endoskeletal prosthesis.**

Orthoses

An orthosis is an externally applied device designed to provide control, correction, and support and decrease of deformity. The orthosis can either resist or assist motion to control deformity, to unweight a body segment by force reduction, and provide corrective measures.

The Task Force on Standardization of Prosthetic-Orthotic Terminology of the Committee on Prosthetic-Orthotic Education, National Research Council, and the AOPA have been largely responsible for the implementation of the terminology generally in use today. In an effort to enhance communication between the prescribing physician and the orthotist, the following descriptive guidelines have been adopted. The standardization is based on indicating those joints and regions that the orthosis is to encompass or control. The orthosis controls the named joint by allowing free, assisted, or resisted motion. Orthosis types are as follows:

AFO: ankle-foot orthosis
AO: ankle orthosis
BFO: balanced forearm orthosis
CO: cervical orthosis
CTLSO: cervicothoracolumbosacral orthosis
CTO: cervicothoracic orthosis
EO: elbow orthosis
EWHO: elbow-wrist-hand orthosis
FO: foot orthosis
HKAFO: hip-knee-ankle-foot orthosis
HdO: hand orthosis
HpO: hip orthosis
KAFO: knee-ankle-foot orthosis
KO: knee orthosis
LSO: lumbosacral orthosis
PRO: pressure-relieving orthosis
PTBO: patellar tendon–bearing orthosis
SEWHO: shoulder-elbow-wrist-hand orthosis
SIO: sacroiliac orthosis
SO: shoulder orthosis
SOMI: sternooccipital mandibular immobilizer
TLSO: thoracolumbosacral orthosis
TO: thoracic orthosis
WAWHO: wrist-action, wrist-hand orthosis

WDWHO: wrist-driven, wrist-hand orthosis
WHO: wrist-hand orthosis

Use of the foregoing terms leaves the materials, design, and components to the discretion of the orthotist, unless otherwise indicated by prescription, as demonstrated in the following examples.

> **Prescription:** AFO to provide dorsiflexion assist. (This simple prescription leaves orthotic management regarding materials for the system to be determined by the orthotist according to patient evaluation.)
> **Prescription:** AFO to provide dorsiflexion assist; double metal uprights, Klenzak ankle joint, calf band, Velcro closure, and shoe attachments.
> **Prescription:** AFO to provide dorsiflexion assist; thermoplastic fabrication.

As demonstrated, this format provides the prescribing physician with various controls over the patient's management.*

Lower-Limb Orthoses

Because all orthoses currently in use are too numerous to discuss, we confine our list to those most commonly prescribed.

Foot Orthoses

club foot o.: consists of a rigid bar riveted or clamped to shoes at either end. The bar provides hip abduction with ratchet adjustments controlling rotation; generally prescribed for treatment of clubfoot, equinovarus, pes planus, or tibial torsion. These systems allow for more independent control and leg movement with infant able to crawl because of jointed bars. Also called **Dobs bar, Ponsetti bar,** and **Denis-Browne bar.**

flexible o. (accommodative orthosis): providing longitudinal arch and metatarsal support; orthosis is removable from shoe. The goal of accommodative foot orthoses are to accommodate and support the current position of the foot, especially regarding rigid deformities.

---

*Those individuals in need of further information in the area of orthotics, see American Academy of Orthopaedic Surgeons, 1975.

hallux valgus o.: a durable medical equipment not fit by orthotists designed for day and night use; reduces bunion pain by decreasing valgus deformity (pulls toe to midline of body).

rigid corrective o.: carbon composite fiberglass and stainless steel designed to provide arch support for pes planus or other related problems of a flexible foot deformity; orthosis is removable from shoe.

UCBL o.: (developed at the University of California Biomechanics Laboratory) similar to the rigid foot orthoses, but trimlines are more proximal to increase stability and correction of the heel.

Ankle Orthoses

elastic o.: provides minimal support, acts as a kinesthetic reminder and helps control swelling.

leather gauntlet o.: leather, canvas, or equivalent material provides substantial immobilization of the ankle to alleviate pain caused by motion.

Ankle-Foot Orthoses

Charcot restraint orthotic walker (CROW): rigid orthotic with rocker bottom foot; inner aspect lined with foam with a dual-density custom insert to stabilize and prevent further deformity of the foot.

conventional o.: fitted ¾-inch distal to head of fibula and is an integral part of the shoe; examples are single or double upright jointed ankle, free motion, limited motion, and dorsiflexion assist; used with calf band, buckle, or hook-and-loop closure and stirrup with shoe attachments. Indicated for patient populations that have edema variance.

double adjustable ankle joint (DAAJ): ankle motion can be adjusted to lock, limit, or provide assistance (via springs) for various flexion and dorsiflexion ranges of motion.

floor reaction o.: most designs mimic a solid-ankle AFO (regarding the ankle), and does not allow plantar or dorsiflexion. Plantarflexion can only be permitted if the orthosis is articulated with adjustable joints. Also called **ground reaction AFO.**

patellar tendon–bearing (PTB) o.: weight-bearing terminates just proximal to the patellar tendon and is fitted around the knee similar to the below-knee prosthetic socket; used with molded foot plate or ankle joints and stirrup with shoe attachments; designed to transmit body weight through the patellar tendon and medial femoral condyle to achieve controlled unloading of weight on the tibia and ankle-foot complex; anteroposteriorly sectioned proximally.

spring wire o.: medial and lateral spring wire uprights attached to calf band proximally and the shoe distally; designed to provide dynamic dorsiflexion assist.

thermoplastic o.: terminates at or near the apex of the gastrocnemius muscle proximally, with molded foot plate fitted into shoe distally; ambulatory, nocturnal, or combination of both; designed to control and correct specific problems of the foot-ankle complex.

Knee Orthoses

dynamic o.: similar to static with the addition of external knee joints with or without locks to allow controlled motion.

elastic knee o.: elastic sleeve encompassing the knee; provides minimal support and stabilization. Variations are the following:

> **medial and lateral contoured knee joints:** similar to elastic knee o., with the addition of joints providing some increased stabilization. Other options include medial and lateral condylar pads, adjustable anterior laces, and additional spiral control straps.
>
> **Swedish knee cage:** metal and leather system allowing flexion but preventing hyperextension of the knee.

ligamentous control o.: commercially available custom-fabricated and custom-fit designs to control special ligamentous deficiencies about the knee.

static o.: Metal, thermoplastic, or equivalent; immobilizes knee in selected degree of flexion or extension.

Knee-Ankle-Foot Orthoses

Legg-Calvé-Perthes disease o.: the following are specialized systems designed for the treatment of Legg-Calvé-Perthes disease.

> **A-frame o.:** when this system is used with an extra-long bar to treat developmental dysplasia of the hips, an A-frame orthosis is sometimes incorporated to control the tendency for genu valgum (knock-knee), which may occur because of extensive hip abduction. The A-frame consists of a metal component fitted medially from the bar up both legs with calf and thigh bands and valgus control pads.

> **Atlanta brace:** a hip abduction brace that allows ambulation without crutch assistance.
>
> **Newington o.:** bilateral and similar in design to the Toronto o.; differs in that flat bars are used, and no joints are incorporated.
>
> **Salter sling:** sling device that holds hip in abduction and internal rotation while the knee is held flexed.
>
> **Scottish-Rite hip o.:** orthosis that includes two thigh bands that are connected by one metal bar that allows the child to walk, maintaining hip abduction.
>
> **Toronto o.:** bilateral proximal high cuffs, center tubular column with universal multiaxial joints at base, outriggers with angled mounting blocks at either end to receive attachment of shoes; ambulatory system providing hip abduction and controlled rotation.
>
> **trilateral o.:** plastic quadrilateral socket fitted at the level of the ischium similar to that of a transfemoral prosthetic socket. Composed of a single upright with shoe attachment and is designed to provide unilateral weight unloading, hip abduction, and internal rotation. Also called **Tachdjian o.**

metal o.: KAFO that can be either single or double upright with an adjustable ankle joint (free motion, limited motion, or dorsiflexion assist). Components include a calf band, distal and proximal thigh bands, and buckle or hook-and-loop closures, with or without lock, stirrup, and shoe attachments.

thermoplastic o.: orthosis fabricated of plastic material with molded foot plate fitted into shoe distally. This type of system has found increased acceptance because of its lighter weight and total contact fitting capabilities.

Other specialized KAFOs include those designed to manage patients with neuromuscular conditions and fractures using plaster or plastic with polycentric knee joints and other sophisticated components.

Hip Orthoses

The following are specialized hip orthoses designed for treatment of developmental dysplasia of the hips or Legg-Calvé-Perthes disease.

abduction o.: bilateral thigh cuffs of plastic, covered metal, or equivalent with adjustable bar to provide hip abduction, and waist belt and/or thoracic section to maintain positioning. Some systems have additional adjustment for hip flexion control. Also called **Ilfeld splint.**

Barlow splint: for dysplastic hips in infants; an abduction, flexion, external rotation splint. Also called **Malmo splint.**

Ferrari o.: for spina bifida patient with high level weakness; a combined thoracic lumbar orthosis with full lower limb orthosis.

Louisiana State University reciprocating gait o.: for spinal cord injuries; a cable-driven brace that allows for support while the flexion of one lower limb drives extension of the other.

Pavlik harness: a series of straps passing over the shoulders, abdomen, and lower limb to properly position the femur head into the acetabulum for proper growth formation. Alignment goal is to provide hip flexion, abduction, and external rotation.

pillow o.: soft splint fitted between the thighs to provide hip abduction with straps over the shoulders to maintain positioning; also called **Frejka o.**

Scottish Rite o.: pelvic band, bilateral free-motion hip joints, proximal thigh cuffs, and adjustable thigh bar with universal joints at inferior medial aspect of cuffs; ambulatory system providing hip abduction for treatment of Legg-Calvé-Perthes disease.

sitting hip, walking hip, standing hip (SWASH) brace: for cerebral palsy; orthosis with a pelvic wrap, rods, and mid-thigh cuffs designed to prevent hip dislocation.

thermoplastic/metal o.: custom-fabricated system designed to maintain the hips in degrees of flexion, abduction, and rotation, as prescribed.

Von Rosen o.: for developmental dysplasia of the hip in infants and very young children; passive motion restraint in abduction and flexion.

Hip-Knee-Ankle-Foot Orthoses

The following orthoses, except for the reciprocating gate orthosis and standing frame type, are described in a unilateral application, although they can be fitted bilaterally.

cable twister o.: pelvic belt with free-motion hip and ankle joint, plastic-covered cable, connecting joints, stirrup, and shoe attachments; calf and thigh bands are incorporated as necessary; adjustable at hip and ankle to provide dynamic control of hip rotation and tibial torsion.

elastic twister o.: rarely used; pelvic belt with elastic straps wrapped around leg and attached to a hook in the shoe; provides dynamic control of hip rotation and tibial torsion.

reciprocating gait o. (RGO): provides support to lower limbs and trunk for paraplegic patients; an orthosis that has a gear box or cable system attached to bilateral knee-ankle-foot o. and contoured lumbosacral section, allowing a lower-level paraplegic to have a reciprocating gait.

standard o.: standard, thermoplastic, metal, or combination of materials used in any of the knee-ankle-foot orthoses to which has been added a pelvic band that is static or with a mechanical hip joint for dynamic control of the pelvis.

standing frame o.: thoracic component, pelvic band, lateral uprights attached to platform base, which has slots to accept patient's shoes, uprights are generally overlapped to allow growth adjustment. Some type of control is used for knee extension. Joints are optional at hips and knees. This system is used to achieve standing and increase awareness in the child with afflictions such as spina bifida.

Steeper advanced reciprocating gait o.: for spinal cord injuries; a cable-driven brace that allows for support while the flexion of one lower limb drives extension of the other.

Components Applicable to Lower Limb Orthoses

ankle, knee, or hip joint: mechanical axis placed anatomically over a joint axis to allow or control motion.

Bail knee lock: posterior spring-loaded ring extending from medial to lateral knee joints with capability of automatic locking and patient activated unlocking for sitting.

calf band: metal covered with leather or equivalent fitted to the calf area on conventional ankle-foot or knee-ankle-foot orthoses.

dial lock: may be set in varying degrees of flexion or extension to accommodate or reduce contractures; other comparable types.

distal thigh band: lower thigh band on knee-ankle-foot orthoses.

double-action ankle joint: anterior and posterior compartments provide infinite adjustment for solid, limited, or dynamic assist with the use of interchangeable pins and springs.

drop-lock ring: rings slide over joint at the knee to maintain extension. Rings allow the joint to be manually unlocked to achieve knee flexion for sitting.

extended steel shank: inserted in sole of shoe to or past metatarsal heads to more effectively reduce force on the plantar aspect of the foot during gait.

floor reaction ankle foot o.: custom thermoplastic orthosis, commonly with plantar flexed position and anterior upper leg bar that forces knee to extension on floor reaction force.

ischial weight-bearing ring or band: metal component covered with soft material and fitted at the level of the ischial tuberosity to partially unload weight from the lower limb; also called **Thomas ring.**

Klenzak o.: dorsiflexion assist or plantar flexion resistance for ankle joint; spring-loaded dynamic assistive control of the foot.

lateral spring-loaded lock: for transfemoral amputees; a spring-loaded ring lock with lever that dynamically locks at full extension. There are also pneumatic and hydraulic extension-assist devices available.

limited- or free-motion ankle joint: permanently adjustable to allow motion as desired.

metal foot plate: similar to New York University insert but fabricated of stainless steel, Monel, or equivalent.

New York University (NYU) insert: metal o. using thermoplastic foot plate attached to ankle joint stirrups; provides correction of the foot and allows various shoes to be worn.

overlapped upright or growth extensions: uprights placed on top of one another to accommodate growth in children.

patellar pad: leather or equivalent; fits over patella with straps around uprights to maintain knee extension.

proximal thigh band: most proximal thigh band on knee-ankle-foot orthoses.

quadrilateral brim: similar to ischial weight-bearing ring but fabricated with thermoplastic.

split stirrup: component mounted in the heel of various shoes to allow interchangeability of conventional (metal) orthoses.

spreader bar: attached medially to both stirrups of bilateral knee-ankle-foot orthoses to prevent uncontrolled abduction.

stirrup: component of conventional lower limb orthoses connected distally in the shoe and attached proximally to the ankle joints of the orthosis.

suprapatellar and infrapatellar straps: small straps above and below knee, continuing around uprights to assist in maintaining knee extension.

upright: metal, plastic, or equivalent used to connect various other components.

varus corrective ankle straps or **valgus corrective ankle straps:** soft, padded leather or equivalent components that wrap around the opposite side. Also referred to as a T strap because of the shape.

varus and valgus knee control pads: leather or equivalent components that wrap around an opposing upright to correct deformity.

valgus control modifications: medial or lateral total contact extension on thermoplastic KAFOs that assist in correcting or stabilizing genu varum or valgum; also called **genu varum control modifications.**

Upper Limb Orthoses

Physiology in design considerations for hand and wrist-hand orthotic systems include the following:

1. Maintain thumb in opposition for prehension.
2. Allow for thumb abduction as may be required.
3. Maintain skeletal stability.
4. Avoid restrictions in use of the orthosis.
5. Prevent or correct contractures.
6. Maintain wrist in the functional 25 to 35 degrees of dorsiflexion.

Because of infinite and intricate variety of systems, only a few common examples are given.

Wrist-Hand and Hand Orthoses

basic hand splint: for muscle weakness in the hand; a dorsal splint that wraps around the ulnar, distal, and volar side of the hand held in place with a strap around the distal wrist.

cock-up splint: one plastic section providing wrist extension with incorporation of a C bar for prehension or a soft hook-and-loop orthosis with palmar bar to extension the wrist.

dynamic finger splint: fitted to individual fingers to dynamically influence flexion or extension of a joint; also called **safety pin o.** and **finger benders.**

externally powered tenodesis o.: through activation of a microswitch, tenodesis graft is achieved using a mechanical muscle.

Galveston metacarpal brace: for distal metacarpal fractures; an adjustable brace that provides dorsally directed pressure on the distal component of the fracture with counter pressure on the middorsum of the hand.

long opponens o.: identical to short opponens with forearm extension for wrist control.

palmar wrist splint: easily removable volar wrist splint that has molded palmar extension that helps hold thumb in functional position.

ratchet tenodesis o.: wrist-hand o. to passively lock hand in a grasp prehension for a partially paralyzed forearm and hand.

reciprocal finger prehension: for severe paralysis of forearm and hand; this orthosis allows patients to use their unaffected hand to adjust and set the fixed position of fingers.

short opponens o.: consists of radial extension, opponens bar, palmar arch, ulnar extension, and dorsal extension; fabricated of plastic or metal. Positions hand and thumb for opposition and does not influence the wrist.

wrist-driven tenodesis o. (WDWHO): opponens bar with jointed radial side with a connection between hand and forearm sections and thumb post. Wrist dorsiflexion produces a lateral prehension pattern using the mechanical axis.

Elbow Orthoses

Elbow orthoses may be static with humeral and forearm sections for immobilization, as in hand orthoses, and external joints to allow motion. Some are designed with turnbuckles or the equivalent to reduce contracture and may be static or dynamic.

dynamic hinged elbow fracture brace: orthotic device to allow graded active range of motion with adjustable, dynamic support to the fracture joint structure to promote healing (Fig. 7-4, *A*).

elbow extension splint: designed to decrease flexion contractures of the elbow and to gain total maximum range of motion and strength (Fig. 7-4, *B*).

FIG 7-4 **A,** Elbow orthosis: dynamic hinged elbow fracture brace. **B,** Santana elbow extension splint. *(Courtesy EC Jeter, OTR, Occupational Therapy Department, National Naval Medical Center, Bethesda, MD.)*

Elbow-Wrist-Hand Orthoses

Elbow-wrist-hand orthoses are adjustable, static systems to provide immobilization. A torsion bar may be incorporated to assist in pronation or supination. They are useful to correct fractures of the forearm.

Shoulder Orthoses

Generally these are static or passive jointed systems used for positioning to correct chronic shoulder dislocation or postoperative stabilization.

Shoulder-Elbow-Wrist-Hand Orthoses

airplane splint: jointed elbow and shoulder, allowing controlled flexion and rotation; glenohumeral joint permits controlled abduction; used for muscle injuries humeral fractures, dislocations, surgery involving

the glenohumeral joint, and brachial plexus nerve injuries. Also called **statue of liberty o.**
gunslinger o.: for shoulder injuries and surgery; a forearm trough mechanically anchored to a hemigirdle on the person's pelvis.
static orthosis: provides controlled positioning.

Components Applicable to Upper Limb Orthoses

C bar: component attached to or an integral part of the palmar arch, designed to maintain the web space between the thumb and hand.
first dorsal interosseous assist: principle similar to that of the spring swivel thumb; designed to hold the metacarpophalangeal joint of the index finger in abduction to provide opposition with the thumb.
flail-elbow hinge: used to overcome muscle deficit at the elbow. Spring assist provides flexion and locks in position for a chosen activity. This is operated with a figure-eight harness, similar to prosthetic transradial harness control, unaffected hand, or nudge control.
joint stabilizer: rigid component extending proximally and distally to a joint of a digit; provides stability or realignment for subluxation.
mobile arm support (MAS): arm trough device with attachment for resting arm on wheelchair.
opponens bars: exert a static holding force on saddle joint of thumb. Keep thumb in palmar abduction, an optimal position for opposition.
outrigger: metacarpophalangeal (MCP), proximal interphalangeal, or distal interphalangeal extension assist; MCP stop (lumbrical bar) positioned just proximal to the interphalangeal joints; holds MCP joints in approximately 15 degrees of flexion.
spring swivel thumb: wire spring attached to radial aspect of orthosis and in turn connected to thumb ring. Patient flexes against this dynamic resistance; in a relaxed state, the thumb is held in abduction.
thumb interphalangeal (IP) extension assist: principle similar to the first dorsal interosseous assist; designed to return IP of the thumb to neutral after flexion and during prehension.
thumb post: static control for prehension achieved by rigid member encompassing thumb.
turnbuckle: adjustable component used to reduce contractures of the elbow.

Specialized Systems for Upper Limbs

For those patients with severe involvement, external power sources are at times used. Electrically powered or carbon dioxide–operated artificial muscle systems are available.

Spine

Sacroiliac Orthoses

cloth binder: material encompassing appropriate region with hook-and-loop closure.
sacroiliac belt: adjustable corset with posterior pad.

Lumbosacral Orthoses

Bennett o.: cloth lumbar corset with reinforced frame consisting of a pelvic and thoracic band with two paravertebral uprights.
chairback o.: posterior frame with lateral and posterior uprights and apron front anteriorly; control restrictions include anterior flexion, extension, and lateral flexion; used for pathologic conditions of the lower back, severe strain, and arthritis. Also called **sagittal control o.** and **sagittal coronal control o.**
lumbosacral corset: custom-fitted corset, generally having rigid paraspinal uprights.
Norton-Brown o.: rigid low-back postoperative brace. The lateral bars extend to cover the greater trochanter to help reduce lateral bending.
sacral belt: for low-back pain; a semirigid or canvas device that is placed across the upper buttocks and fastens near the pubis, over the sacroiliac joint. Also called **SI belt.**
surgical corset: garment encasing the torso and pelvis that is adjustable circumferentially. Adjustment may be made anteriorly, posteriorly, laterally, or in combination. In general, the following statements apply.
  anterior height: superior border 1 inch below xiphoid process; inferior border 1 inch above symphysis pubis.
  fabrication: single or multiple layers.
  function: serves as a kinesthetic reminder to restrict anteroposterior and mediolateral motions; increased intracavitary pressure to reduce axial force on vertebral bodies and disks; restricts some rotary and transverse motions.

materials: nylon, cotton, canvas, elastic, or a combination with metal stays that can be contoured for additional support.

modification possibilities: posterior semirigid or rigid paraspinal uprights, posterior semirigid or rigid plate, posterior inflatable control pads, additional abdominal reinforcements with flexible stays, thoracic extension with shoulder straps and axillary loops, separate frame posteriorly, one-piece garment, special control pads for ptosis (prolapse of any organ), hernia pads, perineal straps, thigh skirt.

posterior height: superior border 1 inch below inferior angle of scapula; inferior border extends to the sacrococcygeal junction or approximately 1 inch proximal to the gluteal fold.

Thoracic Orthoses

clavicle o.: for clavicular fractures; figure-eight harness under the axilla and over the shoulder, crossing posteriorly; control restrictions: glenohumeral flexion.

rib belt: foam padded or elastic with hook-and-loop closure; minimal control and kinesthetic reminder for reducing muscle strain; used for fractures and costochondritis.

Thoracolumbosacral Orthoses

Boston brace: orthotic module customized for scoliosis treatment.

Boston overlap brace (BOB): orthosis for treatment of spondylolisthesis and similar presentations that require reduction in lumbar lordosis and increase in anterior spinal flexion.

Charleston bending brace: for scoliosis; used only at night to hold the patient in maximum side bending correction.

cruciform anterior spinal hyperextension (CASH) o.: a hyperextension TLSO that uses a three-point pressure system to induce spinal extension to decrease weight on the vertebral body. Commonly used for anterior compression fractures.

control o.: used for spondylitis, compression fractures, osteoporosis (reduction in the quality of bone or skeletal atrophy; remaining bone is normally mineralized), arthritis, spinal fusion, adolescent epiphysitis, and osteochondritis; anterior frame with superior and inferior pads; three-point fixation provided by additional posterior pad; control restrictions: maintains hyperextension and tends to increase lumbar lordosis.

dorsal lumbar corset: used for problems related to higher levels of amputation; high corset with shoulder straps and paraspinal uprights; control restrictions: forward flexion. Also called **thoracolumbosacral anterior control corset.**

custom bi-valved (polymer) TLSO: used for conditions such as postsurgical management of fusion, spina bifida, muscular dystrophy, and scoliosis; anteroposterior sectioned, posterior or anterior opening; thermoplastic fabrication; control restrictions: general immobilization and intracavitary pressure; may be designed to provide some distraction. Previously referred to as a *body jacket.*

flexion control o.: used for spondylitis, compression fractures, osteoporosis (reduction in the quality of bone or skeletal atrophy; remaining bone is normally mineralized), arthritis, spinal fusion, adolescent epiphysitis, and osteochondritis; anterior frame with superior and inferior pads; three-point fixation provided by additional posterior pad; control restrictions: maintains hyperextension and tends to increase lumbar lordosis.

lumbodorsal support: lumbar corset with thoracic extension of stays and straps that go over shoulder, pass under axilla, and attach to bottom of thoracic component of the posterior stay; also called **dorsal lumbar o.**

Lyonnaise o.: for treatment of thoracic curves with apices as high as T8.

New York orthopedic front-opening o.: for scoliosis treatment; a prefabricated TLSO.

Rosenberger o.: a TLSO that uses adjustable slings for curve correction; custom-molded polyethylene orthosis for scoliosis, similar to Miami o. and Wilmington jacket.

sagittal-coronal control o.: used for high spinal fusion, lordosis, and osteoporosis; chairback-Taylor combination; posterior and lateral uprights with corset front; control restrictions: anterior flexion, extension, and lateral flexion. Also called **Knight-Taylor o.**

sagittal control o.: used for kyphosis, fractures, arthritis, lordosis, carcinoma (any of the various types of malignant neoplasms derived from epithelial tissue), and after spinal surgery; posterior uprights with shoulder straps and apron front; control restrictions: anterior flexion and extension. Also called **Taylor o.**

triplanar control: thoracic band with supraclavicular extensions (cow horn projections), pelvic band, paraspinal bars, and lateral bars. Triplanar control can also be accomplished with the use of a bi-valved TLSO controlling sagittal, coronal, and transverse motion.

underarm o.: custom-fabricated or modular system; thermoplastic, generally with posterior opening; used for scoliosis. Application is most effective when apex of curve is inferior to T-10.

Wilmington jacket: used in scoliosis in circumstances in which control through the cervical spine is not necessary.

Cervical Orthoses (Fig. 7-5)

Cervical orthoses are used when immobilization is necessary because of whiplash-type injuries, fractures, and surgical fusion. The following provide minimal restrictions.

four-poster o.: same as two-poster o., but uses two bars anteriorly and two posteriorly.

halo brace: structure that includes a ring attached by pins to the outer skull at the level of the forehead and is used in conjunction with a two- or four-poster device (super structure) attached to a rigid vest.

halo traction: skeletal immobilization traction using a pelvic plaster cast or plastic girdle; outriggers to metal ring encircling head; pins are then inserted into skull and outriggers adjusted for distraction.

molded Thomas collar: custom-fabricated leather or plastic over modified cast with adjustable height.

Plastazote collar: unicellular foam, contoured to fit chin and make contact with occiput; hook and loop closure. This configuration is often called a **Philadelphia collar.**

semirigid collar (plastic collar): overlapping plastic sections with hook-and-loop closures; wraps around neck and contacts chin.

soft collar: foam with hook-and-loop closure; wraps around neck.

sternal occipital mandibular immobilizer (SOMI) o.: chin and occiput sections and sternal and posterior sections; may be fitted while patient is supine. The SOMI orthosis can be attached to a thermoplastic body jacket to allow control of the cervical, thoracic, and lumbar spine.

two- or four-poster o.: anterior and posterior bands incorporated into the cervical orthosis. For fractures and postsurgical support, a cervical brace with chest and thoracic extension: one anterior bar with chin rest and chest plate, and one posterior post with thoracic and chest plates attached by shoulder harness (straps) that can be connected to a waist circular support. A thoracic or waist extension can be added for greater neck stability and control. Also called **Dennison brace.**

wire-frame collar: an adjustable, rounded rectangular ring that fits under chin and onto chest, held in place by two straps supported by expansion of material on posterior neck.

When optimal control and restriction are required, the following are prescribed:

Cervicothoracolumbosacral Orthosis

Milwaukee o.: used for spinal scoliosis or Scheuermann kyphosis; leather or thermoplastic pelvic girdle, throat mold, occiput pads, neck ring, and full, connecting superstructure with control pads as necessary.

FIG 7-5 Cervical flexion-extension control orthosis (poster appliance). **A,** Cervical spine in slight extension with head erect. **B,** Cervical spine in flexion with chin depressed. *(From American Academy of Orthopaedic Surgeons:* Atlas of orthotics, *St Louis, 1975, Mosby.)*

Components and Descriptions Applicable to Spinal Systems

Beaufort seating o.: for trunk control in a severely disabled, sitting patient; a large bean bag full of polystyrene beads is molded to patient and then air evacuated to make a firm support.
corset front: cloth anteriorly attached to lateral uprights of spinal orthosis.
matrix seating system: for severely disabled patients; a seating system constructed from interlocking plastic components.
Milwaukee cervicothoracolumbosacral orthoses
  axillary sling: axillary pad with webbing used to maintain alignment of neck ring.
  Friddle low-profile neck rings: function predominantly by reducing the sway of the vertebral column and keeping the upper thoracic spine centered over the sacrum.
  lumbar pad: firm foam or metal and leather incorporated into or attached near posterosuperior edge of girdle on same side as thoracic curve.
  neck ring: metal ring at neck that opens posteriorly for donning and doffing and serves as attachment for throat mold and occiput pads.
  occipital pads: plastic or metal oblong disks fitted bilaterally to the inferior angle of the occiput bones of the head; aligned to provide slight distraction.
  pelvic girdle: custom-fitted section serving as foundation for orthosis.
  shoulder ring: component fitted to axilla and over acromion; attached to the orthosis and used to depress an elevated shoulder.
  superstructure: two posterior and one anterior metal component connecting pelvic girdle and neck ring.
  thoracic pad: floating pad attached to anterior and posterior uprights on same side as thoracic curve.
  throat mold: plastic or equivalent material, attached to neck ring and fitted to within 0.5 cm of throat and just below chin; limits anteroposterior motion.
perineal loops: straps passing between legs to reduce proximal migration of spinal orthosis.
rotary control: modification of rigid spinal orthosis with lateral extension or sternal plate fitted bilaterally into the deltopectoral grooves to restrict rotation.
sternal attachment: component fitted to chest.
thoracic extension: component parts attached to cervical orthosis and fitted to the chest and back regions to provide increased control. Can also be attached at the proximal anterior panel for TLSOs to control anterior spinal flexion when used with shoulder straps.
uprights: metal or plastic extensions or bars to increase stability of the orthosis or aid in correction and management of a deformity. Can be placed on the anterior, posterior, or sides of the orthosis.

Shoe Modifications

Terms for the normal components of shoes are used frequently in describing modifications used in orthopaedic treatment.

counter, heel counter: toe helps hold the heel, firm cup incorporated into the rear of the shoe.
foxing: stripping that adds support to the medial and lateral side of the shoe.
last: three-dimensional model of which the shoe is made, taking the form of the sole of the foot.
shank: reinforcing material that bridges between the ball and heel area of the shoe.
toe box: stiff material that prevents collapse and protects the toes.
tongue: part that protects foot from pressure from the laces.

Shoe modifications are various alterations made in a shoe to complement the orthosis. On occasion, a shoe modification is prescribed by itself to correct a specific problem; for example, leg-length discrepancy is treated by a shoe elevation on the shorter side, and valgus ankles may be treated with medial sole and heel wedging or medially flared heel.

custom-molded shoes: specially and individually constructed shoes designed to fit a patient with multiple foot deformities, as occur with rheumatoid arthritis; also called **space shoes.**
orthopaedic oxford: a hard leather shoe with a leather or rubber sole; sometimes such a shoe has a steel

shank (portion of shoe that lies between the floor of the shoe and the sole), with firmly constructed sides that support the foot in an upright position. This type of shoe is constructed uniformly, allowing for the addition of assistive devices.

surgical shoe or boot: a hard shoe that is constructed of a thick sole, with lacing designed to allow the shoe to be firmly tightened around the foot to reduce motion at the foot during static standing and gait.

Devices for Flat Feet (Pes Planus) and High Arches (Pes Cavus)

ankle corset: a laced leather device that encompasses ankle and rear foot to support arch and subtalar joint.

combined arch support: an interchangeable arch support that has both a tarsal (arch) component and a forward pad to support the metatarsal arch.

extended counter: a piece of leather extending from the inner back side of the shoe to the level of the arch, giving arch support.

lateral heel wedge: wedge of rigid material placed on the lateral aspect of the heel to control pes cavus.

medial heel wedge: small wedge of rigid material placed on the arch side of the heel to control pes planus.

plantar arch support: an interchangeable pad that helps support the tarsal arch.

Plastazote: for a variety of prosthetic and orthotic needs; this is a closed-cell polyethylene foam that, with 280° F heating, can be molded into a force distribution piece of foam.

scaphoid pads: better known as *shoe cookies* or tarsal supports; inserted directly under the arch of the foot in the shoe. Also called **navicular pads.**

Shaffer plate: arch support made of stainless steel; usually for adults.

shoemaker's swan: for molding relief in pressure areas of a shoe; a long-handled device that has a ring on one arm and a ball on the other for stretching shoe material at points of pressure.

Thomas heel: a heel with a curved extension for the arch side of the foot.

Whitman plate: arch support made of stainless steel; for growing feet.

Metatarsal Supports

metatarsal bars: an extra piece of rubber applied externally to the sole, providing support proximal to the metatarsal heads; used in treatment of callosities on the ball of the foot and stiff great toes. Types of metatarsal bars include **Denver metatarsal bar, Flush metatarsal bar, Hauser metatarsal bar,** and **Mayo metatarsal bar.**

metatarsal pads: pads permanently placed in shoe just proximal to the ball of the foot.

metatarsal supports: interchangeable supports that have raised areas just proximal to the ball of the foot.

Devices for Insensitive Feet (Devascularized or Diabetic Neuropathies)

controlled ankle motion (CAM) walker: plastic device incorporating a calf wrap and rigid ankle and foot plate to unweight the foot; to allow healing of an ulcer.

custom-molded shoes: see **space shoes.**

extra-depth shoes: shoes that have increased height to accommodate diabetic (Plastizote) inserts without compromising the fit of the shoe, while decreasing the risk of blistering and ulceration.

Plastizote inserts: to accommodate deformity or heel ulcers; commercially available inserts in which top layers is lined with Plastizote to reduce the risk of callous and ulceration.

rocker sole modification: rigid sole attachment to reduce shear force of metatarsal heads and to prevent a healed ulcer from reoccurring.

Devices for Callosities

Budin splint: splint designed to relieve symptoms caused by hammertoe deformity.

calcaneal spur pad: a heel with a special cutout center designed to redistribute the weight from a painful area of the heel.

heel pad: any soft pad inserted into the shoe to cushion the heel; used for tendonitis, heel spurs, Achilles bursitis, and similar conditions.

sole inserts: known by a variety of trade names, these inserts are made of foam rubber or other material and are designed to cushion the entire walking surface of the foot.

Special Shoes for Infants and Children

equinovarus outflare shoes: used in treatment of clubfoot condition.

inflare last shoes: used to maintain correction for overpronation.

normal last shoes: constructed with normal sole; term used to distinguish this from a reverse or straight last shoe.

reverse last shoes: look as if the left shoe were made for the right foot and vice versa; the side where the arch would normally be is curved out; used in treatment of clubfeet and metatarsus varus. Also called **outflare last shoes.**

straight last shoes: look as if they could be worn on either foot, with a straight sole; used in treating mild forefoot problems such as metatarsus varus; incurring last.

tarsal pronator shoes: used in treatment of clubfoot condition.

torque heels: specially designed heels to make the foot turn in or out, depending on the direction of rubber slits that are arranged to cause torsion on weight-bearing.

Anatomy and Orthopaedic Surgery

Orthopaedic surgery is the branch of medicine concerned with the preservation of the musculoskeletal system. Therefore the goal is to treat diseases and injuries; correct deformities; and make surgical repairs to bone, cartilage, muscles, tendons, ligaments, synovia, bursa, fascia, and nerves of the upper and lower limbs, shoulder, spine, and pelvis. A general list of the types of surgery performed on these tissues is presented in Table 8-1.

Orthopaedic surgery encompasses an overwhelming number of procedures that attempt to alter normal or abnormal anatomic structures. The four-volume *Campbell's Operative Orthopedics** is one of the textbooks of this surgical specialty. Many of the new terms are briefly described in this chapter.

The anatomy of the musculoskeletal system is defined here to correlate with the surgery on specific tissue by anatomic area. Numerous figure illustrations are provided to enhance the understanding of anatomic structures. An associated surgical word list is included at the end of the chapter.

Osteo- (Bone)

Anatomy of Bone

Osseous tissue (bone) constitutes the majority of the skeletal framework consisting of 206 bones of various sizes and shape that are living, hard connective tissue composed of organic (cells and matrix) and inorganic (mineral) components with submicroscopic laminations of protein and crystal layers. The matrix contains a framework of collagenous fibers that are impregnated with the mineral components, mainly in the form of apatite crystals, which give the quality of rigidity to bone. Another function of bone is its hematopoietic ability (i.e., to create and develop blood and other hematopoietic cells in the bone marrow).

If all of the mineral were removed from the bone, the resulting structure would be firm and pliable and have the exact shape of the mineralized bone. The process of **calcification** is not restricted to bones; it may occur in an amorphous form in tendons, bursae, and other tissues. **Ossification** is actual formation of bone tissue, which then calcifies by addition of hydroxyapatite crystals composed of calcium, phosphate, and hydroxyl ions. The following terms relate to the shape, structure, and microanatomy of bone (Fig. 8-1).

apophysis: a tubercle of bone that contributes to its growth but is the point of strong tendon insertion and usually has a ossification center. An example is the greater trochanter.

articular cartilage: epiphyseal covering; thin layer of hyaline cartilage over the articular surface (ends) of bone to provide a bearing surface for joint and respond to shear and compressive forces.

---
* Canale ST, Beaty JH.

TABLE 8-1 Orthopaedic Procedures*

Prefixes/Roots: Tissue Types	Procedures†
Osteo- (bone)	2, 4, 5, 6, 7, 8
Myo- (muscle)	2, 3, 4, 5, 6, 7
Tendo- or teno- (tendon)	3, 4, 5, 6, 7, 10
Desmo- (ligament)	5
Syndesmo- (ligament)	6, 7
Fascio- or fascia- (fibrous bands)	4, 5, 6, 7, 9
Burs- (bursa, sac, pouch)	1, 4, 6, 9
Spondylo- (spine)	3, 6
Myelo- (spinal cord, meninges, bone marrow)	1, 5, 6, 9
Lamin- (lamina)	4, 6
Rachio- (spine)	1, 6
Neur- (nerves)	4, 5, 6, 7, 10
Arthro- (joint)	1, 2, 3, 4, 6, 7, 9, 10, 11
Chondro- (cartilage) (Fig. 8-2)	2, 4, 6
Synov-(synovium)	4
Capsul- (capsule)	3, 4, 5, 6, 7
Condyl- (condyle)	4, 6
Aponeur- (fascial bands)	4, 5, 6

*The left column (prefixes/roots) indicates the anatomy; corresponding numbers in the right column (procedures) describe the types of surgery performed on those tissues.
† 1. **-centesis:** *surgical puncture; perforation or tapping with aspirator, trocar, or needle.*
 2. **-clasis:** *surgical fracture or refracture of bones and other tissue by crushing; refracture of bone in malposition.*
 3. **-desis:** *binding, fixation by means of suture (tendon) or fusion (joints); not to include spine.*
 4. **-ectomy:** *excision of organ or part.*
 5. **-orrhaphy:** *to suture or sew.*
 6. **-otomy:** *surgical incision into a part or organ; cut into.*
 7. **-plasty:** *to form, mold, or shape; surgical shaping or formation.*
 8. **-synthesis:** *putting together, composition, surgical fastening of ends of fractured bones by sutures, rings, plates, or other mechanical means.*
 9. **-gram:** *injection of contrast media for x-ray examination.*
 10. **-lysis:** *dissolution of tissue; decomposition; freeing of scar or adhesions.*
 11. **-oscopy:** *to view by a scope.*

bone marrow: an organ that functions to manufacture the formed elements of blood **(hematopoiesis),** including erythrocytes (red blood cells), lymphocytes (white blood cells), and platelets. It is a network of connective tissue filled with blood vessels that form and develop blood corpuscles and is found in the proximal epiphyses of the humeri and femora, ribs and sternum, and cancellous bone of vertebrae. Yellow bone marrow is found in the medullary cavity in adults and contains fatty marrow.

FIG 8-1 Composition of bone. *(From Young CG, Barger JD: Learning medical terminology step by step, ed 3, St Louis, 1975, CV Mosby.)*

bone matrix: the extracellular substance of bone composed of collagenous fibers embedded in an amorphous ground substance and inorganic salts.

calcium: a necessary mineral that, in combination with phosphorus, forms calcium phosphate (apatite

FIG 8-2 Cartilage on surface of soup bone. Dime for contrasts to strip or removed cartilage. Cartilage within bone is the growth plate cartilage.

crystals), which is the dense, hard material of bones and teeth. It is the most abundant mineral in the body and the skeleton serves as the main center for calcium storage. Calcium is critical in the function of muscles, nerves, blood coagulation, and heartbeat.

cambium layer: loose cellular inner layer of the periosteal tissue; involved in the intramembranous ossification of bone.

canaliculus: communicating, narrow tubular channel between osteocytes in bone.

cancellous bone: spongy, porous, latticelike osseous tissue.

condyle: prominence at the widened end of long bones that function as attachment sites for ligaments, tendons, or muscles. Two examples are the femoral condyles, the inner and outer palpable prominences of the upper knee joint.

cortical bone: the thick, dense outer portion of bone that surrounds the medullary (marrow) cavity; also called **compact bone.**

cut-back zone: in growing bone, the zone just metaphyseal to the growth plate, where the diameter of the bone is being narrowed.

cutting cone: one means of bone remodeling, cone-appearing blood vessel as seen on longitudinal microscopic section; osteoclasts can be seen absorbing bone at the head of the cone.

diaphysis: the thick, compact, midportion of long bones, providing strong support.

enchondral bone: bone that forms by replacing a cartilage precursor, either cartilage growth plate or from cartilage in fracture callus; also called **cartilage bone** and **substitution bone.**

endosteum: the lining of the trabecular and cortical bone that is within the medullary canal or cavity.

epiphysis: the bulbous growth end of a long bone, usually wider than the shaft and entirely cartilaginous or separated from the metaphysic by a cartilaginous disk. The epiphysis is a part of the bone formed from a secondary center of ossification at the ends of long bones, margins of flat bones, and at the tubercles and processes. During growth, the epiphyses are separated from the main portion of bone by cartilage, properly termed the **physis** or **epiphyseal plate.** There are two types of epiphyses:

  pressure e.: a secondary center of ossification in the articular end of a long bone with articular elements subjected to pressure.

  traction e.: a secondary center of ossification at the site of attachment of a tendon and subjected to traction. Contributes to bone shape (e.g., apophysis).

facet: a flat, platelike surface on a bone that acts as part of a joint; facets are seen in the vertebrae and form facet joints and in the subtalar joint of the ankle.

flat bones: bent or curved rather than flat, these bones protect viscera and other soft tissues, and include the pelvis, ribs, and shoulder blade.

haversian canals: one of the minute vascular canals running lengthwise in compact osteonal bone; part of an important system in transporting bloodborne material to widely separated bone cells. This transport system is composed of the haversian canals, surrounding lamellae, connecting canaliculi, and lacunae. The lateral branches of these vessels are called **Volkmann canals.**

Howship lacuna: microscopic area of bone resorption that occurs on the surface of bone, resulting from activity. Microscopically resembles a small pit on the edge of bone surface (resorption pit).

isthmus: narrow portion of the canal in the midshaft of a long bone.

lamellar bone: mature bone that results from the remodeling of immature bone into a highly organized and stress-oriented pattern of collagen.

line: a less prominent ridge on bone—for example, the iliopectineal line—whereas a crest is a more prominent ridge (iliac crest).

medullary canal: the canal in the center of a bone shaft containing soft, fatty marrow elements in adults and cancellous bone.

membranous bone: collagen model bone that is formed directly from the periosteum, without development of cartilage, and develops within a connective tissue membrane. An example is the skull.

metaphysis: the wider portion of a long bone between the diaphysis and the epiphysis. This portion of bone represents the most recently formed bone (growth zone) during the growth process. With closure of physis, it is continuous with the epiphysis.

ossification: process of forming bone (ossifying, adj.). Other related terms include the following:

osseous: general term referring to bony matter.

ossiferous: implies that bone is being produced.

ossific: refers to the presence of bone.

osteoid: refers to the uncalcified bone matrix.

osteoblast: a bone-forming cell; cells that produce osteoid, which is the matrix of bone, composed predominantly of type I collagen and a number of bone proteins.

osteoclast: bone resorbing cell; cells derived from monocellular precursors, which, under the influence of parathyroid hormone and other systemic and local substances, absorb bone. The specific microscopic region of bone resorption is called a **Howship lacuna.**

osteocyte: bone cell; osteoblastic cell that has become encased in bone matrix and has cellular extensions called **canaliculi,** which allow the cell to connect and communicate with other osteocytes and thereby affect bone metabolism.

osteonal bone: a microscopic description of bone seen in mature adults that is highly organized in response to stress-related growth. An **osteon** is the single unit of osteonal bone and represents a central vascular channel surrounded by layers of circumferential lamellar bone.

periosteum: firm, thin, two-layered fibrous outer covering of bone; outer layer contains blood vessels; inner layer contains connective tissue cells and elastic fibers. The periosteum is important for circumferential bone growth and in bone repair because of its bone-forming cells and blood vessels that supply the osteogenic layer. The nerve endings in periosteum are responsible for the sensitivity of bone in trauma. The thin layer of multipotential cells that is immediately next to the bone is called the **cambium layer.**

physis: the cartilage between the apophysis or epiphysis and the shaft of the bone. This cartilage is responsible for the longitudinal growth of the bone. Although the epiphyseal cartilage is called the *growth plate,* as in the previous definition, the term **epiphyseal cartilage** may also refer to the cartilage lining the joint; also called **growth plate** and **epiphyseal plate.** Typically divided into the following zones:

resting zone: zone of cartilage cells with little metabolic activity and no cell division.

proliferating zone: zone of cell replication where cells are stacked in longitudinal rows; also called **columnar zone.**

hypertrophic zone: zone where cells become larger.

zone of provisional calcification: calcium appears in matrix, and beyond this point, invading blood vessels appear with bone cells on surface of calcified cartilage.

Other terms related to epiphyseal growth:

atavistic e.: a bone that fuses naturally to another bone as in the coracoid process of the scapula.

punctum ossificationis: point of ossification (center) where bone begins to form in a specific bone or part; also called **ossification center.**

primary center of ossification: the first site where bone begins to form in the shaft; in a long bone, the diaphysis; also called **punctum ossificationis primarium.**

secondary center of ossification: a center of bone formation that appears later, on the joint side of a growth plate where the center of ossification is a part of bone that has a strong muscle attachment outside of the diaphysis; also called **punctum ossificationis secundarium.**

sesamoid: a small, round bone found in tendons (and some muscles), whose function is to increase movement in a joint by improving angle of approach of tendon into its insertion. The patella is the largest sesamoid bone in the body.

spongiosa: term applied to cancellous or trabecular bone typically in the metaphysis. The term **primary spongiosa** is applied to the **spicular bone** in growth plate that forms on the surface of calcified cartilage on the bone side of the physis. Primary spongiosa remodels into trabecular bone.

subchondral bone: bone directly under any cartilaginous surface.

trabecula: type of bone that is in small interconnected spicules, normally referred to as *trabecular bone* **(cancellous bone)**; predominantly makes up the ends of long bones.

trabecular pattern: refers to the arrangement of the trabeculae of bone such that, when seen on radiographs or in cross-sections, there is a pattern of arches or other designs, like the spokes of a bicycle, providing the structural needs of the bone.

tubercle (small), tuberosity (large): rounded, elevated projection of bone giving attachment to a muscle or ligament; for example, ischial tuberosity or Lister's tubercle (dorsal, of radius).

Volkmann canals: found in osteonal bone; lateral passageways for transporting nutrients from the central haversian canals to bone cells (osteocytes).

woven bone: immature bone seen in very early growth and development, fracture healing, and some disease states. Also called **wormian bone** and **fiber bone**.

> **coarse woven bone:** rapidly developing woven bone with coarse-appearing matrix; also called **burlap bone**.
>
> **fine woven bone:** bone with smooth-appearing matrix but that is not lamellar; also called **linen bone**.

General Surgery of Bone

bone marrow biopsy: surgical or local needle aspiration of bone marrow for microscopic inspection to determine the presence of disease affecting bone, usually drawn from superior iliac crest.

bone marrow transplant: a special procedure done in an effort to treat certain disease conditions of bone marrow. Diseased marrow is chemically destroyed and replaced (transfused) with healthy donor marrow of the same blood type. The transfused cells eventually matriculate to recipient's bone marrow where, in successful transplant, they become established.

bone suture fixation: placement of a peg or screw device to affix a suture to bone for capsular, ligamentous, or tendon repair. There are numerous brands of permanent and absorbable devices.

callotasis: for lengthening a bone; production of fracture and then gradual distraction.

closed reduction: without incision manual manipulation of the fractured part, with return to proper position (called apposition) and alignment.

condylectomy: excision of a condyle at the joint; more specifically, removal of the round bony prominence of the articular end of bone.

condylotomy: surgical incision or division of a condyle or condyles (e.g., toe phalanges).

corticotomy: complete transection of the cortex of a bone without transection of the intramedullary structures. This procedure is basically an osteotomy with care taken to preserve the intramedullary vessels.

diaphysectomy: removal of the shaft of bone, leaving the distal and proximal ends of bone intact.

diaplasis: reduction of a fracture or dislocation.

distraction osteogenesis: lengthening of bone by gradually pulling apart and allowing bone to grow into the created gap.

ebonation: removal of fragments of bone from a wound.

epiphysiodesis: fusion of an epiphysis to the metaphysis of a bone by disruption of the growth plate **(epiphysiolysis)** or by metallic fixation between the epiphysis and metaphysis of bone. An **epiphysiolysis** may also occur traumatically.

fenestration: cutting a window in bone to allow drainage or access to an object covered by the bone, such as a tumor or foreign body.

open reduction: surgical incision and correction of a bone alignment of a fracture; may or may not include stabilization with internal or external fixation.

ostectomy: removal of a portion of bone.

osteoarthrotomy: the excision of the articular end of bone.

osteoclasis: surgical fracture or refracture of bone to bring about a change in alignment in cases of nonunion or malalignment.

osteoplasty: surgical correction by shaping or formation of bone (osteorrhaphy).

osteosynthesis: surgical fixation of bone by the use of any internal mechanical means; usually done in the treatment of fractures.

periosteotomy: incision through the membranous covering of bone; also called **periostomy**.

sequestrectomy: removal of a portion of dead bone.

synostosis: surgical fusion of any two or more bones that would otherwise be separated; may occur in a natural state as well.

Osteotomies

An osteotomy is a cutting or incision of bone, usually to produce a change in bone shape or alignment. It may be considered for correction of a malaligned fracture, osteoarthritis, or other joint conditions. The following procedures are types of osteotomies.

Abbott and Gill o.: for bone growth asymmetry in lower limbs; a distal femoral and proximal tibial epiphysiodesis done through a medial approach. Also, proximal tibial and fibular epiphysiodesis through a lateral approach.

Amspacher and Messenbaugh o.: for cubitus varus with rotatory deformity of the elbow; correction of both deformities is with a distal humeral osteotomy.

Amstutz and Wilson o.: for congenital coxa vara.

Bailey and Dubow o.: for deformities of the femoral shaft; multiple osteotomies held by a telescoping intramedullary rod.

Baker and Hill o.: for heel valgus; lateral opening wedge osteotomy with bone allograft.

ball-and-socket o.: dome-shaped osteotomy.

Bellemore and Barrett o.: for varus deformity of elbow; lateral closing wedge osteotomy of distal humerus; also called **modified French o.**

Bernese o.: for acetabular dysplasia, osteotomy of pubis and ischial-ilial part of acetabulum that allows for more anatomic rotation of entire acetabulum, held in place by internal fixation. Also called **Ganz o.** and **periacetabular o. (PAO).**

Blount o.: for bone growth asymmetry in the lower limbs; epiphyseal growth is arrested using staples across the growth plate.

Blount displacement o.: for hip osteoarthritis.

Blundell Jones varus o.: varus osteotomy of the hip for paralysis.

Borden and Gearen o.: for aseptic necrosis of the hip; an extracapsular transtrochanteric osteotomy.

Borden o.: for coxa vara; see also **Spencer o.** and **Herndon o.**

Brackett o.: ball-and-socket type for the fused hip.

Brett o.: for proximal tibia for genu recurvatum.

closing wedge o.: wedge cut out of bone; the closing of the open space angulates the bone toward the side from which the wedge was removed.

Cole o.: anterior tarsal wedge for cavus deformity.

Cotton o.: for correction of a distal tibial deformity.

Coventry o.: a proximal tibial osteotomy for varus or valgus knees.

Crego o.: for femoral anteversion.

cuneiform o.: a cuneiform-shaped wedge cut in bone allowing for correction of deformities in two planes.

derotation o.: correction of rotational misalignment of a long bone.

dial o.: dome- or circular-shaped osteotomy.

Dickson o.: for malunion of the femoral neck.

Dimon o.: for intertrochanteric fractures; medial displacement of the distal fragment; also called **Hughston o.**

Dwyer o.: for clubfoot and pes cavus deformities; a lateral closing wedge osteotomy that reduces both the cavus and heel varus deformities.

Ferguson-Thompson-King-Moore o.: for long-bone deformity such as malunion; a concave side resection of cortex with replacement after bone is made into chips, careful closure of the periosteum over the chips, and then closing wedge osteotomy on opposite side after sufficient callus formation has taken place.

Fish o.: for fixed slipped capital femoral epiphysis deformity; a cuneiform osteotomy at the base of the femoral head.

French o.: for cubitus varus (elbow); a closing wedge osteotomy.

Gant o.: open-wedge osteotomy for the fused hip.

Ganz o.: for adult acetabular dysplasia; a periacetabular osteotomy.

Ghormley o.: part of a hip fusion procedure.

Hass o.: for dislocation of the hip.

Ingram o.: for fusion of growth plate because of trauma; opening wedge osteotomy with concurrent insertion of fat at growth plate area.

innominate o.: of the pelvis for dislocation of the hip; two common types are **Pemberton o.** and **Salter o.**

Irwin o.: for genu recurvatum; a posterior closing wedge osteotomy of the proximal tibia.

Kramer, Craig, and Noel o.: for fixed slipped capital femoral epiphysis deformity; osteotomy at base of femoral neck.

Langenskiöld o.: to correct partial premature closure of growth plate; an excision of bony bridge across the epiphysis with insertion of fat.

Lorenz o.: for dislocation of the hip.

Lucas and Cottrell o.: notched rotation type of the proximal tibia.

Macewen and Shands o.: for congenital coxa vara.

Martin o.: for fixed slipped capital femoral epiphysis deformity; a closing wedge osteotomy at the base of femoral head and superior neck.

McKay o.: for stabilization of the hip in myelomeningocele; varus osteotomy of the proximal femur with transfer of adductors to the ischial tuberosity and external oblique muscles to the greater trochanter.

McMurray o.: for nonunion of the femoral neck.

Meyer-Burgdorff o.: for recurrent anterior dislocation of the shoulder; a proximal humeral osteotomy.

Moore o.: for long-bone deformity such as a malunion; a three-quarter-width wedge resection with replacement after bone is made into chips, careful closure of the periosteum over the chips, and then closed manipulation after sufficient callus formation.

Müller o.: for osteoarthritis of the hip; an intertrochanteric varus osteotomy.

open-wedge o.: straight cut made across the bone, creating angulation, and leaving an open wedge-shaped gap.

Osgood o.: for correction of malrotation of the femur.

Pauwels o.: for nonunion fracture of the femoral neck.

Pauwels-Y o.: for congenital coxa vara.

Phemister o.: for bone growth asymmetry in the lower limbs; a block of bone is fashioned at the growth plate and then rotated 90 degrees.

Platou o.: for femoral anteversion.

Pott eversion o.: for correction of a distal tibial deformity.

redirection o.: term typically applied to acetabular osteotomy in which the acetabulum is redirected to give more appropriate orientation for the femoral head in cases of dysplasia and in some Legg-Calvé-Perthes disease. Also called **periacetabular osteotomy (PAO), Bernese o., Ganz o., triple o., Steele o.,** and **Wagner o.**

Sarmiento o.: for intertrochanteric fractures; a wedge-shaped piece of bone is resected from the distal fragment to achieve a valgus osteotomy.

Sofield o.: multiple osteotomies of the tibia or femur for bowing deformities caused by osteogenesis imperfecta or nonunions.

Southwick o.: for slipped capital femoral epiphysis; a combination lateral and anterior trochanteric closing wedge osteotomy.

Speed o.: for malunion of the distal radius.

spike o.: creation of a bony spike in a long bone to help hold the fixation of position.

Sugiuka o.: for avascular necrosis of femoral head; the femoral head and neck are rotated to transpose the avascular area away from the weight-bearing portion of the joint.

Thompson telescoping V o.: used in distal femoral deformities.

Weber o.: internal rotation osteotomy of the proximal humerus for recurrent dislocation associated with large posterior humeral head defect.

Whitman o.: closing wedge procedure for the fused hip.

Y o.: for cavus deformity of the foot; also called **Japas o.**

Bone Grafts

Bone grafts are used several hundred thousand times annually in the United States to aid in repair or reconstruction of the skeleton. The scope of applications is associated with congenital (skeletal hypoplasia, pseudarthrosis), developmental (scoliosis), traumatic (fractures, segmental loss), degenerative (osteoarthritis), and neoplastic (benign, malignant) disorders. Bone grafts can be autogenous or allogenic. Advantage of autologous bone graft include maximal biologic potential, histocompatibility, and no potential of transfer of disease from donor to recipient, while allogenic bone grafting avoids donor site morbidity.

In general, autologous bone grafts are removed from one site and transferred to another without direct reestablishment of the blood supply. Consequently, osteogenic cells fail to survive unless they receive sufficient nutrition by diffusion, a circumstance met only by those cells very close to the bone surface. These few surviving cells play an important role in initiation or augmentation of the early phase of bone graft incorporation.

Bone graft repair depends on local factors at and emanating from the recipient site, including ingrowth of new blood vessels and both specialized and multipotential cells required for resorption and new bone formation. The exception to dependence on local tissues occurs with immediate reanastomosis of the blood supply to the graft, often requiring microvascular techniques.

Today, tissue banks have become research centers for bone marrow, stem cell, and growth factor studies. Because all types of blood cells are produced in the bone marrow, research experiments are limitless. Bone marrow collection (harvesting) is still an important part of tissue banking, as is storage and type-matching of bone, tissue, and blood products, but greater emphasis is now being placed on biomedical research of tissue and bone marrow.

General Terminology

histocompatibility: immunologic similarity or identity with respect to cell surface antigens determined by genes of the major histocompatibility complex. There are varying degrees of histocompatibility, some consistent with successful transplantation and some incompatible with this approach unless accomplished with immunosuppression.

immunosuppression: a term applied to any effort directed at lowering the body's natural immune response to foreign substances. In transplant physiology, this is the use of specific chemicals and medications to decrease the body's reaction to transplanted tissues. Nonspecific immunosuppression reduces host responses to most or all antigens and is usually caused by a systemic drug or chemical agent.

implant: a synthetic device or the act of transferring into a host a synthetic device. Some include implants to reflect biologic material without cell viability.

major histocompatibility complex: a sequence of genes that control expression of cell surface glycoproteins that are recognized as foreign when transferred into a genetically dissimilar host. Different terms are used to identify this gene complex, depending on the species, for example, *human leukocyte antigen, histocompatibility-2 in mice,* and *rabbit leukocyte antigen.*

transplant: a tissue or organ transferred from one site to another or the act of accomplishing this transfer. Some use this term to denote the transfer of viable tissue only (versus implant), and others use it to refer to any biologic material.

Classification by Source

allograft: a tissue or organ transferred between nonidentical members of the same species. Also called **allogenic;** formerly called *homograft.*

autograft: a tissue or organ removed from one site and placed in another within the same individual; also called **autogenous.**

isograft: a tissue or organ transplanted between genetically identical members of the same species. Synonymous with **syngraft (syngeneic);** also called **isogenic.**

xenograft: a tissue or organ transferred between species, for example, cow to human, rat to dog. Also called **xenogeneic;** formerly called *heterograft.*

Special Procedures for Preserving Bone Grafts

Most grafts are subject to some form of long-term preservation. The most common storage approaches include deep-freezing, freeze-drying (lyophilization), chemosterilization, and chemical extraction of proteins, or combinations of these techniques. These processing procedures may vary from one tissue bank to another. The methods applied to long-term preservation have some effect on biologic, immunologic, and biomechanical properties of the tissue, but these changes are predictable and often compatible with clinical success. Storage permits time for careful assessment of the donor graft material for potentially harmful transmissible diseases. Graft material should be obtained from tissue banks that use strict processing procedures for allograft processing and donor procurement, under the guidelines of the American Association of Tissue Banks.

Bone Recovery Methods

autolyzed, antigen-extracted allogeneic (AAA) bone: a chemosterilized, autolyzed antigen-extracted, and partially demineralized allogeneic preparation.

chemosterilized grafts: graft material rendered free of microbial organisms by exposure to a chemical, such as ethylene oxide, although thimerosal and alcohol have been used for bacteriostatic properties.

demineralized bone graft: one that has undergone extraction of minerals (superficially or completely) usually by exposure to hydrochloric acid.

freeze-dried grafts: the removal of water from tissue in a frozen state, the same as lyophilized. With respect to bone, usually reflects residual moisture being reduced to approximately 3% or less by weight. Tissues can be stored indefinitely at room temperature in evacuated, sealed containers until required for use. Moisture is then reconstituted by submerging the tissue in water (saline). Also called **lyophilized grafts**.

fresh-frozen grafts: pieces of bone or cartilage that have been frozen without removal of water or cells in an effort to preserve cells.

irradiation-sterilized grafts: exposure of tissues to high-dose ionizing irradiation for the purpose of killing potential pathogens, requiring a dose between 1.5 and 5 megarad.

lyophilized grafts: also called **freeze-dried grafts**.

osteoconductive grafts: graft material that allows for bone ingrowth but does not induce bone growth. This can be applied to some demineralized bone matrix materials as well as synthetics.

osteoinductive grafts: graft capable of stimulating osteoblast formation.

Revascularization of Grafts

The application of immediately revascularized *autografts* is limited by expendability of bone at the donor site, a discrete blood supply to the graft, vessels of sufficient caliber for repair (the fibula, ribs, and iliac crest represent the practical limitations), and microvascular expertise. This approach is especially well-suited for recipient sites compromised by prior irradiation or infection or when rapid repair is mandatory.

The incorporation of devitalized grafts occurs by a lengthy process analogous to creeping substitution, in which the sequence of events includes revascularization of the bone, followed by resorption and new bone formation. Autografts transferred on a vascular pedicle or in which the blood flow is reestablished immediately by vascular anastomoses are incorporated rapidly by a process analogous to fracture repair.

In cases of bone *allografts,* immediate reanastomosis of blood supply is not clinically feasible because it engenders the same immunologic considerations encountered with viable solid organ transplantations, adding the requirement for substantial immunosuppression of the recipient. The following are related terms.

creeping substitution: the process by which a devascularized segment of bone *in situ* or a transferred bone without immediate reanastomosis of its blood supply undergoes repair, beginning with vascular invasion, followed by bone resorption and subsequent new bone formation (incorporation). This is a lengthy process that may take large cortical segments several years to incorporate, and even then, substantial portions of the graft may escape remodeling.

free-revascularized autograft: tissue transferred to a distant site along with its discrete blood supply such that direct reanastomosis of circulation can be accomplished immediately.

incorporation: a process by which recipient site factors grow into and remodel an initially devascularized bone graft. This includes invasion by blood vessels, resorption, and new bone formation. Often used interchangeably with creeping substitution with reference to grafts.

Classification of Grafts by Bone Type

cancellous g.: a bone transplant consisting of cancellous (or medullary) tissue as opposed to cortical bone.

composite g.: a transfer of more than one type of tissue simultaneously, such as bone and muscle transferred at the same time, or bone, muscle, and skin transferred simultaneously; must be accomplished in conjunction with reanastomosis of blood supply at the recipient site. This provides the potential advantage of repairing both bone and soft tissue defects simultaneously.

cortical g.: a transferred bone composed of the cortical (outer) tissue.

    strut g.: cortical bone graft used to give mechanical support in the area of a cancellous bone graft.

corticocancellous g.: transferred bony tissue with both cortical and cancellous elements.

free g.: a bone graft freed of its vascular supply and soft tissue that would encumber its transfer from one location to another. This includes free revascularized autografts as well as other bone graft preparations.

intercalary g.: a segment of transferred bone without an articular surface; usually a portion of diaphysis or diaphysis plus metaphysis, with bone intercalated into bone to reestablish continuity.

intramedullary g.: graft placed in medullary canal. Also called **medullary graft.**

osteoarticular g.: bone graft containing an articular surface.

osteochondral g.: a transplant composed of both bone and cartilage (articular surface).

osteoperiosteal g.: bone graft taken complete with periosteal membrane coverings.

pedicle g.: tissue transferred to another site while retaining (at least temporarily) its required blood supply at the donor site, consequently limiting the distance over which a pedicle can be transferred. The recipient site vascularity can be transected or interrupted following reestablishment of sufficient vascularity at the recipient site.

segmental g.: a portion of transferred tissue representing less than the entire anatomic part being replaced.

Classification by Shape and Bone Grafted

bone block: a bone graft that is inserted next to a joint to prevent a given direction of motion in that joint; also, a bone graft that is shaped in the form of a block and used for fusion of a joint.

chip g.: bone graft broken up into chips.

clothespin g.: coarsely shaped graft used in the spine; resembles a clothespin.

hemicylindric g.: graft cut into the shape of half a cylinder.

inlay g.: any graft that has been cut in a fusion procedure to fit the shape of the graft site.

    diamond inlay g.: graft cut in a diamond shape with recipient site cut to receive that shape.

    sliding inlay g.: a slot of bone cut and moved across the graft site, usually a fracture of a large bone.

massive sliding g.: large graft designed to slide when two portions of recipient bone are compressed.

morcellized g.: cortical or cancellous bone graft that has been finely crushed before implanting.

onlay g.: graft laid directly onto the surface of recipient bone.

    dual onlay g.: two strips of bone laid down on either side of the shaft.

peg g.: cylindric bone graft to be inserted into or through the medullary canal of a bone.

Eponymic Bone Graft Terms	
Albee	Hey-Grooves-Kirk
Banks	Hoaglund
Boyd	Huntington
Campbell	Inclan
Codivilla	McMaster
Flanagan and Burem	Nicoli
Gillies	Phemister
Haldeman	Ryerson
Henderson	Soto-Hall
Henry	Wilson

Osteosyntheses: Internal Fixation Devices for Fracture Healing

Osteosynthesis is a surgical procedure that uses internal fixation devices, especially in the treatment of fractures. This procedure is referred to in context as *open reduction and internal fixation (ORIF)*. It cannot be overemphasized how the orthopaedic surgeon must apply the principles of engineering to biology. The surgeon must be adept in using metal plates, nails, rods, pins,

FIG 8-3 Two internal fixation devices for hip fractures.

bands, screws, bolts, and staples in the correction of skeletal defects (Fig. 8-3). Pegging, pistoning, reefing, shelving, shaving down, shucking, doweling, and saucerization are a few of the shaping and engineering procedures applied within biologic principles. The following internal fixation devices are used or have been used in the past in orthopaedic surgery.

AO: abbreviation for designer of a variety of implant devices. The letters stand for *Arbeitsge-meinschaft für Osteosynthesefragen.*
ASIF: abbreviation for group that studies internal fixation systems and engineering. The letters stand for *Association for the Study of Internal Fixation.*
Asnis screw: for hip cervical fractures; a cannulated screw with reverse cutting thread. (No longer used.)
Badgley nail: for hip fractures; an uncannulated triflanged nail with beveled proximal end that can be attached and inserted through a special side plate.
Bailey-Dubow nail: for osteogenesis imperfecta; an extensible intramedullary nail used in osteotomies.
Basile screw: for hip cervical fractures; a drill point tip screw with pronged washer to be placed over trochanter for compression. (No longer used.)
Benoit-Gerrard: for hip fractures; a spring-loaded sliding nail plate with a proximal outside thread, smooth shaft, and a side plate; provides continuous compression. (No longer used.)
biodegradable fixation: a variety of screws, pins, plates, and other fixation devices made of material that will be absorbed by the body. Such materials include plastic made from single or combined glycolic acid, lactic acid, and other small organic acid capable of forming polymers.
blade plate: general class of plate fixation devices that has a right-angle or nearly right-angle flange.
Blount plate: for fixation of hip fractures and for reconstructive procedures about the hip; a blade plate that can be bent easily to adjust to the correct shape and angle. (No longer used.)
Blount staple: type of staple used around the knee.
Bohler nail: for hip fractures; a triflanged nail with potential use of a side plate. (No longer used.)
Bohlman pin: for hip fractures; a threaded pin with a sharp point and smooth proximal portion. (No longer used.)
bollard: a short, flat-headed, nail-like device that is slotted along a portion of the shaft, used in fixation of ligaments into bone. (No longer used.)
Boyd side plate: to help stabilize trochanteric portion of hip fracture; a plate that could be placed over plate of a Jewett nail. (No longer used.)
Brooker-Willis nail: for unstable femoral fractures; a femoral nail with distal locking screws. (No longer used.)
cable: typically a threaded wire that can be tightened around a piece of bone or the shaft of a bone to maintain apposition or prevent fracture propagation. Often used in association with hip prosthetic surgery.
Calandruccio device: a metallic device for pantalar fusions. (No longer used.)
Calandruccio nail: for hip fractures; a sliding compression screw and plate associated with two to four smaller threaded pins through the plate and into the femoral head for extra fixation. (No longer used.)
cancellous screw: used for trabecular problems near the joints, especially the hip.
cannulated nail or screw: general terms used for nails and screws that have a hole in the center. This hole can be used to direct the nail or screw over a guide wire.
Charnley screw: for intracapsular hip fractures and hip arthrodesis; a compression screw that slides into a barrel and attaches to a side plate. (No longer used.)
cloverleaf nail: used in femoral shaft fractures. (No longer used.)

cobra plate: plate that is shaped like the head of a cobra at the end of a plate used to hold the femur to the pelvis in hip fusion surgery.

cortical screw: used in dense lamellar (cortical) bone. Has smaller thread diameter to diminish chance of cracking hard bone compared with cancellous screws. Similar to machine screws.

Crawford-Adams pin: for hip fracture; use of small threaded pins. (No longer used.)

cruciate screw: screw with cross-shaped head.

Delta nail: for femoral shaft fractures; a nearly triangular nail with interlocking screws. (No longer used.)

Derby nail: for femoral shaft fracture; an intramedullary nail with wings that can be extended at the distal tip, and an antirotation washer at the proximal end. (No longer used.)

Deyerle pin: for intracapsular hip fracture; thick, wide plate with multiple holes to permit the insertion of numerous pins parallel to one another. (No longer used.)

dome plunger: device to facilitate injection of cement into femoral head for better fixation of sliding device.

Dooley nail: for intracapsular hip fractures; a modified Smith-Petersen nail that has an external groove around the base. (No longer used.)

dynamic-compression plate (DCP): plate for fixation of long-bone fractures and osteotomies, with plate fixation designed to allow for compression from muscle and weight-bearing forces.

dynamic hip screw (DHS): for hip fractures; a sliding screw and plate device.

Eggers plate and screw: used in long-bone fractures. (No longer used.)

elastic stable intramedullary nailing (ESIN): for fixation of femoral fractures in children; insertion of a highly elastic intramedullary nail that allows early protected weight-bearing.

Elliott plate: a type of blade plate used mostly in distal femoral procedures. (No longer used.)

encerclage: wiring or banding of bony fragments in the shaft of a bone or for onlay grafts.

Ender nail: intramedullary nail that is curved and can be used to fix intertrochanteric hip fractures through a small incision just above the knee joint; used in a condylocephalic technique.

exchange nailing: use of a larger nail after failure of fixation or union with a smaller nail.

Gamma nail: for hip fractures; a screw and nail device.

Gaenslen spikes: for intracapsular hip fractures; smooth spikes driven from a small incision of greater trochanter. (No longer used.)

Garden screws: for intracapsular hip fracture; large cannulated screws usually used in pairs and inserted at varus and valgus angles. (No longer used.)

Giebel blade plate: blade plate with two screws for fixation of proximal tibial osteotomy. (No longer used.)

Godoy-Moreira stud-bolt: for intracapsular hip fracture; an early model compression screw with external flange and bolt. (No longer used.)

Gore AO screw: AO cortical bone screw modified to affix a ligament replacement implant. (No longer used.)

Gouffon pin: pointed, threaded pin used in the fixation of cervical neck fractures of the hip. (No longer used.)

grommet: a short, flat, hollow cylinder with a head. The device fits over a screw that is considerably narrower than the inner portion of the grommet. Used for fixation of ligaments into bone.

Gross-Kemph nail: for unstable femoral shaft fractures; an interlocking nail system. (No longer used.)

Green-Seligson-Henry (GSH) nail: for supracondylar fractures; nail inserted through intercondylar notch. (No longer used.)

GSU nail: for distal intraarticular fracture of femur; a retrograde nail inserted through joint with nail fixed by transcortical screw. (No longer used.)

Haboush universal nail: for intracapsular hip fractures; a fenestrated plate with a shallow H cross-section; inserted into head and neck of femur, and outside portion bent down over lateral side of femur. (No longer used.)

Hagie pin: used for femoral neck fractures. (No longer used.)

Hansen pin: for intracapsular hip fractures; use of non-threaded, wide pins. (No longer used.)

Hansen-Street nail: used for larger bone fractures. (No longer used.)

Hardinge expansion bolt: for intracapsular hip fractures; a hollow screw with expandable tip and short side plate for femur. (No longer used.)

Harrington rod: used in spinal fixation for scoliosis and some fractures.

Harris nail: intramedullary nail system for intertrochanteric fractures. (No longer used.)

Henderson lag screw: used for hip fractures. (No longer used.)

Herbert screw: for wrist scaphoid fixation; a short screw threaded at both ends; also used in fixation of other small bone fractures or osteotomies such as bunion surgery.

Hessel-Nystrom pin: threaded pin for internal fixation of femoral neck fractures. (No longer used.)

hex screw: hexagon head screw.

Higley side plate: for hip fractures; a side plate that could be attached superiorly for screw fixation into greater trochanter. (No longer used.)

Holt nail: for hip fractures; a one-piece nail-plate combination, with plate fixed by Barr nuts and bolts. (No longer used.)

hook-pin fixation: for femoral neck fractures; a hollow nail has internal hooked pins that can be deployed into the femoral head after introduction of the nail.

Howmedica compression screw: for hip fractures; wide compression screw with side plate and hexagonal shape to cross-section of shaft and barrel to prevent rotation. (No longer used.)

Hubbard side plate: for hip fractures; a wide, long femoral side plate designed to be used with triflanged nail. (No longer used.)

Huckstep nail: for osteotomy of femur with limb lengthening; a nail with holes for cross-screw fixation. (No longer used.)

intramedullary nail: class of nails placed in medullary canal of long bones for fracture stabilization; includes Hansen-Street, Küntscher, Lottes, and Schneider.

Inyo nail: for fractures of the distal fibula, a tapered V-shaped nail made of malleable stainless steel. (No longer used.)

Jewett nail: nail plate used in hip fractures. (No longer used.)

Johansson nail: for hip fractures; a triflanged nail that is cannulated and similar to a Smith-Petersen nail. (No longer used.)

Ken nail: 135-degree sliding nail plate used for hip fractures. (No longer used.)

Kirschner wire (K-wire): small wire used for fixation or traction.

Klemm nail: for femoral shaft fractures; a cloverleaf intramedullary nail with provision for proximal and distal screws. (No longer used.)

Knowles pin: used for hip fractures. (No longer used.)

Küntscher nail: original form was a cloverleaf-shaped nail for simple shaft fractures of the femur. Subsequent modifications are a curved V-shaped nail for valgus reductions of intracapsular hip fractures; a self-locking Y device for hip fractures in which the hip nail has an open base for the passage of a cloverleaf intramedullary nail; and a device for unstable shaft fractures with interlocking proximal and distal screws. Also called **Küntscher rod.** (No longer used.)

Kurosaka screw: special screw designed for fixation of tendon attached to bone in ligament reconstruction.

lag screw: screw with threads at the tip only; used for compression.

Laing H-beam nail: for hip fractures; an H-shaped nail with an adjustable side angle plate. (No longer used.)

Lane plate: plate for long-bone fixation. (No longer used.)

Leinbach screw: long, flexible screw; used often for olecranon fractures. (No longer used.)

less invasive stabilization system (LISS) plate: the screws are locked into the plate.

Lewis nail: intramedullary nail for metacarpal bone fixation.

limited-contact dynamic-compression plate (LC/DCP): plate for fixation of long-bone fractures and osteotomies in which there is only focal point of contact of the plate, with plate fixation designed to allow for compression from muscle and weight-bearing forces.

Lippman screw: for hip fractures; a threaded compression screw with a smooth shaft and threaded base with washer. (No longer used.)

locked intramedullary osteosynthesis (LIFO): for unstable long-bone fractures; a set of flexible 4- or 5-mm diameter pins with a device for proximal interlocking and fixation of two of the pins.

locking plates: plates that act as an internal "external" fixator for long bone fractures. The screws are locked into the plate, helping stabilize the plate without toggling of the screws and with preservation of bone surface circulation.

Lorenzo screw: bone fixation screw. (No longer used.)

Lottes nail: used for tibial fractures. (No longer used.)

Luck nail: several different designs for hip fractures; triflanged nail in which the distal end has multiple perforations to cut off excess length, a proximal pointed nail that can accept a side plate, and a V-shaped nail-plate combination. (No longer used.)

Lundholm screw: for hip fractures; compression screw with proximal washer and nut that could be used with or without side plate. (No longer used.)

Mancini plate: for hip fractures; side plate with multiple-angled screw holes. (No longer used.)

Martin screw: used in hip fractures. (No longer used.)

Massie nail: 155-degree sliding nail used in hip fracture. (No longer used.)

McLaughlin plate or screw: used in hip surgery. (No longer used.)

Medoff sliding plate: for fixation of intertrochanteric and subtrochanteric femur fractures; plate is slotted to allow central portion to slide distally. (No longer used.)

medullary rod: metallic device used in central shaft of bone.

minimally invasive plate osteosynthesis (MIPO): concept of applying plate and screws to fix fractures with small incisions and limited damage to the soft tissue attachments. See also **less invasive stabilization system (LISS) plate.**

Moe plate: for hip fractures; a long lateral plate over femoral shaft and greater trochanter fixed with multiple screws. (No longer used.)

Moore plate or pin: used in hip surgery. (No longer used.)

Morscher plate (AO-Morscher plate): for anterior cervical fusion. (No longer used.)

Müller plate: type of blade plate used in hip surgery. (No longer used.)

Murphy nails: for early attempts at fixation of hip fractures; 8 to 12 penny nails inserted across fracture site. (No longer used.)

Nancy nail: elastic stable intramedullary nails used for pediatric long-bone fractures.

nested nails: a general term for two nails placed side by side in the medullary canal of long bones.

Neufeld nail: for hip fractures in older adults; a V-shaped proximal end portion with short side plate. (No longer used.)

Neufeld pin: for hip fractures; smooth rods with notches easily broken off to adjust length. (No longer used.)

Ogden plate: for fixation of long-bone fractures associated with preexisting intramedullary devices such as rods or the stem of a prosthesis. Long metal plates have slots that are designed to accept encircling bands in locations where screws cannot be easily used. (No longer used.)

olive wire: to help approximate a bone fragment in external skeletal fixation; a small, olive-shaped expansion on a fixation wire can be pulled through the skin to the surface of the small fragment and brought against the main portion of bone.

Parham band: for oblique long-bone fractures; a metal band that can be tightened around the shaft of the bone to achieve fixation by compression. (No longer used.)

Partridge band: for oblique long-bone fracture; a band with ribbed undersurface so that when band is tightened there might be less interference with periosteal and cortical blood flow. (No longer used.)

PGP nail: a flexible nail used in intramedullary fixation of femoral fractures. (No longer used.)

Phillips screw: any screw with a Phillips head.

Pidcock pin: for hip fractures; a small pin that could be passed through a hip nail and into the lateral cortex to prevent shortening. (No longer used.)

Preston screw: for hip fractures; original screw and side plate device. (No longer used.)

Puddu plate: system for fixation of osteotomies that uses a block built into the plate to maintain an opening wedge.

Pugh nail: 155-degree sliding nail used for hip fractures. (No longer used.)

Putti screw: for hip fractures; a compression screw that can be attached to a flange and nut or to a Mancini plate. (No longer used.)

Richards screw: for hip fractures; a sliding compression screw with side plate held by smaller screw to cortex.

Rush nail: stiff intramedullary rod with hooked end used for long bone fixation; also called **Rush rod** and **Rod pin.**

Russell-Taylor nail: intramedullary nail for femur with slots for cross-screw fixation.

Rydell nails: for femoral neck fractures; a four-flanged spring-nail. (No longer used.)

Sage rod: diamond-shaped rod used in forearm fractures. (No longer used.)

Sarmiento nail: for hip fractures, an I-beam with side plate. (No longer used.)

Schanz pins: for external skeletal fixators; screw fixation pins with proximal smooth surface for attachment to the fixation device.

Schneider nail or rod: used in femoral shaft fractures.

Seidel nail: for humeral fractures; a proximal and distal interlocking nail. (No longer used.)

Sheffield rod: for osteogenesis imperfecta; an extensible intramedullary nail used for osteotomies.

Sherman plate: used for long-bone fractures. (No longer used.)

slide plate: used for long-bone fractures.

Smillie nail: small pin used for attachment of the osteochondral fragments in the knee. (No longer used.)

Smith-Petersen nail: flanged nail used in hip surgery. (No longer used.)

Smyth pin: for hip fracture; attachment of two different sized, nonparallel screws through a plate over the greater trochanter. (No longer used.)

Steinmann pin: used in skeletal traction; of larger caliber than a K-wire.

Street medullary pin: used for large long-bone fractures. (No longer used.)

Street nail: split diamond nail for hip fixation. (No longer used.)

Thompson nail: for nondisplaced intracapsular hip fractures; a Z-shaped nail. (No longer used.)

Thornton nail: for femoral neck fractures; a three-flanged spring-nail. (No longer used.)

tibial bolt: used for proximal and distal tibial fractures.

Tieman-Jewett nail: for hip fracture; a one-piece triflanged nail and side plate. (No longer used.)

toggle: a small metallic cylinder with each end slightly larger than the center. Used by tying sutures around it to affix ligaments or tendons to bone.

Tronzo nail: triflanged nail used alone or with side plate. (No longer used.)

True-Flex nail: for fixation of long-bone fractures; fluted intramedullary rods. (No longer used.)

Uppsala screw: for intracapsular hip fracture; multiple, wide, threaded screws. (No longer used.)

Venable screw: original Vitallium screw. (No longer used.)

Veseley-Street nail: for femoral shaft fractures; a splitting of a diamond nail both distally and proximally. (No longer used.)

Virgin screw: for hip fractures; a compression screw using a proximal washer and spring. (No longer used.)

von Bahr screw: for femoral neck fracture; a pin threaded at the tip for multiple screw fixation. (No longer used.)

Watson Jones nail: for hip fractures; a triflanged nail with a small proximal pin through the nail and into lateral cortex. (No longer used.)

Weiss spring: spring device used in some spinal fusions, particularly spondylolisthesis. (No longer used.)

Williams nail: for hip fractures; a modified Küntscher cloverleaf Y nail using a locking nut to secure fixation. (No longer used.)

Williams rod: for pediatric osteogenesis imperfecta deformity or congenital pseudarthrosis of tibia; rod that is inserted through calcaneus into tibia after osteotomy.

Wilson plate: for spinal fusions. (No longer used.)

Zickle nail: a curved 75- and 60-degree nail and screw device for femoral supracondylar fracture; or an intramedullary rod with transfixing nail for subtrochanteric fractures. (No longer used.)

Zuelzer hook plate: commonly used in ankle fractures. (No longer used.)

External Skeletal Fixation for Fractures

The use of external wires transfixed through bone to hold the position of a fracture is not new. Pins in plaster have been used for holding bone fragments in proper position during the healing process. There has been increased use of multiple pins placed through one cortex or both cortices of bone and held by one external device. These external fixation devices are also known as **fixateurs** or **fixators.** This allows easy access to wounds, adjustment during the course of healing, and more functional use of the limb involved. The devices used have increased in number and include the following.

Types by Configuration

articulating frame f.: designed to bridge across a joint and allow joint motion.

bilateral f.: fixation on both sides of bone, pins cross entire limb.

C-clamp f.: occasionally used for emergent treatment of pelvic fractures.

circular f.: circular plates that hold thin through-and-through wires under tension to hold fracture or osteotomy fragments; also called **ring frame f.** and **multiplanar frame f.**

hybrid f.: different techniques are combined such as the combination of a ring system with half pin fixation.

multiplane f.: fixation on multiple sides or surfaces of a bone, used as an index of complexity in procedural coding.

quadrilateral f.: fixation on both sides of bone; pins may or may not cross entire limb; quadrilateral configuration for stability.

semicircular f.: curved plates holding thin through-and-through wires under tension to hold fracture or osteotomy fragments.

Taylor spatial frame f.: multiplanar external skeletal fixation frame that is capable of correcting deformity using a six-axis computer program to create a virtual hinge and determine sequence of correction.

triangular f.: fixation on both sides of bone; pins may or may not cross entire limb; triangular configuration for stability.

unilateral f.: fixation on one side of bone; pins do not cross entire limb.

uniplane f.: fixation on a single side or surface of a bone; used as an index of complexity in procedural coding.

Physical Stimulation of Fracture Healing

The use of direct electric currents, magnetic impulses, and ultrasound waves in the treatment of fractures has been studied for the effect on fracture healing. In the past, the presence of nonunion (extended failure of fracture healing) has often required extensive surgical attention, including bone grafts. Electric and magnetic stimulation in treating fractures has been approved by the Food and Drug Administration for established nonunion of long bones.

capacitive coupling: application of high-frequency surface electrodes that create smaller currents that stimulate fracture healing.

direct electric stimulation: a procedure involving small voltage and amperage electric currents passed through electrodes placed immediately at the fracture site. The source of current is a battery placed external to the body or under the fat, similar to a cardiac pacemaker. For the external battery devices, the electrodes can be placed directly through the skin, eliminating the need for an incision. The limb involved is usually held in a cast.

magnetic stimulation: large magnetic coils applied externally and connected to a specific pulsating current. The home treatment device, used to control the magnetic field, is a small, boxlike apparatus that is plugged into a standard 110-volt outlet; can be used up to 12 hours a day. As in electric stimulation, the affected limb is immobilized in a cast during the treatment period. Because pulsed electromagnetic fields are used, the abbreviation **PEMF** is often used (Fig. 8-4).

ultrasound stimulation: use of low-intensity sound waves applied externally to increase bone healing.

Internal Prostheses

Numerous devices composed mostly of alloys and plastic have been developed to aid in joint replacement efforts. Prosthetic replacements are now available for almost every joint in the body, and even a spinal segment can now be replaced. This field continues to rapidly expand, with a constant influx of new components and the outdating of others. Each is listed in the appropriate section by anatomy. Many of the prostheses listed may already be or soon will be obsolete. They are mentioned because they will still be found in some patients in the future and in their records. Chapter 13 discusses research efforts in internal prostheses.

FIG 8-4 Saddle-shaped coil signal generation device. *(Courtesy EBI Medical Systems, Inc.)*

The advent of a polymer called **methylmethacrylate** led to the development of new types of devices held firmly in place by polymers (not a glue). It is a cement-like substance that forms no chemical bonds but instead holds components to bones by space filling and locking effects. Methylmethacrylate usually has added barium sulfate to make the substance visible on radiographs. When applied, methylmethacrylate is soft and pliable, but it becomes very hard and firm within 15 minutes because of polymerization called **polymethylmethacrylate (PMMA)**. Problems encountered with this method prompted further research and improvement in the development of joint resurfacing techniques.

The cement technique was originally a finger-packing process that was eventually called **first-generation technique**. The use of a gun, a cement-holding device similar to a caulking gun, was used in the **second-generation technique**. The use of a vacuum to help remove bubbles from the cement, thus strengthening the eventual cement construct, has been referred to as **third-generation technique**.

All internal prosthetic devices wear, resulting in the production of microscopic particles that eventually cause a cellular response that leads to bone absorption and prosthetic loosening. The terminology for general material applications for all prosthetics is listed here.

adhesive wear: the most common cause of polyethylene wear in hip replacement; microscopic particles release into joint because of the tendency for adhesion between the opposing surfaces.

alumina: ceramic material used for total joints.

annealing: heating below the temperature of ultra-high-molecular-weight polyethylene.

beaded: tiny cobalt chrome beads bonded to surface of implants for bone ingrowth.

big femoral head (BFH): technology starting with 36-mm size and larger.

computer-aided orthopaedic surgery (CAOS): assists in accurate placement of prosthetic components.

cast components: larger grain size and softer.

ceramic-ceramic bearing: bearing consisting of two like ceramics articulating with each other.

crevice corrosion: breakdown of the metal that affects the grain structure, which ultimately leads to failure of the implant.

cross-linked ultra-high-molecular-weight polyethylene (UHMWPE): increased radiation to 10 megarads and elimination of free radicals causes cross-linking of polyethylene for greater wear resistance.

fibermetal: microtubular-like titanium coating of prostheses for bone ingrowth fixation.

forged components: smaller grain size and greater hardness.

fretting corrosion: corrosion occurring at the junction of two metal interlocking parts that have micromotion.

hemiarthroplasty: only one articular surface is replaced, leaving the native joint on the opposite side intact.

hybrid fixation: the use of cement fixation for one component of a total joint and bone ingrowth for the other component.

hypersensitivity reaction: allergic reaction related to metal ions that become attached to haptens.

keel: portion of prosthesis, typically a tibial tray that has flanges that extend into the metaphysis.

metal-metal bearing: bearing consisting of two metal surfaces articulating with each other. Concern is metal ion levels in blood.

micromotion: when applied to implants, motion of 28–50 μm, which allows for bone ingrowth.

minimally invasive surgery (MIS): procedures done through smaller incisions.

modular components: many prosthetic components, particularly the femoral components of hip replacements, have different-sized interlocking parts to allow for different sizes and shapes of the femur; also called **modularity**.

oxidized zirconium: surface treatment that likely reduces surface wear of ceramic.

polymethylmethacrylate (PMMA): a relatively fast-setting plastic generated from methacrylate that acts as grouting agent in the fixation of prosthetic components.

press fit: design to have a firm fixation based on firm abutment against three points of bone canal margins. Typically these have porous coats for bone ingrowth.

prosthesis of antibiotic-loaded acrylic cement (PROSTALAC): facsimile of a total hip prosthesis that has a very thin polyethylene acetabular cup that is loosely cemented.

remelting: heating above the melting temperature of ultra-high-molecular-weight polyethylene.

resection arthroplasty: removal of joint surfaces without prosthetic replacement; frequently used in the treatment of septic joint infections and prosthetic infections.

resurfacing arthroplasty: used mostly in hips, conserves the femoral head and neck by using a thin-walled acetabular component with typically metal on metal components.

salvage procedure: descriptive of revision procedures with innovative approaches to large bone defects or other anatomic loss.

stress shielding: although more commonly applied to prosthetic devices, this term is applied to the effect of any implant in which there is loss of bone integrity caused by the biologic bone absorption secondary to the shield of stress by the implant.

stripe wear: caused by edge-loading of ceramic during stair climbing.

tantalum: a highly porous material with elastic modulus closer to bone allowing for initial stability.

taper: rounded top of the femoral stem component; designed as a slightly tapered cylinder that will accept a similarly female-shaped portion of the femoral head, which come in various sizes.

  Eurotaper (12/14): taper designed with a 12-mm tip and 14-mm base.

  Morse taper: specific type of taper used to accept femoral head component on the stem component.

third-generation ceramic: small grain size with increased density and each prosthesis proof tested to reduce likelihood of fracture.

third-body wear: wear caused by particle of cement or metal between bearing surfaces.

total joint replacement: both articular surfaces are replaced with a prosthetic component.

two-body abrasive wear: hard surface on opposing soft surface wear.

zirconium: ceramic material used for total joints.

Arthro- (Joints)

Anatomy of Joints (Fig. 8-5)

bursa sac: helps tendons and muscles to glide easily over bones at the joint outside the synovial fluid.

capsule: the general fibrous and ligamentous tissues that act as encasements and enclose the immediate joint area.

cartilage: the strong, smooth covering at the ends of the articular surface of bone. In highly mobile joints like the wrist, fingers, and elbows, this cartilage is called *hyaline*. In less mobile segments,

FIG 8-5 Typical structure of diarthrotic joint. *(From Hilt NE, Cogburn SB: Manual of orthopedics, St Louis, 1980, CV Mosby.)*

such as the intervertebral disk, *fibrocartilage* is present.

meniscus: in the knee, a crescent-shaped fibrocartilaginous disk between the two joint surfaces. There are other menisci and meniscal-like structures in the body. The medial and lateral menisci of the knee receive the most surgical attention.

subchondral bone: named for the bone immediately next to the joint cartilage. Also called **subchondral plate.**

synovium: inner lining of a joint cavity that is a one- or two-layer cell membrane *(synovial membrane)* on a bed of fat. The synovial membrane normally produces and absorbs a clear synovial fluid, which lubricates and feeds cartilage surfaces.

Types of Joints

Joints are the places of union between two or more bones. All joints are not alike in structure and fall into the following categories according to function.

ball-and-socket j.: main points of articulation; femur to acetabulum of hip, humerus to glenoid of shoulder.

hinge j.: located in the elbows, fingers, and knees.

immovable j.: of orthopaedic concern, in the symphysis pubis and sacroiliac region.

synovial j.: two bones connected by fibrous tissue (capsules) with space between them and lined with synovial membrane.

weight-bearing j.: located in the lower spine, hips, knees, and ankles.

General Surgery of Joints

arthrectomy: excision of a joint.

arthrocentesis: needle puncture and aspiration of fluid from a joint.

arthroclisis: surgical breaking down of an ankylosis to secure free movement of a joint.

arthrodesis: a procedure to remove the cartilage of any joint to encourage bones of that joint to fuse, or grow together, where motion is not desired, for example, the spine. Also, an external fusion of a joint by means of a bone graft. The many types of arthrodeses are listed separately.

arthroereisis: a procedure to limit abnormal motion in a joint. Could be in any joint, but frequently referred to in the foot.

arthrokleisis: ankylosis of a joint by closure; production of such ankylosis.

arthrolysis: loosening adhesions in an ankylosed joint to restore mobility.

arthroplasty: reconstructive surgery of a joint or joints to restore motion because of ankylosis or trauma or to prevent excessive motion. This repair and reconstruction may use silicone, metallic, or other implants.

arthroscopy (arthroendoscopy) (Fig. 8-6): a surgical examination of the interior of a joint and evaluation of joint disease by the insertion of an optic device capable of providing an external view of the internal joint area. This technique represents a major advance in orthopaedic technology. The optical system is fiberoptic, giving the surgeon a high-resolution view of a joint, anywhere from a direct forward view to a view at 70 degrees to the end of the microscope, allowing the surgeon literally to see around corners. The arthroscopes vary in diameter from 2.7 to 5 mm. Miniature television cameras are attached directly to the arthroscope, allowing all operating room personnel to view the interior joint. With the advancement of arthroscopic surgery, a wide variety of instruments has made it possible to remove synovium and plicas, repair peripheral tears, excise meniscal tissue, remove loose bodies, shave cartilage, and do many other procedures. The knee receives the most attention in arthroscopic

FIG 8-6 Arthroscope outside of sleeve that is used during surgery; close-up view of 30-degree angle for viewing difficult to see areas. *(Wide-angle arthroscope, 4-mm diameter, 30-degree angle optic. Courtesy Arthrex, Inc., Naples, FL.)*

procedures; however, the arthroscope is now used in almost all joints of the extremities.

arthrotomy: surgical incision into a joint for exploration and removal of joint material; usually refers to knee exploration but can apply to any joint.

arthroxesis: scraping of diseased tissue from the articular surface of bone.

Arthrodeses

Three Basic Categories of Arthrodeses

compression a.: a general class of arthrodeses in which the pins on either side of the joint have some external compression device; the appliance is removed after fusion takes place.

extraarticular a.: fusion of the joint outside the joint capsule; rarely used.

intraarticular a.: fusion of a joint all within its capsule, with or without intraarticular bone grafts.

Specific Arthrodeses

Abbott-Fisher-Lucas a.: two-stage hip fusion that includes a delayed femoral osteotomy.

Baciu and Filibiu a.: intraarticular ankle fusion using dowel bone graft taken from the joint to include the medial and a portion of the lateral malleolus. The graft is rotated 90 degrees and reinserted.

Badgley a.: intraarticular and extraarticular hip fusion, using anterior iliac crest of bone.

Blair a.: a tibiotalar fusion, using an anterior sliding tibial graft.

Bosworth a.: a method of fusing the hip following tuberculosis infection.

Brett a.: extraarticular shoulder fusion, using tibial graft.

Brittain a.: four procedures have this name: (1) intraarticular knee fusion using anterior tibial grafts, (2) extraarticular hip fusion requiring a subtrochanteric osteotomy and tibial bone graft, (3) extraarticular graft to the medial side of the humerus of shoulder, and (4) intraarticular fusion of the elbow using two crossed intraosseous grafts.

Campbell a.: extraarticular fusion of the ankle and subtalar joint.

Chandler a.: intraarticular and extraarticular hip fusion, using the deep portion of the greater trochanter.

Charnley a.: intraarticular type of ankle or knee fusion, using a temporary metallic external compression clamp.

Charnley and Henderson a.: intraarticular and extraarticular fusion of the shoulder, using the glenoid and acromial surface abutting a split humeral head.

Chuinard and Petersen a.: of the ankle, using a wedge of iliac bone.

Compere and Thompson a.: intraarticular hip fusion, using iliac crest and wing for bone graft.

Davis a.: intraarticular and extraarticular hip fusion, accomplished by using a live pedicle of iliac crest.

Ghormley a.: intraarticular and extraarticular hip fusion, using anterior iliac crest graft.

Gill a.: extraarticular and intraarticular fusion, using acromion bone graft from and to the shoulder.

Henderson a.: intraarticular and extraarticular hip fusion, using detached iliac cortical bone graft.

Hibbs a.: intraarticular and extraarticular hip fusion, using greater trochanter as a graft.

Horwitz and Adams a.: ankle fusion, using the distal fibula as a graft.

Key a.: knee fusion, using anterior inlay bone graft.

Kickaldy and Willis a.: intraarticular and extraarticular hip fusion, using iliac crest bone from the ischium to the inferior neck.

King procedure a.: intraarticular hip fusion, using iliac and tibial bone grafts.

Kuntscher modified a.: knee arthrodesis, using a bridging intramedullary rod.

Lucas and Murray a.: knee fusion, using patella for bone graft and held by an internal plate.

Marcus, Balourdas, Heiple a.: chevron-shaped tibiotalar fusion, using inlay graft taken from medial and lateral malleolus.

Müller a.: intraarticular shoulder fusion, using bent plates for fixation.

Potter a.: knee fusion, using a retrograde tibial rod and graft from the distal tibia.

Putti a.: (1) knee fusion, using anterior tibial graft; (2) extraarticular fusion, using the acromion of the scapula; (3) an intraarticular fusion of the shoulder.

Schneider a.: intraarticular hip fusion, using innominate osteotomy with greater trochanter for a bone graft.

sliding a.: anterior ankle fusion, using tibial bone.

Smith-Petersen a.: technique for fusion of the sacroiliac joint.

Stamm a.: intraarticular hip fusion, using free iliac crest bone grafts.

Staples a.: introsseous and extraosseous elbow fusion.

Steindler a.: intraarticular fusion of the shoulder or the elbow, using posterior bone graft.

Stewart and Harley a.: for fusion of ankle, using lateral and medial malleoli as grafts.

Stone a.: intraarticular hip fusion, using a split acetabulum and bent plate from the ilium to the femoral neck.

Trumble a.: extraarticular hip fusion, using a tibial graft from the ischium to the femur.

Watson-Jones a.: intraarticular and extraarticular hip fusion, using a nail and iliac crest graft; also, a shoulder fusion, using a piece of acromion.

White a.: intraarticular hip arthrodesis, using posterolateral approach and iliac bone graft.

Wilson procedure a.: extraarticular fusion of the elbow.

Wolf blade plate a.: ankle arthrodesis performed with a specifically designed blade plate internal fixation device.

John C. Wilson a.: intraarticular and extraarticular hip fusion, using an iliac side graft.

Chondro- (Cartilage)

Cartilage (L. *gristle*) is a fine, glistening, resilient, *nonvascular fibrous connective* tissue that absorbs shock and facilitates the mechanics of joint motion. All mobile joint surfaces contain cartilage. *Perichondrium* is a connective tissue that covers cartilage in some places. Cartilage cells *(chondrocytes)* are widely separated and surrounded by matrix, also *(chondromucoid)* known as *ground substance,* composed of collagen and mucopolysaccharides. In the embryo, cartilage forms the temporary skeleton and is important to growth in providing the model in which most of the bones develop. Then it is called *ossifying* or *precursory cartilage*.

Cartilage cannot be seen on radiographs; if open space is apparent between two bones on radiography, cartilage is present. However, if the radiograph shows two bones touching at a joint, such as the femur on the tibia, osteoarthritis and dissolution of the cartilage in that joint may have occurred.

Types of Cartilage

articular c.: thin layer of hyaline cartilage on articular surface of bones in synovial joints; also called **arthrodial c.** and **diarthrodial c.**

calcified c.: in which granules of calcium phosphate and calcium carbonate are deposited in interstitial substance; seen adjacent to subchondral bone and at the terminus of the physis.

cellular c.: composed almost entirely of cells with little interstitial substances.

connecting c.: connects surfaces of an immovable joint; also called **interosseous c.**

elastic c.: yellow opaque flexible substance (more so than hyaline) in which cells are surrounded by a territorial capsular matrix, outside of which is an interterritorial matrix containing elastic fiber networks, collagen fibers, and ground substance; also called **reticular c.** and **yellow c.**

fibrocartilage: contains types I and II collagen fibers with a strongly basophilic ground substance in area of chondrocytes; seen in the meniscus, labrums, some tendon attachments.

floating c.: detached piece of cartilage on medial or lateral condyle of femur or on patella.

hyaline c.: somewhat elastic, semitransparent cartilage, characterized by type II collagen and proteoglycan aggrecans. Seen in movable joint surfaces and the physis (growth plate).

Surgical Procedures on Cartilage

articular cartilage implant (ACI): cells harvested from a non–weight-bearing portion of the joint are suspended in cell culture for cell division. Weeks later, the expanded mass of cells are placed in the defect with a covering of neighboring periosteum. Also called **articular cartilage transfer (ACT)**.

chondrectomy: surgical removal of cartilage.

chondrodiastasis: for limb-length discrepancy; closed, gradual, and progressive distraction of the growth plate by using an external bone fixation device.

chondroplasty: plastic surgery on cartilage by repair of lacerated or displaced cartilage.

chondrosternoplasty: surgical correction of funnel chest.

chondrotomy: dissection or surgical division of cartilage.
  synchondrotomy: incision and division of an articulation that has no appreciable mobility and in which cartilage is the intervening connective tissue.

microfracture: piercing of the subchondral bone base of a cartilage defect to promote development of a hematoma and healing with fibrocartilage.

mosaicplasty: removal of plugs of cartilage and bone from a limited–weight-bearing portion of the joint to be placed in the area of a defect.

shell osteochondral allograft: donor-intact cartilage and subchondral bone is harvested from the same location as similar-sized donor and implanted in defect site. The term *shell* refers to the relatively thin 5-mm shell of bone that distinguishes this procedure from larger bony segments.

Capsulo- (Capsule)

A capsule is the circumferential sleeve surrounding a joint composed of a tough band of fibrous and ligamentous tissues. It may be referred to as a joint capsule or a capsular ligament.

Surgical Procedures on the Capsule

capsulectomy: excision of a joint capsule; most commonly done on the hip.

capsulodesis: imbrication of a capsule (see Chapter 10).

capsuloplasty: plastic surgery on a joint capsule.

capsulorrhaphy: suturing of a joint capsule. If used by itself, the term implies a procedure on the shoulder (glenohumeral joint) because this joint commonly has soft tissue reconstructions.

capsulotomy: incision into a joint capsule; also called **capsotomy**.

Bursae

A bursa (sac or saclike cavity) is filled with viscid fluid and situated in places in tissue where friction would otherwise develop. Bursae act as cushions, relieving pressure between moving parts such as an **anserine bursa**, a goose-foot sac found between tendons of the sartorius, gracilis, and semitendinous muscles and the tibial collateral ligament. A bursal sac is easily recognized during surgery and is involved in only four procedures.

bursectomy: excision of a bursa.

bursocentesis: puncture and removal of fluid from a bursa.

bursoscopy: endoscopic visualization of a bursa, most commonly hip or shoulder.

bursotomy: incision into a bursa.

Other Specific Tissues

The entire musculoskeletal system is made up of connective tissues, that is, cellular and organic materials that establish structure and shape. Bones and joints receive the most attention in orthopaedic surgery and are, therefore, listed separately.

All connective tissues have, to some degree, cohesion that is supplied by a protein structure called **collagen**.

Collagen, in its most familiar form, is a household product, gelatin. However, when combined with other chemical and cell elements, it is the basic molecular matrix of bone, cartilage, tendons, and many other tissues. The connective tissue cells are the following.

adipose tissue: fatty tissue.
chondroblasts: cells that form cartilage.
chondroclasts: cells that remove cartilage.
chondrocytes: cartilage cells.
fibroblasts: cells that predominantly form collagen.
fibrocytes: cells seen in tendons, ligaments, and similar structures.
histiocytes: cells involved in removal of cellular or chemical debris; a type of phagocyte.
myoblasts: muscle-forming cells.
myocytes: muscle cells, voluntary (striated) and involuntary (nonstriated).

Myo- (Muscle)

Muscle is the contractile tissue essential for skeletal support and movement. The anatomic features of muscles with associated tissues and surgery are presented here.

Muscle fibers are composed of small bundles of cells combined to form distinct muscular units. Terms often related to muscle include *actin, myosin, sarcomere, nerve spindle, motor unit, neuromuscular junction,* and *spindle cell.*

The smooth, coordinated way in which muscles work together in the execution of a movement is called **synergy** (syn- [together] + ergon- [work]). In particular, the muscles that play the part of **synergists** during any particular movement are concerned with obviating any unwanted movement that might result from the action of the **prime movers** or **agonists.** Muscles that pull in the opposite direction are called **antagonists.** Synergist muscles are usually classified as **corrective** if they obviate such unwanted movements, and **fixative** if they fix the point proximal to that at which the movement is taking place. **Muscle insertion** is the attachment of a muscle or its tendon to the part of the skeleton that the muscle moves when it contracts. **Muscle origin** is a fixed attachment or anchor of muscle allowing a muscle to exert power when it contracts. The many muscle groups are named and illustrated in Fig. 8-7.

Surgical Procedures on Muscles

myectomy: excision of a portion of muscle.
myoclasis: intentional crushing of muscle; rare.
myomectomy (myomatectomy): surgical removal of tumors with muscular tissue components.
myoneurectomy: surgical interruption of nerve fibers supplying specific muscles; used for patients with cerebral palsy.
myoplasty: plastic surgery on muscle in which portions of partly detached muscle are used for correction of defects or deformities.
myorrhaphy (myosuture): muscle repair by suture of divided muscle.
myotenontoplasty: surgical fixation of muscles and tendons.
myotenotomy: surgical division of a tendon from muscle.
myotomy: incision or dissection of muscle or muscular tissue.

Aponeuroses

Aponeurosis is the name given to the end of a muscle that becomes a tendon. This muscular component is a white, flattened, ribbonlike tendon expansion that connects muscle with the parts it moves.

Surgical Procedures on Aponeuroses

aponeurectomy: excision of the aponeurosis.
aponeurorrhaphy: repair and suture of muscle and tendon; **fasciorrhaphy.**
aponeurotomy: surgical incision into the aponeurosis.

Teno- (Tendons)

The extension of muscle into a firm, fibrous cord that attaches into a bone or other firm structure is a tendon. Some muscles have a tendon at both ends, some have direct attachment to bone at one end, and a few attach directly to bone at both ends and have no tendon.

A **common tendon** serves more than one muscle, such as a **conjoined tendon** that is found in the inguinal region. The tendons that receive the most attention are the following:

Achilles t.: the common tendon of the gastrocnemius and soleus muscle inserted into the medial posterior

FIG 8-7 Muscular system, **A,** Anterior view.

FIG 8-7, cont'd B, Posterior view. *(From* Mosby's medical and nursing dictionary, *ed 2, St Louis, 1986, CV Mosby.)*

surface of the calcaneus; also called **calcaneal t.** or **tendo calcaneus, heel t.**

hamstring t.: one of the tendons that cross the popliteal fossa laterally and medially. The inner hamstring includes tendons of the gracilis and sartorius muscles, and the outer hamstring is the tendon of the biceps flexor femoris muscle.

patellar t.: anterior or inferior ligamentum patellae.

rotator cuff t: tendons of muscles that surround the shoulder joint

Sharpey fibers: fibers of a tendon attached to bone that actually penetrate the periosteum and cortex of bone, and thus make a very strong attachment.

Surgical Procedures on Tendons

The nomenclature of surgical procedures on tendons has a certain amount of overlap, because several prefixes are used: *teno-, tendo-,* and *tendino-*. Therefore the same surgical procedure may have several spellings. The preferred term for a surgical procedure is listed first, with the related term appearing after the definition.

tendon release: surgical transection of a tendon, with or without repair.

tenectomy: excision of a lesion (ganglion or xanthoma) of a tendon or of a tendon sheath.

tenodesis: tendon fixation by suturing proximal end of a tendon to the bone or by reattachment of the tendon to another site.

tenolysis: surgically freeing a tendon from adhesions; also called **tendolysis.**

tenomyoplasty: procedure involving repair of tendon and muscle; also called **tenontomyoplasty.**

tenomyotomy: excision of a portion of tendon and muscle.

tenonectomy: excision of a portion of tendon with or without excision of a portion of tendon to shorten it.

tenontomyotomy: incision into the principal tendon of a muscle, with partial or complete excision of that muscle.

tenoplasty: surgical repair of a ruptured tendon; also called **tendoplasty, tendinoplasty,** and **tenontoplasty.**

tenorrhaphy: union of a divided tendon by a suture; also called **tenosuture** and **tendinosuture.**

tenosuspension: surgical repair that fashions a soft tissue sling to hold the tendon in a specific place.

tenosynovectomy: resection or excision of excessive synovial lining within the tendon sheath.

tenotomy: incomplete or complete division of a tendon, as in clubfoot; also called **tendotomy.**

Desmo- (Ligaments)

Ligaments are bands of strong fibrous connective tissue that bind together the articular ends of bones and cartilage at the joints to facilitate, stabilize, or limit motion. Also, they give support and attachment to fascia, viscera, and muscles. An **accessory ligament** supports another ligament on the lateral surface outside the joint capsule where excessive motion occurs. In the knee, elbow, and wrist, the **medial, lateral,** and **collateral ligaments** provide additional support. There are many others, but the knee receives the most attention. Because ligaments tie bones together, the prefix *syn-* (together) is used with *desmo-* (ligament) for ligament surgery. **Syndesmosis** is the name for an articulation in which the bones are united by ligaments (e.g., the distal tibiofibular articulation).

Surgical Procedures on Ligaments

desmotomy: surgical division of a ligament or ligaments.

ligamentotaxis: use of strength of ligaments to bring about reduction of fracture fragments by using external skeletal fixation.

syndesmectomy: excision of a ligament or portion thereof.

syndesmopexy: surgical fixation of a dislocation by using the ligaments of a joint.

syndesmoplasty: ligaments sutured together.

syndesmorrhaphy: suture or repair of ligaments.

syndesmotomy: dissection or cutting of ligaments.

Fasciae

Fasciae (pronounced fash'-e-e) (fascia, sing.) are sheets of dense connective fibrous tissue that act as a restricting envelope for muscular components and bind groups of muscles, blood vessels, and nerves into bundles. Generally, the fascia does not play any role in the movement of joints and bones. The exception to this is the *fascia lata* of the outer thigh; this fascia has its own muscle, the *tensor fascia lata*, that, when tightened, will pull through the fascia to points across the knee.

Surgical Procedures on Fasciae

fasciaplasty: plastic surgery of fascia; also called **fascioplasty.**
fasciectomy: excision of strips of fascia.
fasciodesis: suturing a fascia to another fascia or tendon.
fasciorrhaphy: suturing and repair of lacerated fascia; also called **aponeurorrhaphy.**
fasciotomy: surgical incision or transection of fascia, commonly done for forearm and leg injuries, in which the pressure in the compartment surrounded by the fascia has become very high.

Neuro- (Nerves)

Nerves are cordlike structures that convey electrical impulses between a part of the central nervous system and some other region of the body. Structural components of the nerves include epineurium, perineurium, nerve sheath, axon, Schwann cell, and myelin. **Innervation** refers to the nerve supply to any tissue. Nerves are usually named for the anatomic area involved. Hilton law states that a nerve trunk that supplies any joint supplies the muscles moving that joint and the area over the skin over that joint.

Orthopaedic Surgical Procedures on Nerves

Mellesi cable graft: for neuroma excision and replacement with grafts of specific length of fascicular gap.
neurectomy: resection of a segment of a nerve.
neurolysis: destruction of a perineural adhesion by a longitudinal incision to release the nerve sheath.
neuroplasty: plastic repair of a nerve.
neurorrhaphy: suture of a severed nerve; repair.
neurotomy: division of a nerve or nerves.
neurotripsy: surgical crushing of a nerve.
rhizotomy (radicotomy, radiculectomy): procedure dividing the nerve roots close to their origin from the spinal cord; *rhizo-* refers to root of the spinal cord. Typically performed to decrease muscle tone in cerebral palsy patients

Vascular (Blood Vessels) System
(Fig. 8-8)

There are thousands of miles of blood vessels in the human body and approximately 2000 gallons of blood per day coursing through these vessels, likened to a road map with its major arteries, tributaries, and branches. The **arteries** are the major pipelines that distribute oxygenated blood from the heart to the various organs. In each group, the main artery resembles a tree trunk that gives off numerous branches and these branches form smaller vessels called **arterioles**, which branch again, forming microscopic vessels called **capillaries.**

The **veins** are an extension of the capillaries in that capillaries unite into vessels of increasing size to form **venules** and eventually **veins.** Their function is to carry deoxygenated blood from the various organs back to the heart. Veins differ from arteries in that they have **valves** that create a unidirectional flow. Arteries and veins often have the same name for their location in the body, for example, *femoral artery* and *femoral vein*. The following terms relate to blood vessels.

adventitia: loose outer lining of a blood vessel; outermost wall of artery.
artery: blood vessel that carries oxygenated blood away from heart on its way to various organs and tissues in the body.
arterioles: smallest vessels considered arteries (0.2 mm diameter) made mostly of smooth muscle; blood flows through arterioles and moves to capillaries.
capillaries: tiny network of blood vessels supplying oxygen directly to cells of body. At this level, oxygen and other nutrients are delivered to cells, and carbon dioxide and waste materials are passed from the tissues back to the bloodstream.
cardiovascular: pertaining to blood vessels (arteries and veins) and the heart.
cerebrovascular: pertaining to blood vessel circulation of the brain and to the brain.
collateral circulation: named and unnamed secondary vessels supplying blood to an organ or extremity through indirect channels. These collateral vessels become particularly important when the main artery

FIG 8-8 A, The arteries of the body distribute oxygenated blood from the heart to the body. The name of each artery corresponds to the organ or region served. The pulmonary arteries pumps deoxygenated blood to the lung.

FIG 8-8, cont'd B, The major veins are named to correspond to the regions of the body they drain: blood is returned by these veins to the heart. The oxygenated blood returns to the heart via the pulmonary vein. *(From Thibodeau GA, Patton KT: Anatomy and physiology, ed 6, St Louis, 2006, Mosby.)*

is damaged (occluded), for example, genicular arteries around the knee in support of an occluded popliteal artery.

diastole: heart chamber filling or relaxation phase of the heart cycle.

intima: the innermost lining of the arterial wall.

lipid: one of many chemical compounds normally found in blood that are considered fats and have a relationship between the amount and kinds of lipids in the blood and hardening of the arteries.

lumen: the space inside a blood vessel, duct, or hollow viscus.

patency: refers to an open blood vessel (artery or vein) in which blood is flowing.

systole: contraction phase of cardiac cycle.

vascular: pertaining to vessels. Can also refer to amount of blood supply to an organ, such as a vascular tumor, that is, a tumor with a good blood supply.

vein: blood vessel that carries blood from the various organs in the body back to the heart. Veins usually have valves creating a unidirectional flow, whereas arteries do not. Small veins are then called **venules**.

vena cava: either of the two main veins (superior and inferior) that convey blood from other veins to the right atrium of the heart.

Vascular Surgical Procedures (Arteries and Veins)

Peripheral vascular surgery procedures center around the treatment of disorders of the blood vessels, that is, the arteries and veins (not including the heart), and may be performed in conjunction with orthopaedic procedures, such as the repair of a disrupted popliteal artery following knee dislocation. An understanding of peripheral vascular surgery is also necessary in diagnosing patients with vascular disease who come to the orthopaedic surgeon. For example, a patient may see an orthopaedic surgeon for a painful foot believing it to be a bony problem, only to find it is rest pain from occluded arteries in the thigh and calf. In this case, the patient is referred to the vascular surgeon for further evaluation and treatment. Because these two specialties overlap in diagnosis, treatment, and surgery, vascular procedures are included for reference.

Most peripheral vascular surgical procedures performed today are done to correct the problem of arteriosclerosis (hardening of the arteries). In this regard, the problems can usually be corrected by a bypass, by replacing the artery, or by cleaning it out (endarterectomy). The terms relating to blood vessel surgery follow.

aortofemoral bypass (AFB): surgical procedure whereby the narrowing or occlusion of the abdominal aorta and iliac arteries (from arteriosclerosis) is bypassed with a graft (usually Dacron) going from just below the renal arteries down to the femoral arteries in the groins. This is considered one of the bigger vascular procedures; it requires opening the abdomen and takes from 3 to 6 hours. Separate bypass grafts may be taken off the main aortofemoral graft to increase the blood supply to the kidneys, intestines, or pelvic viscera to include the male genitalia.

aortoiliac bypass: a bypass graft going from just below the renal artery down to the iliac arteries. This procedure is usually performed for abdominal aortic aneurysms.

aneurysmorrhaphy: a repair of an aneurysm in which it is left in place, but disconnected from the circulation, and a graft is sewn in its place. Following this, the aneurysm wall can either be wrapped around the graft or left in place. (Totally removing the aneurysm is rarely done because it may jeopardize adjacent organs.)

arthrectomy catheter: a vascular procedure for a localized endarterectomy in which a device is passed percutaneously or intraoperatively to an area of stenosis, using a small circular knife blade.

autogenous saphenous vein graft (ASVG): the greater saphenous vein of the lower extremity is removed and used to either bypass or replace a diseased segment of artery or vein elsewhere in the body. When the vein is removed and placed in a different location, care must be taken to ensure that the valves of the vein are either destroyed or that the vein is put in a reversed fashion so that the arterial blood will flow unimpeded.

axillofemoral bypass (AxFem): an extraanatomic bypass whereby either Dacron or polytetrafluoroethylene graft is used to carry blood from the axillary artery (under the arm) down to one or both common femoral arteries. This procedure is usually performed in lieu of an aortofemoral bypass because the abdomen is inaccessible resulting from infection in the abdomen, for example, infected aortofemoral graft, severe cardiac disease, or severe pulmonary disease. The patency rate for these grafts is not nearly as good as that for a usual aortofemoral bypass graft.

balloon angioplasty: a procedure whereby a balloon catheter is passed up to an area of stenosis in an artery to widen vessel, a balloon is inflated, and the area of the stenosis (stricture) is dilated. This procedure is augmented by adding a stent or wire mesh inside the artery to support the dilated segment; also called **percutaneous transluminal angioplasty (PTA).**

carotid endarterectomy: an opening up and cleaning out of the common carotid and internal carotid artery in the neck. During this procedure, the diseased intima and portions of the media are removed to open and smooth out the channel of blood flow to the brain. The procedure removes the roughened irregular buildup of atherosclerosis and is done to prevent transient ischemic attacks and strokes.

carotid subclavian bypass: procedure involving either vein or prosthetic material whereby a bypass graft is placed between the carotid artery and subclavian artery. It is done to improve the blood flow in the subclavian artery to the arm and hand by bringing blood up the carotid artery and down into the subclavian, bypassing a narrowing at the origin of the subclavian artery; also called **subclavian carotid bypass.**

coronary artery bypass graft (CABG): procedure on the blood vessels of the heart whereby narrowed areas in the arteries leading to the heart muscle itself are bypassed with a vein graft going directly from the aorta to more distal portions of the coronary (heart) arteries. This procedure, performed by cardiac surgeons, is done while the patient is on a cardiac bypass machine.

distal bypass: procedure performed with either synthetic material or vein whereby blood is brought from either the common femoral or superficial femoral artery down to the small named blood vessels below the knee. The procedure is usually performed to prevent amputation of an extremity from severe ischemia. The patient frequently has severe pain and skin breakdown before the operation.

endarterectomy: an opening up and cleaning out of blood vessels diseased by hardening of the arteries, which begin in the intima and progress down through the media. In this procedure, the diseased intima, fatty deposits, and much of the media are removed; the roughened irregular surface of the blood vessel can produce a surface on which blood clots will collect and break off, moving downstream, or a surface on which more clot can form and occlude (close off) the artery.

endovascular grafting: reconstruction of aneurysms and, in some cases, occlusive disease by passing balloon expandable synthetic grafts into the aneurysm and opening the graft. The graft is held in place with stents or other devices. Fluoroscopy and angiography ensures proper positioning. Limitations and complications (early and late) are the focus of current active development.

endovascular therapy: catheter-based endovascular approach to quickly dissolve clots and blockages. An ultrasound-enhanced drug delivery system is used that is composed of tiny transducers situated on hair-thin wires (catheters) that dissolve blood clots in the pelvis and limbs, and stroke-causing blood clots in the brain. More recently clot-busting drugs are infused at the site of the clot in the pelvic arteries or limbs.

end-to-end anastomosis: a joining of two vascular structures—arteries, graft and artery, or vein and artery—to bypass an occluded or damaged segment; the end of one structure is sewn to the end of the other.

end-to-side anastomosis: a joining of the end of an artery or vein or prosthetic material to the side of another vein, artery, or prosthetic material to bypass an occluded or damaged segment.

extraanatomic bypass: bypass graft in which prosthetic material or vein is used to route blood between the two arteries or two veins. The route of the graft is other than a usual anatomic position, such as axillofemoral or femoral-femoral bypass.

extracranial-intracranial bypass (ECIC): a procedure performed by neurosurgeons whereby severely narrowed or occluded blood vessels within the brain are bypassed. The usual procedure is to take the superficial temporal artery, which is a branch on the scalp, make a bone flap in the skull, and move the distal end of this artery down into the brain to supply blood flow directly into the brain.

femoral-femoral bypass (fem-fem bypass): a bypass procedure using a synthetic or vein graft material whereby one femoral artery is used to supply the blood to both lower extremities. This could be done to bypass an infection, or to provide blood flow from one undiseased iliac femoral system to another femoral system. It is considered an extraanatomic bypass.

femoral popliteal bypass (FPB): bypass graft from the femoral artery to the popliteal artery. The distal end of the graft can go to a portion of the popliteal artery above the knee or the popliteal artery below the knee. May be performed with vein or prosthetic material. It is done to correct an occluded superficial femoral artery. Indications for this procedure are claudication, rest pain, or threatened limb loss.

vena cava filter: for venous thromboembolic disorders, an umbrella-shaped metallic device that is inserted into the inferior vena cava to prevent clot from breaking off from legs or pelvis and going into the lungs (pulmonary emboli), for example, **Greenfield filter.**

in situ bypass: instead of removing the greater saphenous vein and reversing it, it is left in place and the valve destroyed through a variety of techniques. The proximal end is sutured into the inflow artery, and the distal end of the vein is sutured into the recipient artery. The side branches of the vein are ligated in distal artery of leg. This technique provides better patency than taking the vein out and reversing its course.

laparotomy: a procedure whereby the abdomen is opened for exploration or to conduct another surgical procedure.

limb salvage: a general category of procedures performed on a lower extremity to improve the blood supply and prevent amputation. Skin ulceration and gangrene are often present.

patch angioplasty: a local procedure whereby the artery is opened, the inside of the vessel is cleaned out and a patch of vein or prosthetic material is used to widen that area of the artery. This procedure is also done in the repair of traumatic injuries.

polytetrafluoroethylene (PTFE): a plastic graft that has gained popularity in bypassing and replacing occluded arteries throughout the body.

reversed vein bypass graft: a technique in which a vein, usually the greater saphenous, is removed and used as a bypass. The small end of vein is sutured to proximal artery (inflow) and distal (large) end of vein is sutured to outflow artery. The vein must be turned around in this fashion to obviate the function of valves.

sympathectomy: division of sympathetic chain to allow some dilatation of small extremity blood vessels. Not considered adequate treatment of claudication but may be a useful adjunct in limited situations. Sometimes helpful in upper extremity vasospastic disorders (Raynaud's or reflex sympathetic dystrophy).

thrombolytic therapy: a dissolution of thrombus in an artery or vein with urokinase or streptokinase. Has been most useful in recent thromboses, but some contraindications must be considered.

Specific Anatomy and Surgery by Location

The Shoulder

Shoulder separations and shoulder dislocations are very distinct injuries and involve two different joints. Palpating the collar bone (clavicle) and working the fingers laterally, a distinct bump is felt—the acromioclavicular (AC) joint, which is the junction between the collar bone and shoulder blade (Fig. 8-9). The acromion is the part of the shoulder blade that connects with the collar bone. Injury of this joint is often called a *shoulder separation*. However, a person dislocating the shoulder has disrupted the ball-and-socket joint between the arm and the shoulder blade (glenohumeral joint). The orthopaedist may not be able to feel this joint dislocation under the numerous muscles, but its presence is apparent through pain and an inability to place the arm behind the back or raise it over the head.

Anatomy
Bones

clavicle (cleido-): collar bone.
　　AC joint: between clavicle and scapula.

FIG 8-9 Shoulder joints. *(From Hilt NE, Cogburn SB: Manual of orthopaedics, St Louis, 1980, CV Mosby.)*

sternoclavicular joint: at the junction of the clavicle and breast bone.
humerus: arm bone between the shoulder and elbow.
  anatomic neck: point of attachment of shoulder capsule (humerus).
  biceps groove: groove for the long head of the biceps muscle; also called **bicipital groove.**
  greater and lesser tuberosity: points of attachment for the rotator cuff.
  humeral head: half-circle-shaped portion of the humerus for the shoulder joint.
  surgical neck: most common point of fracture of the humerus.
rhomboid fossa: an inconsistent feature on the medial side of the clavicle. It is the attachment of the costoclavicular or rhomboid ligament and has importance only because it may be mistaken for a tumor.
scapula: shoulder blade.
  acromion process: outermost tip of the shoulder.
  coracoid: knob of bone attached to the anterior scapula just medial to the shoulder.
  glenoid fossa: saucer-shaped depression of the scapula that has direct contact with the humerus and glenohumeral joint.
  glenoid labrum: ring of fibrocartilage of connective tissue attached to rim of margin of bony glenoid cavity of shoulder blade to increase its depth.
  scapular spine: outcropping portion of the posterosuperior scapula.
  spinoglenoid notch: small, fingernail-sized, V-shaped groove in the superior border of the scapula through which the suprascapular nerve courses.

Muscles Around the Shoulder

axilla: also known as the *arm pit*, the axilla is bordered in the front by the pectoral muscle and in the back by the latissimus dorsi.

coracobrachialis: from the coracoid of the scapula to the inner distal humerus; pulls the arm across the midline.

deltoid: triangular muscle arising from the acromion that attaches to the lateral arm; elevates, flexes, and extends the arm.

infraspinatus: from the posterior upper scapula to the posterior superior humerus; externally rotates the arm.

latissimus dorsi: from the lower thoracic and lumbar spine to the anterior upper humerus; pulls the arm down and helps depress the humeral head.

levator scapula: from central midneck to the superior medial scapula; controls scapular elevation and rotation.

pectoralis major and minor: from the clavicle (major) and coracoid (minor) to the anterior chest wall; pulls the scapula forward.

rhomboideus major and minor: from the midline of the thoracic spine to the medial scapula; pulls the scapula back toward the midline.

rotator cuff: arrangement of four muscles from the scapula to the humerus, which, with the capsule and glenoid labrum (a cartilaginous margin of the joint), stabilize the shoulder. The four muscles of the rotator cuff are supraspinatus, infraspinatus, teres minor, and subscapularis. The supraspinatus and infraspinatus are the tendons most commonly addressed during a cuff repair procedure.

serratus anterior: from the medial scapula to the chest anteriorly; holds the scapula into the body during shoulder motions.

shoulder girdle: a general term for the soft tissue around the glenohumeral joint.

sternocleidomastoid: from the base of the skull to the sternum and medial clavicle; turns head and flexes the neck.

subscapularis: from the anterior scapula to the lesser tuberosity; strong internal rotator of the shoulder.

supraspinatus: from the top of the scapular spine to the greater tuberosity of the humerus; abducts the arm and depresses the humeral head.

teres major and minor: from the lateral scapula to the humerus; pulls the arm in with the minor externally rotated as a part of the rotator cuff.

trapezius: kite-shaped muscle from the base of the neck to lower spine to scapular spine; controls scapular motion.

Ligaments Around the Shoulder Region

At the sternoclavicular joint, the **sternoclavicular l.**

At the AC joint, the **AC l.** and **coracoclavicular l.** (the **conoid l.** and **trapezoid l.**).

At the glenohumeral joint:

anteroinferior glenohumeral l.: lower of the three anterior glenohumeral l.

anteromedial glenohumeral l.: most substantial of the three anterior glenohumeral l.

anterosuperior glenohumeral l.: most superior of the three anterior glenohumeral l.

conjoined tendon: the common origin of two tendons from the coracoid process of the scapula leading to the arm and forearm. In surgery it is detached temporarily to gain access to the shoulder joint.

coracohumeral l.: starting at coracoid and crossing over humeral head.

glenoid labrum: meniscus-like rim of cartilage that deepens the glenohumeral joint.

rotator interval: area of thin tissue under coracohumeral l. and between the subscapularis and supraspinatus tendons.

superior suspensory complex: a combination of the glenoid, coracoid process, coracoclavicular ligaments (conoid and trapezoid), distal part of the clavicle, AC joint, and acromion process; maintains suspension of the glenohumeral joint.

transverse humeral l.: covering long head of biceps tendon over the bicipital groove.

Main Arteries, Veins, and Branches Around the Shoulder

axillary artery: a continuum of the subclavian artery in the axillary area that branches into highest thoracic, lateral thoracic, anterior humeral circumflex, posterior humeral circumflex, thoracoacromial, and subscapularis.

brachial artery: a continuum of the axillary artery and main artery of the arm. The branches are listed in "Surgery of the Arm and Forearm" later in this chapter.

cephalic vein: large vein between the deltoid and pectoralis muscles.

subclavian and axillary vein: the continuous vessel running alongside the subclavian and axillary arteries. The branches are not consistent and are rarely described in orthopaedic procedures.

subclavian artery: main artery from the chest leading down through the arm that branches into internal thoracic, vertebral, thyrocervical, transcervical, superior intercostal, and suprascapular.

Nerves

anterior thoracic n.: from the lateral cord, supplies the pectoral muscles.

axillary n.: arising from the posterior cord, supplies the upper arm, particularly the deltoid and teres minor.

brachial plexus: a large complex of nerves from the lower cervical and upper thoracic (C5 to T2) spinal segments. This nerve plexus includes:
Superior, medial, and inferior trunk
Anterior and posterior division
Medial, lateral, and posterior cord
Lower and upper subscapular nerve
Musculocutaneous nerve
Radial nerve
Ulnar nerve
Dorsal scapular nerve
Axillary nerve
Medial nerve
Scapular nerve
Long thoracic nerve

dorsal scapular n.: from the fifth nerve root; supplies the rhomboids.

long thoracic n.: from the fifth, sixth, and seventh cervical root; supplies the serratus anterior. Also called **n. of Bell.**

lower scapular n.: from the posterior cord; supplies the lower scapular and teres major muscles.

median n.: from the lateral and medial cord; supplies the finger and wrist flexors, except the fourth and fifth profundus and flexor carpi ulnaris, and the thumb intrinsics, except the adductor.

musculocutaneous n.: from the lateral cord, supplies the biceps coracobrachialis, brachialis, and lateral cutaneous nerve of the forearm.

radial n.: from the posterior cord, supplies the triceps, anconeus, supinator, and hand and wrist extensors.

suprascapular n.: from the superior trunk, supplies the supraspinatus and infraspinatus.

thoracodorsal n.: from the posterior cord, supplies the latissimus dorsi muscle.

ulnar n.: from the medial cord, supplies the fourth and fifth profundus and flexor carpi ulnaris along with the hand intrinsics including the thumb adductor, but not the other thumb intrinsics.

upper subscapular n.: from the posterior cord, supplies the subscapularis muscle.

Eponyms

The following list of eponyms for surgical procedures is arranged according to the area of injury or deformity. In most instances, the arthroplasties can be referred to as capsulorrhaphies of the shoulder.

Arthroplasties for Acromioclavicular Separations

Bosworth
Dewar and Barrington
Mumford-Gurd
Neviaser

Arthroplasties for Anterior Shoulder Dislocations

Bankart
Bristow
Cubbins
de Toit and Roux
Eden-Hybbinette
Magnuson-Stack
Nicola
Putti-Platt
Speed
Trillat

Arthroplasties for Posterior Shoulder Dislocations

McLaughlin
Scott
Wilson and McKeever

For High-Riding Scapulae (Sprengel Deformity)

Chang and Farahvar
Green
Inclan-Ober
Robinson
Schrock
Woodward

Arthrodeses for Shoulder Stabilization

Brittain
Gill
Putti
Steindler
Watson-Jones

Muscle Transfers for Paralysis of Scapula

Chaves His-Haas
Chaves-Rapp
DeWar and Harris
Dickson
Henry
Whitman
Saha
Vastamäki

Posterior Bone Block Elbow

Boyd
Putti
Putti-Scaglietti

Shoulder Procedures

acromionectomy: excision of all or part of the acromion, usually in cases of rotator cuff injuries.

acromioplasty: repair or partial removal of the acromion.

Armstrong p.: for rotator cuff impingement; resection of entire acromion.

Bankart p.: capsular repair in the glenoid for chronic anterior dislocation of the shoulder.

Bateman p.: for paralysis of the deltoid; a trapezius muscle transfer to the greater tuberosity.

Bosworth p.: screw fixation of the clavicle to the coracoid for AC separations.

Boyd and Sisk p.: for stabilization of recurrent posterior shoulder dislocation; transfer of long head of biceps to posterior glenoid.

Braun p.: for partial ankylosis of the shoulder; open tenotomy of the subscapularis. Also, for painful shoulder in stroke patients; section of subscapularis and pectoralis major tendons.

brisement p.: a closed manipulation of a stiff shoulder.

Bristow p.: coracoid process transfer for chronic anterior dislocation of the shoulder; also called **Bristow-Laterjet p.**

Brittain p.: extraarticular fusion of the shoulder.

Brooks and Saddon p.: for paralysis of biceps; transfer of pectoralis major tendon to biceps.

Bunnell p.: for paralysis of elbow flexion; transfer of triceps anterior to radial tuberosity. Also, for paralysis, biceps transfer of sternocleidomastoid to long head of biceps.

Burrows p.: for dislocation of sternoclavicular joint; use of subclavian muscle to hold reduction.

Chaves-Rapp p.: for long thoracic nerve palsy; transfer of the pectoralis major to inferior scapula.

clavicectomy: excision of all or part of the clavicle.

clavicotomy: surgical division of the collar bone.

Cofield p.: for rotator cuff tear; resection of distal clavicle, acromioplasty, and V-Y repair of rotator cuff or subscapularis substitution.

Copeland and Howard p.: for shoulder paralytic instability; fusion of scapula to ribs using tibial cortical grafts.

coracoacromial veil: a filmy piece of tissue that arises from the AC ligament and affects the position of the humerus in relation to the glenoid through a range of motion.

costectomy: excision of part or all of a rib for purposes of either a bone graft or approach to thorax.

costotransversectomy: excision of the transverse process of a vertebra and the neighboring rib for approach to the spine or cord.

Cubbins p.: passage of the coracohumeral ligament through the humeral head for an old anterior dislocation of the shoulder.

Das Gupta p.: technique of excision of scapula.

Debeyre p.: for repair of rotator cuff tear; superior approach to supraspinatus to advance tendon.

Dewar and Barrington p.: transfer of the coracoid tip to the clavicle for AC separations.

du Toit and Roux p.: a stapling procedure of the anterior shoulder capsule for chronic anterior dislocation of the shoulder.

Eden-Hybbinette p.: a bone block to the anterior glenoid for chronic anterior dislocation of the shoulder.

Eden-Lange p.: for spinal accessory nerve palsy; transfer of levator scapulae, rhomboid major, and rhomboid minor.

Eyler p.: for paralysis of elbow flexor; transfer of flexor wad of five proximally on humerus facilitated with tendon fascia lata graft.

Fairbanks and Sever p.: for internal rotation and adduction contraction of shoulder; resection of tendinous portion of pectoralis major and minor, coracobrachialis, and short and long head of the biceps.

Gill p.: intraarticular and extraarticular fusion of the shoulder.

girdle resection: various resections of proximal humerus or scapula in an attempt to preserve the shoulder in ablative tumor surgery.

Green p.: soft tissue release and repair for high-riding scapulae.

Harmon p.: for partial paralysis of deltoid; transfer of posterior origin to anterior part.

His-Haas p.: for long thoracic nerve palsy; transfer of teres major from humerus to chest wall.

Hitchcock p.: tenodesis of long head of biceps into biceps groove.

Hovanian p.: for paralysis of biceps; transfer of latissimus dorsi to radial tuberosity. Also for triceps weakness; transfer of latissimus dorsi to triceps muscle.

Inclan-Ober p.: soft tissue release and repair for high-riding scapulae.

Janecki and Nelson p.: for scapular malignancy; radical resection that includes a portion of the clavicle, proximal humerus, and entire scapula.

Jobe and Kvitne p.: for recurrent anterior dislocating shoulder; a criss-cross and overlapping imbrication of capsule to help re-create a labrum.

Kristiansen and Kofoed p.: for proximal humeral fractures; percutaneous pin is used to reduce fracture, and an external fixation is then applied.

L'Episcopo Zachary p.: for internal rotation and adduction contracture of the shoulder; resection of anterior capsule and tendon of pectoralis major with transfer of triceps and latissimus dorsi tendon.

Magnuson-Stack p.: stapling of the subscapularis for chronic anterior dislocation of the shoulder.

Marcove, Lewis, Horos p.: for scapular malignancy; radical resection that includes a portion of the clavicle, proximal humerus, and entire scapula.

McKeever p.: for open fixation of clavicle fracture, using a threaded wire.

McLaughlin p.: for rotator cuff injury of shoulder, a technique of repair; a transfer of the subscapularis into a hatchet head deformity of the humerus for old posterior dislocation of the shoulder.

McShane, Leinberry, and Fenlin p.: for rotator cuff impingement; excision of 50% of the inferior surface of the anterolateral acromion.

Moberg p.: for paralysis of triceps; posterior transfer of deltoid.

B. H. Moore p.: for muscle imbalance in shoulder caused by stroke; posterior transfer of part of deltoid muscle.

J. R. Moore p.: for posterior dislocation of humeral head in stroke; multiple anterior tendon and anterior capsule resection with bone graft to glenoid.

Mumford-Gurd p.: resection of the distal clavicle for a chronic AC separation or arthritis.

Neer p.: for recurrent multidirectional anterior dislocating shoulder; capsular lateral advancement with superior placement of distal flap.

Neviaser p.: transfer of the coracoacromial ligament to the clavicle for AC separation. Also a Knowles pin fixation of the clavicle, especially for nonunion of a fracture.

Nicola p.: transfer of the long head of the biceps tendon through humeral head for chronic anterior shoulder dislocation.

Ober and Barr p.: for weakness of triceps; transfer of brachioradialis.

O'Brien p.: for multidirectional anterior dislocating shoulder, superior and inferior placement of laterally based flaps in capsular repair.

Phelps: for tumor; technique of partial resection of the scapula.

Putti p.: fusion of the shoulder by two different methods.

Putti-Platt p.: subscapularis muscle and capsular repair for chronic anterior dislocation of the shoulder.

remplissage procedure: in addition to a Bankart procedure, the attachment of the intact infraspinatus tendon in a large Hill-Sachs defect.

Rockwood p.: for chronic AC separation; resection of distal clavicle and repair with AC ligament, and 12-week fixation with a lag screw to coracoid.

Roger p.: for paralytic internal rotation deformity of the shoulder; a proximal derotation osteotomy of the humerus.

Rowe and Zarins p.: for chronic anterior shoulder dislocation; open reduction and fixation by a number of temporary means including sling.

Saha p.: for paralysis of deltoid; transfer of trapezius and distal acromion to humerus below greater tuberosity. Also, for paralysis of subscapularis; transfer of two superior digitations of serratus anterior or transfer of pectoralis minor. Also, for paralysis of supraspinatus; a transfer of levator scapulae or sternocleidomastoid. Also, for paralysis of infraspinatus or subscapularis; a transfer of latissimus dorsi or teres major.

scapulectomy: excision of all or part of the scapula.

Schrock p.: soft tissue release and repair for high-riding scapulae.

Scott p.: wedge bone block procedure for chronic posterior dislocation of the shoulder.

Speed p.: ligamentous repair for sternoclavicular joint separations. Also for chronic dislocation of the elbow; reduction and stabilization using a folded expansion of triceps muscle.

Spira p.: for paralysis biceps; transfer of pectoralis minor.

Steindler p.: intraarticular fusion of the shoulder.

Stewart p.: for AC joint separation; resection of distal clavicle with repair of coracoacromial ligament.

Swafford and Lichtman p.: for suprascapular nerve entrapment; release of ligamentous tissue at the suprascapular notch.

Tikhoff-Linberg p.: for scapular malignancy; radical resection that includes a portion of the clavicle, proximal humerus, and entire scapula.

Trillat p.: for anterior shoulder dislocation; osteotomy of coracoid with attachment to glenoid to act as bone block.

Watson-Jones p.: shoulder fusion using a piece of acromion.

Weaver and Dunn p.: for AC separation; transfer of coracoacromial ligament to distal clavicle.

Weber osteotomy: for recurrent shoulder dislocations associated with large posterior humeral head defects; internal rotation osteotomy of proximal humerus.

Whitman p.: for long thoracic nerve palsy; stabilization of scapula with fascial strips attached to spinous processes.

Wilson and McKeever p.: Kirschner wire (K-wire) fixation after open reduction of an old posterior shoulder dislocation.

Woodward p.: soft tissue release and repair for high-riding scapulae.

Zeir p.: for long thoracic nerve palsy; pectoralis minor transferred to scapula using a tensor fascia lata graft.

Surgery of the Shoulder: Prosthetic Procedures

Bechtol p.: for replacement of the glenohumeral joint.

designed after natural anatomy (DANA) total shoulder: a plastic component for glenoid associated with metallic-stemmed prosthesis for humerus.

Gristina and Webb p.: nonarticulated, semiconstrained shoulder prosthesis.

Michael Reese p.: replacement for shoulder joint involving an interlocking device.

Neer p.: shoulder replacement prosthesis.

reverse shoulder: for degenerative arthritis of the shoulder with cuff insufficiency, a socket is on the humeral side with a ball attachment to the glenoid. The **glenosphere** is the glenoid component of a reverse shoulder arthroplasty.

Roper-Day p.: an unconstrained metal on plastic shoulder replacement.

The Arm, Elbow, and Forearm

Specifically, the arm is the portion of the upper limb between the shoulder and the elbow, and the forearm is between the elbow and the wrist. Most surgical procedures on the arm and forearm are of a general type, that is, nerve and vessel repairs and fracture fixations. Most forearm tendon transfers are considered in Chapter 10.

Anatomy
Bones

humerus: the humerus, the arm bone, extends from the shoulder to the elbow (Fig. 8-10).
  capitellum: provides articulation with the radial head.
  epitrochlea: medial epicondyle.
  medial and lateral epicondyles: large prominences on either side of the elbow.
  olecranon fossa: thin portion of the bone with an opening above the elbow joint.
  spiral groove: groove in the bone for the radial nerve.
  trochlea: provides articulation with the ulna.

radius: The radius is the bone on the thumb side of the forearm (Fig. 8-11).

FIG 8-10 Right humerus. **A,** Anterior view. **B,** Posterior view. *(From Seeley RR, Stephens TD, Tate P:* Anatomy and physiology, *St Louis, 1989, Times Mirror/Mosby College Publishing.)*

---

biceps tuberosity: point of insertion of biceps tendon.
Lister tubercle: a prominence on the distal dorsum of the radius.
radial head: the articular portion of the radius to the elbow.
styloid process: the most distal portion of radius.
ulna: The ulna is the bone of the forearm on the little finger side of the wrist, prominent at the elbow (see Fig. 8-11).
  coronoid process: anterior part of the ulna at the elbow joint at the brachialis insertion.
  olecranon: prominent ulnar portion at the elbow.
  styloid process: the most distal portion of the ulna, prominent on turning the wrist downward.

Muscles of the Arm

arcade of Struthers: a fibrous expansion of the medial distal triceps muscle; a potential area of entrapment for the ulnar nerve.

biceps m.: a two-belly muscle that flexes the elbow; extends from the scapula to the radius.
brachialis m.: flexes the elbow from the arm to the ulna.
coracobrachialis m.: pulls the arm in and up; extends from the scapula to the arm.
triceps m.: a three-belly muscle that extends the elbow; its origin is at the scapula, down the arm to the ulna.

Muscles of the Forearm

Many muscles of the forearm that affect hand function are discussed in Chapter 10. Others that relate to forearm function are the following.

anconeus: small muscle on the ulnar side of the elbow.
extensor wad of three: muscles that extend the wrist and flex the elbow.
  brachioradialis muscle: located on the lateral side of the forearm; helps flex the elbow.

extensor carpi radialis brevis: short muscle that extends the wrist.
extensor carpi radialis longus: long muscle that extends the wrist.
flexor wad of five: muscles that flex the wrist and fingers and pronate the forearm—flexor carpi ulnaris, palmaris longus, flexor digitorum superficialis, pronator teres, and flexor carpi radials; see Chapter 10.

Gantzer's m.: (accessory head to flexor pollicis longus) can cause anterior interosseous nerve compression.
pronator quadratus: flat muscle at the distal forearm that turns the palm down in pronation.
supinator muscle: located at the proximal forearm; brings the palm up in supination.

Blood Vessels (Fig. 8-12)

basilic vein: branches upward and laterally from ulnar side of forearm to front of elbow, winding around ulnar border of forearm to join the brachial vein, which becomes the axillary vein.
brachial artery: main artery of the arm that divides at the elbow into the radial and ulnar arteries.
brachial vein: branches off axillary.
cephalic vein: branches off from an axillary artery and vein on radial side; runs upward and medially to front of elbow and winds around and enters the axillary vein.
median cephalic vein: near elbow area (where blood is drawn).
median basilic vein: near elbow area.
profundus: deep anterior brachial artery of the arm.
radial artery: one that travels deep into the muscle on the thumb side of the forearm.
radial vein: branches off from cephalic vein.
ulnar artery: one that travels deep into the muscle on the little finger side of the anterior forearm.

Other Blood Vessels of the Elbow

Ulnar collateral
Anterior and posterior ulnar recurrent
Anterior and posterior radial recurrent

Other Blood Vessels of the Forearm

Anterior and posterior interosseous

Nerves

The nerves leading to the forearm and hand are all listed in the section on shoulder anatomy. Some specific branches to the arm and forearm are listed here.

anterior interosseous n.: branch of the median nerve; supplies the radial-sided deep finger flexors, thumb flexor, and pronator quadratus.
cutaneous n. of the arm: posterior, medial, and lateral; also called **brachial cutaneous n.**

FIG 8-11 Ulna and radius of the right forearm. *(From Seeley RR, Stephens TD, Tate P:* Anatomy and physiology, *St Louis, 1989, Times Mirror/Mosby College Publishing.)*

cutaneous n. of the forearm: posterior, medial, and lateral; also called **antebrachial cutaneous n.**

posterior interosseous n.: branch of radial nerve that passes through supinator muscle and then supplies some of the deep muscles of the posterior forearm.

superficial radial n.: does not go through supinator; supplies no muscles but supplies sensation for the dorsal radial side of the hand and thumb.

Ligaments

arcade of Frosche: tunnel for posterior interosseus nerve that travels through the supinator.

cubital tunnel: expansion of fibers from medial epicondyle to proximal dorsum of forearm; is a potential source of entrapment of ulnar nerve. Also called **arcade of Struthers.**

interosseous membrane: thick, fibrous tissue between most of the length of the radius and ulna.

FIG 8-12 Blood vessels of the upper limb. **A,** Veins of the upper limb—the subclavian vein and its tributaries. The major veins draining the superficial structures of the limb are the cephalic and basilic veins. The brachial veins drain the deep structures. Blood vessels of the upper limb.

Continued

FIG 8-12, cont'd B, Arteries of the upper limb—the brachiocephalic, subclavian, axillary, and brachial arteries and their branches. *(From Seeley RR, Stephens TD, Tate P: Anatomy and physiology, St Louis, 1989, Times Mirror/Mosby College Publishing.)*

lacertus fibrosus: expansion of fibers of the biceps tendon at the elbow; becomes an important structure in some injuries.

ligament of Struthers: fibrous band extending from the humerus supracondylar process to the median epicondyle where the median nerve and the brachial artery are enclosed. Not to be confused with **arcade of Struthers.**

oblique ligament: a part of the radial collateral ligament of the elbow.

orbicular ligament: surrounding the radial head and holding it to the ulna at the elbow.

Osborne fascia: covering fascia over the ulna nerve between the medial humeral epicondyle and the olecranon.

ulnar and radial collateral ligament: on the medial and lateral side of the elbow.

Surgery of the Arm and Forearm
Prostheses

The classification of elbow prostheses is similar to that used for knee prostheses. They are generally categorized as constrained, semiconstrained, or unconstrained. Because there is such a long list of manufacturers' names for these devices, they are not listed. These are typically specific to individual hospitals and the trade names can be found in the operating room supply section.

Eponymic

Amspacher and Messenbaugh p.: for malunion of humeral fracture; a distal rotation osteotomy.

Aronson and Prager p.: for supracondylar fracture in children; percutaneous pin fixation.

Baumgard and Schwartz p.: for lateral epicondylitis; percutaneous or small open incision release of origin of extensor carpi ulnaris and extensor carpi radialis brevis and longus.

Blount p.: for supination deformity of forearm; closed osteoclasis of both bones of forearm setting at 45 to 90 degrees of pronation.

Bosworth p.: resection of a portion of the radial head ligament and muscle attachment for tennis elbow.

Bowers hemiresection: for radioulnar joint arthritis; resection of distal radial side of ulna with interposition of fascia.

Boyd and Anderson p.: for biceps distal tendon rupture; a method of reattachment.

Boyd and McLeod p.: for tennis elbow; excision of a part of the orbicular ligament.

Brady and Jewett p.: for proximal cross-union of radius and ulna; resection of radial head and 4-week screw fixation to separate radius and ulna.

Campbell p.: for arthritic radial capitellar joint; resection of capitellum and radial head with imbrication of capsule over bone. Also for malunited Colles fracture; resection of distal ulnar side of ulna to use as graft correcting radial deformity.

Campbell and Akbarnia p.: for tumor of distal radius; resection of distal radius with replacement using tibial bone graft.

capitellocondylar p.: an unconstrained elbow prosthesis designed to allow greater supination and pronation.

De Rosa and Graziano p.: for varus deformity in elbow; closing step-cut osteotomy of distal humerus.

Ellis p.: for reduction of intraarticular volarly displaced wrist fracture; a technique of screw plate fixation.

Feldon wafer resection: for radioulnar joint arthritis; resection of thin portion of bone and joint of distal ulna, preserving the styloid.

Fernandez p.: for dorsal and radial shortening of a radius fracture; dorsal wedge resection with radial replacement to correct both deformities.

Flynn p.: for nonunion or delayed union of minimally displaced lateral condylar fractures in children; open reduction, peg bone graft, and fixation.

Fowles p.: for chronic posterior dislocation of elbow; a posterolateral approach with detachment of all tight structures and possible V-Y plasty of triceps.

French p.: for malunion of ulna; distal ulnar osteotomy with screw and wire fixation.

Froimson and Oh p.: for chronic tendonitis of long head of biceps; a keyhole is fashioned in the bicipital groove and then used to insert a knotted portion of biceps tendon. Also called **keyhole p.**

Gaille p.: for recurrent anterior dislocation shoulder; use of fascia lata graft to replace anterior capsule.

Gill p.: for nonunion of ulna; a massive sliding graft technique.

Hall and Pankovich p.: for midhumeral fracture; use of multiple small Ender nails in antegrade or retrograde fashion.

Hassman, Brunn, and Neer p.: for recurrent elbow dislocation; plastic repair of lateral capsuloligamentous structures.

Hirayama p.: for chronic dislocation of the radial head with ulnar deformity in a child; osteotomy of the proximal ulna.

Hitchcock p.: for rupture of the long head of biceps; a method of reattachment.

Hovanian p.: for restoring elbow flexion; transfer of latissimus dorsi to olecranon.

Hohmann p.: for tennis elbow.

JS Speed p.: for old dislocation of radial head; fashioning of sling from a portion of triceps expansion.

Kapel p.: triceps and biceps tendon formed into ligaments for a chronic dislocated elbow.

Liebolt p.: for subluxing distal radial/ulnar joint; using tendon graft.

MacAusland p.: arthroplasty of the elbow for a recurrent dislocation.

Manktelow p.: for loss of forearm flexor muscle mass; free neurovascular pedicle transfer of pectoralis major. Also called **Ikuta p.**

McKeever and Buck p.: for olecranon fracture with adequate remaining joint surface; excision of olecranon fragment and reattachment of triceps mechanism.

Milch p.: for radial shortening; an ulnar shortening by step cut resection of distal shaft of ulna. Also, for pronation deformity; an osteotomy of distal ulna with fixation in supinated position. Also humeral osteotomy for cubitus valgus deformity.

Milch shortening o.: for radioulnar joint arthritis; resection of circular section of distal ulnar shaft with plate fixation and resultant shortening of ulna.

Mital p.: for spastic muscle contracture of elbow; Z-plasty of biceps tendon and release of brachialis sheath and joint capsule.

Mizuno, Hirohata, and Kashiwagi p.: for displaced distal humeral epiphysis; posterior open reduction and pin fixation.

Nirschl p.: for chronic lateral epicondylitis; excision of hypercapsular tendon segment of extensor carpi radialis brevis and decortication of anterolateral condyle.

Osborne and Cotterill p.: capsular reefing for a chronic dislocated elbow.

Outerbridge-Kashiwagi p.: for osteoarthritis of the elbow; debridement arthroplasty using posterior approach and fenestration of olecranon fossa.

Reichenheim-King p.: transplantation of the biceps tendon into the coronoid process for a chronic dislocated elbow.

Sauve-Kapandji p.: distal radioulnar joint arthritis; fusion of distal radius and ulna with creation of an ulnar pseudoarthrosis proximal to the fusion.

Sherk and Probst p.: for proximal humeral epiphyseal fracture; reduction and percutaneous pinning.

Speed and Boyd p.: for irreducible Monteggia fracture; reconstruction of orbicular ligament and plating of ulnar fracture.

Spittler p.: for forearm amputations; a biceps muscle cineplasty.

Staples arthrodesis p.: arthrodesis of the elbow; see also **Steindler arthrodesis.**

Steindler arthrodesis p.: arthrodesis of the elbow; see also **Staples arthrodesis.**

Steindler flexorplasty: transfer of the flexor wad of five muscles in the elbow to a higher level for loss of voluntary elbow flexion; **Eyler flexorplasty** is a variation of this procedure.

Stewart p.: for radial navicular arthritis; excision of radial styloid.

Tommy John p.: for laxity in pitchers and other throwing athletes, ulnar collateral ligament repair of the elbow

Weber-Vasey p.: for comminuted olecranon fracture; combined use of bent pin and figure-eight wire fixation.

Wilson p.: for extraarticular ankylosis of elbow in flexion; release of anterior structures with Z-plasty of biceps tendon.

Zancolli p.: for supination deformity of forearm; suturing of biceps tendon after lengthening.

(The anatomy and surgery of the hand and wrist are found in Chapter 10.)

The Pelvis and Hips

The pelvis is a large, basinlike structure that supports the lower abdominal viscera, contains the birth canal, and acts as a weight-bearing bridge between the spine and the lower extremities. It is often referred to as the **pelvic girdle.** It is composed of a bilateral set of three bones that are completely fused and are on either side of the sacrum. The largest and uppermost bone is the **ilium,** the lowermost and strongest is the **ischium,** and the anteriormost is the **pubis.** In the outer center of these fused bones is the hip socket, called the **acetabulum,** the true anatomic hip and socket for the ball-and-socket joint.

Most hip surgical procedures involve structures immediately neighboring the acetabulum. The anatomic structures involving the pelvis that are occasionally encountered in hip procedures are listed first, followed by anatomic structures directly related to hip procedures.

Anatomy of the Pelvis
Bones

ala of the ilium: the outer flair of the ilium; resembles a wing.

anterior inferior iliac spine: prominence in the deep ilium just above the hip is origin of rectus femoris.

arcuate ligament: *arcuate*, meaning "arch-shaped." The arcuate line of the pelvis is the iliac continuation of the iliopectineal line; the arched inferior edge of the posterior layer of the rectus sheath.

calcar: a spur; **calcar femorale** is a bundle of cancellous laminae of bone in the neck of the femur, serving to strengthen it.

greater sciatic notch: the large notch on the posterior surface of the ilium below the posteroinferior iliac spine where the sciatic nerve exits.

gluteal lines: refers to the three curved lines across the outer surface of the ilium, anteriorly, posteriorly, and inferiorly.

iliac crest: the outer uppermost margins of the ilium, two of the four iliac spines arise from the crest; the

anterior superior iliac spine is the origin of the oblique abdominal muscles and sartorius; the **posterior superior iliac spine** is a part of the origin of the gluteus maximus.

iliopectineal line: a ridge inside the pelvis that denotes the entrance into the birth canal, with a concave inner surface called the **iliac fossa.**

ilium: wide platelike bone that forms the top of the pelvis just below the waistline; generally referred to as the *hips.*

inferior pubic ramus: lower portion of the pubic bone.

innominate bone: composed of three fused bony subunits, called the ilium, pubis, and ischium, that are attached to the sacrum and coccyx to form the pelvis.

ischial spine: prominence of bone of strong ligamentous attachment above the tuberosity; main significance is in obstetrics.

ischial tuberosity: the prominent, hard portion of bone at the base of the ischium, felt when sitting erect.

ischium: a U-shaped bone of the lower part of the pelvis, which forms a ring.

obturator foramen: refers to the large opening of the innominate bone almost entirely occluded by the obturator membrane. Bordered by the pubic ramus superiorly and the ischial ramus inferiorly. Two muscles cover the membrane: obturator internus and externus; also pertains to the nerves and vessels penetrating this orifice.

pelvic girdle: a general term that denotes the entire bilateral bony pelvis; the ring that the pelvis makes with its articulation to the sacrum (sacroiliac joint) is called the **pelvic ring.**

posterior inferior iliac spine: prominence of posterior inferior lower margin of the joint with the sacrum; attachment of ligaments.

pubis: the anterior increased shape of bone of the pelvis, which meets its counterpart from the other side at a point called the **symphysis pubis.** Also called **pubic bone.**

sacroiliac: joint space between the sacrum and the ilium on each side; junction of the pelvis to the spine.

superior pubic ramus: top portion of the pubic bone.

symphysis pubis: the junction of the two pubic bones just above the genital area.

Muscles

Most of the pelvic muscles affect the hip or abdominal motion and are described in this section. However, those muscles of the lower abdominal wall surrounding the bladder, uterus, and rectum are sometimes encountered in orthopaedic procedures; they are the levator ani, pubococcygeal, transverse urethral, and cremaster (in scrotum).

sphincter ani: muscle that controls defecation; loss of control of this muscle is a serious sign of herniated disk disease.

Ligaments

anterior sacroiliac l.: large ligament between the sacrum and the ilium.

Poupart inguinal l.: anterior ligament at the groin fold from the anterosuperior iliac spine to the pubic tubercle.

sacrospinous l.: from iliac spine to sacrum.

sacrotuberous l.: ligament from the sacrum to the ischial tuberosity; small sacrosciatic.

Blood Vessels

Most large blood vessels within the pelvis are not encountered in orthopaedic practice. The aorta divides into the common iliac arteries at about the level of the fourth lumbar vertebra. Branches within the pelvis include the hypogastric, superior and inferior gluteal, iliac (which becomes the femoral to the inguinal ligament), and pudendal.

Nerves

cluneal n.: inferolateral, inferomedial, and superior sensory nerves of the buttocks and thighs.

lumbar plexus: arises from the second through fourth lumbar vertebrae, with two major nerves.
 femoral n.: arises from L2, L3, and L4, and supplies most of the knee extensors.
 obturator n.: arises from L2, L3, and L4, and supplies many of the thigh adductors.

pudendal n.: arising from just below the sacral plexus, traveling along the ischium (Alcock canal), and supplying the lower pelvic muscles that do not affect hip motion but affect sexual function.

sciatic n.: the large nerve developed by the sacral plexus supplying the hip rotators, knee flexors, and entire leg and foot muscles and most of the sensation.

sciatic plexus: the major plexus of nerves arising in the pelvic area to include nerves from L4 and L5 and nerves of the first three sacral levels. Major injuries or disorders of this plexus are rare, but it is important to understand that this plexus forms the sciatic nerve, which eventually becomes the tibial and common peroneal nerves. Most sciatica is actually a nerve root irritation in the spinal column.

Miscellaneous Terms

inguinal: refers to the area of the groin. The precise line is from the anterosuperior iliac spine to the pubis; this is the line of the natural fold of skin in the groin. Terms relating to the area include *inguinal nerve, hypogastric nerve, ilioinguinal nerve,* and *inguinal canal.*

peritoneum: inner membrane lining of the abdominal cavity.

Anatomy of the Hip

The average person refers to the prominent part of the pelvis that flares out just below the waistline (iliac crest) as the *hip*. However, the hip portion of the pelvis is the lesser part of the entire pelvic mass; it is 5 inches below the iliac crest and is called the *acetabulum,* or *true hip.* The three bones of the pelvis merge to form the cup-shaped depression of the hip joint, which holds the femoral head in place. The proximal femur (thigh bone) and its components are described here as the major elements of the hip function and not as part of the lower extremities.

Bones

acetabulum: cup-shaped depression in the mid-outer pelvis known as the *hip;* this is the socket of the ball-and-socket joint of the hip.

acetabular notch: a notch at the inferior margin of the fovea centralis.

  fovea centralis: central depression in the center of the acetabulum and origin of the ligamentum teres.

  posterior lip: posterior part of the acetabulum, which sometimes breaks off in a dislocation of the hip.

pseudo acetabulum: a cup-shaped defect in the lateral iliac wall above the acetabulum in which the femoral head rests in congenital hip dislocation, false acetabulum

superior dome: the weight-bearing portion of the acetabulum.

triradiate cartilage: growth center for the acetabulum and pelvis; the meeting point physis of the ischium, ilium, and pubis.

digital fossa: a deep depression on the inner surface of the greater trochanter; the site of the insertion of the obturator externus and posterior aspect of the superior border of the greater trochanter.

femoral head: the ball and topmost part of the ball-and-socket joint of the hip; in a growing child may be referred to as the **capital epiphysis.**

femoral neck: the area below the femoral head where the bone narrows into a tubelike structure approximately 2 inches long.

femur: when the term is related to the hip, is considered the upper, proximal 4-inch segment of bone.

greater and lesser trochanters: part of the femur just distal to the neck where the bone widens into two large prominences, the lower, smaller, and medial of which is the lesser trochanter; the greater trochanter is the larger, lateral prominence. In thin individuals, the greater trochanter can be felt at approximately the level of the palm of the hands when the arms are resting by the sides. It is often used as a landmark in physical and x-ray examinations.

intertrochanteric: refers to any region between the two trochanters; a large number of fractures of the hip occur in this region.

piriformis fossa: small, shallow depression located at the tip of the greater trochanter; site of insertion of the piriformis tendon.

subtrochanteric: refers to the femoral shaft just below the lesser trochanter.

Muscles

adductors: a group of five muscles that pulls the thigh inward (adduction); these include the adductor magnus, adductor longus, adductor brevis, pectineus, and gracilis muscles.

external and internal rotators: a group of muscles originating at the pelvis around the hip, helping to control internal and external rotation; these muscles are the internal and external obturator gemelli (superior and inferior gemellus), quadratus femoris, and piriformis.

gluteus maximus m.: the large buttock muscle that helps to extend the hip.

gluteus medius and minimus muscles: the deeper significant muscles (**hip abductors**) that abduct the hip and prevent a waddling or Trendelenburg gait.

iliopsoas m.: a combination of the iliacus and psoas muscles arising from the anterior lumbar processes and inner pelvis inserting into the lesser trochanter. These large hip flexors are often involved in hip reconstructive procedures.

rectus femoris m.: anterior thigh muscle of the quadriceps group; attaches across the hip joint.

sartorius m.: the muscle stretching from the anterolateral pelvis (anterosuperior iliac spine) to the medial tibia, crossing two joints; it enables the person to assume a cross-legged position.

tensor fascia lata m.: the most lateral hip abductor muscle.

Ligaments

Bigelow l.: major ligamentous expansion of the capsule covering the femoral neck; also called **anterior iliofemoral l.**

labrum: fibrocartilaginous rim that surrounds the outer margin of the acetabulum, particularly prominent in the superoanterior portion.

ligamentum teres: the round ligament between the middle of the femoral head and the center of the acetabulum (fovea centralis).

Arteries

femoral a.: the major artery from the point of exit from the pelvis to the point of exit behind the knee. Near the hip, it gives off a branch called the **deep femoral a. (profundus a.).** The **lateral circumflex a.** arises from the lateral profundus and supplies the lateral and anterior femoral neck. This is the major blood supplier to the femoral head in late childhood and adult life. Another branch of the profundus artery is the **medial circumflex a.,** which arises from the deep femoral artery and supplies the posterior femoral head.

inferior gluteal a.: large artery from the internal iliac artery within the pelvis; supplies the gluteus medius and minimus.

obturator a.: a branch from within the pelvis that supplies some of the adductor muscles after exiting through the obturator foramen.

superior gluteal a.: a large artery from the internal iliac artery within the pelvis supplying the gluteus maximus and lesser muscles outside the pelvis.

Nerves

All three nerves supplying the thigh and leg also supply the hip. As a result many patients with hip problems complain of thigh, calf, and even foot pain. The large nerves passing near the hip are the following.

femoral n.: supplies sensation to the anterior thigh, medial leg, and the muscle for knee extension.

obturator n.: supplies sensation to the medial side of the thigh and the muscles for pulling the thigh inward (adducting).

sciatic n.: supplies sensation to the posterior thigh and hip extensors; the more distal branches (common peroneal and posterior tibial) are discussed under nerves of the lower limbs.

Surgery of the Pelvis and Hips

Most of the surgery performed on the hip is directed toward making the hip a mobile, painless, weight-bearing joint. Surgical procedures designed to remodel the hip or replace the parts involved are described in this section. Surgical procedures to fuse the hip or to change the direction of alignment of the femur or pelvis are defined in the following sections.

Hip Arthroplasty

A hip arthroplasty is a procedure designed to directly change the contour of or to replace the hip joint (acetabulum) or femoral head. This term is so general that it includes most procedures for developmental dysplasia of the hips (DDH) and all procedures that involve prosthetic replacement. For example, the term **total hip arthroplasty** is used often to denote the total joint replacement procedure. Nonprosthetic procedures are listed first.

shelf procedure: an extension of the outer acetabulum (hip joint) so it more completely covers the femoral head. This is commonly done for DDH in which the acetabulum is not well rounded and allows the femoral head to displace. It is necessary, in many instances, to reduce the hip and then perform a shelf procedure, using a bone graft to maintain a new position of the lateral acetabulum. Some types of operative shelf procedures are listed. This term specifically means the creation of a bony shelf at the edge of the acetabulum. However, femoral head coverage is sometimes accomplished by pelvic osteotomy with or without the addition of a bone graft to create a shelf.
Albee
Bosworth
Chiari
Colonna
Eppright Wagner
Frank Dickson
Ghormley
Gill (type I, II, III)
Hall Kalamchi
Hay-Groves
Lance
Lowman
Pemberton
Salter
Steel
Sutherland
Weston
Wiberg

Joint Replacement Surgeries

Short, straight-stem femoral components designed to replace the femoral head are now obsolete. The original effort to replace the hip joint was centered around the femoral head component. One of the first femoral head components was made of acrylic attached to a metal stem (Judet). These became loose fairly rapidly. As bone remodeling and response to stress became better understood, the devices were no longer used. This led to the development of single femoral canal stem devices. Although the cartilage on the acetabular side would often disappear over time, many of these prostheses lasted for years. In addition, they were fairly easy to replace. These prostheses are still used in some cases for femoral head replacement in hip fractures. Because of loosening problems and loss of articular cartilage in the hip socket, total joint replacement surgery was developed. The names of these devices can be found for historical reference in previous editions of this dictionary. The range of manufacturer's brand names for joint replacement devices is so large that incorporation here is not practical. Related terms specific for hip replacement surgery follow (Fig. 8-13).

bipolar hip replacement: large femoral head on a stem in which there is a head within a head using a high-molecular-weight polyethylene interface. No acetabular component. These can be used for primary femoral neck fractures and some salvage circumstances.

cage: typically used in hip socket (acetabular) replacement where large bone defects or poor bone stock exists to obtain improved acetabular fixation; this is a metal device with a larger surface area than traditional acetabular cups, designed to hold multiple screws and other fixation components. The acetabular component is then cemented into the cage.

composite beam model: stem is held in place with collars and roughened surface finish, designed to load the proximal femur.

constrained liner: for prosthetic hip instability, locks femoral head inside of acetabular component.

cup arthroplasty: surgical remodeling of the femoral head and the acetabular socket with the insertion of a metal cup. This procedure was usually reserved for younger persons with severe deforming diseases of the hip after trauma; replaced with resurfacing procedures. Also called **mold arthroplasty.**

distal coated stem: term usually applied to porous coating where the coating is on the entire stem.

double bubble: term applied to acetabular hip components designed to accommodate bone defects.

dual geometry: radius of acetabular component is larger at the periphery than the dome and designed to maximize rim fit.

equatorial contact: seen in metal on metal articulations in which equal contact is made over entire femoral head.

femoral head prosthesis: insertion into the femoral shaft of a metallic or synthetic component that resembles the femoral head. In present use, it replaces

Anatomy and Orthopaedic Surgery 257

FIG 8-13 Development of the total hip prosthesis in the past seven decades has shown remarkable improvement in fixation and biologic acceptance. Lined areas are cartilage, grossly stippled areas are cement (methylmethacrylate), finely stippled areas are plastic, and solid black areas are metal. More recent alternative bearing surfaces are porocoated with metal on metal, ceramic on plastic, and ceramic on ceramic. Current metal on metal not shown.

the femoral head in an older person who has a normal acetabulum, but a recent fracture of the hip. This may be unipolar or bipolar.

first-generation cementing: the use of methylmethacrylate by finger-packing into the femoral canal though the exposed neck.

matte finish: roughened finish on stem.

mid-coated stem: term usually applied to porous coating in which the coating is only on the proximal and mid-part of the stem.

polar contact: seen in metal on metal articulations in which top portion of head has a higher amount of contact.

proximal coated stem: term usually applied to porous coating in which the coating is only on the proximal part of the stem.

resurfacing procedures: method of arthroplasty attempting to replace only the joint surfaces of the ball and socket in order to minimize the amount of normal bone that has to be removed. Sometimes used in young patients to preserve bone stock for anticipated later revisions.

safe zone of Lewinnek: for position of the acetabular cup in total hip arthroplasty; the best orientation to reduce risk of dislocation is 5–25 degrees cup anteversion and 30–50 degrees for cup inclination.

second-generation cementing: the use of methylmethacrylate by lavage of the canal, plugging canal, and retrograde filling of the canal.

surface finish: range of finish from smooth, mirrorlike finish to roughened (mat) finish.

tantalum: chemical element with porous form increasingly used as a metal component in arthroplasty, especially in revision.

taper slip design: stem subsides in cement mantle, taking advantage of viscoelastic properties of cement.

third-generation cementing: the use of methylmethacrylate by lavage of the canal, plugging canal, and retrograde filling of the canal pressurization, vacuum mixing, and proximal and distal centralizers to center the prosthesis with the best possible cement mantle.

total hip arthroplasty: a joint replacement involving an internal prosthesis by removing the diseased joint and replacing the acetabular component with either metal or plastic materials and a metal prosthesis of the femoral segment. This type of procedure is usually reserved for older individuals who are suffering from osteoarthritis, avascular necrosis, or other degenerative diseases of the hip. Bearing surfaces include metal on plastic, ceramic on plastic, metal on metal, and ceramic on ceramic. Fixation can be by bone ingrowth or methylmethacrylate. Also called **low-friction arthroplasty.**

unipolar: large single unit design of a femoral head on a stem without acetabular component, which lacks an artificial articulating bearing in the femoral head (as seen in bipolar head replacements)

Closed Hip Reduction Procedures for Developmental Dysplasia of the Hip

These are manipulations in an infant or child to reduce a dislocated hip. The method of reduction, followed by the casted position after reduction, varies.

Crego: use of skeletal traction until a closed manipulation with minimal force becomes possible.

Lange: positioning the hip in abduction, internal rotation, and extension after a closed reduction.

Lorenz: both a method of reduction and the frogleg position cast applied following the reduction.

Ridlon: method of reducing a congenitally dislocated hip and then using a Lorenz cast.

Wingfield frame: used in a gradual method of closed reduction.

Open Hip Reduction

An open hip reduction is a procedure that, when listed by itself, implies the need to reduce a hip under direct surgical vision. Some open techniques include **Calandriello p., Ferguson p., Howorth p., Scaglietti p.,** and **Somerville p.** More often described by direction of approach: *medial o., anterior o,* and so on.

Iliopsoas Transfers

This strong hip flexor is sometimes transferred to act as a hip abductor in conditions of muscle imbalance and hip dislocation. Two such procedures are the **Mustard p.** and the **Sharrard p.**

Osteotomies

The osteotomies of the hip are listed here for reference, but some are defined more fully in "Osteotomies" earlier in this chapter.

Amstutz and Wilson
Bernese
Blount
Blundell Jones
Borden, Spencer, and Herndon
Brackett
Chiari
derotation
dial
Dimon
Gant
Ganz
Ghormley
Hass
Irwin
Langenskiöld
Lloyd-Roberts
Lorenz
MacEwen and Shands
McCarroll
McMurray
Müller
Osgood
Pauwels
Pauwels Y
Pemberton
Platou
Salter (innominate)
Sarmiento
Schanz
Schede
Southwick
Steel-triradiate
Sutherland-Greenfield
Whitman

Arthrodeses

The arthrodeses are listed for reference but some are defined more fully in "General Surgery of Joints" earlier in this chapter.

Abbott
Abbott-Fisher-Lucas
Albee
Badgley
Blair
Brittain
Chandler
Davis
Gant
Ghormley
Henderson
Kickaldy and Willis
Schneider
Stamm
Trumble
Watson-Jones
John C. Wilson

Other Pelvic and Hip Procedures

acetabuloplasty: any surgical remodeling of the cup side of the hip joint.

Asnis p.: for mild chronic slipped capital femoral epiphysis; fixation with a cannulated screw.

Baxter and D'Astous p.: for hip contracture in myelomeningocele; resection of proximal femur and interposition of muscle mass.

Bleck p.: for excessive hip internal rotation when walking; a recession of the iliacus and psoas tendon to anterior capsule of hip.

Campbell p.: for abdominal and hip flexion contracture; excision of a part of the anterior ilium after a soft tissue release.

Canale p.: for mild chronic slipped capital femoral epiphysis; cannulated screw fixation.

capsular arthroplasty: many procedures for a dislocation of the hip involve soft tissue manipulation only and include curetting of the acetabulum and muscle transfers but do not involve bony osteotomies such as are seen in the shelf procedures. One of these procedures is the **Colonna capsular arthroplasty.**

Castle and Schneider p.: for spastic cerebral palsy hip dislocation; interposition of muscles over joint following resection of femur proximal to subtrochanteric line.

Chandler p.: for hip adduction gait; intrapelvic obturator neurectomy.

Couch, DeRosa, and Throop p.: for hip adduction gait; transfer of the adductor tendon to ischial tuberosity.

coxotomy: surgical opening of the hip joint.

Dimon and Hughston p.: for comminuted intertrochanteric hip fracture; a method of reduction with valgus placement and use of a high-angle nail.

Dunn p.: for displaced slipped capital femoral epiphysis, removal of hump and fusion of epiphysis.

Fish p.: for chronic slipped capital femoral epiphysis; resection of dome-shaped wedge at femoral head.

Girdlestone resection: excision of the femoral head and neck for infection or nonhealing intertrochanteric hip fracture

Graber-Duvernay p.: boring holes leading to the center of the femoral head for the purpose of promoting circulation.

hebosteotomy: incision into the pubis; also called **hebotomy.**

Heyman-Herndon p.: for displaced slipped capital femoral epiphysis, a shortening of the femoral neck with correction of deformity.

ischiectomy: surgical excision and removal of a part of the ischium.

ischiohebotomy: surgical division of the ischiopubic ramus and ascending ramus of the pubis.

ischiopubiotomy: incision into the ischial pubic junction.

Karakousis and Vezeridis p.: for malignancy of pelvis; resection of hemipelvis and head of femur, preserving neurovascular structures.

King and Richards p.: for posterior acetabular fracture; oblique screw fixation.

Kramer, Craig, and Noel p.: for chronic slipped capital femoral epiphysis; osteotomy and wedge resection at base of femoral neck.

Legg p.: for paralysis of gluteus maximus; posterior portion of tensor fascia lata muscle is transferred to a more posterior position.

Lyden p.: for mild chronic slipped capital femoral epiphysis; use of cannulated screw; also called **Lehman p.**

Lynne and Katcheria p.: for spastic cerebral palsy subluxation of hip; ipsilateral iliac crest used as a graft in pelvic osteotomy.

Martin p.: for chronic, severe slipped capital femoral epiphysis; a closed-wedge osteotomy at base of femoral head.

Malta and Saucedo p.: for sacral fracture; reduction and fixation with posterior screws placed lateral to medial.

McCarty p.: for chordoma of sacrum; resection of a portion of sacrum.

Menson and Scheck p.: for osteoarthritis of the hip; release of the pericapsular muscles. Also called **hanging hip p.**

Morrisay p.: for mild chronic slipped capital femoral epiphysis; percutaneous single-screw fixation.

Ober-Barr p.: for paralysis of gluteus maximus; a fascia lata graft still attached to fascia lata and flap transferred to erector spinae m.

pubiotomy: surgical incision and division in the pubic bone.

Radley, Liebig, and Brown p.: for malignancy of ischium; resection of tuberosity and lower portion of pubis.

Root p.: for spastic cerebral palsy with tight hip adductors; transfer of adductors to ischial tuberosity.

Root and Siegel p.: for valgus and internal rotation deformity of hip; varus derotational osteotomy of proximal femur.

Sarmiento p.: for intertrochanteric fracture of the hip; use of osteotomy cut in the distal fragment to achieve valgus nail plate fixation.

Selig p.: for hip-adducted gait; intrapelvic obturator neurectomy.

Soutter p.: for abdominal and hip flexion contracture; release of the soft tissues about the iliac crest.

Staheli p.: for developmental hip dysplasia; shelf procedure using iliac crest bone graft for buttress.

Stee p.: for spastic cerebral palsy internal rotation and flexion hip deformity; transfer of gluteus medius to vastus intermedius.

Stener and Gunterberg p.: for chordoma of sacrum; resecting portion of sacrum.

Sutherland p.: for internal rotation deformity of the hip; transfer of semitendinosus and semimembranosus to lateral posterior septa of thigh.

Taylor, Townsend, and Corlett p.: technique of vascularized free iliac crest graft.

Thomas, Thompson, and Straub p.: for gluteus medius paralysis; transfer of external abdominal oblique to the tensor fascia lata.

trochanteric slide: an osteotomy of the outer portion of the greater trochanter done from an anterior direction so that it and the attachment of the gluteus medius and vastus lateralis can be retracted posteriorly as a single flap and then replanted with wire fixation following a hip procedure.

trochanterplasty: surgical excision of a ridge of bone to form a new femoral neck.

Veleanu, Rosianu, and Lonescu p.: for hip adduction gait; combination of adductor tenotomy and obturator neurectomy.

Ward, Thompson, and Vandergriend p.: for vertical shear fracture of pelvis; posterior iliac to sacral screw fixation after reduction.

Webb p.: for separation of symphysis pubis; two-screw and plate fixation after reduction.

Weber, Brunner, and Freuler p.: for displaced hip fracture in children; cancellous screw fixation after initial fixation with Kirschner wires; also called **Boitzy p.**

The Lower Limbs

Anatomy
Bones

adductor tubercle: the knobby prominence of the medial femoral condyle, which is easily felt by pressing on the medial side of the knee 5 cm above the joint. Also called **adductor tuberosity.**

anterior and posterior tibial spines: tibial prominences of bone inside the knee joint; attachment for the anterior and posterior cruciate ligaments.

anterior tibial tubercle: the large knob just below the anterior knee joint; the point of insertion for the quadriceps (knee extensors) muscles.

Chaput tubercle: the anterolateral tubercle of the distal tibia at the ankle joint for the strong attachment of the anterior tibiofibular ligament; also called **tubercle of Tillaux-Chaput.**

femoral condyles: the two prominences at the distal end of the femur, called the **medial** and **lateral femoral condyles.** The space between the condyles, called the **intercondylar notch,** contains the cruciate ligaments within the knee.

femur: thigh bone; largest bone in the body (Fig. 8-14).

fibula: the smaller bone on the lateral side between the knee and ankle (Fig. 8-15).

fibular facet (proximal tibiofibular facet): the flat portion of bone on the lateral side of the proximal tibia for articulation with the fibula.

fibular neck: narrow part of the fibula just below the proximal enlargement of the bone.

Gerdy tubercle: prominence of bone superior and lateral to the anterior tibial tuberosity; used as reference point in some knee surgery.

lateral malleolus: the distal end of the fibula, which is the outer prominence of the ankle.

linea aspera: a line of prominent bone on the lateral side of femur in the posterior proximal and middle femur for insertion of the gluteus maximus.

medial malleolus: the large prominence on the inner side of the ankle and part of the tibia.

patella: the kneecap, a round to ovoid bone within the quadriceps (knee extensor) tendon (Fig. 8-16). It has a posterior cartilaginous surface for articulation with the femoral condyles known as the **medial facet** and **lateral facet.**

posterior malleolus: a structure that cannot be seen or felt but is the posterior joint aspect of the tibia. It may fracture by itself or, more commonly, in association with other ankle fractures.

tibia: the large leg bone on the medial side between the knee and ankle (see Fig. 8-15).

tibial eminence: prominence of bone for attachment of anterior cruciate ligament on tibial plateau.

tibial plateau: the surface that articulates with the femur; may be subdivided into the medial and lateral plateaus.

trochlea: the groove that holds the patella in line on the distal femoral joint surface.

Muscles

adductor m.: the medial muscle of the thigh responsible for pulling the thigh toward the midline.

hamstring m.: three posterior thigh muscles, originating mostly at the pelvis and posterior femur, that help flex the knee. They are given this common name because when they reach the knee joint they are mostly tendinous. The three hamstring muscles are:
biceps femoris: outer hamstring
gracilis: inner hamstring
semimembranosus: inner hamstring
semitendinosus: inner hamstring

FIG 8-14 Right femur. **A,** Anterior view. **B,** Posterior view. *(From Seeley RR, Stephens TD, Tate P: Anatomy and physiology, St Louis, 1989, Times Mirror/Mosby College Publishing.)*

pes anserinus: the distal tendon portion of the gracilis, sartorius, and semitendinosus muscles, which at their attachment on the proximal medial tibial side are similar to a goose's foot in appearance.

popliteus m.: a muscle in the posterior superior tibia that has its tendon insertion into the posterior femur. It is important in lateral injuries of the knee in that the structure may be involved or encountered on arthrographic examination or as a part of surgical procedure.

quadriceps m.: muscle group with four divisions that are the bulk of the anterior thigh that become a tendon that surrounds the patella and ends on the tuberosity of the tibia. They function in extending the knee and, in the case of the rectus femoris, help to flex the hip. The quadriceps femoris group of muscles includes the **vastus lateralis, vastus medialis, vastus medialis obliquus (VMO),** **vastus intermedius,** and **rectus femoris (direct head rectus femoris** and **indirect head rectus femoris).**

Muscle Compartments

Muscles act in groups to bring about movements, primarily as agonists, antagonists, synergists, and prime movers. There are many muscle groups and compartments throughout the body. The most commonly referred to muscle groups are in the leg, because swelling within the compartments can lead to irreversible muscle change and loss of motor function. Therefore the four compartments of the leg are defined here and the function and names given of the muscle groups of the lower extremity.

Achilles tendon: the tendinous heel cord that is the extension from the **triceps surae** group of muscles.

FIG 8-15 Right tibia and fibula, anterior view. *(From Seeley RR, Stephens TD, Tate P: Anatomy and physiology, St Louis, 1989, Times Mirror/Mosby College Publishing.)*

anterior c.: contains the muscles responsible for dorsiflexion of the ankle and the large and lesser toes; included are the **tibialis anterior, extensor hallucis longus, extensor digitorum longus,** and **peroneus tertius.**

deep c.: contains the flexors of the toes and ankle and are known as the **tibialis posterior, flexor digitorum longus,** and **flexor hallucis longus.**

gastrocsoleus muscle: refers to the combination of the two largest muscles contributing to the Achilles tendon.

lateral c.: contains the muscles that evert or plantar flex the ankle; they are the **peroneus longus** and the **peroneus brevis.**

posterior c.: contains the **triceps surae** muscles, which make up the bulk of the calf; included are the following:

  gastrocnemius: the most posterior muscle of the calf, leading to the Achilles tendon, that flexes both the ankle and knee.

  plantaris: the smaller ankle flexor that leads to the Achilles tendon over the medial side.

  soleus: the larger deep ankle flexor of the calf leading to the Achilles tendon.

Ligaments

The knee is an encapsulated joint that has several layers of fascial tissue. The deeper layer is referred to as the **joint capsule,** but numerous ligaments and tendons make up this capsule (Fig. 8-17).

anterior and posterior cruciate l.: the two deep, intraarticular ligaments within the knee that are crossed near the knee's center.

arcuate ligament: curved ligament in posterolateral corner of the knee.

FIG 8-16 Right patella. **A,** Anterior view. **B,** Posterior view. *(From Seeley RR, Stephens TD, Tate P: Anatomy and physiology, St Louis, 1989, Times Mirror/Mosby College Publishing.)*

FIG 8-17 Major joints in terms of disease and surgical sites. **A,** Hip. **B,** Knee. *(From Hilt NE, Cogburn SB: Manual of orthopedics, St Louis, 1980, CV Mosby.)*

---

fabellofibular l.: between fabella in lateral head of gastrocnemius and posterior fibular head.

infrapatellar l.: is often referred to as the *infrapatellar tendon,* but because this tendon bridges two bones and not a muscle to bone, it is more correctly referred to as the *infrapatellar ligament.* Its bursa is the infrapatellar bursa.

lateral collateral l.: strong fibrous ligament of the lateral knee joint with fibers from the femur to the tibia and fibula. This ligament is sometimes called the **tibial collateral l.,** but caution should be taken to distinguish this from the ankle ligaments.

ligaments of Henry and Wrisberg: small ligaments of attachment for the meniscus in the posterior knee.

ligamentum mucosa: not a true ligament but the thin, filmy membrane that sometimes divides the knee joint.

medial collateral l.: strong fibrous ligament on the medial side of the knee connecting the femur with the tibia. There is a **superficial ligament** and a **deep ligament** in most knees. The posterior oblique ligament

FIG 8-18 Blood vessels of the pelvis and lower limb. **A,** Arteries of the pelvis and lower limb—the internal and external iliac arteries and their branches. The internal iliac artery supplies the pelvis and hip, and the external iliac artery supplies the lower limb through the femoral artery. **B,** Veins of the pelvis and lower limb—the right common iliac vein and its tributaries. *(From Seeley RR, Stephens TD, Tate P:* Anatomy and physiology, *St Louis, 1989, Times Mirror/Mosby College Publishing.)*

---

is composed of fibers that arise from the medial collateral ligament and attach more posteriorly in the joint.

meniscofemoral ligament: contribution of meniscal margin to medial collateral ligament leading to femur.

meniscotibial l.: contribution of meniscal margin to medial collateral ligament leading to femur.

proximal tibiofibular l.: ligament between the fibular neck and tibia.

tibiofibular l.: when used without distinction as to distal or proximal, refers to the ligaments just above the ankle; these ligaments are divided into the anterior, middle, and posterior tibiofibular ligaments.

Arteries and Veins (Fig. 8-18)

anterior tibial a.: main artery of the anterior leg supplying the extensors and peroneal muscles.

deep femoral a.: the largest branch of the femoral artery in the upper thigh that travels closely to the femur and gives off numerous circumferential branches around that bone; the branches are referred to as the **perforating arteries.**

femoral artery and vein: large artery and vein of the thigh that originate in the groin area; they penetrate posteriorly through fascia above the knee (Hunter canal) and become the popliteal artery and vein.

highest genicular a.: large branch from the femoral artery supplying the muscles and joints on the medial aspect of the knee. Branches above the knee may be referred to as *medial* and *lateral superior genicular, medial* and *lateral inferior genicular, anterior* and *posterior tibial recurrent,* and *fibular arteries.*

other arteries near the ankle: perforating, anterior, and posterior medial malleolar, and anterior and posterior lateral malleolar arteries.

peroneal a.: travels along the posterior fibula supplying deep calf muscles and collateral circulation of the leg.

popliteal artery and vein: continuation of the femoral artery and vein as they emerge behind the knee, dividing distally to that joint and giving off the anterior and posterior tibial artery.

posterior tibial a.: large artery of the posterior leg supplying most of the muscles of the calf and deep spaces; a major branch is the peroneal artery.

saphenous vein: large vein of the subcutaneous tissue in the medial thigh; continuous to the medial side of the ankle.

venae communicantes: complex of communicating subcutaneous veins associated with an artery. The association can be useful for preparation of vascular-based pedicle grafts.

Other Structures

infrapatellar fat pad (retropatellar fat pad): a distinct mass of fat behind the patellar tendon extending into the anterior joint of the knee. Also called **Hoffa fat.**

medial and lateral meniscus: referred to as the **semilunar cartilages,** which are fibrocartilaginous structures interfacing the medial and lateral rim of the femorotibial joint; serve to help distribute the weight load on the two cartilaginous surfaces by changing shape and position during motion.

interosseous membrane: a very strong fibrous membrane between the fibula and tibia, extending throughout most of the length of the bones.

plica: a fold, pleat, band, or shelf of synovial tissue; minor structures but may be large enough to produce symptoms and demand surgical attention. Specific locations include the transverse suprapatellar, medial suprapatellar, mediopatellar (also called medial patellar shelf), and infrapatellar plica (also called ligamentum mucosa, which does not produce symptoms).

prepatellar bursa: a bursa in the fat in front of the kneecap.

suprapatellar pouch: the extension of the anterior knee joint to approximately 12 cm above the joint line.

Nerves of the Lower Limbs

common peroneal n.: a brief segment of nerve that divides into the superficial and deep peroneal nerve just distal to the fibular head.

deep peroneal n.: nerve that supplies voluntary function of the toe and ankle extension; the sensory branch is between the first and second toes.

posterior tibial n.: nerve of the posterior leg that supplies the outer and deep calf muscles and eventually the muscles of the foot and sensation on the sole of the foot.

saphenous n.: nerve branch from the femoral nerve; supplies only sensation to the medial leg.

sciatic n.: nerve of the posterior thigh, supplying muscles of the posterior thigh and dividing into the common peroneal and posterior tibial nerves.

superficial peroneal n.: nerve that supplies the voluntary muscle function that turns the ankle out; also supplies sensation on the dorsum of the foot.

sural n.: large sensory nerve of the calf deriving branches from both the peroneal and posterior tibial nerves.

Surgery of the Lower Limbs: Eponymic and Named Procedures of the Femur and Tibia

Caldwell and Durham p.: for quadriceps rupture; a transfer of the biceps femoris tendon to quadriceps tendon.

D'Aubigne p.: for tumor of femoral condyle or tibial plateau; use of attached patella to act as graft for joint surface.

Enneking p.: for malignancy of distal femur or proximal tibia; resection of affected bone and use of graft taken from healthy bone and fixation with rod and patellar screws.

Gage p.: for spasticity of hamstring muscle; transfer of semitendinosus to rectus femoris.

Grant, Surrall, and Lehman p.: for spastic flexion contracture of knee; anterior closing wedge osteotomy of distal femur.

Lewis and Chekofsky p.: for malignant tumor of proximal femur; resection of proximal femur.

Moore p.: for malunion of distal femur in child; excision wedge of bone, using fragments as a graft after correcting deformity.

Sage p.: for hamstring spasticity with dislocating patella and internal rotation deformity of hip; lengthening of rectus femoris.

Sutherland p.: for hamstring spasticity with weak quadriceps muscle; transfer of semitendinosus and semimembranosus to patellar extensor mechanism.

Tachdjian p.: for hamstring spasticity in a child; lengthening of semitendinosus, semimembranosus, and biceps femoris.

Wagner p.: for correction of leg-length discrepancy; a method of shortening the femoral or tibial diaphysis, shortening the metaphysis of the femur or tibia, or lengthening the femur or tibia.

White p.: for leg-length discrepancy; a method of shortening the femur.

Surgery of the Knee

Knee injuries account for a large percentage of the surgical procedures of the lower limbs because many muscles arising in the thigh and leg affect that joint. Often more than one procedure is indicated at the same time. Over the years, some of the combinations of procedures have acquired eponymic designations. To give a general purview of surgery of the knee, the single procedures and their modifications are listed first, and the combined procedures are listed last.

Knee Surgery for Internal Derangement

anatomic anterior cruciate ligament reconstruction: uses a tendon or tendons to re-create the anterior-to-medial and posterior-to-lateral relationship that the normal anterior cruciate ligament has from proximal tibia to distal femur; also called **double-bundle repair.**

Andrews p.: for anterior cruciate laxity; extracapsular tenodesis by using iliotibial band.

Campbell p.: use of fascial strip from quadriceps tendon to replace anterior cruciate ligament.

Cho p.: for anterior cruciate deficiency; intraarticular use of semitendinosus tendon.

Clancy p.: for anterior cruciate–deficient knee; use of midpatellar tendon with attached patellar and tibial bone. Also, for posterior cruciate laxity; use of midpatellar tendon graft.

double bundle repair: for anterior cruciate rupture; a tendon is harvested from the patient or a donor and is folded to replicate the anteromedial and posterior lateral bundle of the anterior cruciate ligament.

Drez p.: for anterior cruciate replacement; use of patellar tendon.

Ellison p.: extraarticular repair to replace anterior cruciate function; rerouting iliotibial band under the lateral collateral ligament.

Engebretsen p.: for anterior cruciate ligament deficiency; use of semitendinosus tendon with an ligamentous anterior dislocation prosthetic graft as augmentation.

Ericksson p.: for anterior cruciate instability; midportion of patellar tendon and portion of bone redirected through tibia and into posterior lateral femoral condyle.

five-in-one repair: five procedures for severe ligamentous injuries to the knee; includes a medial meniscectomy, medial collateral ligament repair, vastus medialis advancement, semitendinosus advancement, and a pes anserinus transfer. Also called **Nicholas p.**

Fox-Blazina p.: extraarticular repair to replace anterior cruciate function by rerouting the iliotibial band under the lateral collateral ligament and placing it distal to original attachment.

Hey-Groves p.: a reconstruction of the anterior cruciate ligament using tensor fasciae latae graft.

Hughston and Degenhardt p.: for posterior cruciate–deficient knee; use of medial head of gastrocnemius.

Hughston and Jacobson p.: for posterolateral instability; advancement of bony attachment of fibular collateral ligament and popliteus tendon to a superior and anterior direction.

Insall p.: for anterior cruciate laxity; use of iliotibial band and bone block as replacement.

Insall and Hood p.: for posterior cruciate ligament laxity; use of medial gastrocnemius and bone block as replacement.

Jones p.: repair of the anterior cruciate ligament using a portion of the patella and patellar ligament.

Lam modification is a modification of the Jones anterior cruciate transfer procedure.

ligamentous advancement: implies a soft tissue procedure only. The ligament is detached and then pulled up or down and reattached to bone. This is done for the medial and lateral collateral ligaments.

Lindeman p.: for anterior cruciate ligament rupture; gracilis tendon transfer as a replacement.

Loose p.: for anterior cruciate instability with pivot shift; portion of iliotibial band is redirected through lateral femoral condyle and around lateral joint.

MacIntosh p.: using infrapatellar and quadriceps tendon for transfer over posterior lateral femoral condyle for anterior cruciate ligament replacement. Also, iliotibial band used in reconstruction to provide anterior cruciate stability.

Marshall p.: for anterior cruciate ligament laxity; portion of patellar tendon and fascia is directed through notch and over lateral femoral condyle.

Mauck p.: detachment of a segment of the tibia containing the medial collateral ligament and replacement of that block of bone in a position that tightens the ligament.

meniscectomy: excision of the medial or lateral meniscus. There are other menisci in the body, but meniscectomies are usually done on the knee. A **partial meniscectomy** is the removal of the torn portion only or a definite attempt to leave meniscal margins of an even width.

Muller p.: for posterolateral instability; reinforcement with iliotibial band graft.

over-the-top p.: for anterior cruciate deficiency; any procedure that places the transferred ligament over the lateral femoral condyle rather than through the condyle.

Pagddu p.: for anterior cruciate–deficient knee; intraarticular use of gracilis and semitendinosus tendons.

Paulos p.: for anterior cruciate–deficient knee; use of medial patellar tendon and retinaculum through tibial grove.

reverse Mauck p.: detachment of a segment of the femur containing the medial collateral ligament and insertion of this block of bone into a position that tightens the ligament.

Slocum p.: a pes anserinus transfer (pes transfer). This is commonly done in association with other procedures and involves a change in the direction of pull of tendons inserting just below the medial knee joint; designed to help replace dynamic stability in ligamentous laxity.

triad knee repair: a repair involving the anterior cruciate ligament, medial collateral ligament, and a medial meniscectomy; also called **O'Donoghue p.**

vastus medialis advancement: tightening of the vastus medialis muscle. The procedure is rarely done by itself, but more commonly in association with procedures for ligamentous laxity of the knee or chronic subluxing patella.

Wirth Jager p.: for posterior cruciate ligament deficiency; use of proximally based semitendinosus and gracilis tendon for replacement.

Yount p.: for severe contracture of posterior knee; division of iliotibial band and biceps tendon.

Zaricznyj p.: for anterior cruciate–deficient knee; use of double strand semitendinosus for replacement.

Zarins and Rowe: for anterior cruciate–deficient knee; simultaneous over the top of semitendinosus and iliotibial band with posteromedial and posterolateral capsular reefing.

Knee Surgery for Chronic Subluxation of the Patella

Campbell p.: fascial tissue transfer and vastus medialis reefing.

Elmslie-Trillat p.: medial displacement of anterior tibial tuberosity on a bone pedicle for subluxing patella.

Galeazzi p.: for chronic lateral subluxing patella; use of fold of medial strip of parapatellar capsule, strip is brought across inferior to superior patella and back again.

Hauser p.: inferomedial displacement of a block of bone with the infrapatellar tendon attached.

Hughston p.: lateral release with quadricepsplasty and patellar tendon transfer as needed.

Insall p.: lateral retinacular release and lateral advancement of vastus medialis.

Maddigan, Wissinger, and Donaldson p.: for chronic lateral subluxing patella; wide lateral advancement of vastus medialis.

Maquet p.: anterior tibial tuberosity displacement on bone pedicle for patella alta.

Roux-Goldthwait p.: medial displacement of the lateral portion of the infrapatellar tendon.

Sargent p.: lateral release and advancement of vastus medialis over patella with attachment to exposed, bleeding patellar surface.

Silfverskiöld p.: for knee flexion contracture (in cerebral palsy); transection of medial and lateral head of gastrocnemius muscle and motor branch to medial gastrocnemius.

Southwick slide p.: medial displacement of bony attachment of the patellar tendon, replacing the lateral defect with bone from the medial side.

Stanisavljevic p.: for congenital dislocating patella; massive patellar tendon and quadriceps refashioning.

West and Soto-Hall p.: patellectomy and medial advancement of the quadriceps mechanism for patellar osteoarthritis.

Patellar Surgery

Cave and Rowe p.: for osteoarthritis of the patella; partial patellectomy with fold of infrapatellar fat sewn onto the posterior patella.

Codivilla p.: for neglected quadriceps tendon rupture; direct repair and advancement of fold from superior quadriceps mechanism.

Houston and Akroyd p.: for sleeve fracture of patella; tension band wire fixation with two Kirschner wires.

Magnuson p.: for unstable fracture of the patella; arthroplasty of the knee (fascia) in an attempt to remodel, and use of encircling metal wire.

Martin p.: for patellar fracture; fixation with a wire loop.

McLaughlin p.: for quadriceps or patellar tendon rupture; a reinforcing encircling wire is attached to patella or tibia, respectively.

Miyakawa p.: patellectomy with fabrication of a fold taken from the thick tissue well superior to the patella and reinforcing the patellar area to provide better mechanical force.

patellar or femoral condylar shaving (skiving): direct removal of diseased cartilage from the patella and femoral cartilage, usually done in combination with treatment of other chronic knee injury problems.

patellectomy: removal of the kneecap; this procedure has two different meanings: (1) total removal of cartilage from the patella or entire patella, and (2) removal of a portion of the bone following a fracture, which is also called **partial patellectomy.**

Scudari p.: for fresh quadriceps rupture; repair with reinforcing flap from superior quadriceps mechanism.

Quadricepsplasty

Any repair or reapproximation of the quadriceps mechanism is called a **quadricepsplasty.**

Judet quadricepsplasty: for knee fibrosis; parapatellar and intraarticular adhesion release with intraoperative manipulation.

Thompson quadricepsplasty: for knee fibrosis; isolation of vastus lateralis and medialis from rectos femoris and capsular incision.

Total Knee Arthroplasty

Total knee arthroplasty (TKA) is the replacement of both sides of the knee joint by metal or plastic components. See "Internal Prostheses" earlier in this chapter for various types of prostheses.

Knee Prostheses (Fig. 8-19)

Knee prostheses are designed to replace portions or all of the knee joint. The original attempts involved solid metal to replace one side or the other of the joint. Metal with plastic interfacing, better joint mechanical design, and superior attention to detail in surgical applications have improved the relative success of knee joint replacements.

The listing of total knee devices is not practical because of the number of manufacturers and their variety of trade names. Previous editions of the dictionary list names of those devices that are possibly remaining in some joints or are still being used. Most hospital operating rooms have a limited list of devices and are a good resource for location of specific terminology. The following are general terms that describe the basic types of knee replacement devices.

FIG 8-19 A, Total knee prosthesis showing accumulated wear that occurred over years of use. **B,** Total knee. *(A, Courtesy Orthopaedic Research Laboratory, Good Samaritan Medical Center, West Palm Beach, FL.)*

bicompartmental replacement: the medial and lateral side of the joint is replaced but there is no patellar-trochlear resurfacing. The breakdown of the patellar mechanism resulted in disuse of this design.

cruciate retaining: designs that retain the posterior cruciate ligament.

cruciate sacrificing (cruciate substituting): designs that remove the posterior cruciate ligament and replace with a plastic post on the polyethylene component.

constrained: the prostheses are not necessarily totally constrained. Some are nonhinged, prevent posterior subluxation with a post, and limit varus and valgus to less than 5 degrees. The term **fully constrained** implies no motion and actually denotes a block of anteroposterior shifting on lateral motion. Because there is restriction in at least one plane of motion, there are forces that produce high stresses on the bone. These devices are more likely to become loose as the bone breaks down or the prosthesis itself fails. One design is a **hinged knee** design that locks components in place with a hinge and prevents any anterior posterior shift or varus-valgus motion.

high flex design: total knee replacements designed to allow up to 160 degrees of flexion.

meniscal bearing: plastic able to move anterior to posterior on a smooth groove on the tibial tray.

monoblock: one piece tibial component; metal-based plate is bonded to polyethylene liner.

patellar button: typically all plastic, dome-shaped devices to replace articular surface of the patella. Previously used devices were **fixed anatomic,** which was an anatomically shaped piece of plastic on metal backing. Another device was **rotating,** which is an anatomically shaped piece of plastic attached to a metal backing in such a way that the plastic can rotate during knee motion.

rotating platform knee: plastic fitted on a smooth tibial metal surface with central hole for the plastic insert, which allows rotation of the plastic on the tibial surface.

semiconstrained knee: the degree of constraint ranges from minimal to nearly full in any given plane. This is the design of many of the current prostheses.

tricompartmental knee: most knee replacements entail a design that replaces both tibial-femoral surfaces and the patella.

unconstrained knee: the most minimally constrained prosthetics with the maximal freedom of motion of the knee joint. These devices require good soft tissue stability.

unicompartmental knee: the unicompartmental design has evolved into a metal unicondylar component for the femur making contact with a plastic or plastic on metal tibial component. There are few patients for whom this limited procedure is appropriate.

Tendon Transfers

Surgical releases for muscle imbalance or knee contractures are referred to as **tendon transfers.**

Baker p.: patellar tendon advancement; semitendinosus transfer for knock-kneed gait caused by internal rotation deformity of the hip.

Bickel and Moe p.: translocation of the peroneus tendon.

Caldwell and Durham p.: for quadriceps paralysis; transfer of biceps femoris to quadriceps mechanism.

Chandler p.: patellar tendon advancement.

Ecker, Lotke, and Glazer p.: for neglected infrapatellar tendon rupture; transfer of gracilis and semitendinosus for reinforcement.

Eggers p.: transfer of the biceps femoris tendon associated with capsular releases and soleus neurectomy.

Galleazzi p.: for chronic subluxation of the patella; transfer of the semitendinosus.

Hughston p.: for chronic subluxation of the patella; patellar tendon transfer fixed by staple and redirection of vastus medialis.

Kelikian p.: for old patellar tendon rupture; transfer of the gracilis tendon.

Sutherland p.: for internal rotation deformity in hip affected by cerebral palsy; lateral transfer of medial hamstring.

Tachdjian p.: for hamstring tightness in cerebral palsy; plastic lengthening of hamstring sheaths and tendons.

Genu Recurvatum Procedures

Brett and Campbell p.: tibial osteotomies.

Heyman p.: reinforcement of posterior capsule using multiple tendon transfers; soft tissue release and transfers.

Perry p.: posterior capsular repair with multiple tendon transfers.

Surgery Below Knee and Above Ankle

Anderson p.: for unequal leg lengths; tibial lengthening using an external skeletal fixator.

Anderson and Hutchins p.: for unstable tibial fractures; a method of skeletal pins and casting for fixation.

banana peel p.: for total joint revision; peeling off the patella tendon intentionally with the capsule as a construct to attempt to preserve quadriceps function without rupture.

beefburger p.: for failed TKA; debridement with interposition of acrylic cement between leveled edges of femur and tibia, followed by brace immobilization.

Bosworth p.: for anterior tibial epiphysitis; insertion of bone pegs into the tibial tubercle.

Brett p.: for malunited proximal tibial fractures with knee recurvatum; bone graft applied to opened anterior tibial plateau hinged posteriorly.

Brown p.: for congenital absence of tibia; transfer fibula to femoral intercondylar notch.

Carroll p.: bone graft replacement of the distal end of the fibula for tumors.

d'Aubigne p.: for tumors; a method of excision of femoral condyle or tibial plateau.

Fahey and O'Brien p.: for excision of tumor; technique of excision of a portion of the shaft of a bone.

Forbes p.: for nonunion tibial fracture; iliac bone graft to tibia.

Gilbert p.: technique of obtaining vascular fibular graft by using lateral approach; also called **Tamai p.**

Gill p.: for long-bone nonunion; a half diameter slide graft of a 10- to 15-cm portion of bone.

Gruca p.: for congenital absence of the fibula; construction of an ankle mortise by splitting of the fibula.

Hsu and Hsu p.: for ankle flexion contracture in muscular dystrophy; percutaneous tendocalcaneus lengthening.

Irwin p.: for paralytic genu recurvatum; a closing wedge osteotomy of the proximal tibia.

Langenskiold p.: for partial absence of fibula; fusion of distal tibia and fibula.

Lee p.: for depressed tibial plateau fracture; anterosuperior iliac spine used to replace joint surface.

Malawer p.: for malignancy of proximal fibula; resection of proximal fibula.

Nicoll p.: for tibial or other long-bone nonunion; dual onlay bone graft with cancellous bone in the middle.

Russell p.: for central depression lateral plateau; proximal portion of fibular head is used to support depression of joint surface.

Taylor p.: technique of obtaining vascular pedicle fibular graft through posterior approach.

Van Ness p.: for proximal focal femoral deficiency; a derotation osteotomy of the tibia to fit the limb more readily with a prosthesis.

Wagner p.: for leg-length disparity; shortening of proximal tibia or distal femur.

Weber p.: for persisting acute valgus deformity tibial shaft fracture in children; open reduction and removal of tissue.

Weiland p.: technique of obtaining vascular fibular graft by using lateral approach.

Wilson and Jacobs p.: for comminuted tibial plateau fractures; replacement technique for the lateral side using iliac crest graft.

The ankle and foot procedures are covered in Chapter 11.

Skin Grafts

Skin grafts are of three major categories: split-thickness skin graft (STSG), full-thickness skin graft (FTSG), and pedicle and rotational flaps.

Split-Thickness Skin Graft

An STSG is 0.015 inch or 0.4 mm thick. Taking a graft this way leaves viable skin from the donor site and living cells in the graft. However, both donor site and the graft will appear different from normal surrounding skin. Names associated with skin grafts are **Blair-Brown skin graft, Douglas skin graft (mesh skin graft), Dragstedt skin graft,** and **Ollier-Thiersch skin graft.**

Full-Thickness Skin Graft

An FTSG is a procedure that, throughout the entire surface of the graft, includes all the epidermis and therefore all the smooth skin coverage. This leaves behind a donor site that will need some form of closure or an STSG; for example, if a small necrosed area on a finger needs full skin coverage, a small ellipse of skin could be removed from the forearm; this is called a pinch graft, and the wound edges are closed.

Names associated with full-thickness skin grafts are **Braun skin graft, Davis skin graft, Esser skin graft (Stint skin graft), Krause-Wolfe skin graft, Reverdin skin graft,** and **Wolfe skin graft.**

Pedicle Grafts and Rotational Flaps

A pedicle graft is a layer of fat, dermis, and epidermis raised from a portion of the body having a sufficient blood supply to keep it alive. Pedicles are often used to cover large tissue defects, areas of exposed tendons, or areas where there will be considerable wear on the skin. The intended purpose of a pedicle is to eventually transfer this loose piece of skin and fat to cover another portion of the body. A *flap* is another name for *pedicle*, although the term connotes a local use in some cases; for example, a **rotational flap skin graft** is a rearrangement of the skin and fat in one area to cover a local defect. Pedicles may include muscle or bone.

A **delayed flap skin graft** is used for stimulation of the blood supply. An incision in the skin and fat with approximation of the wound margins into their original position is carried out. In a second or third procedure the flap is raised on a pedicle that is still attached, but now the distal part of that flap can be laid on another portion of the body. For example, a U-shaped incision is made in the leg and closed; 3 weeks later that skin is raised through the same incision and the flap that develops is laid on an open area of the opposite leg. This is called a **cross-leg pedicle skin graft.**

Other terms referring to pedicle grafts and flaps are **bilobed, compound, compound lined, double pedicle, Verdan, jump, marsupial, tumbler, Tait,** and **island pedicle.**

Surgical Blocks

The term **local anesthesia** is sometimes used to indicate a regional anesthesia. In precise parlance, **local anesthesia** indicates the injection of anesthetic agents at the site of the procedure. **Regional anesthesia** is infiltration of anatomic structures proximal to the location of the procedure. Those used for orthopaedics are the following.

axillary b.: injection of anesthetic agent into the nerves immediately around axillary artery, approached from the axilla; used for elbow, forearm, and hand procedures.
epidural b.: infiltration of anesthetic agent into spinal canal but outside of the dura; can be used for so-called continuous drip anesthesia, in which a catheter is left in place during procedure so that if more anesthesia is required it can be administered without repositioning the patient.
intravenous b.: application of double tourniquet and the infiltration of anesthetic agents directly into vein to produce anesthesia in the limb below the tourniquet. Also called **Bier block.**
scalene b.: injection of anesthetic agent into brachial plexus at the point of scalene muscles; used for shoulder and other upper limb procedures.
spinal b.: infiltration of anesthetic agent into the spinal canal within the dura in the lumbar region. The proper positioning of patient during anesthetic infiltration is important in ensuring correct and sufficient anesthesia for procedures on the pelvis and lower limbs.

American Society of Anaesthesiologists Physical Classification System

For anesthetic risk classification based on comorbidities.

1. Healthy person
2. Mild systemic disease
3. Severe systemic disease
4. Severe systemic disease that is a constant threat to life
5. A moribund person who is not expected to survive without the operation
6. A declared brain dead person whose organs are being removed for donor purposes

---

Surgical Approaches

A surgical approach implies the type of incision made by the surgeon to do a particular procedure. Many surgical approaches have been described by various surgeons whose names are applied to those approaches. However, those approaches are not all original and have been modified and improved over the years. Anatomically, the direction of the incision may be modified by another surgeon, whose name then becomes attached to that incision, although in fact it is designed for accessing the same area of the body. In many instances, an experienced surgeon may decide to plan an individualized approach in a given situation.

This prior consideration to surgical intervention may be described by the anatomic location and direction of the incision, for example, anterolateral or posterolateral approaches. More frequently, the anatomic terms are favored in describing where an incision is to be made, even though the eponyms are also used for a particular anatomic area described.

Approaches are listed by anatomic location, eponyms, and common uses for the incision. Those interested in the technique of an incision will use other references. At the end of this section is a list of common incision shapes.

Shoulder Approaches

anterior axillary a.: usually used for repair of anterior dislocations; also called **Roberts a.**
anteromedial shoulder a.: used for repair of shoulder and AC joint injuries; also called **Cubbins a., Callahan and Scuderi a., Roberts a., Thompson and Henry a.,** and **saber-cut a.**
deltoid splitting a.: used to approach the rotator cuff and subacromial bursa.
deltopectoral a: for anterior shoulder repairs and prosthetic replacement; separation of deltoid muscle from pectoral muscle is part of the approach.
posterior shoulder a.: used for repair of a posterior dislocation of the shoulder and lateral scapula; also called **Abbott and Lucas a., Bennett a., Harmon a., Kocher a., McWhorter a., Rowe a.,** and **Yee a.**
transacromial a.: used to approach the rotator cuff and bursa; also called **Codman a., Darrach-McLaughlin a.,** and **saber-cut a.**

Humerus Approaches

anterolateral humerus a.: an approach to the bone and radial nerve; also called **Thompson a.** and **Henry a.**
anteromedial humerus a.: an approach to the median and ulnar nerves.
deltopectoral a.: an approach to the proximal humerus using the interval between the deltoid and pectoralis m.
posterior humerus a.: an approach used to visualize the humerus, triceps, and radial nerve; also called **Henry a.**

Elbow Approaches

anterior elbow a. and anteromedial elbow a.: for exploration of the median nerve, brachial artery, and other soft tissues; often associated with fractures.
anterolateral elbow a.: for exploration of the radial nerve; also called **Henry a.**
medial elbow a.: for exploration of the ulnar nerve and medial epicondyle; also called **Campbell a., Molesworth a.,** and **Campbell a.**
posterior elbow a.: for fractures of the distal humerus; also called **Bryan a.** and **Morrey a.**
posterolateral elbow a.: for elbow dislocations, radial head and distal humeral fractures, and arthroplasties; also called **Kocher a.**

Forearm Approaches

anterior forearm a.: used for visualization of most of the forearm muscles that flex the fingers and for internal fixation of fractures of the radius; also called **Henry a.**
distal a.: used for some distal forearm fractures, tendon transfers, and excision of the distal ulna; also called **Gordon a.**
posterior forearm a.: in the proximal forearm used for fixation of proximal ulnar fractures and an approach to radial fractures; also called **Thompson a.**
posterolateral forearm a.: approach used for radial head fractures, some ulnar fractures, and exploration of the deep radial nerve; also called **Boyd a.**

Pelvis Approaches

Avila a.: anterior approach along the iliac crest to reach the anterior sacroiliac crest.
ilioinguinal a.: anterior approach to the pelvis that extends from the iliac crest to the pubic symphysis.
Radley a., Liebig a., and **Brown a.:** to the ischium.

Stoppa a.: for pelvic ring fractures, an ilioinguinal approach that allows access to pubic body and multiple deep structures.

Hip Approaches

anterior hip a.: using interval between sartorius and rectus muscle in front of hip; also called **Smith-Peterson a.**

anterolateral hip a.: for ORIF of the femoral neck, prosthetic replacement, and some congenital dysplasia surgery; also called **Smith-Petersen a., Van Gorder a., Wilson a., Watson Jones a., Cave a., Callahan a.,** and **Fahey a.**

Hardinge a.: splitting gluteus medius and reflecting anterior portion of that muscle with part of vastus lateralis.

Heuter approach a.: anterior hip exposure technique for arthroplasty techniques; also called **direct lateral a.**

lateral hip a.: for internal fixation of hip fractures and prosthetic replacement; also called **Callahan a., Charnley-Müller a., Fahey a., Harris a., Hay a., McLaughlan a., Murphy a., Ollier a.,** and **Watson-Jones a.**

medial hip a.: for congenital dysplastic hip surgery and other iliopsoas tendon approaches; also called **Ludloff a.** and **Young a.**

posterior hip a.: for prosthetic replacement and repair of some pelvic fractures; also called **Abbot a., Gibson a., Guleke-Stookey a., Kocher a., Langenbeck a., McFarland a., Osborne a., Moore a.,** and **Osborne a.** The **Kocker-Langenbeck a.** is a more extensive approach for access to pelvic fractures.

Senegas a.: for acetabular fractures; an extensive exposure of the involving detachment of the greater trochanter. Also called **modified Ollier a.**

trochanteric slide: removal of trochanter and portion of lateral proximal femoral shaft for improved access in prosthetic revision surgery.

two-incision anterior a.: a combination approach in which the anterior approach is used for cup placement and percutaneous posterior approach for the stem.

Femur Approaches

anterolateral femur a.: used for rod or plate fixation fractures; also called **Thompson a.**

lateral femur a.: used for fracture fixation; also called **Eycle-Shymer a.** and **Shoemaker a.**

posterior femur a.: used for some muscle surgery and fixation of fractures; also called **Bosworth a.**

posterolateral femur a.: used for muscle procedures, fracture fixation, and nerve explorations; also called **Eycle-Shymer a., Shoemaker a.,** and **Henry a.**

Knee Approaches

All approaches to the knee are for ligamentous and bony reconstruction, meniscectomies, and vascular explorations. The posterior approaches are more specifically devoted to neurovascular surgery but may also be used in ligamentous and bony reconstructive procedures.

anterior knee a.: Coonse and Adams a., Bosworth a., Putti a., Jones and Brackett a., Insall a.

anterolateral knee a.: Kocher a., Henderson a.

anteromedial knee a.: Abbott and Carpenter a., Langenbeck a.

lateral knee a.: Bruser lateral a., Aufranc a., Henry a., Hoppenfeld a., deBoer a., Pogruna and Brown a.

medial knee a.: Aufranc a., Cave a., Henry a., Bosworth a.

midvastus a.: vastus medialis muscle fibers are split in their midsubstance.

parapatellar a.: typically medial for knee approach in knee replacement.

posterolateral knee a.: Henderson a.

posterior knee a.: Abbott a., Osgood a., Bracket and Osgood a., Putti and Abbott a.

posteromedial knee a.: Banks and Laufman a., Henderson a.

quad snip a.: for difficult joint replacement knee approaches; cutting the quadriceps tendon proximal to the patella at a 45-degree angle.

quad sparing a.: avoidance of cutting the quadriceps in the approach.

transverse a.: Cave a., Charnley a., Cozen a., Sir Henry Platt a., McConnell a.

trivector retaining a.: for extensive knee surgery such as a total joint replacement; an incision that is medial to the standard parapatellar incision cutting into a portion of the vastus medialis muscle.

Lower Limb Approaches

anterior leg a.: for internal fixation of fractures; this is an exploration of the anterior deep spaces.

posterior leg a.: approach to the superomedial region of the tibia and gastrocnemius muscle; also called **Banks a.** and **Laufman a.**

posterolateral leg a.: for peroneal nerve and muscle surgery and for some bone grafts; also called **Harmon a., Henry a.,** and **Huntington a.**

posteromedial leg a.: for neurovascular exploration and internal fixation of fractures; also called **Phemister a.**

Surgical Incisions Described by Appearance	
J shaped	curvilinear
L curved	double
S-flap	linear
T shaped	longitudinal
T-tube saber-cut	saber-cut
U shaped	split
Y incision	transverse
Z-plasty	

Replantation Microsurgery

Microsurgery, the use of a binocular microscope to assist in intricate surgery, is another challenge for the skilled orthopaedic surgeon and is adapted to a variety of orthopaedic conditions. Microtechniques are applied to nerve and vascular repair, replantation, and free tissue transfers, as well as knee and spine surgery.

The integration of this technique provides the surgeon with a three-dimensional telescopic view of the operating field at magnifications of structures 2½ to 25 times the size. Nylon sutures of high tensile strength, finer than human hair, are used to reattach small blood vessels and nerves. To keep vessels open and carefully avoid constriction are the goals of this procedure. Use of the technique requires extreme patience and perseverance on the part of the microsurgical team.

Replantation of traumatically severed extremities has become a common practice in orthopaedic surgery and in musculoskeletal trauma management. The reintegration of tissues by way of microsurgical techniques has successfully restored functional use and eliminated the need for amputation in many cases. Hand surgery has benefited greatly from microsurgery.

Replantation is truly a team effort, involving many hours of work with no room for compromise. The surgeon must spend many hours practicing and developing the skill, applying extreme patience and good judgment during application. The team approach is used to allow replacements during the long procedures.

Although other tissues heal in a short time, the regeneration of nerves may take from 1 to 2 years. Other technologic developments, such as the **laser scalpel,** are also useful in surgical procedures.

Treatment of Tumors

The prognosis for musculoskeletal tumors has improved with the addition of various chemotherapies and other interventions. Some of these therapies are used in conjunction with amputation and wide excisions.

adjuvant therapy: a method of treatment (i.e., radiation or chemotherapy) combined with another treatment (surgery) to improve therapeutic success. **Neoadjuvant therapy** specifies the adjuvant therapy (usually chemotherapy) is given prior to surgical intervention.

chemotherapy: the use of drugs to treat tumors.

intralesional resection: surgical removal of tumor from within the surrounding capsule; often piecemeal as opposed to en bloc.

marginal resection: surgical removal of tumor through the capsule or reactive zone.

radiation therapy: the use of ionizing radiation to treat tumors.

radical resection: removal of an entire anatomic compartment, which includes tumor, tumor capsule, and all muscle, bone, nerve, and artery found within that compartment.

wide resection: surgical removal of tumor capsule and surrounding margin of normal tissue.

Amputations

An **amputation** is the removal of a part through bone, and a **disarticulation** is the removal of a part through a joint space. Both of these terms are interpreted by most as the same procedure, but there is a distinction.

Most amputations take place in the lower limbs and may be indicated for traumatic injury, burns, infection, loss of blood supply, or malignancy. Amputation may also be indicated when a nonfunctioning limb could be replaced by a functional prosthetic device or when a congenital defect could be improved cosmetically or functionally by the removal of a part.

In the case of dysvascular and traumatic indications, the level of amputation is often based on preservation of as much of the residual limb as would heal well with the vascular and peripheral circulation intact. In the case of neoplasm, the level of amputation is often determined by the most proximal extent of the tumor. The most common levels fall into the following categories: above elbow, above knee, below elbow, and below knee. The terminology used by prosthetists for limb replacement have a recent terminology for each level based on prosthetic design.

In the present nomenclature, the description for limb absences can be reversed, that is, a leg, complete, is a complete-leg amputation; if there is a partial amputation, it can be stated as to the level, for example, partial arm (upper one-third). Any amputation through an epiphysis or closer to a joint is considered a complete amputation; an amputation of the distal third to the distal growth plate (growth plate scar in an adult) is considered a complete leg amputation (Tables 8-2 and 8-3).

Following such a procedure the patient is often fitted right away with an artificial limb for the residual limb. The after treatment of the residual limb is most important for the adjustment and rehabilitation of the amputee, as well as for the psychologic aspects.

Before and after a prosthesis (artificial limb) is prescribed for an amputee, the physical medicine and rehabilitation team is an important link in teaching the patient prosthetic training. Prostheses have come a long way in appearance, fit, and functional use, and often it is not evident that a person is using a prosthesis. Chapter 7 discusses the many types of prostheses available. The following list of general terms applies to amputations.

TABLE 8-2 Amputation Levels, Upper Limbs

New Terms (with Abbreviations)	Current Terms	Eponyms
Shoulder (Sh), complete	Forequarter	Littlewood
Arm (Arm), complete	Shoulder disarticulation	Larrey, Dupuytren, Lisfranc
Arm (Arm), partial (upper ⅓)	Short (upper-third) AE	
Arm (Arm), partial (middle ⅓)	Medium (mid-third) AE	
Arm (Arm), partial (lower ⅓)	Long (lower-third) AE	
Forearm (Fo), complete	Elbow disarticulation	
Forearm (Fo), partial (upper ⅓)	Short (upper-third) BE	
Forearm (Fo), partial (middle ⅓)	Medium (mid-third) BE	
Forearm (Fo), partial (lower ⅓)	Long (lower-third) BE	
Carpal (Ca), complete	WD	
Carpal (Ca), partial	WD, with some carpals still present	
Metacarpal (MC), complete	Partial hand amputations, usually without precise differentiation	
Metacarpal (MC), partial		
Phalangeal (Ph), complete		Kutler
Phalangeal (Ph), partial		

AE, Above elbow; BE, below elbow; WD, wrist disarticulation.
Note: An amputation at the metacarpophalangeal joints of the ring and little fingers would be designated as Ph, 4,5, complete; an amputation of the same two fingers at the proximal interphalangeal joints would be Ph, 4,5, partial.
(From Kay HW: A nomenclature for limb prosthetics, Orthot Prosthet J 28(4):37-47, 1974. Reprinted with permission of the American Orthotic and Prosthetic Association.)

General Amputations

cineplastic a.: amputation that includes a skin flap built into a muscle (the biceps being the most common); a portion of the prosthetic mechanism is activated by the muscle. Also called **kineplastic a.**

circular a.: a perfectly circular incision is used.

closed a.: any amputation in which the wound is closed at the time of initial or secondary surgery.

disarticulation: any amputation in which the limb is severed through a joint.

TABLE 8-3 Amputation Levels, Lower Limbs

New Terms (with Abbreviations)	Current Terms	Eponyms
Pelvic (Pel), complete	Hemicorporectomy	
Hip (Hip), complete	Hemipelvectomy	King and Steelquist, Jaboulay, Gordon-Taylor, Sorondo-Ferré
Thigh (Th), complete	Hip disarticulation	Béclard, Boyd, Pack
Thigh (Th), partial (upper ⅓)	Short (upper-third) AK	Alouette
Thigh (Th), partial (middle ⅓)	Medium (mid-third) AK	
Thigh (Th), partial (lower ⅓)	Long (lower-third) AK	Kirk
Leg (Leg), complete	Knee disarticulation	Gritti-Stokes, Morestin, Callander, Pollock, Carden, Batch, Spittler and McFaddin
Leg (Leg), partial (upper ⅓)	Short (upper-third) BK	
Leg (Leg), partial (middle ⅓)	Medium (mid-third) BK	
Leg (Leg), partial (lower ⅓)	Long (lower-third) BK	Came
Tarsal (Ta), complete	Ankle disarticulation	Syme, Pirogoff, Guyon, Hancock, MacKenzie
Tarsal (Ta), partial		Chopart, Le Fort, Malgaigne, Vladimiroff-Mikulicz, Tripier
Metatarsal (MT), complete	Known collectively as partial foot amputations	Lisfranc, Hey
Metatarsal (MT), partial		
Phalangeal (Ph), complete		
Phalangeal (Ph), partial		

AK, Above knee; BK, below knee.
(From Kay HW: A nomenclature for limb prosthetics, Orthot Prosthet J 28(4):37-47, 1974. Reprinted with permission of the American Orthotic and Prosthetic Association.)

guillotine a.: amputation making a straight cut through the limb; also called **chop a.**

Marquardt technique: to broaden bone support for below-knee stump, an iliac crest bone graft is inserted in the distal tibia.

open a.: any amputation in which the wound is left open for drainage, as opposed to a closed amputation.

skew flap a.: for below-knee amputation, creating better coverage of anteromedial tibia with a fish mouth in which the axis of amputation creates a posterolateral flap.

stump revision: any surgery designed to revise the shape or scar of a residual limb.

Syme a.: the term is used to describe a special method of incision and closure for amputations at other locations but most commonly the term is used for an amputation through the ankle where the heel pad is closed over the tibial and fibular stump to give a firm walking surface.

Associated Surgical Terms

ablate: to completely excise or amputate; the surgical removal of a part is referred to as **ablative surgery,** for example, the excision of a large tumor mass and the surrounding soft tissue.

advancement: surgical or traumatic detachment of muscle, tendon, or ligament structure followed by reattachment at a more advanced point.

anastomosis: restoration of continuity of any vessel or organ; usually refers to the suturing of a tubular structure such as a blood vessel creating the passage between two distinct parts, such as end-to-end anastomosis.

anesthesia: loss of sensation with or without loss of consciousness as a direct result of the administration of a systemic drug agent. The term also describes the local or systemic loss of sensation caused by trauma or other injury.

antibiotic beads: methylmethacrylate impregnated with antibiotics and place on a suture for later removal, used in the treatment of deep wound infections and osteomyelitis.

approximate: to bring together or into apposition; this term is commonly used to refer to suturing of tissues or the repositioning of fractures.

aseptic: free from bacteria; aseptic technique is any technique designed to prevent contamination by bacteria.

aspiration: withdrawal of fluid from any open or closed space.

attenuate: to make thin, small, or fine; reduce in size.

autopsy: a postmortem and pathologic examination of the body by dissection; also called **necropsy.**

biopsy: the excision of a section of living tissue for microscopic examination and diagnosis. This may be performed on any tissue; for example, a bone marrow biopsy is performed by closed method (use of a needle or trocar) to sample bone marrow. The terms **needle biopsy, closed biopsy,** and **percutaneous biopsy** are often used to denote tissue sampling performed through a minimally invasive approach. An **open biopsy** is performed with a skin incision. The purpose of a biopsy is to determine the cause of the lesion and test for systemic, neoplastic, or reactive conditions.

brisement: the forcible breaking up of joint capsule, usually for conditions of partial fibrous ankylosis such as frozen shoulders (pronounced breezmaw).

broaching: the act of widening a bone medullary canal in such a fashion that it will accept the stem of a specific implant. The instrument used to do this is a **broach.**

callotasis: for limb-length disparity, a transverse section of the bone of the short limb is stabilized with an external skeletal fixator and then the limb is gradually lengthened over a period of weeks.

catheterization: insertion of a tube into a cavity or blood vessel for drainage.

cauterization: the use of an electric current to stop local bleeding. This term also denotes the use of caustic materials such as silver nitrate to reduce local tissue granulation, as seen in open wounds.

cautery: an instrument designed to stop bleeding by destroying tissue through heat, electricity, or corrosive chemicals.

chamfer: applied to the act of smoothing off soft edges or rounding the end of a bone by making small cuts.

computer assisted orthopaedic surgery (CAOS): using fiduciary (specific markers placed in bone) reference laser light beams allows for more accurate position of bone cutting jigs used to prepare surfaces for total joint components.

costoplasty: correction of rib deformity by osteotomies of rib, often used for correction of scoliosis deformities.

curettage: procedure in which a sharp, scraping instrument is used to remove abnormal tissue, to obtain diagnostic specimens, or to obtain donor bone or marrow.

curette: sharp, scraping, spoon-shaped instrument used in curettage.

damage control orthopaedics: named for the immediate reaction to a severely damaged ship at sea, damage control orthopaedics is the timing of immediate and follow-up care for the severely injured orthopaedic patients with a design to reduce the maximum effect on vital life functions.

débridement: cleansing a wound of devitalized, contaminated, or foreign material.

decompression: surgical relief of pressure to any structure.

dehiscence: a separation or splitting of the edges of a surgical wound, in which the expectation was for the wound to remain closed.

delayed primary closure: the closure of an open wound by intention after the initial surgery or injury; this is often done when the risk of infection is very high. Also called **secondary closure.**

diaplasis: obsolete term for the reduction of a fracture or dislocation by surgical means.

dismemberment: amputation of a limb.

dissection: separation of tissue for any reason. **Sharp dissection** is the use of a sharp instrument to facilitate dissection. **Blunt dissection** refers to the separation of tissues along natural lines of cleavage by the use of the fingers or other blunt instruments.

drainage: removal of fluid from a cavity. This term is often used to refer to material arising from open surgical wounds. **Dependent drainage** is an active effort to position a patient so that gravity will carry fluid away from the wound via catheterization.

ebonation: stripping of one tissue from another. In orthopaedics, this refers to a surgical or pathologic removal of hard, bony loose cartilage from the surface of bone.

electrocautery: surgical instrument used to control bleeding of a surgical wound. The use of this instrument is called **electrocauterization.**

enucleate: to remove whole and clean in its entirety an organ, tumor, or cyst by shelling out.

evacuate: to empty a cavity.

excise: to cut out.

exploration: the examination by direct surgical visualization; surgery done for the express purpose of examining tissue is called **exploratory surgery.**

extirpation: the removal in its entirety of diseased tissue, a structure, or mass; also called **excision.**

extraction: process of removal by pulling out.

extubation: the removal of a tube; used to refer to the tube inserted into the windpipe during anesthesia.

fixation: as applied to orthopaedics, implies the use of internal or external fixation, which is the use of metallic devices inserted into or through bone to hold a fracture in a set position and alignment while it heals.

fulguration: the use of high-frequency electrocautery to destroy tissue during surgical procedures.

fusion: the uniting of two bony segments, whether a fracture or a vertebral joint.

granulation: the proliferation of numerous small blood vessels at a wound site to give the general appearance of a raw, red tissue. This is a normal healing process in that this rich vascular bed can modulate into normal tissue or act as a base for skin grafts or primary closure. **Granuloma** is a pathologic reaction to a foreign body or organism and should not be confused with *granulation.*

imbrication: the overlapping of tissue structures in closure of a wound and in repair of defects to improve the tightness of a structure.

implant: any substance inserted into the tissue for an indefinite period; this includes all internal prostheses, internal fixation devices, and other materials not absorbed by the body.

incision and drainage (I&D): surgical incision into a cavity, usually for purpose of removing purulent (infected) material; most common example is the lancing of an abscess.

infiltration: usually refers to local injection of anesthetic solutions or fluids that then permeate soft tissue; may be a result of failure of intravenous fluids to go into the vein correctly.

infusion: introduction of any solution such as saline into a blood vessel or cavity.

injection: introduction of material, nutrients, or medicine into tissues of the body by the use of a syringe and needle.

in situ: in orthopaedics, the fixation of a fracture in the position that it presents at the time of injury, usually a nondisplaced fracture; also used to describe a lesion that is highly localized.

in toto: in total; removal of an organ, cyst, or tumor in its entirety.

intubation: insertion of a tube into the trachea for entrance of air during surgical procedure; for example, endotracheal intubation.

in vitro: cells or tissue maintained in an artificial environment such that they can survive outside the living body usually for experimental purposes. (This term is sometimes italicized in the literature.)

in vivo: within the living organism, such as an experimental drug being used on an animal or human subject. (This term is sometimes italicized in the literature.)

irrigation: washing out of a wound or cavity with a solution. In this context **Closed suction irrigation** is a specific system by which irrigating tubes are surgically implanted in a wound and used continuously after the time of surgery.

lavage: the copious washing out or irrigation of a wound or cavity.

ligation: tying off; used particularly in reference to the tying of blood vessels at a surgical wound.

ligatures: sutures used to tie off blood vessels.

light amplification by stimulated emission of radiation (laser): a device used in surgical procedures consisting of a resonant optical cavity in which a substance is stimulated to emit light radiation and a mirror that reflects the rays back and forth so molecules will emit more radiation. Finely directed laser light sources can be used to cut tissue, coagulate vessels, or cause the adhesion of one tissue surface to another.

locking plates: plates that act as an internal "external" fixator for long bone fractures. The screws are locked into the plate helping stabilize the plate without toggling of the screws and with preservation of bone surface circulation.

manipulation: the planned and carefully managed manual movement of a joint or fracture to produce increased joint motion or better position and alignment of the fracture. This term is sometimes used to denote a precise sequence of movements of a joint to determine the presence of disease or to reduce a dislocation.

marsupialization: incision into a cystic lesion with incorporation of the walls of the cyst to the exterior edges of the skin to produce constant drainage.

matte finish: a fine-ground-glass-appearing finish, designed for better cement to metallic surface fixation of internal prosthetics.

morcellation: breaking up or subdividing tissue for easier removal; also, to leave in place but in a refashioned shape such as cortical or cancellous bone graft material.

paddle: term applied to a patch of skin and subcutaneous tissue that can be transferred on its vascular pedicle.

palliative: surgical procedure or use of medications to treat the symptoms without curing the disease process; used relative to the treatment of terminal conditions such as cancer.

paracentesis: needle puncture into a cavity to aspirate fluid; usually done in the abdominal and thoracic cavities.

parenteral: the introduction (injection) of substances into the body by way of intravenous, intramuscular, subcutaneous, or intramedullary route, other than through the alimentary canal.

per primam: the healing of a surgical or traumatic wound by first intention, after closure. This means that the closure of the wound is successful and that there is no reopening of the wound resulting from failure of healing.

-pexy (suffix): fixation by solid tissue attachment. In orthopaedics, the most common term using this root is **scapulopexy,** a procedure whereby the scapula is fixed directly to the ribs.

phantom pain: the sensation of pain following amputation that seems to be in the part that has been removed. Eventually, the patient is able to localize the pain to the stump and loses the sense of the presence of the amputated part.

plication: taking tucks in a structure to shorten it; folds.

polyacetyl rod: synthetic polyester rod used for fracture fixation. The rod is bioabsorbable.

portal: small stab incision used for introduction of arthroscope or instrument into a joint.

primary closure: the closure of the wound edges at the time of trauma or surgery.

prosthesis: this term has a very broad meaning and includes all artificial limbs as well as materials implanted in the body to replace the structure, function, or appearance of the missing structure.

reefing: a folding in or overlapping of soft tissue by surgical suture designed to make that structure tighter.

reflect: in the surgical sense, to fold back tissue such as a muscle belly to expose deeper structures.

regimen: a system of therapy regulated to achieve certain results (e.g., diet, exercise following surgery).

release: incision into any soft tissue to produce relaxation of that tissue, for example, tendon release.

resection: partial excision of soft tissue or segment of bone; also, the removal of a portion of diseased nerve tissue, called a **nerve resection.**

retraction: a pulling back of tissue, whether done mechanically at the time of surgery or by scar formation after surgery; for example, a scar that is indented inward toward the body is considered a retracted scar.

revision: any surgical reconstruction of soft or hard tissue. A revision may be done at the time of initial trauma if damaged tissue is removed and normal structures are repositioned to compensate for that destruction. The term is more commonly used to describe a later surgical effort to reposition various tissues.

rongeur: to cut into bone with a sharp biting instrument called a *rongeur,* usually to remove bone that is diseased or obstructing visualization of deeper structures.

saucerization: creation of a saucerlike depression in bone in an effort to remove diseased bone. This is most commonly done for bone infections, and the wound is usually left open for drainage; it is also a saucerlike collapse of a crushed vertebrae on the horizontal surface.

scaffold: a support, usually of an absorbable construct such as fiber, for the ingrowth of tissue.

second hit: surgical or other insult that occurs after an initial severe and life-threatening set of injuries.

secondary closure: closure of a wound that had been left open after previous trauma or surgery. This is also called **delayed primary closure** and is done often when there was initially a high risk of infection.

sepsis: the presence of bacterial infection in blood or tissue from any source. This term is often used to describe the systemic condition resulting from an infection, for example, septicemia.

septic: contaminated with bacteria. A septic wound, otherwise known as a **dirty wound,** is one in which there is an existing infection with purulent material.

-stasis (suffix): to control flow or progression (e.g., hemostasis).

stasis: condition arising from a static circumstance. For example, a stasis ulcer is one that is created in a patient kept in the same position for any length of time in which blood or fluids stagnate.

stent: a support, flexible or rigid, usually biodegradable, designed to relieve excessive strain during graft or other tissue repair and remodeling.

subcutaneous: the fatty and fibrous tissues beneath the thick layers of skin.

subcuticular: the thick layer of skin below the epidermal layers. A subcuticular suture is used to close the skin by a continuous suture that pulls the deep layer of skin together, with the suture exiting at each end of the wound only.

sulcus: any normal groove or depression in bone or soft tissue.

suspension: usually refers to a soft tissue procedure designed to help hold some anatomic structure in a more functional position; tenodesis.

suture: any threadlike, pliable material such as catgut or nylon that is used to close soft tissue.

tamponade: method to control bleeding by direct pressure.

-tome (suffix): any instrument that cuts.

tourniquet: any instrument used to compress blood vessels to slow or stop circulation. If light pressure is applied by tourniquet, there will be congestion in the venous system. This is often used to help draw blood for laboratory testing. More secure tourniquet pressure, designed to stop all blood flow to a part, is used to prevent bleeding.

toxic: poisonous. This term is often used to describe the systemic condition of a patient with infection.

transect: to cut across the long axis of a tissue. For example, a tendon transection is often done to release the pull of that tendon at its point of insertion.

transfusion: term commonly used to describe the intravenous infusion of whole blood or blood components; however, any solution may be transfused.

transposition: the repositioning of an intact and attached tissue segment from one place to another. This term is often used in describing soft tissue and bone graft procedures.

-tripsy (suffix): surgical crushing, for example, an osteotripsy is a procedure done in the foot to relieve a corn or callus caused by prominence of bone under the skin.

vest-over-pants closure: closure of fascia, particularly near joints, in which one layer is closed on top of another to produce tightening or pull on the joint capsule.

viable: alive or capable of living; used to describe healthy tissue that appears to be intact.

The Spine

The spine consists of three basic elements: bones, joints, and neural tissue. Together these components allow the spinal column to perform a variety of functions in the human body. The weight of the body is transferred through the vertebrae and disks; motion occurs through the intervertebral joints and disks; and the brainstem, spinal cord, and spinal nerves that travel in and around these bones and joints are allowed to function in a protected environment.

The body has three main neural components: the central, peripheral, and autonomic nervous systems. The **central nervous system** consists of the brain, brainstem, and spinal cord. Protecting the spinal cord and spinal nerves are the meninges, composed of the dura mater, pia mater, and arachnoid. These protective layers help protect and isolate the central nervous system from the outside world. The brainstem and spinal cord travel within a tunnel-like structure called the **spinal canal.** The spinal cord gives rise to 31 pairs of spinal nerves or nerve roots that branch off along the length of the spinal cord and exit from the spinal canal through a tunnel called the foramen. After these nerve roots exit from the spine, they join other nerves to become **peripheral nerves.** Peripheral nerves contain the sensory fibers, voluntary muscle fibers, and fibers of the autonomic nervous system. The **autonomic nervous system** is composed of small nerve branches arising from the central nervous system and supplying **ganglia,** which are clusters of cells near but outside the bony limits of the vertebrae. The **sympathetic nervous system** and **parasympathetic nervous systems** are subdivisions of the autonomic nervous system, which is involved in the control of visceral organs and blood vessels. Most spinal nerves and peripheral nerves contain a mixture of sensory and motor fibers that supply specific muscles and provide sensation in particular locations in the body. By treating the anatomy of the spinal cord and its peripheral branches like a road map, a physician can often determine the cause of numbness, tingling, or weakness found on a sensory and motor examination.

The spine is made of bony segments known as **vertebrae.** These are separated by intervertebral disks and **facet joints** that permit motion. A complex arrangement of ligaments and muscles provide stability and motion of the spinal column. Neural elements exit and enter the spinal column through openings called **foramina.**

Each component of the spinal column depends on the others to function normally. If one part of the spine changes in character, such as in a fracture or a disk herniation, other structures can be affected, leading to arthritis, muscle fatigue, nerve or spinal cord damage, or irritation resulting in pain, numbness, weakness, or even paralysis in severe cases.

General Anatomy of the Spine

The 32 vertebrae composing the spinal segments are divided into five regions, with the segments numbered from top to bottom. There are 5 cervical, 12 thoracic, 5 lumbar, 5 sacral, and several coccygeal vertebrae (Fig. 9-1).

A **vertebra** is labeled by segment such as C-5, L-4, and S-1. The **intervertebral disk** is labeled for the level of the vertebrae between which the disk exists.

cervical spine: seven spinal segments (C1–C7) and eight cervical nerve roots (C1–C8) between the base of the skull (occiput) and the thoracic spine. The cervical spine differs from the rest of the vertebrae in one major aspect: the numbered nerve roots exit the spinal canal above the correspondingly numbered vertebra's pedicle instead of below it.
thoracic spine (dorsal spine): 12 spinal segments (T1–T12) incorporating the 12 ribs of the thorax. Other than a slight increase in size from top to bottom, they are fairly uniform in appearance.
lumbar spine: five mobile segments of the lower back (L-1 to L-5). These are the largest of the vertebral segments.
sacral spine: five fused segments of the lower spine that connect to the pelvis and have four foramina on each side; also called **sacrum.**
coccygeal spine: remaining three or four, somewhat fixed, fused segments at the end of the spine (tailbone) that articulate with sacrum above; also called **coccyx.**

Except for the coccyx, sacrum, and the first cervical spine, there are anatomic parts that are common to all 32 spinal segments. Moving from anterior to posterior (front to back), the main vertebral parts are the following.

facet joint: small articular cartilage-surfaced joints connecting the posterior elements of one spine to the posterior elements of the neighboring spine; also called **zygapophyseal joint.**
foramen: an opening allowing for the egress of spinal nerve roots from between two vertebrae.
intramedullary: refers to medullaris, marrow; (1) within the medulla oblongata of the brain, (2) within the spinal cord, and (3) within the marrow cavity of bone.
lamina: the posterior part of the spinal ring that covers the spinal cord or nerves.
pars interarticularis: the posterior continuation of the spinal arch from the pedicle; the superior and inferior facets are connected to each other by the pars interarticularis.

FIG 9-1 Diagram showing the relation of the segments of the spinal cord and nerves to the segments of the vertebral column. *(From Hamilton WJ, editor:* Textbook of human anatomy, *ed 2, London, England, 1976, The Macmillan Press, Ltd.)*

FIG 9-2 Vertebral body and posterior elements.

pedicle: the first portion of the posterior spine arising from the vertebral body.
spinous process: the most posterior extension of the spine arising from the laminae.
transverse process: bony process arising from midportion of the spinal ring just posterior to the pedicle and pars interarticularis.
vertebral body: from a lateral view, it is the main rectangular portion; from an overhead view, oval (Fig. 9-2).

Cervical Spine Anatomy

Bones and Landmarks

atlas: the first cervical vertebra (C1), lying directly under the skull, through which the head articulates with the neck. The main connection to the vertebra below is a pivot around the odontoid process that is an upward projection of the body of the second cervical vertebra. The atlas is held to the odontoid by a ligament complex attaching it to the odontoid anteriorly and facet joints posteriorly, allowing rotation, flexion, and extension between C1 and C2.
axis: the second cervical vertebra (C2), about which the first cervical vertebra rotates, allowing head movement. It bears the **odontoid process,** the projecting part of the second cervical vertebra, which allows the first cervical vertebra (atlas) to rotate.
carotid tubercle: prominence of the transverse process of C6 felt on the lateral side of neck.
chondrum terminale: in young children, a cartilaginous epiphysis at the tip of the odontoid. The fusion takes place at 10–12 years, and is the weak point at the C1–C2 junction in younger children.
cricoid ring: cartilage ring above the trachea and below the thyroid cartilage; the first cricoid ring is at the level of C6.
hyoid bone: small, vertically oriented bone lateral to trachea, located at the level of C3.

joints of Luschka: unique to the cervical spine, these jointlike structures are formed by the apposition of posterolateral portions of adjacent vertebral bodies; forms the anterior portion of the canal where nerves pass through; also called **uncovertebral joints.**

lateral mass: the lateral expansion of the spinal ring in the cervical spine, consisting of the facet joints and intervening bone as well as a tunnel through which the vertebral artery travels in the second through seventh cervical vertebra.

occiput: the base of the skull.

thyroid cartilage: widening expanses of cartilage above the trachea; the top marks the level of C4, and the bottom C5.

Muscles

longissimus colli: long muscle immediately anterior to the cervical spine.

platysma: thin, outermost muscle layer of the anterior neck.

posterior neck muscles: splenius m., spinalis m., and **semispinalis m.**

scalenus: the deep lateral muscles of the anterior neck, including anterior scalene m. (scalenus anticus), middle scalene m. (scalenus medius), and posterior scalene m. (scalenus posticus).

sternocleidomastoid: large, externally visible muscle of the anterior neck, enabling head to turn to either side.

strap muscles: a general term applied to the ribbonlike muscles in the anterior neck; they include omohyoid, sternohyoid, sternothyroid, and thyrohyoid.

Arteries and Veins

carotid artery: main artery to the head that divides into external and internal carotid arteries.

jugular vein: large, obvious vein in the neck.

other arteries and veins: transcervical, facial, superior thyroid, and inferior thyroid.

vertebral artery: large artery that travels in the lateral masses of the cervical spine and eventually supplies the lower brainstem.

Nerves

cervical plexus: plexus of nerves that supply the neck muscles with branches named by muscles supplied, a portion of which is called the **ansa cervicalis.**

facial nerve: supplies some facial muscles and sensation; also called **seventh cranial n.**

laryngeal n. and **recurrent laryngeal n.:** branches of the vagus nerve important in anterior neck surgery.

occipital n.: nerve from the back of the neck that supplies motor function and sensation to the forehead; two parts—greater and lesser.

phrenic n.: nerve arising from three cervical nerve roots (C3–C5); supplies the diaphragm.

spinal accessory n.: the nerve from the brainstem that supplies the sternocleidomastoid muscles; also called **eleventh cranial n.**

vagus n.: the long nerve in the anterior neck traveling with the carotid artery; responsible for many organ functions in the chest and abdomen; also called **tenth cranial n.**

Other Structures

esophagus: portion of the gut between the mouth and stomach in the anterior neck.

interspinous ligament: ligament between each of the spinal processes.

nuchal ligament: large posterior midline ligament in the neck from the base of the skull to the seventh cervical vertebra.

thyroid gland: near the Adam's apple; responsible for secretion of hormone that is involved in regulation of the rate of the metabolism.

trachea: the windpipe.

triangles: for surgical approaches and other considerations, the anterior half of the neck is divided into triangles—anterior, digastric, posterior, submental, and carotid.

Thoracic Spine Anatomy

costo-: combining form denoting relation to ribs.

costochondral junction: junction of the rib into cartilage in the anterior chest. NOTE: Most of the ribs have attachment to the cartilage rather than a direct junction with the breast bone.

costovertebral angle: juncture of tissue inferior and lateral to the twelfth rib and vertebral body.

costovertebral joint: junction of the rib with the thoracic spine.

diaphragm: the muscle between the abdomen and thorax; main muscle of normal breathing.

intercostal m.: the muscles between the ribs.

latissimus dorsi m.: large muscle arising from posterior thoracic spine and attaching at proximal humerus.

pectoralis m.: from sternum and ribs to humerus.

rotator cuff muscles: include **supraspinatus m., infraspinatus m., subscapularis m.,** and **teres minor m.**

sternum: the breast bone; further divided into three segments.

    manubrium: upper portion, proximal end

    sternum: main portion, medial portion

    xiphoid: the daggerlike tip of the sternum, distal end

thorax: the chest or rib cage; also refers to the space containing the lungs and heart. There are 12 vertebral segments and ribs; the lower two are called **floating ribs.**

Lumbar and Lower Spine Anatomy

Bones

coccyx: the three, and sometimes four, segments of bone just below the sacrum; referred to as the **tailbone**; the end of the spinal column.

lumbar spine: the five movable spinal segments of the lower back and largest of the spinal segments.

sacral ala: lateral portions of the sacral bone.

sacral spine (sacrum): the five segments fused together as a solid bone and below the last lumbar segment position.

sacroiliac joint: the junction between the sacrum and the ilium; resembles a large ear.

Disk and Spinal Canal

intervertebral disk: the structure that normally occupies the space between two moving vertebrae, and acts to distribute forces through surrounding structure such as the facet joints, subchondral plate, and ligaments. It is more prominent in the cervical and lumbar spines. The centermost portion of the disk (**nucleus pulposus**) is normally composed of a gelatinous material that varies in consistency from a firm jelly material to a very thick and less pliable substance. This core is then surrounded by numerous layers of fibrous (fibrocartilaginous) material called the **annulus fibrosus.** That structure goes to the normal margins of the vertebral body, called the **anterior longitudinal ligament,** and to those on the spinal canal side posteriorly, the **posterior longitudinal ligament.** Also called **interspinal disk.**

ligamentum flavum: a band of yellow elastic tissue that runs between the laminae from the axis to the sacrum; it assists in maintaining or regaining erect position and serves to close in the spaces between the arches. It is important as a surgical structure in that a portion is usually removed during an exploration of the spinal canal.

spinal canal: the space between the vertebral body anteriorly and the lamina and spinal process posteriorly. The spinal cord extends to the level of the second lumbar segment in adults and the second sacral segment in infants. Below this level are numerous spinal nerves from the spinal cord. This lower portion resembles a horse's tail and is referred to as the **cauda equina** ("horse's tail" in Latin). The lower tip of the spinal cord is attached to the end of the spinal canal by a single filament called the **filum terminale.** The brain, spinal cord, and spinal nerves float in a waterlike substance called the **cerebral spinal fluid.** This fluid is contained in a thin sac called the **meninges.** The thick, outer portion of that sac is called the **dura** or **dura mater.** The more flimsy inner coverings are the **arachnoid** (Latin for "spiderlike") and **pia.** The dura extends over the nerve roots out into the foramina. This saclike covering is called the **nerve root sleeve.** The dura also extends within the spinal canal down to the level of the second sacral segment. Any space within the dura from the first cervical to the second sacral level is considered **intradural.**

spinal cord: the part of the central nervous system below the level of the brainstem and above the cauda equina in the regions of the cervical, thoracic, and upper lumbar spines. Usually, the orthopaedist does not deal with the spinal cord—that is for the neurosurgeon. Based on training, both the orthopaedist and neurosurgeon deal with spinal cord problems. Many of these conditions can result in peripheral neuromuscular disorders.

    dorsal column: the main, normal sensory tract to the brain.

dorsal lateral column: the main tract of position and tone to the brain.
gray matter: the nerve cell bodies to muscle and sensory outflow and input, respectively; also called **anterior and posterior horns.**
long tracts: the nerve fibers that connect the spinal cord with the brain; main spinal nerve pathways.
pyramidal tract: carries the voluntary muscle messages from the brain.
spinal thalamic tract: the main tract of pain to the brain.

Muscles

abdominal muscles: important for support of the spine; these muscles are the **rectus abdominis m., external oblique m., internal oblique m.,** and **transversus m.**
iliopsoas muscle: large muscle starting at L1 and becoming wider as it picks up segments from the lower lumbar spine; combines with the iliacus m. muscle before attaching to the lesser trochanter of the hip.
posterior spinal muscle segments: upper and lower posterior serratus m., spinalis m., semispinalis m., and rotators.
quadratus lumborum m.: a muscle lateral to the iliopsoas muscle of the spine running from the lower ribs to the ilium.

Artery

artery of Adamkiewicz: an important source of blood supply to the lower portion of the spine, usually occurring at the levels of T9 to T11; however, it is not the only blood supply to the cord at that level.

Diseases and Structural Anomalies

Back and Neck Diseases

The spine is a complex organ that is a series of joints with attending bone, nerve tissues, muscles, and ligaments. In addition, there are two elements not common to other joints, namely, intervertebral disks and the spinal cord and nerves in the bony spinal canal. The nerves may be affected by either bone or disk disease; therefore this section is divided into discussions of diseases affecting bone, nerves, spinal cord, vertebral disks, and congenital disorders.

Diseases of the spine may be treated by other medical specialties, particularly neurosurgery in the case of spinal cord and nerve lesions and injuries. However, the orthopaedist treats many diseases and conditions of the spine such as scoliosis, spina bifida, and degenerative disk disease. Treatment may last for years in the correction of some deformities.

General Bone Diseases of the Spine

The Latin word *vertebra* and the combining form *spondylo-* both denote the bony spinal segments. In some word combinations, the root word is assigned only to a specific part of the vertebra, such as spondylolysis in which the defect is always at the pars interarticularis. However, *spondylo-* in general means "vertebra."

Spondylo- Root Diseases

spondylalgia: pain in vertebrae.
spondylarthritis: arthritis of the spine.
spondylarthrocace: tuberculosis of the spine; also called **spondylocace.**
spondylexarthrosis: dislocation of a vertebra.
spondylitis: inflammatory disease involving the spine with inflammation of vertebrae, including types such as ankylosing, rheumatoid, traumatic, spondylitis deformans, Kümmell, and Marie-Strümpell d.
spondylizema: depression or downward displacement of a vertebra, with destruction or softening of one below it.
spondylocostal dysostosis: a rare autosomal recessive growth disorder characterized by potentially severe malformations of the vertebrae and ribs.
spondylodynia: pain in vertebrae.
spondyloepiphyseal dysplasia: disorder of growth affecting both the spine and the ends of long bones.
spondylolisthesis: usually an anterior displacement of one vertebra on the adjacent lower vertebra. When the superior segment is posterior to the inferior one, it is called a **retrolisthesis.** Many, but not all, patients with spondylolisthesis have spondylolysis. Spondylolisthesis is a general term with multiple distinctions:
  anterior displacement: forward movement of the superior segment on the inferior one.

lumbar lordosis: angle made by lines drawn from the superior surface of the first and fifth lumbar vertebra.

lumbosacral joint angle: angle between the inferior surface of the fifth lumbar vertebra and the top of the sacrum.

rounding of the cranial border: relationship of the height to the width of the rounded portion of the superior sacrum.

sacral inclination: relationship of the sagittal plane of the sacrum to the vertical plane.

sacrohorizontal angle: angle between the top of the sacrum and the horizontal line.

sagittal rotation: denotes an abnormal angular relationship between the body of the fifth lumbar vertebra and the sacrum; also called **sagittal roll, lumbosacral kyphosis,** and **slip angle.**

wedging of olisthetic vertebra: measure obtained by dividing the height of the anterior border of the fifth vertebra by the height of its posterior border, multiplied by 100.

spondylolysis: a fracture or defect in the pars interarticularis (a portion of bone between each of the joints of the spine), allowing one vertebral body to slide forward on the next (Fig. 9-3). May be referred to as **pars interarticularis defect.** Patients with spondylolysis do not always have spondylolisthesis.

Spondylolysis and Spondylolisthesis Classification System
I. **dysplastic:** congenital abnormalities of the arch of the sacrum or the arch of L5 that permit the slipping to occur.
II. **isthmic:** the lesion is in the pars interarticularis. Three types occur: 　1. lytic, fatigue fracture of the pars interarticularis 　2. elongated, but intact pars interarticularis 　3. cute fracture of the pars interarticularis, not to be confused with traumatic
III. **degenerative:** the lesion results from intersegmental instability of long duration.
IV. **posttraumatic:** results from fracture in other areas of the bony hook than in pars interarticularis.

Wiltse Classification of Spondylolisthesis
I. dysplastic (congenital)
II. isthmic lytic, fatigue fracture of the pars interarticularis elongated but intact pars acute fracture of pars (not to be confused with "traumatic")
III. degenerative
IV. posttraumatic
V. pathologic

Marchetti and Bartolozzi Classification of Spondylolisthesis
A cause-based classification system that divides spondylolisthesis into two categories: development and acquired.
Development:
High dysplastic with lysis or with elongation
Low dysplastic with lysis or with elongation
Acquired:
Traumatic (acute fracture or stress fracture)
Postsurgical (direct or indirect)
Pathologic (local or systemic)
Degenerative (primary or secondary)

pathologic: generalized or localized bone disease is present.

spondylomalacia: softening of vertebrae; also called **Kümmell disease.**

spondylopathy: any vertebral disorder.

spondylopyosis: infection in vertebrae.

spondyloschisis: congenital fissure (splitting) of vertebral arch.

spondylosis: bony replacement of ligaments around the disk spaces of the spine, associated with decreased mobility and eventual fusion; also called **marginal osteophyte.**

Rachio- Root Diseases

Rachio-, as relating to spine, is less frequently used than more specific combining forms.

rachialgia: pain in the vertebral column.
rachiocampsis: curvature of the spine.
rachiochysis: effusion of fluid within the vertebral canal.
rachiodynia: pain in the spinal column.
rachiokyphosis: humpbacked curvature of spine; kyphosis.
rachiomyelitis: inflammation of the spinal cord.

FIG 9-3 A, Oblique view: *A,* Articular facet joint; *I,* isthmus or pars interarticulars; *T,* transverse process; *L,* lamina; *P,* pedicle. The oblique view visualizes the so-called Scottie dog. Spondylolysis occurs through the isthmus *(arrow).* **B,** Bony defect *(arrow)* in the isthmus or neck of the Scottie dog present in spondylolysis (oblique view). **C,** Meyerding's classification of spondylolisthesis. The amount of slippage is graded 1–4. Grade 1 represents 25% forward displacement; grade 2, 25%–50%; grade 3, 50%–75%; and grade 4, greater than 75%. **D,** Spondylolisthesis of the lumbosacral junction. *(From Mercier LR: Practical orthopaedics, ed 5, St Louis, 2000, Mosby.)*

rachioparalysis: paralysis of the spinal muscles.
rachiopathy: any disease of the spine.
rachioplegia: spinal paralysis.
rachioscoliosis: lateral curvature of the spine.
rachisagra: pain or gout in the spine.
rachischisis: congenital fissure of the spinal cord.

Miscellaneous Spinal Disorders

alar dysgenesis: abnormality in development of the sacroiliac joint.
anisospondyly: different abnormal shapes of the vertebral bodies.
ankylosing spinal hyperostosis: arthritic disorder in which bridging osteophytes located anteriorly and posteriorly on the vertebral body bind two or more vertebrae together; also called **Forestier disease.**
anterior spurring: ligament turning to bone on anterior side of vertebral body.
Baastrup d.: false joint formed by wide posterior spinous processes of the lumbar spine. This may become a source of pain. Also called **kissing spine.**
camptocormia: severe forward flexion of upper torso, usually an excessive psychologic reaction to back pain.
cervical rib: riblike structure in the seventh cervical vertebra that may cause nerve root irritation.
coccyalgia: pain in the coccyx region; also called **coccygodynia, coccyodynia,** and **coccydynia.**
crankshaft phenomenon: progressions of a spinal curve caused by continued growth of the unfused anterior aspect of the spine following a posterior spine fusion for scoliosis in children. The deformity can be severe with increased lordosis and rotation despite little change in the curve as measured on an anterior-posterior radiograph.
dysraphism: any failure of closure of the primary neural tube. This general category includes the disorder **myelomeningocele.** This definition includes the conditions in which there is an abnormal midline structure in the neural axis. Hence, **diastematomyelia,** in which the midline structure has fused, but the term also implies a bony spike from the anteriorlying vertebral body.
facet tropism: asymmetrical orientation of the facets comparing right to left side.

Grisel syndrome: subluxation of the atlantoaxial joint from inflammatory ligamentous laxity caused by infection. Can result in neurologic complications.
interspinous pseudarthrosis: formation of a false joint between two spinous processes.
limbus annulare: a mass of bone situated at the anterosuperior margin of a vertebra. Arises from failure of fusion of the primary and secondary ossification centers.
lumbarization: partial or complete formation of a free-moving first sacral segment so that it looks like a lumbar vertebra.
marginal osteophytes: excess bone formation at the margin of the vertebral body; also called **spondylosis.**
olisthy: slipping of bones from normal anatomic site; for example, a slipped disk.
paravertebral muscle spasm: spasm in the muscles on either side of the spinous processes (midline of the back); the term may be used to describe a physical finding or improperly used to define a disease process.
pseudoclaudication: increased pain and decreased strength in lower limbs associated with physical activity. Complaints are similar to those caused by an insufficient blood supply to the limb but are caused by diminished blood supply to the nerves in a narrowed spinal canal.
retrolisthesis: posterior displacement of the vertebra on the one below.
Redlund-Johnell: an alternative method for measuring vertical dislocation of C1 and C2 vertebrae in rheumatoid arthritis based on the distance from lower endplate of C2 to the palatooccipital or McGregor's line.
rudimentary ribs: nubbins of ribs seen below the level where the last rib normally occurs.
sacralgia: pain in the sacrum.
sacralization: fusion of L5 to the first segment of the sacrum, so that the sacrum consists of six segments; this abnormality is called **Bertolotti syndrome.**
sacralized transverse process: one or both of the lumbar spinous transverse processes abnormally joining with the sacrum; also called **sacralization.**

sacrodynia: pain perceived to be in the area of the sacrum but may originate elsewhere.

sacroiliitis: inflammation of the sacroiliac joint. A very painful, often one-sided sacral area pain that follows delivery, is not due to sepsis, and will subside gradually and completely. A form is **acute postpartum sacroiliitis.**

sciatica: pain radiating down the sciatic nerve into the posterior thigh and leg; can be caused by irritation of a nerve anywhere from the back to the thigh.

scoliorachitis: disease of the spine caused by rickets; abnormal bone mineralization.

Spinal Deformities

Spinal deformity is the abnormal angulation of the spinal column when a person is viewed from the back or the side. It can occur from a variety of causes and at any age. An **inclinometer** is a device used to measure the amount of trunk rotation on examination.

Structural Anomalies

Scoliosis is a general term that applies to any side-to-side curve in the back, that is, a lateral and rotational deviation of the spine from the midline. Such a curve may be termed **fixed curve,** which means that any attempt to eliminate the curve by motion is not successful. Curves may be C-shaped or S-shaped (Fig. 9-4).

A **compensatory curve** has a flexible segment above or below the fixed curve; this compensation will place the spine (above or below) into a vertical position with the head at the midline. The rotation of the spinous process is away from the apex of the curve. **Levorotatory scoliosis** means that this rotation of the most dorsal element of the spine is to the left if one is looking at the patient from behind. **Dextrorotoscoliosis** is the opposite condition. The apex of a curve is called the *convex side,* for example, a right lumbar scoliosis is a lateral deviation of the spine in the lumbar region, with the apex of that curve to the right; the *concave side* of the curve is the opposite side.

Scoliosis may be associated with vertebral anomalies (missing parts of the vertebrae) and with forward bending (round back); the latter is called **kyphoscoliosis.** Scoliosis may occur at birth *(congenital),* occur from known causes or diseases *(acquired),* or occur from unknown causes *(idiopathic).* An example will best illustrate the terminology. In a right thoracic, left lumbar, **uncompensated rotatory scoliosis,** viewed from behind, the upper back curves to the right and the lower back to the left; there is rotation of the spine, which may or may not be in both curves (unless so stated); and the center of the head is not in the midline when the patient is standing.

FIG 9-4 Scoliosis. **A,** Normal. **B,** Right convex curve, uncentered. **C,** Right convex curve, centered. *(From the American Orthopaedic Association: Manual of orthopaedic surgery, ed 5, Chicago, 1979, The Association.)*

Spinal Deformities and Conditions

Lenke Classification of Adolescent Idiopathic Scoliosis

Classification system for scoliosis that helps to determine the appropriate regions of the spine to be fused. The classification scheme consists of three steps:

Step 1: Identification of the primary curve (Type 1–6):

Measure the regional curves.
Identify the major curve.
Determine whether the minor curve is structural or not.
Type 1: Main Thoracic
   Proximal Thoracic: Nonstructural
   Main Thoracic: Structural (Major)
   Thoracolumbar/lumbar: Nonstructural
Type 2: Double Thoracic
   Proximal Thoracic: Structural
   Main Thoracic: Structural (Major)
   Thoracolumbar/lumbar: Nonstructural

Type 3: Double Major
  Proximal Thoracic: Nonstructural
  Main Thoracic: Structural (Major)
  Thoracolumbar/lumbar: Structural
Type 4: Triple Major
  Proximal Thoracic: Structural
  Main Thoracic: Structural (Major)
  Thoracolumbar/lumbar: Structural
Type 5: Thoracolumbar/Lumbar
  Proximal Thoracic: Nonstructural
  Main Thoracic: Structural
  Thoracolumbar/lumbar: Structural (Major)
Type 6: Thoracolumbar/Lumbar-Main Thoracic
  Proximal Thoracic: Nonstructural
  Main Thoracic: Structural
  Thoracolumbar/lumbar: Structural (Major)

Step 2: Assignment of lumbar modifiers

Identify the apical lumbar vertebrae (inferior lumbar body falling outside the curve).
Draw a central sacral vertical line (CSVL) and examine its relationship with the pedicles of the apical lumbar vertebrae.
  A: CSVL falls between the pedicles of the apical lumbar vertebrae
  B: CSVL touches the pedicles of the apical lumbar vertebrae
  C: CSVL does not touch apical lumbar vertebrae

Step 3: Assignment of sagittal thoracic modifier

Measure Sagittal Cobb angle from T5 to T12.
Assign the modifier:
  "−": Hypokyphotic: if < 10 degrees
  "N": Normal: 10–40 degrees
  "+": Hyperkyphotic: if > 40 degrees

An example of a classification is "1B+"

adolescent scoliosis: lateral curvature of the spine occurring during adolescence.

adult scoliosis: scoliosis occurring after skeletal maturity.

chin-on-chest deformity: seen in ankylosing spondylitis, a marked kyphosis with fixed posturing of chin on chest.

Cobb syndrome: cutaneous vascular marking associated with spinal vascular formation within the same metameric (segmented) region.

compensatory curve: a curve located above or below a rigid structural curve to maintain normal overall body alignment.

congenital scoliosis: scoliosis caused by bony abnormalities present at birth involving either failure of formation of a vertebra or separation of adjacent vertebrae.

double curve: two lateral curves in a single spine; **double major curve** is two lateral curves of equal magnitude, and **double thoracic curve** is two thoracic curves.

exotic scoliosis: early onset spinal deformity that is more complex.

flattening of normal lumbar curve: condition in which the hollow of the back becomes shallow or even straight.

functional scoliosis: any scoliosis that is caused by leg length or other functional disorder and not by a primary curvature of the spine.

gibbus: most commonly used for spine deformity; a hump or exaggerated convexity.

idiopathic scoliosis: structural lateral curvature of an unknown cause.

infantile scoliosis: lateral curvature of the spine that begins before age 3.

juvenile scoliosis: begins between the ages of 3 and 10 years of age.

kyphoscoliosis: lateral curvature of the spine associated with forward inclination of the spine.

kyphosis: round shoulder deformity, humpback, dorsal kyphotic curvature; may refer to any forward-bending area or deformity of the spine.

lordoscoliosis: lateral curvature of the spine associated with backward bending of the spine.

lumbar curve: curve with apex between the first and fourth lumbar vertebrae.

lumbar kyphosis: reverse of the normal curve of the low back.

lumbosacral curve: a lateral curve with its aspect at or below the fifth lumbar vertebra.

neuromuscular scoliosis: scoliosis caused by a muscle or central nervous system disorder.

pelvic obliquity: slanting of the pelvis that can be caused by leg length inequality, contractures about the hips, a structural scoliosis, or as a combination of two or more of these disorders.

reversal of cervical lordosis: change in the normal curvature of the cervical spine as seen on lateral radiograph. This is usually a straightening of the normal lordotic curve or an actual reversal and is most commonly caused by muscle spasm, indicating cervical disk abnormality.

structural curve: a fixed lateral curve of the spinal column.

thoracic curve: a spinal curvature with its apex between the second and eleventh thoracic vertebrae.

thoracolumbar curve: a spinal curve with its apex at the first lumbar or twelfth thoracic curve.

segmental instability: abnormal response to applied loads characterized by motion in the motor segment beyond normal constraints.

spinal stenosis: general term denoting narrowing of the spinal canal in the lumbar area leading to nerve root compromise; term often used for developmental abnormality that leaves a narrow, bony canal. There are four subgroups of this condition:
   achondroplastic stenosis: increased vertebral thickness, marked concavity of the vertebral body, and short pedicles.
   constitutional stenosis: normal-stature individuals with congenital variance in vertebral structure leading to a narrow canal.
   degenerative stenosis: gradual hypertrophy of the vertebral body margin, facet joints, and ligamentum flavum leading to stenosis.
   combined stenosis: for congenital or developmental reasons, the midsagittal diameter is decreased.

temporomandibular joint (TMJ) syndrome: complex of symptoms often seen in cervical sprain conditions. Symptoms include clicking in the jaw on opening and closing the mouth, soreness in the jaw, headaches, buzzing sounds, changes in hearing, stiffness in the neck and shoulders, dizziness, and swallowing disorders. It is believed that much of the reason for this symptom complex relates to change of the mandibular posture and the resultant change in cervical posture, or vice versa; also called **craniomandibular cervical syndrome.**

thoracic outlet syndrome: mechanical problem related to the exit of arteries and nerves at the base of the neck leading down the arm, and can also involve the vein bringing blood back from the arm. Compression of these structures as they pass through a narrow space between the anterior scalene (scalenus anticus) muscle and first rib. Problem may be exacerbated by congenitally present additional cervical rib. An early sign is pain in the hand or shoulder. Arteries may be damaged in the process and cause an aneurysm in the area with possible break-off of clot from the aneurysm.

traction spur: bony excrescence appearing on the anterolateral surface of the vertebral body near but not at the body margin that arises as a result of disk degeneration.

transitional vertebra: vertebra whose structure features some of the characteristics of the two adjacent vertebra. A common example is the fifth lumbar vertebra that has partial sacral components.

wedging: deformity of vertebral body, caused by trauma or gradual collapse, resulting in wedge-shaped vertebra; can also occur congenitally.

Eponymic Spinal Disorders

Andersson lesion: lesions that have mixed patterns of disk plate sclerosis or bone absorption in some patients with ankylosing spondylitis

Marie-Strümpell d.: inflammation of the spine, occurring as a rheumatoid-type disease in children.

Pott d.: tuberculosis of the spine, usually in the lower thoracic segments.

Scheuermann d.: inflammation of the anterior cartilage of the bodies of the lower thoracic and upper lumbar segments, causing pain in some older, growing children. There is more than 5 degrees of wedging of at least three adjacent vertebrae as seen on radiographs.

Schmorl nodes: developmental change resulting in inferior or superior extension of the intervertebral disk into the vertebral bodies.

Nerve Root Diseases of the Spine

The nerve roots in the spinal canal lie in close contact with the vertebrae and emerge through openings called **foramina.** In the neck, nerve root irritation may be localized at the place where it exits through the foramen, whereas in the lumbar spine, nerve root irritation usually occurs one level above the point of nerve exit.

Vertebrae and nerve roots of the spine are the same in number, except for the cervical spine. There are seven cervical vertebrae and eight cervical nerve roots (see Fig. 9-1). This occurs because the first cervical nerve exits between the skull and the first cervical vertebra. Therefore between C-7 and T-1 the eighth cervical nerve makes its exit. After this level, all nerves exit in conformance with the vertebra above the point of exit. When the examiner speaks of the *nerve roots* of the spine, it is recorded singularly as C1 or C2, whereas if the examiner is speaking of the *intervertebral disk* between the vertebrae, it is recorded in combination as C1-2 or C2-3. The vertebrae are recorded individually as C1 or L4.

This section is concerned with the local spinal processes and the wide range of neurologic diseases seen by an orthopaedist and especially by a neurosurgeon.

cauda equina syndrome: sufficient pressure on the nerves in the low back to produce multiple nerve root irritation and commonly loss of bowel and bladder control.

compression of nerve root: mechanical process resulting from a tumor, fracture, or herniated disk; the resultant irritation is called **radiculitis** if there is actual inflammation around the nerve. Pain from this type of disorder is called **radicular pain.** A common lay term for pressure on the nerve is **pinched nerve,** as sometimes used by examiners. After surgery and a normal healing process, the patient may still have some irritation of the nerve, which is often referred to as **residual nerve root irritability. Sciatica** and **neuritis** may be used in describing these disorders, but the terms are not discrete in that the irritation of the nerve is not necessarily from within the spinal canal.

dermatome: refers to the distribution of sensory nerves near the skin that are responsible for pain, tingling, and other sensations (or lack of). The afferent nerve fibers (leading to the spinal cord) and cutaneous branches arise from a single posterior spinal nerve root and contain sensory fibers. Loss of sensation in a **dermatomal** distribution may indicate damage to a nerve root that is caused by a disk prolapse.

  referred pain: sclerotomic in distribution and felt distant from its origin (e.g., bursitis in the shoulder produces pain in the lateral arm, and sciaticlike leg pain can be referred from the low back area).

  sclerotomal pain: more diffuse and ill-defined pain arising from voluntary muscles in spasm, also called **myotomic distribution.**

neurofibroma: fibrous tumor of a nerve, which may affect a nerve root and thus give the appearance of herniated disk disease.

radiculopathy: disease of the nerve roots in or near the spinal canal as a result of direct pressure from a disk or inflammation of the nerve roots caused by disk or spinal joint disease.

root sleeve fibrosis: scar tissue surrounding a nerve in the spinal canal or neural foramen.

sacral cyst: abnormality in the spinal fluid sac in the sacrum.

Disk Diseases

A disk is described as having a soft or fluidlike center called the **nucleus pulposus** and is surrounded by radial, circular, and longitudinal fibers that are firm, like gristle in meat. These intervertebral (IV) disks are situated between the vertebrae and act as shock absorbers. Any portion of the disk may herniate or extrude into the spinal canal, causing irritation and pressure on a nerve (Fig. 9-5).

cartilage space narrowing: narrowing of any cartilage space; also called **disk space narrowing.**

degenerative disk disease: gradual or rapid deterioration of the chemical composition and physical properties of the disk space. This may involve a simple increase in the rigidity of the nuclear material to be more involved with cellular removal of abnormal tissue and an inflammatory response. If the ligaments around the disk space ossify, they are often referred to as **bony spurs.** Because the disk changes its physical properties, some clinicians describe the condition as a **disorganized disk;** that is, the normal property of a soft center surrounded by more rigid, fibrous tissue is disrupted. The inflammation and muscle

FIG 9-5 Diagram of herniated nucleus pulposus (*HNP*) as seen from back with spinous processes and laminae removed from pedicles (*P*). Note that disk protrusion between fourth and fifth lumbar vertebrae impinges on fifth lumbar nerve root. *(From Brashear RH, Raney BR:* Shand's handbook of orthopaedic surgery, *ed 9, St Louis, 1978, Mosby.)*

spasm that may result over a prolonged period are often referred to as **chronic cervical sprain,** reflecting the abnormal stresses on the ligaments.

discitis: inflammation or infection of the disk space.

discogenic pain: back pain resulting from the disk itself. This pain is mechanical in nature and worse with sitting rather than standing. May be due to annular tears.

disk space infection: infection in the space normally occupied by an intervertebral disk.

herniated intervertebral disk (HID): outpouching of a disk.

herniated nucleus pulposus (HNP): fibrous extrusion of semifluid nucleus pulposus through a ruptured intervertebral disk; damage results from pressure on the spinal cord or nerve roots, causing pain and disability; also called **herniated intervertebral disk (HID), ruptured disk, slipped disk.** There are four recognized degrees of disk displacement:

  intraspongy nuclear herniation: bulge of the disk within the annulus fibrosus.

  protrusion: displaced nuclear material causes a discrete bulge in the annulus, but no material escapes through the annular fibers.

  extrusion: displaced material reaches the spinal canal through disrupted fibers of the annulus, but remains connected to the central disk material.

  sequestration: displaced material escapes as free fragments, which may migrate elsewhere.

intervertebral disk narrowing: narrowing of the space between any two vertebral bodies.

Naffziger syndrome: intervertebral disk disease, cervical rib, or some other disorder causes the scalene muscles to go into spasm, resulting in pressure on the major nerve plexus of the arm, causing pain in the neck, shoulder, arm, and hand; also called **scalenus anticus syndrome.**

sequestered disk herniation: portion of intervertebral disk that is completely extruded into spinal canal.

Diseases of the Spinal Cord

Because *myelo-* is the Greek root for marrow, and because it was originally thought that the spinal cord was a part of the bone marrow, many words seem to denote bone diseases but actually refer to an affliction of the spinal cord. For that reason, the term *myelitis* is not used alone in this discussion; for example, it may be used to denote a disease of the bone marrow (osteomyelitis) or a disease of the spinal cord (poliomyelitis). This section contains a mixture of terms, some of which may not necessarily relate to the spine. Disorders that are most commonly congenital problems are discussed in a following section.

Myelo- Root Diseases, Acquired

myelalgia: pain in the spinal cord.

myelanalosis: wasting of spinal marrow; also called **tabes dorsalis.**

myelapoplexy: hemorrhage within the spinal cord.

myelasthenia: loss of nerve strength caused by some disorder of the spinal cord.

myelatrophy: atrophy (wasting away) of spinal cord because of lack of nutrition, causing it to diminish in size.

myelauxe: abnormal increase in size of spinal cord.

myeleterosis: abnormal alteration of the spinal cord.

myeloencephalitis: inflammation of spinal cord and brain; also called **myelencephalitis.**

myelomalacia: softening of the spinal cord. A term that may be used to describe a whitish magnetic resonance imaging finding on T2 images, which are related to ischemic changes in the cord.

myelomeningitis: inflammation of spinal cord and meninges (spinal membranes).

myeloneuritis: inflammation of spinal cord and peripheral nerves.

myeloparalysis: spinal paralysis.

myelopathy: functional disturbance and pathologic changes in the spinal cord. The myelopathies are defined as follows:

Nurick Classification Scale for Spinal Cord Compression Caused by Spondylosis

Grade 0: signs and symptoms of root involvement but without evidence of spinal cord disease.

Grade 1: signs of spinal cord disease but no difficulty in walking.

Grade 2: slight difficulty in walking but does not prevent full-time employment.

Grade 3: severe difficulty in walking that requires assistance and prevents full-time employment and avocation.

Grade 4: ability to walk only with assistance or with the aid of a frame.

Grade 5: chair-bound or bedridden.

Modified Frankel Classification for Cord Damage Caused by Any Cause
Grade A: complete motor and sensory involvement.
Grade B: complete motor involvement, some sensory sparing including sacral sparing.
Grade C: functionally useless motor sparing.
Grade D: functional motor sparing.
Grade E: no neurologic involvement.

myelophthisis: wasting of the spinal cord; reduction of cell-forming function of bone marrow.

myeloplegia: spinal paralysis.

myeloradiculitis: inflammation of spinal cord and nerve roots.

myeloradiculopathy: disease of spinal cord and spinal nerve roots.

myelorrhagia: spinal hemorrhage.

myelosclerosis: hardening of the spinal cord.

myelosyphilis: syphilis of the spinal cord.

Other Spinal Diseases or Conditions, Acquired

American Spinal Injury Association (ASIA) Impairment Scale:
A standard method of assessing the neurologic status of a person who has sustained a spinal cord injury.
A Complete: No motor or sensory function is preserved in the sacral segments S4-S5.
B Incomplete: Sensory, but not motor function, is preserved below the neurologic level and includes the sacral segments S4-S5.
C Incomplete: Motor function is preserved below the neurologic level, and more than half of key muscles below the neurologic level have a muscle grade less than 3.
D Incomplete: Motor function is preserved below the neurologic level, and at least half of the key muscles below the neurologic level have a muscle grade of 3 or more.
E Normal: motor and sensory function are normal.

Subaxial Injury Classification Scale:
The subaxial injury classification scale is a novel classification system for subaxial cervical spine injury based on three injury axes: morphology, integrity of the discoligamentous complex, and neurologic status. The purpose of this classification system is to categorize the injury and predict treatment. The higher the number of points a patient receives, the more severe the injury and the more likely surgery is needed. In the case of injury to multiple cervical levels, separate scores should be calculated for each level.

Morphology	
No Abnormality	0 points
Compression	1 point
Burst	1 point
Distraction	3 points
Rotation/translation	4 points
Discoligamentous Complex	
Intact	0 points
Indeterminate	1 point
(Isolated interspinous widening, MRI signal changes only)	
Disrupted	2 points
Neurologic Status	
Intact	0 points
Root injury	1 point
Complete cord injury	2 points
Incomplete cord injury	3 points
Continuous cord compression	(+1 point)

MRI, *Magnetic resonance imaging.*

central cord syndrome: most common of the incomplete traumatic cervical spinal cord syndromes characterized by motor impairment that is proportionately greater in the upper limbs than in the lower, with bladder dysfunction and a variable degree of sensory loss below the level of the cord lesion.

ependymoma: tumor of the spinal cord.

hematomyelia: effusion of blood (hemorrhage) into the substance of the spinal cord.

hematorrhachis: spinal apoplexy; hemorrhage into vertebral canal.

hyperlordosis: increase in the normal anterior concavity of the cervical or lumbar spine.

leptomeningitis: inflammation of the pia mater and arachnoid of the brain and spinal cord.

leptomeningopathy: disease of the arachnoid or pia mater of the brain and spinal cord.

lordosis: not a disease state, but the normal anterior concavity of the neck or low back.

meningioma: tumor arising from meninges, usually benign, does not recur if totally removed.

meningismus: apparent irritation of brain or spinal cord in which symptoms simulate meningitis but in which no actual inflammation of the membranes is present; also called **meningism.**

meningitis: inflammation of the meninges of the brain or spinal cord caused by infectious agents such as bacteria, fungi, or viruses.

meningocele: local cystic protrusion of meninges through a cranial fissure; may be congenital or acquired.

meningoencephalomyelitis: inflammation of brain and spinal cord and their membranes.

meningomyelitis: inflammation of spinal cord, its enveloping arachnoid and pia mater, and sometimes the dura mater.

piriformis syndrome: a clinical diagnosis based on complaints of pain and abnormal sensations in the buttocks region with extension into the hips and posterior thigh as is seen in sciatica. This is due to tightness of the piriformis muscle with pressure on the sciatic nerve.

SCIWORA: acronym for "spinal cord injury without radiographic abnormality." Seen more commonly in younger children

syringomyelia: cavities filled with fluid in spinal cord, usually involving upper segments initially and involving the shoulder muscles.

Thoracolumbar Injury Classification and Severity Score

For fractures and dislocation of the thoracic and lumbar spine. Less than 4 is nonoperative, 4 is nonoperative or operative, and more than 5 is operative.

Injury Morphology

Compression without burst	1
Compression with burst	2
Rotation/translation	3
Distraction	4

Neurologic Status

Intact	0
Nerve root	2
Spinal cord, conus medullaris incomplete	3
Spinal cord, conus medullaris complete	2
Cauda equina	3

Posterior Ligamentous Integrity

Intact	0
Suspected, intermediate	2
Disrupted	3

Congenital Disorders of the Spine

Myelo- Root Diseases, Congenital

myelatelia: imperfect development of the spinal cord.

myelocele: herniation and protrusion of substance of spinal cord through defect in the bony spinal canal.

myelocystocele: cystic protrusion of substance of the spinal cord through a defect in the bony spinal canal.

myelocystomeningocele: cystic protrusion of substance of the spinal cord, with meninges, through a defect in the spinal canal.

myelodiastasis: archaic term for softening or other destruction of the spinal cord.

myelodysplasia: defective development of any part of spinal cord.

myelomeningocele: herniation of cord and meninges through a defect in the vertebral column.

Other Spinal Disorders, Congenital

diastematomyelia: congenital defect associated with spina bifida in which the spinal cord is split in half by bony spicules or fibrous bands, each half being surrounded by a dural sac.

failure of segmentation: failure of a portion or all of two or more adjoining vertebrae to separate into normal units.

hemivertebra: incomplete development of one side of a vertebral body, resulting in a wedge shape. If two hemivertebrae are near each other, they may be **balanced,** that is, the two wedges point in opposite directions, and a lesser curve or no curve results. **Unbalanced** means that there is no opposing wedge for one or more hemivertebrae, and the net result is an abnormal curve.

interspinous pseudarthrosis: formation of a false joint between two lumbar spinous processes caused by the congenitally large size of those processes; also called **Baastrup d.**

sacral agenesis: failure for normal development of the sacrum.

Renshaw Classification for Sacral Agenesis

Type I: partial or total unilateral agenesis.

Type II: partial sacral agenesis with a partial but bilateral symmetric defect and a stable articulation between the ilia; first sacral vertebra is normal or hypoplastic.

Type III: variable lumbar and total sacral agenesis; ilia articulate with the sides of the lowest vertebra present.

Type IV: variable lumbar and total sacral agenesis; caudal end plate of the most distal vertebra rests above either fused ilia or an iliac amphiarthrosis.

segmental spinal dysgenesis: a rare set of distinct spinal anomalies including focal stenosis at the level of the dysgenesis with the spinal segments below that point being normal.

spina bifida: congenital defect common in the low back (lumbosacral region) of infants in which part of a vertebra does not fully develop (and in severe cases, nerve tissue) leaving a portion of spinal cord exposed. There are four forms of spina bifida:

encephalocele: rare.

meningocele: not as severe.

myelocele: severe form; also called **meningomyelocele.**

spina bifida occulta (SBO): congenital defect consisting of the absence of a vertebral arch of the spinal column; normally, there are no symptoms.

symmetric fusion: equal fusion throughout the vertebral body.

tethered cord: neurologic disorder associated with failure of filum terminale to detach from the sacrum during fetal or early postnatal development growth.

unsegmented bar: fusion on one side or the other of the vertebrae, which may involve the posterior elements or vertebral bodies; may occur at multiple levels and skip vertebral segments and may result in severe curves.

Eponymic Congenital Spinal Disorders

Arnold-Chiari syndrome: congenital combination of brain herniation and exposed spinal cord in the lower back. Two types are described:

Type I: cerebellum displaced caudally, brainstem normal, hydrocephalus occasionally present, onset of symptoms in adolescence.

Type II: commonly associated with myelomeningocele, caudal displacement of entire brainstem, cerebellar dysplasia, hydrocephalus in 90%, symptoms in infancy.

Jarcho-Levin syndrome: extensive defects of the spine with associated defects in the ribs leading to a small, stiff thorax and pulmonary compromise.

Surgery of the Spine

The two types of back surgery as applied to orthopaedics are the removal of disk fragments, bone, or ligaments causing pressure on neural elements from the spinal canal and fusion of two or more vertebral segments. The definitions of disk surgery are given to present some important distinctions between procedures of the cervical spine as compared with those of the lumbar spine and to clarify the misuse of terms related to spinal surgical procedures.

Before **invasive spine surgery** takes place, such as removal of a herniated disk, conservative measures are often initially taken in the form of medications, physical therapy, activity modifications, and often interventional blocks (i.e., epidural corticosteroid injections, root injections, facet blocks). Tests to determine the cause of the symptoms are usually performed prior to interventions. These can include plain radiographs (x-rays), myelography followed by computed tomography (CT), magnetic resonance imaging (MRI), and occasionally discography.

For **myelography,** the patient is placed on a tilting table, and a needle is introduced into the subarachnoid space in the lower lumbar spine or upper cervical spine. Cerebrospinal fluid can be withdrawn for analysis and then one of several types of radiopaque contrast material injected. Currently, this material is water soluble. The contrast material infiltrates up and down the spinal canal to outline the nerve roots, nerve sleeves, dural sac, and, at higher levels, the spinal cord.

Multiple plain radiographs can be obtained at different angles and any given level to best outline the offending structure. A CT scan is then taken to obtain better definition of the areas in question. MRI is often used as a substitute for myelography and CT scanning because it does not require injection of contrast material into the spinal column. MRIs are performed and images reconstructed in axial or sagittal views. This examination can be performed in different modes or spins to give labels such as T1 and T2 images and can be done with contrast such as gadolinium to assess vascular tumors or scar tissue.

The following spinal surgical procedures are performed by orthopaedic surgeons.

chemonucleolysis: a little used, but once common procedure for lumbar disk herniation. Under direct radiographic control, a chemical that denatures the protein or protein sugar complex in the disk space is injected. The injected disk tends to dissolve itself, and the remaining cartilage cells repopulate the disk and produce ground substance similar in composition to normal nucleus pulposus, or continued degeneration and scar formation takes place. This procedure is designed to speed up the process of relief of compression of the nerve root without surgery. The procedure carries a risk similar to standard discectomy via laminectomy.

costotransversectomy: excision of the transverse process of a vertebra and the neighboring rib for approach to the spine or cord.

decompression: in relation to the spine this procedure is carried out to relieve pressure on the spinal cord or nerve roots. The pressure may result from fracture fragments, disk fragments, tumors, or infections. The approach may be anterior, lateral, or posterior.

decompressive laminectomy: a decompression done by removing the lamina and spinous process.

discectomy: the removal of intervertebral disk material placing pressure on neural elements. If the annulus of the disk is torn, the disk is protruded. If the fragment of the disk material is torn through a hole in the ligament, it is called an **extruded fragment** or **extruded disk.** If the fragment has migrated completely through the ligament, it is termed a **sequestered disk** or **free fragment.** The term **herniated nucleus pulposus (HNP)** is a catchall phrase for all of these conditions. In the neck, a fresh (soft) disk excision is sometimes done through a posterior approach (laminotomy). However, many cervical disk problems are approached anteriorly and include a spinal fusion.

foraminotomy: a procedure carried out alone or in conjunction with disk surgery. The foramina (tunnels or openings for the individual nerves to pass from the spine) may become narrowed because of disk impingement, intervertebral collapse, and spondylolisthesis. This surgical widening of the foramen is an attempt to relieve pressure on the nerve roots from a variety of causes.

kyphoplasty: for osteoporotic collapse fractures of the spine; a minimally invasive procedure with vertebral reduction using an inflatable balloon tamp, and space is then injected with methylmethacrylate.

laminectomy: removal of the lamina, the bony element covering the posterior portion of the spinal canal. This procedure removes the lamina on both sides of and including the spinous process. It may be performed at more than one level to approach the spinal cord and nerves for conditions including tumors and herniated disks. The spinal canal is approached from both sides of the spinous process, and the term is often inappropriately used in reference to the following two lesser procedures.

   hemilaminectomy: the excision of only one side of the lamina (right or left) relative to the spinous process.

   laminotomy: formation of a hole in the lamina without disrupting the continuity of the entire lamina to approach the intervertebral disk or neural structures (see Fig. 9-5). This is the most common approach to a herniated disk and is often mistakenly called a laminectomy when in fact it is a **partial laminotomy.**

laminoplasty: the lamina are hinged laterally, opened like a door, and secured in their new position with suture or bone to enlarge the spinal canal. Most often used in the cervical spine.

less invasive spine surgery (LISS): surgery done through smaller incisions using special retractors or access systems. Also an acronym for a less invasive stabilization system in which the screws are locked into the plate for long bone fracture fixation.

microsurgery: microdiscectomy using a microscope during the surgical procedure or to accomplish the procedure.

minimally invasive spine surgery (MISS): often described as being done with minimal disruption to surrounding tissue yet still getting access to a surgical site. This type of surgery may be accomplished with special retractor systems, endoscopes, or done percutaneously.

> **Spino-Pelvic Tumor Resection Classification for Reconstruction Following Combined Resection of Spinal and Pelvic Segments**
>
> **Type 1 resection:** total sacrectomy +/– lumbar spine resection and bilateral iliac wings; posterior stabilizing fusion lumbar spine to pelvis; fibular struts lumbar spine to pelvis
>
> **Type 2 resection:** hemisacrectomy +/– lumbar hemivertebrectomy and unilateral medial ilium; posterior stabilizing fusion lumbar spine to pelvis with unilateral strut lumbar spine to pelvis
>
> **Type 3 resection:** hemisacrectomy +/– lumbar hemivertebrectomy and external hemipelvectomy; none versus posterior stabilizing fusion remaining lumbar spine to remaining hemipelvis
>
> **Type 4 resection:** total sacrectomy +/– lumbar spine and external hemipelvectomy +/– medial ilium on retained side; femur of amputated leg used to connect lumbar spine to remaining hemipelvis

vertebroplasty: for vertebral fracture and collapse in osteoporosis, in which methylmethacrylate is percutaneously injected through a pedicle directly in defect to stop the pain caused by movement at the fracture site.

Spinal Fusions

A procedure in which two or more adjacent vertebrae are induced to grow together as a single, solid bone by destroying the intervening joints or disks and adding bone or bone substitutes that eventually heal into a solid bone bridge between the vertebrae. The fusion can be done anteriorly, posteriorly, or both. Spinal hardware or instrumentation is often used to stabilize the vertebrae, which helps with bone growth between them. The indications for fusion are spinal instability (caused by disease or iatrogenic from extensive decompression), arthritis, deformity correction, and in some instances pain. The excision of an intervertebral disk does not necessarily lead to symptomatic chronic degenerative arthritis or instability and is not in itself an indication for spinal fusion. However, it is often the case that disk surgery and spinal fusions are done concurrently for a variety of reasons. Fusions are sometimes done to restore adequate stability when it has been disturbed by a fracture, tumor, infection, or surgery. The lumbosacral region is the most common area for spinal fusions.

anterior spinal fusion: approaching the spine from the front, the intervertebral disk or vertebral body is removed and bone graft is inserted. Some variations of this procedure include the **Smith-Robinson p.**, **Cloward p.**, and **dowel p.**

cervical spinal fusion: spinal fusion involving the seven cervical segments. This may include the base of the skull, the occiput, and the first thoracic spine. The fusion may be anterior or posterior, with or without bone graft, and with or without fixation.

- **Aebi, Etter, and Cosica f.:** anterior approach to inferior C2 to fractured dens with screws.
- **Bohman p.:** posterior triple spinous process wiring technique in the cervical spine to secure bone graft.
- **Brattstrom p.:** use of acrylic cement for C1 to C2 fusion.
- **Brooks and Jenkins f.:** loops of wire around lamina of C1 and C2 to hold bone graft between lamina.
- **Callahan p.:** individual wire fixation of a strut bone graft to involved facets.
- **de Andrade and MacNab f.:** anterior approach for cervical occipital fusion.
- **Gallie f.:** wire around lamina of C1 and spinous process of C2.
- **Halifax f.:** clamp across lamina of C1 and C2.
- **Mageri f.:** wire looped around lamina of C1 and C2.
- **Magerl f.:** transarticular facet screw fusion for posterior C1 on C2 with the use of bilateral screws directed from inferior posterior lateral mass to anterior superior C1.
- **McAfee f.:** anterior retropharyngeal approach to upper cervical spine; often used for fusion, allowing excision of tumor.
- **Meyer f.:** for C1 on C2 instability, posterior fusion using vertical strut grafts and wires.
- **Newman f.:** C1 to C2 posterior fusion without fixation.
- **Overton f.:** a dowel graft that is applied across facet joints.
- **Robinson and Riley f.:** an extensive anterior approach for fusion of C1 to C3 or lower.
- **Roy-Camille f.:** for stabilization between the skull and C2; posterior bone graft with wire and parallel vertical screw plate fixation from occiput to C3.

Simmons f.: use of keystone-shaped graft in anterior fusion.

Spetzler f.: approach to anterior C1 to C3 by using a transoral approach for fusion following excision of tumor.

Wertheim Bohlman f.: for occipital cervical fusion; use of iliac crest graft and wire fixation from occiput to C2.

Whitecloud and Larocca f.: anterior technique for cervical spine fusion using fibular graft.

Hibbs spinal f.: a lumbar spinal fusion that includes fusing the spinous process, lamina, and facet for stabilization.

posterior cervical spinal f.: spinal fusion done from the back, using the lamina, facets, and spinous processes of the neck.

Roger f.: posterior cervical fusion using iliac cortical and cancellous grafts.

Southwick f.: a posterior fusion with wire attaching bone graft to the facet joints.

posterior lumbar spinal f.: spinal fusion done from the back using the lamina, the facets, and spinous processes of the lower back.

Albee f.: fusion of the spine using grafts across the spinous processes in spondylolisthesis.

Bosworth f.: fusion using an H-shaped bone graft in spondylolisthesis.

Dwyer-Hartsill f..: for failed lumbar degenerative disk disease; pedicle screws wired to a rectangular frame along with posterolateral fusion.

Gill f.: removal of the posterior spinal arch in spondylolisthesis.

Gill, Manning, and White f.: a procedure sometimes combined with a posterolateral spinal fusion.

posterior spinal f.: a fusion of the cervical, thoracic, or lumbar regions primarily fusing the lamina and sometimes the facet joints, using iliac or other bone graft.

posterolateral f.: a fusion of both the lamina and transverse process, using the iliac bone for graft, usually in the lower lumbar and first sacral segments.

posterolateral interbody f. (PLIF): lumbar spine fusion that involves an interbony fusion accomplished through the posterior approach.

transforaminal lumbar interbody f. (TLIF): approaching the spine in a similar manner as the posterolateral interbody f. but more from the side of the spinal canal through a midline incision in the patient's back. This approach reduces the amount of surgical muscle dissection and minimizes the nerve manipulation required to access the vertebrae, disks and nerves.

extreme lateral interbody fusion (XLIF): incision that traverses the abdomen and also avoids cutting or disrupting the muscles of the back. In this fusion technique, the disk space is accessed from a very small incision on the patient's side (flank) approximately two inches in length

Material Used for Bone Grafting in Spinal Fusion

For bone to grow between two vertebrae, one must provide material. The material can be **osteoinductive,** which means it can induce bone to form, that is, like autograft, which contains precursor cells that form bone. Or the material can be **osteoconductive,** which means it works as a scaffolding for bone to grow through. Autograft or bone from the patient is both osteoinductive and conductive. Several sources and types of graft are important in spine surgery.

autograft: bone taken from the patient. The sites of graft harvest can be the bone from the local area, that is, bone removed during decompression, or from separate sites, which may include additional incisions such as from the iliac crest, fibula, tibia, or occasionally from a vertebral body.

structural graft versus **morselized graft:** the material can be structural or morselized. Structural graft is needed to hold up disk spaces or replace vertebrae that may be removed. Morselized graft is used in posterior or posterolateral fusions where structural support is not required. It can also be used to fill a structural device such as a cage. (See "Spinal Instrumentation" later in this chapter.) The problems with autograft usually have to do with insufficient quantities for large surgeries, morbidity or problems at the site where it was harvested (i.e., fracture or infection), or pain at that site, which is most common.

allograft: human bone harvested from cadavers that can be processed into several types of usable forms. It can be made into morselized graft, putties, or granular material. It can also be made into spacers for the lumbar, thoracic, or cervical spine to fit into disk spaces or replace vertebral bodies. Most allograft used today is processed to prevent disease transmission. The lumbar replacements are often made of femoral rings and can be called **femoral ring allograft (FRA)**. The cervical spacers are made of fibulas, ulnas, or from the radius cut into rings. Allograft is osteoconductive and osteoinductive by the presence of proteins, which can induce bone formation as the cells are dead. Not as effective as autograft but quantity is not limited by what you can harvest and there is no graft site pain or complications.

xenograft: graft material from other animals such as bovine (cow bone) used in the past. Better products are now available.

Calcium phosphates are inert materials that are osteoconductive and can be used to expand the graft, that is, to make it more bulky when there is insufficient quantities, or on its own.

bone marrow aspirate: syringe of blood withdrawn from the marrow areas such as the iliac crest containing cells that can form bone, that is, osteoinductive. This is often added to allograft.

bone morphogenic proteins (BMP): osteoinductive proteins included in the superfamily of transforming growth factor–beta. Human BMP was discovered several decades ago by Marshall Urist at the University of California–Los Angeles. Since then, human BMP extracted and purified from cadaver bones has been used to accomplish fusions. Human BMP is of limited quantities. Through the use of recombinant genetic technology, a set of proteins, designated rhBMP-1 through rhBMP-9, have been produced to obtain unlimited quantities. One of these recombinant proteins, rhBMP-2, was found to promote new bone and cartilage growth. They are osteoinductive and are often used with a osteoconductive collagen scaffold, which also binds the proteins.

rhBMP-2: recombinant human bone morphogenic protein number 2, sold as INFUSE commercially, and is Food and Drug Administration approved for anterior interbody fusions with a lumbar-tempered (LT) cage.

rhBMP-7: sold as OP-1 is approved for use in posterior lumbar fusions.

platelet gels: by centrifuging blood there is a buffy coat layer that is rich in platelets and platelet derived factors. This also has osteoinductive ability and is used to form bone often with local graft or allograft.

trabecular metal: this is an implant made of tantalum with a porous structure that allows bone to directly grow into it. Ideally in this case two vertebra could be fused together by simply attaching on both sides of this device, obviating the need for graft material.

Spinal Instrumentation

Spinal instrumentation is composed of metal, plastic, carbon fiber, or resorbable devices that are used to stabilize the spine, correct deformity, take the place of removed elements such as disks or vertebral bodies, and now attempt to replicate spinal function. The commonest types of instrumentation systems are listed and defined with respect to where they are used.

screws: usually used in conjunction with a plate or rod system to hold vertebrae stable. Screws are the anchoring devices into vertebrae and then they are connected to the rods or plates with connecting devices. Screws can be used on their own in the spine in several situations: as compression screws during the treatment of type 2 odontoid fractures, isthmic screws in hangman fractures, translaminar screws, or facet screws in lumbar fusions.

anchoring screws: these screws are placed into the vertebral body, occiput, or pelvis and secured to a rod or plate system, which holds them and the vertebral bodies they attach to together.

cervical pedicle screws: are placed in C2 or C7 most commonly and connected to a rod screw construct.

iliac screws: often used to fix long spinal fusions with rods to the pelvis. In the Galveston technique, the rods themselves are bent and placed into the iliac wings to secure the system to the pelvis on each side.

lateral mass screws: usually used from C2–C6 and connected to a rod or plate construct.

occipital screws: placed in the midline at the back of the skull during occipital cervical fusions.

pedicle screws: for placement in thoracic and lumbar spines.

sacral screws: can be pedicle screws often in S1 or S2 or alar screws, which angle out into the sacral ala.

Other anchoring devices include wires such as Luque wires, which are placed around the lamina and secured to long rods during scoliosis surgery by twisting the wires. This type of fixation is most commonly used for neuromuscular scoliosis.

plates and screws: used for anterior fusions to buttress interbody fusions or vertebral replacements. The plates are commonly locking plates, which means the screw can be fixed to the plate and make the construct rigid. Posterior fusions sometimes use a plate and screw device such as the Steffi plate in the lumbar spine or lateral mass plates in the cervical spine. For occipital cervical fusion, plate devices are still used in the occiput.

cages: spacers that provide structural support to nonstructural bone grafting material until it heals into solid bone. Cages can be described by:
- **what they replace:** removed disks, that is, intervertebral spacers or vertebral body replacements.
- **what they are made of:** metals, such as titanium, tantalum, or steel, and in the past, plastics such as polyetheretherketone, carbon fiber, or even resorbable materials, which disappear once bone has grown through them.
- **how they are inserted:** anterior lumbar interbody fusion cages, posterior lumbar interbody fusion cages, transforaminal lumbar interbody fusion cages.
- **by their shape:** box cages, cylindrical cages.
- **by what they do:** that is, expandable cages.

Nonfusion Devices

New implants are being designed to replace anatomic elements of the spine but trying to maintain the original function unlike fusion devices.

disk replacements: currently metal-backed devices that try to mimic the function of the intervertebral disk once it has been removed for pathologic examination. Designed primarily for the lumbar and cervical spine. Their use has increased dramatically during the last 10 years. Currently the Charite disk, Bryan, Prestige and ProDisc-C are the only Food and Drug Administration–approved devices, but a multitude of companies and artificial disks may be available in the future.

ligament replacement devices: often anchored by pedicle screws to the vertebral body; also called **nonrigid stabilization devices.**

nucleus replacement: a technology not yet perfected but designed to replace the nucleus pulposus after herniation or degeneration; to reconstruct the springlike component of the intervertebral disk, which is lost once the disk has been damaged.

Names of Instrumentation Systems

AO fixateur interne: a posteriorly placed spinal fixation device.

Banks-Dervin rod: for scoliosis fixation; a multiple-level rod fixed with oblique spinous process to contralateral lamina screws.

Cotrel-Dubousset: posterior fixation device for spinal deformity, fracture, tumor, and degenerative conditions.

Dwyer: anteriorly placed screws and band device for correction of spinal deformities.

Edwards: a posterior rod and sleeve device used in stabilization of traumatic spinal conditions.

Harrington rod: an instrumentation and fusion using a straight, stiff rod for distraction or compression; associated with a posterior spinal fusion in the thoracic or thoracolumbar spine for scoliosis or trauma.

Isola: a posterior fixation device.

Jacobs locking hook: thick, threaded rods for fixation of various spinal deformities.

Kaneda: an anteriorly placed fixation device for spinal deformities.

Knodt distraction rod: for distraction stabilization of thoracic and lumbar spine.

Kostuick-Harrington: anteriorly placed device for spinal deformity correction.

Long Beach pedicle screw: posterolateral fusion screw and rod device.

Luque: a posterior method of fixation.

Luque interspinal fusion (ISF): for posterolateral fusion fixation; a pedicle screw and plate device.

Rogozinski: a combined anteroposterior device used in correction of spinal deformities.

Roy-Camille: posterior pedicle screw and plate device for spinal stabilization.

Steffee plate: for posterolateral fusion fixation; plate and screw device.

Texas Scottish Rite Hospital: instrumentation used anteriorly and posteriorly.

Vermont (Krag): posteriorly placed internal fixation device.

Wiltse plate: screw plate device for posterior spinal stabilization.

Wisconsin interspinous segmental spinal: series of wires, rods, and buttons for multisegmental spine stabilization also called **Drummond interspinous segmental spinal.**

Zielke: a method of fracture treatment with transpedicular fixation.

Miscellaneous Procedures on the Spine

Bradford p.: for kyphoscoliosis deformity; staged anterior and posterior approach for interbody fusion and correction of deformity.

Capner p.: draining of thoracic spinal abscess through an anterolateral approach.

coccygectomy p.: excision of the coccyx (tailbone).

coccygotomy p.: incision into the coccyx (tailbone).

commissural myelorrhaphy p.: a longitudinal division of the spinal cord to sever crossing fibers.

cordotomy p.: transverse incision into the spinal cord.

corpectomy p.: excision of vertebral body usually combined with interposition of prosthesis or bone graft.

Dunn p.: for myelomeningocele spinal deformity; use of contouring L-rod for posterior stabilization.

eggshell p.: excavation of vertebral body for correction of deformity that is combined with spinal fusion.

facetectomy p.: excision of an articular facet of a vertebra.

Getty p.: for decompression of lumbar spinal stenosis; excision of lamina and portion of facet.

Goldstein p.: for scoliosis deformity graft incorporating posterior elements, including facet joints and ribs.

Hodgson p.: anterior approach to C1 and C2 area for drainage of tuberculous abscess.

kyphectomy p.: for kyphotic deformity in myelodysplasia; excision of kyphotic portion of lumbar spine combined with spinal fixation.

Leeds p.: for scoliosis, segmental wiring of a contoured square-ended Harrington rod.

Localio p.: for sacral tumor; a method of partial excision of the sacrum.

Loughheed and White p.: for drainage of lower abdominal abscess; coccygectomy and drainage from space anterior to sacrum.

MacCarthy p.: for sacral tumor; a method of excision of the sacrum.

myelotomy p.: a procedure for severing tracts in the spinal cord.

Ponte osteotomy p.: for kyphotic deformity in patients with Scheuermann's kyphosis; the anterior column is lengthened and the posterior column shortened.

rachicentesis p.: lumbar puncture for examination of the spinal fluid; rachiocentesis.

rachiotomy p.: incision into a vertebral canal for exploration.

rachitomy p.: surgical or anatomic opening of the vertebral canal.

radiculectomy p.: excision of a rootlet or resection of spinal nerve roots.

rhizotomy p.: division of the roots of the spinal nerves.

Risser p.: for scoliosis deformity; particular attention to fusion of facet joints and use of cast stabilization.

Roaf, Kirkaldy-Willis, and Cattero p.: drainage of thoracic spinal abscess through dorsolateral approach.

Schollner costoplasty: for rib deformity or scoliosis; multiple rib partial excisions.

Scott p.: use of cross-wire fixation transverse process to inferior pedicle in stabilization of spondylolysis fusion.

Seddon p.: drainage of thoracic spinal abscess through anterolateral approach with partial resection of rib.

Simmons p.: for cervical spinal kyphosis; a posterior osteotomy.

Smith Peterson p.: for correction of kyphotic deformity in ankylosing spondylitis; lumbar spine osteotomy.

Speed p.: for spondylolisthesis spine fusion and anterior interbody fusion by using tibial cortical graft; also called **Kellogg Speed p.**

spondylosyndesis: surgical immobilization or ankylosis by fusion of the vertebral bodies with a short bone graft in cases of tuberculosis of the spine; also called **spondylodesis** and **Albee p.**

spondylotomy p.: incision into a vertebra or vertebral column; also called **rachiotomy p.**

Tsuli p.: for severe cervical spondylosis; an expansive, multiple laminectomy.

Wiltse p.: a bilateral lateral spine fusion for spondylolisthesis.

Winter p.: for hemivertebra deformity; anterior and posterior approach with stabilization. Also a procedure for correction of congenital kyphosis, by using an anterior approach and strut bone grafts.

Spinal Approaches

anterior a.: when used to approach the cervical, cervicodorsal, dorsal, and lumbar spines, it is designed to provide sufficient surface for multiple segmental spinal fusions; also called **Hodgson a.** and **Roaf a.**

anterior a.: for specific cervical spinal explorations and fusions; also called **Southwick a.; Robinson a.; Bailey a.; Badgley, Whitesides, and Kelly a.;** and **Henry a.** (to the vertebral artery).

anterolateral a.: an approach to the dorsal spine by rib resection to explore the spine anteriorly and in some cases to do spinal fusions and decompressions of the spinal cord.

dorsolateral a.: an approach to the dorsal spine by costotransversectomy, usually done for fractures and other affections of the spinal cord.

Lehmer a.: for adult isthmic spondylolisthesis using a paramedian retroperitoneal approach

posterior a.: used for laminectomies and spinal fusions at any level; also called **Hibbs a.** and **Wagoner a.**

The Hand and Wrist

10

Where is there available a precision instrument that can either gently pick up eggs or lift 200 pounds? That can detect the weight of only four grains of sand, temperature differences of 1 degree, and the distance between two points less than 0.1 inch? That is remote controlled, self-powered, and transportable to any part of the world? This priceless tool is available at no cost to almost all humankind—the hand.

A description of the intricate anatomic features of the hand and wrist is presented with illustrations. The sequence of definitions given here will help to define the basics of hand control, kinematics, and function. The chapter reflects changes in the anatomy format, with an explanation of zones, pulleys, and other miscellaneous names specific to the hand.

There are many abbreviations used in hand anatomy because of the lengthy Latin names, for example, flexor pollicis longus (FPL) tendon or metacarpophalangeal (MCP) joint. Usually the Latin name is spelled out initially and abbreviated subsequently. Appendix A, Orthopaedic Abbreviations, lists the many hand abbreviations used to simplify the terminology.

Anatomy of the Hand and Wrist

Bones (Fig. 10-1)

accessory bone: an extra bone that may develop in the carpus of the wrist as seen on radiographs; an anomaly.

carpal bones: the eight bones of the anatomic wrist, arranged in a proximal and distal row, and held firmly together by ligaments. The proximal row from lateral to medial (radial to ulnar) includes the **scaphoid (navicular), lunate (semilunar), triquetrum (triangular),** and **pisiform.** The distal row leading from the thumb side is composed of the **trapezium (greater multangular), trapezoid (lesser multangular), capitate (os magnum),** and **hamate (unciform).**

carpus: the wrist; term applied to the structures of the wrist including the carpal bones.

DRUJ: acronym commonly used to describe the distal radial ulnar joint (pronounced *drudge*).

fossae (fossa, sing.): the scaphoid and lunate fossae are normal recesses in the articular surface of the distal radius that allow articulation of the scaphoid and lunate, respectively.

hamulus: not a separate bone; this term is used to describe the hook of the hamate in the wrist.

metacarpals: the five long bones of the hand in the palm area. The bases of the metacarpal bones articulate proximally with the distal row of carpal bones.

phalanges (phalanx, sing.): the bones of the thumb and fingers. Each phalanx has a proximal base, shaft, neck, and distal head. There are two phalanges in the thumb (proximal and distal) and three phalanges in each of the four digits (proximal, medial, and distal).

sesamoids: small bones on the medial and lateral side of the base of the proximal phalanx of the thumb (metacarpophalangeal [MCP] joint). The sesamoids

FIG 10-1 Bones of the right hand and wrist, dorsal surface. *(From Anthony C, Kolthoff N:* Textbook of anatomy and physiology, *ed 9, St Louis, 1975, Mosby.)*

articulate with the head of the metacarpal bone to which muscles are attached. A sesamoid bone may also be found on the lateral side of the MCP joint of the index finger and medial side of the MCP joint of the little finger.

sigmoid notch: the articular surface on the distal radius that accepts the ulna in the distal radioulnar joint.

styloids: bony protuberances off the radius and ulna that act as attachment sites for the radial and ulnar collateral ligaments, respectively. The ulna styloid base is also an attachment for the triangular fibrocartilage complex.

tubercles: bony prominences that provide ligamentous attachment. In the hand, these include the scaphoid, trapezium, Lister tubercle, and the hook of the hamate.

tuft: the terminal bony expansion of the distal phalanx.

Joints

The joints of the hand are remarkable for the variability of motion that supports the fingers and thumbs in many tasks (e.g., the carpometacarpal [CMC] joint of the thumb can move in all planes). The joints of the phalanges are the proximal, medial, and distal joints and are referred to as follows:

    Carpometacarpal (CMC)
    Distal interphalangeal (DIP)
    Interphalangeal (IP)
    Metacarpophalangeal (MCP)
    Midcarpal (MC)
    Proximal interphalangeal (PIP)
    Radiocarpal (RC)

volar plate: a thickening of the joint capsule of the volar aspect of the MP and IP joints that prevent hyperextension of these joints. Proximally, these begin with the check-rein ligaments.

Muscles

There are large muscles in the forearm that insert into the bones of the hand by means of their tendons (Figs. 10-2 and 10-3). These **extrinsic muscles** cause the hand and fingers to flex and extend (close and open). The **intrinsic**

FIG 10-2 Muscles of the anterior aspect of the human hand; the palmar aponeurosis has been removed. *(From DiDio LJA: Synopsis of anatomy, St Louis, 1970, Mosby.)*

FIG 10-3 Muscles of the anterior aspect of the human hand. *(From DiDio LJA: Synopsis of anatomy, St Louis, 1970, Mosby.)*

muscles are small and originate within the hand. These control positioning, and, to a large extent, functional coordination of the fingers. In normal hand function, all these groups work together in intricate unison.

Extrinsic Muscle Function

wrist flexors: flexor carpi ulnaris (FCU), palmaris longus (PL), flexor carpi radialis (FCR); insert on the metacarpals, carpal bone, and ligaments. They cause strong wrist flexion.

wrist extensors: extensor carpi radialis longus (ECRL), extensor carpi radialis brevis (ECRB), extensor carpi ulnaris (ECU); insert on the metacarpals.

finger flexors: flexor digitorum profundus (FDP), flexor digitorum sublimis or flexor digitorum superficialis (FDS), flexor pollicis longus (FPL) (thumb); insert on either the distal or the middle phalanges of the digits and cause powerful finger or thumb flexion.

finger extensors: extensor digiti quinti proprius (EDQP), extensor digitorum communis (EDC), extensor indicis proprius (EIP); insert on the bones and extensor hoods of the fingers and cause extension of the digits.

thumb extensors: extensor pollicis longus (EPL) and **extensor pollicis brevis (EPB).**

thumb abductors: abductor pollicis longus (APL) and **abductor pollicis brevis (APB).**

thumb adductors: extensor pollicis longus (EPL) and **adductor pollicis (AdP).**

Intrinsic Muscle Function

hypothenar muscles: opponens digiti quinti (ODQ) or **opponens digiti minimi (ODM), flexor digiti quinti brevis (FDQB), abductor digiti quinti (ADQ)** or **abductor digiti minimi (ADM);** a less important group of intrinsic muscles that arise from the carpal bones and insert on the little finger, metacarpal, and proximal phalanx.

intrinsic muscles: lumbricals, dorsal interossei, volar interossei; arise from the metacarpals or from the flexor tendons and insert into the finger dorsal (extensor) mechanism and base of the proximal finger bone. They are responsible for spreading and bringing together the fingers and for firm coordination of motion at each finger joint.

thenar muscles: opponens pollicis (OP), abductor pollicis brevis (APB), flexor pollicis brevis (FPB) deep and superficial head (the deep head is sometimes called *first palmar interosseous* [intrinsic muscles of the thumb]); arise from the carpal bones and ligaments at the base of the palm and insert on the proximal phalanx or on the thumb metacarpal. They function to bring the thumb out and away from the palm and to oppose it to the other fingers. One intrinsic muscle arises from the metacarpals and crosses deep in the palm to the thumb. This adductor pollicis muscle pulls the thumb forcefully back in toward the palm (adduction).

Associated Forearm Muscles and Tendons

other muscles in the forearm: brachioradialis, pronator teres (PT), supinator, anconeus, and **pronator quadratus (PQ);** these do not extend to the hand but affect the position of the hand by actions such as rotation of the forearm (pronation and supination).

aponeurosis: term usually used to denote the whitish or silvery thick membranes that separate muscles, but in the hand is a description of the entire extensor apparatus of the digits distal to the MCP joint to its insertion on the proximal end of the distal phalanx.

extensor carpi radialis intermedius: an anatomic variant (a third radial wrist extensor) that can be used to restore thumb function in paralytic disorders when present.

extensor digitorum brevis manus muscle: an anatomic variant of the extensor indicis proprius muscle originating from the dorsal lip of the distal radius inserting on the extensor indicis proprius.

flexor wad of five: five muscles with a common origin in the medial elbow: **pronator teres (PT), flexor digitorum profundus (FDP)** and **flexor digitorum sublimis (FDS), palmaris longus (PL),** and **flexor carpi radialis (FCR).**

flexor tendons of the wrist: flexor carpi radialis (FCR) is the radial wrist flexor that travels in its own tunnel and inserts at the base of the second metacarpal. The **flexor carpi ulnaris (FCU)** (the ulnar wrist flexor) is the more important and powerful. It has a primary insertion on the pisiform but will send fibers distally to intermesh with the hypothenar muscle fascia. These tendons, with a synovial lining, glide back and forth through the tunnel as the fingers and wrist are moved.

radial sagittal bands: transverse tendinous structures on the radial side of the central extensor tendon slip in the region of the MCP joint to prevent ulnar subluxation of the extensor digitorum communis with flexion of the MCP joint.

retinacular ligament: fibrous bands that cover tendon tunnels such as extensor retinaculum and flexor pulleys.

Flexor Zones

A surgical zone system has been established for the fingers, hand, wrist, and forearm. The anatomic zones are important in determining technical considerations for each zone, surgical approaches, and corrections for different disorders. The clinical importance of anatomic zones is that, if an area is left unrepaired, specific deficits will occur in the extensor or flexor tendon zones.

zone I: from flexor digitorum profundus insertion to flexor digitorum sublimis insertion, anatomic structures found distal to the insertion of the sublimis tendon into the middle phalanx.

zone II: the anatomic structures found in the region just proximal to the A1 pulley up to zone I; also called **no-man's land.**

   Camper chiasm: a bifurcation of the flexor digitorum sublimis (FDS) in zone II that allows passage of the flexor digitorum profundus through it. This occurs just proximal to the insertion of the FDS in the middle phalanx; also called **chiasma tendinum.**

zone III: anatomic structures at the origin of the lumbricals in the region of the arterial arch, from the carpal tunnel to zone II.

zone IV: the carpal tunnel.

zone V: anatomic area of the wrist proximal to the carpal tunnel.

Pulleys

Pulleys are thickened portions of flexor tendon sheaths that hold tendons in place. They are labeled as *annular* or *cruciate*, depending on the orientation of the fibers of the pulley. The most proximal pulley is located on the distal metacarpal and is labeled annular 1 (A1) and then annular 2 through 4. The cruciate pulleys are similarly labeled C1 through C3 (Fig. 10-4).

A1	zone II	C1	zone II
A2	zone II	C2	zone I
A3	zone II	C3	zone I
A4	zone I	A0	zone IV (palmar fascia)

Ligaments and Fascia

There are numerous ligaments named for the bones to which the ligaments are attached.

deep transverse metacarpal l.: specific distal ligaments between the second, third, fourth, and fifth MCP volar plates.

juncturae tendinum: tendinous interconnection between extrinsic extensors over the dorsum of the

FIG 10-4 This anatomic diagram of various parts of flexor sheath is helpful in understanding gliding of tendon. Maintenance of second annulus (A2) and fourth annulus (A4) is essential to retain appropriate angle of approach and prevent bowstringing of flexor tendons or tendon graft. *(From Doyle JR, Blythe W: In American Academy of Orthopaedic Surgeons:* symposium on tendon surgery in the hand, *St Louis, 1975, Mosby.)*

hand. These allow synchronized digital extension; also called **connexus intertendineus.**

transverse carpal l.: the strong ligamentous band that lies across the arch of the carpal bones forming the roof of the carpal tunnel. It covers the median nerve and binds down the nine long flexor tendons of the thumb and fingers.

triangular l.: interconnecting fibers that join the two lateral bands dorsally and hold them in place. They are located over the proximal end of the middle phalanx just distal to the insertion of the central slip of the extensor tendon; also called **triangular fibrocartilage complex.**

Vickers ligament: volar fibrous band that runs from radius to the lunate, implicated in Kienböck disease.

vincula longa and breva: vascular and fibrous connections from the floor of the flexor tunnel to each of the two flexor tendons. The vincula breva lie close to the tendon insertions.

volar carpal l.: the ligament that spans and covers the median nerve and canal of Guyon and runs from the transverse carpal ligament radially to the hypothenar fascia ulnarly. This ligament binds down the nine long flexor tendons of the thumb and fingers.

Extrinsic Wrist Ligaments

dorsal intercarpal l.: connects radial distal row to ulnar proximal row.

dorsal radiocarpal l.: radiolunatotriquetrum.

volar l.: deep radioscaphocapitate, long radioscapholunate, short radioscapholunate, and radiolunate and ulnar lunate.

Intrinsic Wrist Ligaments

arcuate l.: a major stabilizer of the MC joint; ulnar arm (triquetrocapitate l.), radial arm (distal to scaphocapitate l.); also called **deltoid l.**

deep transverse intermetacarpal l.: fibrous interconnections between metacarpal heads II through V.

intermediate l.: lunatotriquetrum, scapholunate, and scaphotrapezium.

long l.: volar intercarpal deltoid arcuate.

short l.: interosseous.

space of Poirer: a weak area of the MC joint, that is, the arcuate ligament volar and distal to the lunate because the capitolunate l. is either absent or attenuated.

superficial transverse intermetacarpal l.: the expansion of the palmar fascia in the region of the distal metacarpals; also called **natatory l.**

Collateral Ligaments

The collateral ligaments of the elbow and wrist are supportive ligaments providing stability on the medial and lateral side of the wrist joint.

radial collateral l.: scaphocapitate l. (radial arm).
ulnar collateral l.: triquetrocapitate l. (ulnar arm).

Digital Collateral Ligaments

accessory l.: originates volar and deep to the main collateral ligaments and runs to the volar plate.

beak l.: volar ulnar ligament that stabilize the CMC joint of the thumb; originates on the volar aspect of the triscaphe joint and inserts on the volar ulnar surface of the proximal thumb metacarpal.

dorsal extensor compartments: the six fascial compartments on the dorsum of the distal radius for the wrist extensors numbering from radial to ulnar; these are defined by extensor retinacular tunnels over the wrist.

   I: abductor pollicis longus and extensor pollicis brevis.
   II: extensor carpi radialis longus and brevis.
   III: extensor pollicis longus.
   IV: extensor indicis proprius and extensor digitorum communis II-V.
   V: extensor digiti minimi or quinti.
   VI: extensor carpi ulnaris.

dorsal radial l.: primary stabilizer for thumb CMC joint.

main l.: runs from the center of rotation of the metacarpal or phalangeal head to the proximal metaphyseal flair of the phalanx adjoining.

Palm

Palmar Fascial Compartments

flexor and extensor retinacula: special thickening of deep fascia where muscles of forearm become tendons and pass into the hand into a broad band of superficial fascia over the dorsum of the wrist; help to restrain the extensor tendons and prevent tendons from bowstringing away from wrist.

digital retinaculum: the covering fascia of the finger flexors.

hypothenar eminence: prominence caused by intrinsic muscle mass on little finger side of the palm.

hypothenar space: deep space overlying the fifth metacarpal that may or may not be connected to the thenar space proximally.

Kanavel spaces: two fascial spaces of the palm, one thenar and one midpalmar, lying deep to the long flexor tendons and separated by a septum.

Landsmeer l.: fibrous tissue bands on the lateral side of the fingers that help to synchronize the motion of the two distal joints; also called **oblique retinacular ligaments.**

midpalmar space: a deep potential pace that runs from the third to fifth ray.

natatory l.: another name for the superficial transverse intermetacarpal l.

palmar fascia: complex interwoven fascia in the palm of the hand that is a part of the expansion of the palmaris longus and protects the delicate structures in the hand.

palmar skin crease: the creases in the palm caused by natural folds in the skin. These are labeled as **distal palmar crease (DPC), midpalmar crease (MPC),** and **thenar palmar crease (TPC)** (the life line). The digital skin creases are labeled *proximal, middle,* and *distal.*

septae (septa, sing.): two fibrous septae pass deeply from sides of palmar aponeurosis and separate muscles of the thenar and hypothenar deep spaces from midpalmar space.

thenar eminence: the prominence caused by intrinsic muscle mass on the thumb side of the palm.

thenar space: the potential space on the thumb side of the hand deep to the tendons and nerves.

web l.: expansion of the palmar fascia between the base of the fingers.

Bursa

All bursae (bursa, sing.) are lined with synovial sheaths (tenosynovium). Following are the important ones in the hand.

intermediate bursa: occasionally seen anatomically as the bursa containing the index finger flexor tendon sheath.

radial bursa: sac containing the FPL tendon sheath in the palm and thumb.

ulnar bursa: sac in the palm containing tendon sheaths of the index, long, ring, and little fingers and extending to the end of the little finger.

Miscellaneous

anatomic snuff box: the area of the lateral wrist formed between the extensor pollicis longus tendon medially, and abductor pollicis longus and extensor pollicis brevis tendons laterally. With the thumb abducted and extended, a triangular depression is made on the dorsum of the wrist at the radial border.

arcade of Frohse: tunnel through supinator muscle for the deep radial nerve; anatomic series of arches.

carpal tunnel: space in the wrist created by the volar carpal ligament. This space contains the flexor tendons of the fingers and thumb, as well as the median nerve.

Guyon canal: space between the hamate and pisiform bones at the wrist for the ulnar artery and nerve, covered by the ulnar side of the volar carpal ligament. Floor is the pisohamate ligament.

hook of hamate: bony prominence (tubercle) that provides ligamentous attachment; **hamulus.**

ligamentum subcruentum: the loose, richly vascularized connective tissue that sits near the ulnar styloid in between the limbs of the distal radial ulnar joint ligament.

Lister tubercle: bony prominence on the distal dorsal radius for ligamentous attachment.

radial lunate angle: an angle created by the line perpendicular to the line connecting the distal tips of the lunate on the lateral x-ray with the long axis of the radius. This is used to estimate dorsal intercalated segment instability and volar intercalated segment instability deformities in wrist injuries.

slider crank mechanism: an engineering model of scaphoid motion in carpal kinematics.

The Fingers

central slip: the portion of the extensor tendon that inserts into the middle phalanx; also called **tendon.**

cutaneous l.: ligaments that restrain the skin during finger motion and include the following:

Cleland l.: fibrous tissue bands on the lateral side of the fingers that stabilize the skin during finger movement, dorsal to Grayson l.

Grayson l.: fibrous tissue bands of the finger extending from the volar DIP and PIP joints to the lateral skin.

distal pulp: the mass of tissue of the volar distal finger. It is the soft cushion of the palmar surface of the distal phalanx.

dorsal expansion: the fibers spreading laterally at the base of the dorsal hood.

extensor hood: the fanlike expansion of the extensor communis tendon over the dorsum and sides of the MCP joints. This complex structure brings together intrinsic and extrinsic tendons to control IP joint extension and MP joint flexion or extension.

interdigital commissure: floor of the webspace between two digits, which follow a very specific anatomic pattern and must be carefully reconstructed in syndactyly surgery.

knuckle pad: the thick skin over the dorsum of the DIP and PIP joints of the finger.

lateral bands: the portions of the intrinsic muscle tendons that run laterally across the proximal phalanx to the dorsum of the DIP and PIP joints.

septa: fibrous tissue structures in fat pad of the fingertips.

skin creases: indentations in the skin at the point of natural motion points of the finger. The digital skin creases are labeled *proximal, medial,* and *distal.*

webspace: the skin web area between the base of the fingers.

The Nail

cuticle: the skin edge immediately covering the base of the fingernail.

eponychium: thin skin covering (epidermis) at the base of the nails on the dorsal surface; also called **cuticle.**

germinal matrix: the cells that generate the tissues that eventually form the nail from the base of the nail; primitive stage of development.

hyponychium: the thickened epidermis immediately under the distal portion of the nail; also called **subungual tissue.**

lunula: the white crescentic (half-moon shaped) area at the base of the nail.

nail matrix: the proximal portion of the nail bed from which growth mainly proceeds; also, the tissue on which the deep aspect of the nail rests; also called **matrix unguis** and **nail bed.**

nail plate: the hard plate of the distal end of the dorsum of the fingers and thumbs. This rigid outer covering extends approximately 8 mm under the nail fold (perionychium) and arises from the nail bed (matrix unguis).

paronychium: a fold of skin (nail folds) that surrounds the nail at the base; the epidermis bordering the nail; also called **perionychium.**

subungual space: the potential space between the nail and nail bed; common site for a hematoma.

unguis: the horny cutaneous plate on the dorsal surface of the distal end of a finger; also called the **finger nail.**

Nerves and Arteries

antebrachial cutaneous n.: medial-lateral and sensory to the thumb.

axolemma: a column of neuronal cytoplasm enclosed by cell membrane including cell body, dendrites, and the axon.

common digital arteries and nerves: the main branch of the various nerves or arteries in the palm; these then divide into the proper digital arteries and nerves (Fig. 10-5).

dorsal digital artery and nerve: common and proper, the branches of artery and nerve in the dorsum of the finger.

intercompartmental supraretinacular arteries: these are series of arteries that branch off of the radial artery and supply the dorsal aspect of the distal radius, and are described by the relationship to the extensor compartment of the wrist and the extensor retinaculum. These are generally fairly superficial in nature, and are used in the formation of vascularized pedicle-based bone grafts.

intercostal nerves: an array of nerves that run between the ribs and are occasionally used in brachial plexus reconstruction.

interscalene triangle: an anatomic space defined anteriorly by the anterior scalene, posteriorly by the middle scalene, and inferiorly by the first rib. This space facilitates the exit of the subclavian vein and brachial plexus in thoracic outlet syndrome.

ANTERIOR (PALMAR) VIEW

FIG 10-5 Major arterial and nerve supply to the hand. Note the median nerve crossing under the carpal tunnel and the separate structure of the Guyon canal. *(Netter illustration from www.netterimages.com. © Elsevier Inc. All rights reserved.)*

---

lateral cutaneous nerve of forearm: sometimes provides sensation to the lateral side of the thumb metacarpal area.

Martin-Gruber connection: a connection between the median and ulnar nerve in the forearm in which fibers that normally travel with the ulnar nerve from the brachial plexus distally travel with median nerve until the midforearm and only enter the median nerve at that connection; also called **Martin-Gruber anastomosis**.

median n.: the nerve that conducts sensations from the hand to the central nervous system and crosses under the small volar carpal ligament. Supplies some of the small muscles of the thumb, including the opponens, the superficial head of the flexor pollicis brevis (FPB), and the abductor pollicis brevis, but not the adductor and the deep head of the FPB; provides sensation for most of the palm and volar thumb, long and index fingers, and thumb side of the ring finger. The motor branch controls muscles surrounding the thumb.

Meissner corpuscles: pressure receptors at nerve endings in the skin.

proper volar digital nerve and artery: the nerves and arteries after they have divided in the palm and travel along the two volar sides of the finger.

radial a.: major artery on the thumb side of the palm and wrist.

Riche-Cannieu connection: the deep motor branch of the ulnar nerve may send a branch to join the motor branch of the median nerve. The relevance is that in injuries to the median nerve at the wrist, one may still retain motor function at the wrist.

superficial and deep palmar arterial arches: the superficial and deep connecting arcades of the radial and ulnar artery in the palm.

superficial branch of radial nerve: this nerve supplies sensation only; sensory distribution is over the dorsum of the thumb, index finger, long finger, and radial side of the ring finger.

ulnar a.: artery on the little finger side of the palm and wrist.

ulnar n.: the nerve crossing the wrist through the Guyon canal and supplying the adductor pollicis, deep head of the flexor pollicis brevis, and all small muscles of the hand, except the thumb and first two lumbricals. The sensation supplied is to the little finger and the little finger side of the ring finger.

Vater-Pacini corpuscle: pain pinpoint receptor.

vinculae: blood vessel bridges to the flexor tendons having a **vinculum breve** and **vinculum longum.**

Diseases and Structural Anomalies

Most of the diseases that affect the bones and joints of the hand are described in Chapter 2. The specific terminology for deformities caused by rheumatoid arthritis, nerve injuries, and congenital defects related to the hand is listed here. The terminology for diseases of the hand comprises many words not specific to other parts of the anatomy and is divided as follows.

Arthritic Deformities

arthritis mutilans: a form of inflammatory arthritis manifesting extreme loss of bone stock; medullary, cancellous bones and markedly same with cortices, characteristic of psoriatic arthritis.

attenuation of tendons: erosion and eventual rupture of tendons by diseased synovium or bony spurs; also called **attrition attenuation of tendons.**

crystalline arthropathy: with chronic crystal formation there is recurrent joint inflammation, typically with fever and leukocytosis that affects fingers, wrists, and elbows; medical and surgical treatment indicated.

> **gout:** caused by hyperuricemia, increased blood levels of uric acid.
>
> **pseudogout:** the deposition of calcium pyrophosphate crystals with episodic inflammation of wrist and MP joints; also called **chondrocalcinosis.**

degenerative arthritis: commonly seen in the following joints: DIP Heberden nodes; PIP Bouchard nodes; MCP posttraumatic or infection; CMC digits associated with CMC bossing; trapeziometacarpal (thumb); intercarpal (triscaphe, radiolunate, triquetrohamate, lunatotriquetral), radioscaphoid (seen in postscaphoid nonunions or with scapholunate advanced collapse wrist).

scapholunate advanced collapse (SLAC): after untreated scaphoid nonunion or untreated scapholunate dissociation, there is rotatory subluxation of the scaphoid. Typically will have radioscaphoid arthritis, sparing the radiolunate joint with proximal migration of the capitate.

grind test: a diagnostic test to clinically determine the presence of basal joint arthritis of the thumb by exerting axial pressure on the thumb metacarpal to the trapezium.

inflammatory arthritis: rheumatoid hand deformities that include the following: flexor or extensor tenosynovitis, tendon ruptures, caput ulnar syndrome (Vaughn-Jackson syndrome), intercarpal collapse or volar carpal subluxation, MP volar collapse with ulnar deviation, thumb digits, boutonnière deformity, swan-neck deformity, carpal tunnel syndrome, and intrinsic contractures.

progressive systemic sclerosis (PSS): typically scleroderma, Raynaud subcutaneous calcinosis, resorption of the distal tufts. Diffuse hand involvement with skin thickening and fibrosis.

psoriatic arthritis (PA): typically of the DIP, but any joint can be affected. Joint pain and stiffness can have similar clinical picture to rheumatoid arthritis.

pyogenic arthritis: bacterial infection of a joint.

systemic lupus erythematosus (SLE): deformity similar to rheumatoid arthritis with pain and swelling in the mid-PIP joints and the wrists. Usually systemic, there is relative sparing of articular cartilage until late.

Deformities (Specific)

boutonnière deformity: a fixed deformity of the finger consisting of flexion of the PIP joint and extension of the DIP joint. A result of rheumatoid destruction of the extensor tendon mechanism at the PIP joint and also secondary to trauma without arthritis. Can be moderate to severe and indicates that a separate classification system exists.

diabetic cheiroarthropathy: hand arthritis associated with diabetes; characterized by flexion contracture of the MCP and PIP joints of the fingers, with thickening, induration, and a waxy appearance of the skin.

mallet finger: drop of the distal phalanx caused by traumatic or arthritic avulsion to the extensor tendon over the DIP joint; also called **drop finger.**

opera-glass hand: a rare, advanced stage of arthritis, such as psoriatic arthritis, in which the joints are destroyed and the bones become thin, fragile, and shortened; also called **arthritis mutilans.**

radial drift: the position toward which the metacarpals tend to drift in rheumatoid arthritis—the alignment of the hand deviates toward the thumb; may apply to the thumb but usually specified.

swan-neck deformity: a static or dynamic position of the finger that exhibits DIP flexion and PIP hyperextension. Seen in posttraumatic or rheumatoid patients. Anatomically, there is failure of the distal extensor mechanism, tightness of the central slip, and PIP volar plate laxity. In rheumatoid arthritis, the classification system is as follows:

Type I: PIP joint flexible in all positions of MP joint.
Type II: PIP joint is limited in certain positions.
Type III: PIP joint is limited in all positions.
Type IV: stiff PIP with gross articular destruction.

tophus: accumulation of any crystalline material in the soft tissue; seen commonly in gout.

trapeziometacarpal arthritis: an arthritis at the base of the thumb; often occurs in the absence of systemic disease or previous trauma. Most common in women.

ulnar drift: the position of the fingers in rheumatoid arthritis; the fingers point away from the thumb and are often associated with radial drift at the wrist.

Neuropathies

allodynia: a perception of nonpainful stimulus as painful. This is a symptom of complex regional pain syndrome.

complex regional pain syndrome: syndrome of abnormally intense, inappropriately prolonged pain, not a reflection of actual or impending tissue damage commonly seen after trauma, in a variety of neurogenic and vascular sequelae; formerly called **reflex sympathetic dystrophy.**

compressive neuropathy: loss of motor or sensory nerve function, acute or chronic, caused by extrinsic compression. Entrapment can occur within tight fibroosseous tunnels or as a result of tumor, hemorrhage, or metabolic changes, causing swelling of soft tissues around the nerve.

dysesthesia: an unpleasant spontaneous sensation occurring in patients with chronic regional pain syndrome.

Halstead maneuver: a compression test of the thoracic outlet by moving the shoulders downward and backward with the chest protruding to draw the clavicle closer to the first rib, thus narrowing the thoracic outlet.

Horner syndrome: strongly correlated with avulsion of the C8 and T1 nerve root in brachial plexus injury. This includes ptosis, meiosis, and anhidrosis.

hyperesthesia: increased sensitivity to a stimulus that would normally not be painful; seen commonly in chronic regional pain syndrome.

hyperpathia: a state of exaggerated and painful response to stimulation seen in complex regional pain syndrome.

Jeanne s.: hyperextension of the MCP joint of the thumb doing key pinch or gross grip caused by paralysis of the adductor pollicis muscle, which acts as a first metacarpal adductor seen commonly in ulnar nerve palsy.

Klumpke palsy: a paralysis caused by isolated injury to the C8 and T1 nerve roots either in birth plexus injuries or traumatic injuries later in life.

phantom limb pain: a sensation after amputation of a limb. The patient may still have sensation that the amputated part is still present. This may be painful and may be due to representation of the limb in the terminal neuromatous stumps in the amputated part.

Pitres Testut s.: an inability to actively move the long finger in radial and ulnar deviation with palm placed flat on the table. Demonstrating paralysis of the second and third dorsal interosseous muscles in ulnar nerve palsy.

Pollock s.: loss of extrinsic power with inability to flex the distal joint of the ring and little fingers because of the weakness of the flexor digitorum profundus through the fourth and fifth fingers in ulnar nerve palsy.

posttourniquet syndrome: characterized by edema, stiffness, pallor, and weakness without paralysis, and subjective numbness without objective anesthesia caused by prolonged use of tourniquet in upper-extremity surgery.

reflex sympathetic dystrophy (RSD): usually posttraumatic (major or minor) pain dysfunction syndrome. Thought to be due to abnormal modulation of afferent pain signals with possible short-circuiting of somatic and autonomic nerve fibers. Attendant autonomic nervous system hyperactivity will produce abnormal peripheral small vessel response to cold and heat stimulus. Symptoms include hyperpathia (increased pain at rest), allodynia (painful response to a nonpainful stimulus), erythema (brawny edema), joint stiffness, and loss of skin elasticity. Osteoporosis and complete loss of dexterity result. Bone scan and tomography are diagnostic, and treatment includes physical therapy, oral medications, and a sympathetic ganglion blockade; also called **autonomic dystrophy, chronic regional pain syndrome (CRPS), shoulder-hand syndrome, Sudeck atrophy, causalgia,** and **sympathetic maintained pain syndrome (SMPS).**

Roo classification: classification of thoracic outlet syndrome depending on the segment of the brachial plexus involved, either upper, lower, or combined compressions.

Roo test: a clinical test to diagnose thoracic outlet syndrome in which the patient abducts both arms 90 degrees and flexes with 90 degrees of elbow flexion, repeatedly opening and closing the hands to elicit numbness, tingling, or weakness in both hands.

Semmes-Weinstein monofilament tests: an array of monofilaments placed perpendicular to wooden or plastic rods that are held against the skin in progressive thickness and progressive skin resistance used to test innervation and density at the fingertips in nerve injury areas.

Spurling test: a clinical test for cervical nerve root compression by compressing the nerve root at the foraminal exit in the cervical spine. Compression is applied to the patient's head. A positive test represents a spray of numbness and pain shooting down the ipsilateral arm.

Sunderland Classification for Grades of Nerve Injury

I neuropraxia: local conduction block, nerve in continuity, no Wallerian degeneration, all have elements intact. No Tinel sign.

II axonotmesis: axonal damage; Wallerian degeneration distally; endoneurium, perineurium, and epineurium intact; nerve sprouting; progress excellent.

III axonotmesis: axon and endothelium are disrupted, perineurium intact. Nerve mismatching with regeneration. Recovery depends on degree of neural matching, unpredictable; advancing Tinel sign and Wallerian degeneration distally.

IV axonotmesis: axon, endoneurium, and perineurium violated. Nerve is grossly in continuity held by epineurium; advancing Tinel sign, regenerative units trapped in scar; requires surgical intervention.

V neurotmesis: complete nerve transection requiring surgical intervention by repair graft or conduit.

---

traction injury: refers to injury to nerve tissue from an over-pull that exceeds 10% of resting length, resulting in neuronal dysfunction, which is commonly seen in brachial plexus injuries. This injury may also pull the nerve root out of the cervical spine resulting in pseudoceles.

Median Neuropathy

anterior interosseous nerve syndrome: anterior elbow and forearm pain and motor weakness of the flexor digitorum profundus II, FPL, and pronator quadratus. Electromyography may be helpful. Conservative therapy may be tried for several months, and, failing that, surgical decompression of the nerve is indicated.

carpal tunnel syndrome (CTS): a median nerve compression at the wrist caused by chronic synovitis surrounding the flexor tendons with repetitive finger motion or squeezing. Maximum pressure elevation occurs 3 to 4 cm distal to the volar wrist crease. Thenar motor loss may be included if untreated. Patient describes numbness, tingling, and dysesthesia in the hand at the median nerve distribution. Conservative therapy is indicated in chronic cases, and, failing that, surgical decompression of the carpal tunnel is necessary. Electromyograms and nerve conduction studies are usually diagnostic.

pronator syndrome: entrapment of the median nerve in the elbow causes anterior elbow and forearm pain, with numbness, tingling, and paresthesias in the median nerve distribution. Electrodiagnostics are occasionally helpful. Conventional therapy is tried for several months, and, failing that, decompression of the median nerve is indicated.

Radial Neuropathy

posterior intraosseous nerve syndrome: compression of the motor branch of the radial nerve near the arcade of Froshe that causes weakness of the finger and wrist extensors. Electrodiagnosis and conservative treatment are not helpful. Surgical release of the radial nerve may improve function, but tendon transfers may be necessary.

radial sensory nerve entrapment (Wartenberg syndrome): the radial sensory nerve can become entrapped in the distal third of the forearm as it emerges between the brachioradialis and the extensor carpi radialis longus. Patient experiences numbness and dysesthesia in the dorsoradial hand and wrist, provoked by hyperpronation of the forearm. Sensory nerve conduction studies are helpful, and surgical release is curative in most cases; also called **brachialgia statica paresthetica.**

radial tunnel syndrome: usually misdiagnosed as **resistant tennis elbow,** it is posterolateral elbow pain accentuated on resisted supination of the forearm or extension of the middle finger. Electromyography and nerve conduction studies are helpful. Treatment includes rest, splinting, and avoiding stressful activities.

wrist drop: a radial nerve palsy with loss of muscle control for wrist extension. This can be due to a variety of central and peripheral nerve conditions but is most commonly associated with radial nerve palsy; also called **posterior intraosseous nerve syndrome.**

Ulnar Neuropathy

cubital tunnel syndrome: entrapment of the ulnar nerve at the elbow caused by fibrous tissue in the fibroosseous arcade and the two heads of the flexor carpi ulnaris as a result of prolonged elbow flexion. Early on, symptoms are sensory and involve the fourth and fifth digits; later, intrinsic motor weakness predominates. Surgical compression or ulnar nerve transposition is necessary.

Charcot-Marie-Tooth disease: in the hand, spontaneous deterioration of the neuromuscular complex will affect the ulnar nerve and cause severe intrinsic wasting with a characteristic clawhand deformity; also called **intrinsic minus deformity.**

double crush syndrome: compression of a peripheral nerve (i.e., median or ulnar nerve) in two or more locations. There is cervical root compression at C-6 or C-7 and carpal tunnel syndrome. Three types exist: multiple anatomic regions along a peripheral nerve, multiple anatomic structure access to peripheral nerve with anatomic region superimposed on a neuropathy, or a combination of these. These complex conditions require a multifactorial approach. Prognosis is guarded. Also called **multiple crush syndrome.**

focal dystonia: a condition whereby muscles become imbalanced when some muscles are used more than others. This is due to repetitive motions of the hand, such as seen in musicians (pianists, string, or brass instrumentalists). The brain does not send proper signals to the affected muscles, resulting in spasms and seizures of the hand. Sometimes the arm is affected. Treatment is in the form of electrical stimulation, ultrasound, exercise, or surgery.

intrinsic minus hand: in low ulnar nerve palsy, will cause intrinsic palsy with a characteristic MCP hyperextension and PIP and DIP sensory deformity. Results from any interruption of intrinsic function; intrinsic minus deformity, intrinsic plus deformity; also called **clawhand deformity.**

intrinsic plus hand: loss of extrinsic muscle function or intrinsic contracture will cause MP flexion and IP extension.

monkey paw: an adduction and extension of the thumb in which it cannot be opposed. It is unable to touch the tips of the fingers because of weakness of the opposing muscles of the thumb, as in a lesion of the median nerve.

peripheral neuropathy: intrinsic axonal or myelin pathologic condition usually caused by an underlying metabolic malfunction or toxic state (i.e., diabetes, renal failure, alcoholic neuropathy).

Saturday night palsy: localized pressure palsy (e.g., in an alcoholic who falls asleep on a rested arm on a hard object); a first-degree neuropraxia occurs, which is worsened by an underlying alcoholic neuropathy.

tardy ulnar palsy: delayed chronic ulnar neuropathy secondary to chronic stretching of the nerve in the cubital tunnel caused by cubitus valgus deformity at the elbow.

thoracic outlet syndrome: a constellation of signs and symptoms with multiple etiologic factors. Common complaints include aching pain and heaviness in the neck, shoulder, and upper arm with numbness and tingling mainly to the fourth and fifth fingers. Symptoms worsen with arm elevation to include chest pain, tightness, and headaches. Thoracic outlet syndrome is believed to be caused by compression of the brachial plexus over the cervical rib and between the scalenus anterior and scalenus medius muscles; in early adult life with shoulder sagging, brachial plexus traction can result. Initial treatment must include physiotherapy. Surgery may be indicated if symptoms persist for more than 1 year. Related conditions are *brachial plexus compression, scalenus anticus syndrome,* and *hyperabductor syndrome.*

- **ulnar tunnel syndrome:** entrapment of the ulnar nerve at the wrist (Guyon canal). Could be acute or caused by repetitive trauma. Electrodiagnostics studies are helpful. Surgical release may be necessary.
- **vibration white finger syndrome:** digital arterial or nerve injury in the hand from using tools with at least 2000 to 3000 cpm; characterized by Raynaud phenomenon: cold intolerance, numbness, tingling, and weakness with loss of dexterity.

Congenital Anomalies

Classification of Upper Limb Anomalies

The International Federation of Societies for Surgery of the Hand Classification System for Anomalies Affecting Hand Function
I. Failure of formation of parts
Transverse congenital amputations, constriction band syndrome (amniotic Streeter bands)
Longitudinal (radial, ulnar) hemimelias, phocomelias, hypoplastic digits
II. Failure of differentiation of parts (incomplete morphogenesis)
Shoulder: Sprengel deformity
Arm and forearm synostosis: humeroradial, humeroulnar, radioulnar
Hand synostosis: syndactyly, camptodactyly, congenital trigger digit, clinodactyly
III. Duplication.
Polydactyly triphalangism, central polydactyly (polysyndactyly, mirror hand)
IV. Overgrowth (gigantism)
Macrodactyly, lipofibromas, hamartoma of nerve, limb hypertrophy, hemihypertrophy
V. Undergrowth
Brachydactyly
VI. Constriction ring syndrome (amniotic Streeter bands)
VII. Generalized skeletal anomalies
Dwarfism, arthrogryposis, chromosomal anomalies (i.e., Madelung deformity); also called **Klippel-Feil syndrome**

Agenesis

acheiria: absence of the hand.

acquired thumb flexion contracture: in children, a thumb flexion contracture that usually develops *after* birth, and, if present for more than a year, can be relieved by release of the A1 pulley at the volar base of the thumb. The thumb rarely catches or snaps. Hence the term **congenital trigger thumb** is not appropriate for this condition.

acrosyndactyly: terminal interconnection of the syndactylyzed digits. These may or may not be connected proximally. The connection may be simple (skin) or complex (bone or other associated structures). These are commonly seen in Apert syndrome.

adactyly: absence of the digits.

amelia: total absence of the upper limb (congenital amputation).

amniotic bands: congenital circumferential crease rings that may be present at a fingertip or at upper arm level, or anywhere in between. This can be isolated or in conjunction with associated anomalies such as clubfoot or cleft palate. Neurovascular embarrassment depends on the depth of the crease and may be complete if the crease goes down to the bone. Four types are evident: (1) simple constriction rings, (2) rings associated with distal lymphedema or deformity, (3) rings associated with soft tissue fusion of distal parts, and (4) intrauterine amputations. If there is any question of neurovascular compromise, Z-plasty releases are initiated in at least two stages; also called **constriction bands, Streeter bands,** and **Streeter dysplasia.**

Apert syndrome: hand anomalies that include delta phalanx, metacarpal synostosis, complex syndactyly, and other anomalies including skull and facial.

Digits are usually short, deformed, stiff, and at the tips spoon hand.

aphalangia: absence of phalanges.

arachnodactyly: long, spiderlike fingers seen commonly in Marfan syndrome.

arthrofibrosis: joint capsular thickening and scarring with resistant stiffness seen in either posttraumatic situations, chronic spasticity, or an arthrogryposis.

arthrogryposis: joint contractures present at birth; cause is not yet known. Muscle weakness with immobility leads to contractures. Absent skin lines give it a waxy appearance. Also called **arthrogryposis multiplex congenita.** There are three groups:

- **single localized deformity (in upper extremity):** forearm pronation contracture, palm clutched thumb, selected loss of wrist and finger extensors, and intrinsic muscle contracture.
- **whole upper extremity involvement:** no shoulder girdle musculature; thin, tubular arms and forearms; straight, stiff elbows; flexion and ulnar deviation of the wrist; and stiff fingers and adducted thumbs.
- **global rigidity with associated deformities:** polydactyly or windblown deformity (intrinsic plus hand).

Bayne classification: for radial longitudinal congenital deficiencies describing the spectrum of deficits on the radial side of the forearm from hypoplastic thumb to complete absence of all radial structures including the radial bone.

Beal syndrome: a system to categorize the different types of camptodactyly and congenital contractures in fingers.

Bell classification: spectrum of inherited anomalies that include brachydactyly as the dominant feature.

bifid thumb: a generic term for thumb duplication or preaxial polydactyly. Wassel classification (see p. 323) is the most commonly used.

brachydactyly: digital hypoplasia may result from an arrest of development and it may affect any or all component tissues in a digit. It can be isolated or in conjunction with other congenital anomalies; also called **short fingers.**

camptodactyly: congenital nontraumatic flexion contracture in the sagittal plane of the PIP joint of the little finger, usually accompanied by MCP joint hyperextension. This is usually associated with other anomalies; causes are multifactorial, treatment is difficult, and outcome is uncertain. Also called **bent finger.**

carpal coalition: a congenital fusion or synostosis between two carpal bones, most commonly lunate and triquetrum or capitohamate. These are usually asymptomatic.

clasped thumb: refers to a spectrum of congenital thumb abnormalities resulting from deficiency of the thumb extensor mechanism. Overactivity of thumb extrinsic and intrinsic flexors.

cleft hand: a central ray deficiency (ectodactyly, oligodactyly) secondary to failure of formation of parts. High association with extraskeletal (i.e., cardiac) defects that may be metacarpal and carpal anomalies or deficiencies. These present deep clefts that may extend down to the carpus. Despite the cosmetic appearance, function may be surprisingly good; also called **lobster-claw hand** (archaic).

clinodactyly: radial or ulnar deviation of the digit tip in coronal plane. Usually this is expressed as radial deviation of the little finger at the DIP joint and is associated with other anomalies. Also called **bent finger.**

congenital trigger thumb: a congenital locking or clicking of the thumb with flexion posture of the IP joint. Nodular formation on the FPL tendon or tendon sheath thickening is common. Tendon sheath release is curative.

congenital ulnar drift: ulnar deviation of the digits at the MCP joint with PIP joint flexion deformity. Thumb webbing is also present. General muscular hypoplasia in the arm is present. Associated with craniofacial deformities and a markedly narrowed mouth; also called **windblown hand, whistling face syndrome,** and **Freeman-Sheldon syndrome.**

delta phalanx: a triangular-shaped bone interposed in the digit between two normal phalanges. A C-shaped physis is common and will cause a sharp angular digital deformity.

Ellis-Van Crevel syndrome: a form of ulnar polydactyly that is postaxial (multiple digits coming out of the ulnar aspect of the hand).

Fanconi anemia: pancytopenia, hematophoretic anomalies associated with radial hemimelia (autosomal recessive).

flipper hand: congenital absence of the arms; the hands appear to arise directly from the shoulder. Also called **phocomelia**.

floating thumb: an unstable hypoplastic thumb that may be connected to the hand by skin and a simple neurovascular pedicle. These digits are generally useless and are best removed. Also called **pouce flottant**.

hemimelia: absence of the forearm and hand.

heart-hand syndrome: cardiac septal defects, autosomal dominant, and seen with radial ray deficiency; also called **Holt-Oram syndrome**.

hereditary multiple exostosis: autosomal dominant inheritable disease characterized by multiple osteochondromas growing from the physis of long bone, pelvis, rib, scapula, and vertebra. This commonly appears in forearm bones and short tubular bones of the hand.

hyperphalangism: an extra (fourth) phalanx interposed between the phalanges of a finger. There are no extra digits. The digits are usually short.

hypoplastic thumb: an incompletely developed thumb that can range from a short thumb to complete absence. This is usually seen in conjunction with many associated abnormalities. There are five types: short thumb, adducted thumb, abducted thumb, floating thumb, and absent thumb.

Kirner deformity: parrot-beak convexity of the nail bed caused by volar bending of the distal phalanx. This may not be obvious until age 12.

macrodactyly: a disproportionately large digit apparent at birth or early childhood. In a "true" case, all structural components may be enlarged, including vessels and nerves. Commonly, there is a marked increase in subcutaneous fiber or fatty tissue.

Madelung deformity: congenital growth plate disorder of the volar ulnar physis of the distal radius. This will cause a severe volar and ulnar bowing of the radius, initially normal at birth, and the deformity becomes evident by 8 to 12 years of age.

Marfan syndrome: a disease of connective tissue that causes arachnodactyly (long, pencil-like fingers) without flexion contractures. Patients with this condition also have loose ligaments in their finger joints.

mirror hand: the forearm contains two ulnas and has no radius. Typically, the patient presents with eight digits. This is a rare spontaneous genetic mutation that, when present, can be passed down in an autosomal dominant fashion. Also called **ulnar dimelia**.

monodactyly: a single-digit hand that may also be seen as part of a spectrum of cleft hand disease.

Poland syndrome: thumb ray or finger deformity associated with absence of pectoral muscle head.

polydactyly: extra digits that may be complete or partially formed. These can be postaxial (ulnar side of the hand) or preaxial (on the thumb).

polysyndactyly: polydactyly of the index and ring fingers, usually associated with complex syndactyly. These are usually bilateral. Also called **central polydactyly**.

radial clubbed hand: total or partial absence of radial structures of the hand and forearm (preaxial). There are four types: (1) short distal radius, (2) hypoplastic radius, (3) partial absence of the radius, (4) total absence of the radius. These may be accompanied by thumb, index, or long-finger anomalies. Muscle or neurovascular anomalies can be isolated as part of a syndrome complex (i.e., vertebral defects, imperforate anus, tracheoesophageal fistula, and radial and renal dysplasia, Holt-Oram syndrome). Hand is radially deviated; also called **talipomanus**.

radial deficiency: a series of congenital malformations affecting the radial aspect of the hand, wrist, and forearm with varying degrees of hypoplasia of the bones, joints, muscles and tendons, ligaments, nerves, and blood vessel. This may be associated with other systemic conditions.

radio-ulnar synostosis: a congenital or posttraumatic fusion of the radius and ulna seen generally near the proximal radial ulnar joint of the elbow, but it can occur distally as well.

supernumerary digits: extra nubbins of fingers and thumb with no function.

symbrachydactyly: literally shortened, stiff digits. Seen commonly in the spectrum of cleft hand disease.

syndactyly: a congenital joining of two or more digits; the connection may be complete or incomplete, simple or complex. Simple-shared element of skin and subcutaneous tissue. Complex shared element of skin, subcutaneous tissue, tendon, bone, and neurovascular structures.

synostosis: fusion between two adjacent parallel bones (i.e., metacarpals or radius and ulna). Term may also be used for humeral-radial fusion.

synphalangism: heredity dysplasia and ankylosis of distal joints, most notably the PIP joint. There may be partial or total bone bridging.

synpolydactyly: a congenital anomaly resulting in the formation of extra phalanges or digits within an conjoined digital nerve with syndactyly of skin and bony structures.

thrombocytopenia, absent radius (TAR) syndrome: complete absence of the radius may be present (autosomal recessive).

trident hand: typical hand appearance of an achondroplastic dwarf in which there is a persistent space between the ring and long fingers.

triphalangeal thumb: interposition of an extra phalanx between two normal phalanges of the thumb; can at times be functionally normal or cause marked deformity or malfunction. The extra phalanx can be normal or be a delta phalanx. Often seen with congenital heart disease.

triplicate thumb: a variant form of preaxial polydactyly involving three thumbs; all are markedly diminished in size and may lack one or more tissue elements.

ulnar deficiency: usually isolated with severe limitation of elbow function; hypoplasia of ulna, partial aplasia of the ulna (absence of distal or middle third of the ulna), total aplasia of the ulna; also called **postaxial deficiency** and **radiohumeral synostosis.**

ulnar variance: relative position of the distal ulnar joint referred to the level of the ulnar side of the distal radial joint, as determined on an anteroposterior radiograph that is obtained with neutral pronation and supination. A longer ulna is called a **positive variance,** and a shorter ulna is called a **negative variance,** measured in millimeters.

Wassel Classification of Thumb Polydactyly
I: bifid distal phalanx (DP)
II: duplicated DP
III: bifid proximal phalanx (PP)
IV: most common type with duplication of distal and PPs that rest on broad MC
V: bifid MC
VI: duplicated MC
VII: triphalangism

VATER syndrome: acronym referring to vertebral anomalies, anal atresia, tracheoesophageal fistula, renal and vascular anomalies, accompanied by a radial clubhand.

whistling face syndrome: an autosomal dominant condition affecting the hands and feet with a characteristic facial appearance in the form of arthrogryposis, which is a congenital and pathologic stiffness of the arms or legs down to the hands or feet in characteristic postures; also called **Freeman-Sheldon syndrome.**

Muscle and Tendon Disorders

trigger finger: entrapment of finger flexor tendons usually under the proximal A1 pulleys; usually caused by a disproportion between the flexor tendon and the flexor tendon sheath. Usually, the cause is obscure, with thickening of the pulley tissues or nodular formation about the tendon. This can be acquired secondarily (e.g., resulting from diabetes, rheumatoid arthritis, or gout). Conservative measures and steroid injections may help, but surgery is usually curative.

boutonnière deformity: usually caused by a central slip rupture of the middle phalanx with an injury to the triangular ligaments. Volar subluxation of the lateral bands below the flexion axis of the PIP joint will cause a fixed flexion attitude of the PIP joint.

carpal pedal spasm: an intrinsic plus position with wrist flexion usually seen in hypercalcemia.

de Quervain disease: stenosing tenosynovitis of the first dorsal extensor compartment, usually involving the extensor pollicis brevis and abductor pollicis longus.

intersection syndrome: pain and swelling over the place where the muscles of the first dorsal extensor compartment cross over the muscles of the second compartment. This is believed to be a tenosynovitis of the second dorsal compartment.

Landsmeer test: a test that elicits a tight oblique retinacular ligament of Landsmeer as seen in boutonnière's deformity, in which passively extending the PIP joint sends the IP joint into a tight, fixed-extension posture. Also, the particular anatomy of Landsmeer ligament is volar to the PIP joint and dorsal to the DIP joint.

lumbrical plus finger deformity: a condition in which there is overactivity of the lumbricals, creating a paradoxical extension of the PIP and DIP joints with attempted flexion of the fingers.

"no man's land": usually refers to an injury to the digital flexor tendons at zone II (under the tendon sheath and pulleys). Until recently, injury to this area was fraught with technical difficulty and poor results.

peritendinitis stenosans/digitus saltans: an archaic term used to describe conditions of stenosing tenosynovitis such as those found in de Quervain disease, flexor carpi radialis tendonitis, and trigger digits.

quadriga: in a setting in which the profundus tendon to a digit is contracted or repaired too tightly, there will be a limitation of proximal excursion of the remaining flexor digitorum profundus (FDP), causing a weak grip (as all the FDP tendons usually share a common muscle belly).

tendovaginitis: form of tendon entrapment seen in trigger digits and de Quervain tenosynovitis by tight retinaculum or tenosynovitis obliterating the space between the tendons and the overlying retinaculum.

tetraplegia: neurologic injury secondary to cervical spine trauma. Altered functional capacity of the hand, depending on the level of injury. This will also dictate operative and nonoperative intervention. A system has been devised:

International Classification for Tetraplegia	
Functional Group	**Root Level Intact**
Brachioradialis	C-5, C-6
Extensor carpi radialis longus	C-7 (possibly C-8)
Extensor carpi radialis brevis	C-7, C-8
Pronator teres	C-7, C-8
Flexor carpi radialis	C-8
Extensor digitorum communis	C-8
Extensor pollicis longus	T-1
Partial digital flexion	T-1
Lacks intrinsics only	T-1
Miscellaneous (i.e., Brown-Séquard syndrome or syringomyelia)	

Volkmann contracture: contracture affecting the volar forearm musculature as a result of scarring after an ischemic insult. This is the usual sequela of an untreated volar muscle compartment syndrome (seen in muscle crush injuries or forearm fracture). Circulation is usually impaired in the center of the forearm. The flexor digitorum profundus and FPL muscles are most severely affected. There is a mild, moderate, classic, or severe type.

Vaughn–Jackson syndrome: rupture of ring and little finger extensors caused by synovitis at the distal radial ulnar joint.

washer woman's sprain: an archaic description of de Quervain tenosynovitis, tendinopathies of the tendons of the first dorsal extensor compartment.

Vascular Disorders

acrocyanosis: seen in Raynaud phenomenon. With exposure to cold, the fingers become deep blue and cold. This is usually caused by peripheral vasospasm.

Buerger disease: an inflammatory thrombosis seen in smokers, usually in men. Digital arteries are affected. The disease is progressive, leading to digital loss and possibly loss of the whole hand. Also called **thromboangiitis obliterans.**

hypothenar hammer syndrome: an ulnar artery aneurysm or thrombosis caused by repetitive striking of the hypothenar eminence and the hook of hamate region against a hard, blunt object; typically, localized pain, digital pallor, and cold sensibility are common symptoms.

Kienböck disease: a posttraumatic, vascularly mediated avascular necrosis of the lunate with subsequent collapse, dislocation, and arthrosis. Magnetic resonance imaging and bone scan have fine-tuned the classification; also called **isolated dislocation.**

Lichtman Classification for Keinböck Disease
Stage I: normal radiographic findings, positive bone scan, questionable linear fractures.
Stage II: lunate sclerosis without collapse. Magnetic resonance imaging subclassification:

IIA: T2 focal signal intensity increase.
IIB: T2 focal signal intensity loss.
IIC: T2 generalized signal intensity increase.
IID: T2 generalized signal intensity loss.

Stage III: lunate sclerosis, fragmentation, and collapse.

IIIA: without rotatory subluxation of the scaphoid.
IIIB: fixed scaphoid rotation and carpal collapse.

Stage IV: stage III plus degenerative changes of the carpus.

Traumatic Disorders

annulus fracture: fractures of the hook of the hamate usually caused by compression force as a direct blow.

Barton fracture: an intraarticular fracture involving either the dorsal or the volar lip of the distal radius resulting in either dorsal or volar subluxation of the lunate.

chauffeur's fracture: displaced fracture of the radial styloid accompanied by ulnar translocation of the carpus.

dye punch fracture: a type of intraarticular distal radius fracture involving the compression of the lunate facet of the distal radius.

factitious edema: history of minor trauma followed by persistent dorsal forearm pain, swelling, and tenderness caused by repeated self-inflicted trauma; also called **secretan edema.**

fragment specific fixation: a method of repairing the distal radius using a small plate to fix small fractures to the main body of the bone.

gamekeeper's thumb: an abduction laxity of the thumb at the MCP joint caused by acute or chronic disruption of the ulnar collateral ligament of the finger joint.

Herbert's Classification of Scaphoid Fractures
A four-part classification describing scaphoid fractures:
stable acute fractures
unstable acute fractures
delayed union
established nonunion

Holstein-Lewis fracture: a fracture of the distal humerus in which the radial nerve is in particular jeopardy. The proximal spike of the spiral fracture breaks through the lateral cortex of the humerus near where the radial nerve is most grossly opposed to the bone.

Hotchkiss fracture: a classification system describing fractures of the radial head and neck in trauma situation.

hypothenar hammer syndrome: a rare occupational or recreational condition that may be due to repetitive microtrauma to the ulnar artery at the level of the Guyon canal.

interdigital contracture: results from extensive scarring about the hand resulting in cicatrix forming in between the digits and preventing digital abduction; seen commonly in severe burns of the hand.

Jahss maneuver: a method of closed reduction of metacarpal neck fractures flexing the MCP joint and the PIP joint and pushing upward on the flexed PIP joint while applying a cast, flexing the MCP joint into maximal flexion. The PIP joint is usually then brought out into extension.

lunotriquetral dissociation: a condition whereby a lunate becomes volar-flexed in sagittal plane because of a dissociation between it and the adjacent triquetrum.

malrotation: a condition whereby there is a mismatch between the proximal and distal ends of a fracture of a tubular bone in which the distal end of the fracture rotates relative to the proximal end on its long axis. This can cause finger overlap.

Melone classification: a four-part classification of distal radius fractures that identifies specific intraarticular fragments of the distal radius and ranks them in order of severity based on displacement.

negative pressure therapy: a technique that uses a suction apparatus on a mangling high-energy wound. This technique removes exudates, decreases edema, closes the dead space, and promotes wound healing commonly seen in the treatment of wartime injuries. Also called **vacuum assisted closure (VAC).**

Palmer Classification
For triangular fibrocartilage complex (TFCC) injury:
Class 1: traumatic
Type A: central perforation
Type B: medial avulsion (ulnar attachment), with or without distal ulnar fracture
Type C: distal avulsion (carpal attachment)
Type D: lateral avulsion (radial attachment) with or without sigmoid-notch fracture

> **Class 2:** degenerative (ulnocarpal impaction syndrome)
> **Stage A:** TFCC wear
> **Stage B:** TFCC wear with lunate or ulnar chondromalacia
> **Stage C:** TFCC perforation with lunate or ulnar chondromalacia
> **Stage D:** TFCC perforation with lunate or ulnar chondromalacia and lunotriquetrial-ligament perforation
> **Stage E:** TFCC perforation with lunate or ulnar chondromalacia and lunotriquetrial- ligament perforation, and ulnar carpal arthritis

peritendinous fibrosis: scarring around a tendon.

pseudoclawing: an intrinsic minus position with MCP hyperextension and PIP joint flexion caused by flexion malunion of metacarpal neck fractures.

radial styloidectomy: the excision of the radial styloid done usually in conjunction with scaphoid excision and four-poster fusions in the reconstruction of scapholunate advanced collapse wrist.

Rolando fractures: comminuted intraarticular fractures of the base of the thumb metacarpal.

scaphoid ring sign: a scapholunate dissociation in which the scaphoid collapses into flexion and has a foreshortened view on the anteroposterior x-ray. The distal end of the scaphoid appears to have radial band with a ring superimposed on it.

scaphoid shift test: a test that determines the integrity of the scapholunate ligament by mobilization from pressure supply to the palmar tuberosity of the scaphoid while the wrist is moved from ulnar to radial deviation. A positive test is seen in a patient with scapholunate dissociation. The scaphoid no longer can strain proximally and subluxes out of the scaphoid fossa of the distal radius. When the pressure is released, the scaphoid goes back into position and a typical snapping occurs.

scapholunate ballottement test: with the lunate stabilized with the thumb and index finger and the scaphoid held over the other hand, a dorsal volar alternating pressure between the scaphoid and the lunate elicits pain and crepitance as well as instability of the joint in scapholunate dissociation.

Secretan syndrome: rare disorder characterized by woody edema of the dorsum of the hand seen typically in association with a crush injury or self-induced injury.

sheer testing for lunotriquetral dissociation: a ballottement test for lunotriquetral dissociation secondary to interosseous injury. The lunate and triquetrum are held stably by the thumb and index fingers of both hands shifted dorsally and volarly relative to one another. A positive test elicits crepitance, pain, and increased movement between the lunate and triquetrum.

skier's thumb: an acute rupture of the ulnar collateral ligament of the MCP joint of the thumb seen commonly in skiers, but generally seen in fall on outstretched hands, hyperabducting the thumb at the MP joint.

Stener lesion: in a complete tear of the ulnar collateral ligament of the MCP joint of the thumb, the ligament may avulse distally and roll up proximally, causing an interposition of the adductor aponeurosis. Nonoperative treatment usually results in a chronically unstable thumb.

turret exostosis: a painful mass on the dorsal aspect of the middle phalanx seen on lateral x-ray as an exostosis; also called **bone spur.** This is believed to be traumatic in origin.

ulnar impaction syndrome: excessive pressure from the ulnar aspect of the carpus, notably the lunate onto the distal end of the ulna in those situations in which the distal radius has been shortened leaving an ulnar positive variance.

Specific Dislocations

Wrist Dislocations and Instability

In a distal radius dislocation, the radius is dislocated in reference to the ulna. However, the standard terminology describes the position of the ulna in relationship to the radius.

carpal instability dissociative (CID): a carpal collapse pattern caused by a ligamentous disruption in the proximal carpal row (i.e., scapholunate lunotriquetral pattern); also called **Linsheid instability.**

carpal instability nondissociative (CIND): a carpal collapse pattern caused by disruption of ligaments connecting the proximal and MC row or by other extrinsic factors (e.g., radial malunion).

Desault d.: involves the RC joint with dorsal displacement of carpus and ulnar styloid process.

dorsal intercalated segment instability (DISI): a zigzag collapse pattern seen best on the lateral views of the wrist. The lunate appears to send its distal face dorsally. This can occur as a result of displaced scaphoid fractures, scapholunate instability, a nondissociated carpal instability. Commonly, the lunate follows the triquetrum volarly without the scaphoid to contract its movement. The capitolunate angle is greater than 20 degrees and the scapholunate angle is greater than 70 degrees when the wrist is held in neutral posture.

lumbrical plus finger: posttraumatic contracture of the lumbrical will cause a paradoxical extension of the PIP and DIP joints each time an attempt is made to flex the digits.

lunate d.: volar semilunar dislocation in the wrist; a type of dislocation often not recognized.

perilunate d.: involves all carpals, which are shifted posteriorly, leaving the lunate in proper position; may be associated with a scaphoid fracture, in which case it is termed a **transscaphoid perilunate d.** Rarely do other carpi dislocate singularly or in association with fractures about the wrist. Wrist instabilities may be associated with fractures but specifically relate to ligamentous instabilities of the carpal bones. A devastating injury in which all the connecting ligaments between the lunate and its surrounding carpal bones are severed. Commonly, the capitate sits dorsal to the lunate. The lunate may dislocate volarly as part of the spectrum.

transscaphoid perilunate d.: similar to the perilunate dislocation except that the stress lines extend through the body of the scaphoid itself rather than the scapholunate ligament. The radial styloid may be fractured as well.

volar-flexed intercalated segment instability (VISI): a zigzag collapse pattern with the lunate distal face turned volarly. This is seen best on lateral x-rays of the wrist. These can follow triquetral lunate instability or nondissociated instability patterns. An average reduced scapholunate angle of more than 35 degrees.

Hand Dislocations

Dislocation can occur at all the small joints of the hand. Dislocations at the CMC and MCP joints generally occur in a dorsal direction. Dislocations at the MCP joints can sometimes be reduced without surgery. Dislocations in the hand are often associated with intraarticular fractures. Fracture-dislocations often require surgical reduction and fixation to realign joint surfaces.

Bennett d.: lateral or dorsal displacement of the first CMC joint.

boutonnière deformity: flexion contracture of the PIP joint that may progress to subluxation. It is associated with hyperextension contracture of the DIP joint. Deformity begins with rupture of the extensor tendon insertion of the PIP joint and later becomes a fixed deformity.

carpal instability: partial or complete dislocations between individual wrist bones, causing a click-clunk with wrist movement. Most often occurs at the scapholunate joint, but can occur at the triquetrolunate, MC, and even the RC joint.

gamekeeper's thumb: a hyperabduction injury with partial subluxation and instability of the thumb MCP joint caused by traumatic rupture of the ulnar collateral ligament. Commonly caused by a ski-pole-strap injury; also called **skier's thumb.**

Nail and Skin Disorders

acanthosis nigricans: dull, gray, friable nails with leukonychia; can be an external marker of an internal malignancy.

acquired digital fibrokeratoma: benign tumors of fibrous tissue usually found on the hands and feet. These are flesh-colored with thornlike projections with a raised erythematous skin rash at the base. These are otherwise known as **acral fibrokeratomas.**

acrolentiginous melanoma: an unusual variant of melanomas found on the palmar surface of the hand and nail apparatus.

beak nail deformity: with amputation of the tip of the distal phalanx, the nail may grow over the edge of the finger. It is unsightly and occasionally painful. Also called **hook nail** and **nail horn.**

Bowen disease: the eponym given to intraepidermal squamous cell carcinoma known as **squamous cell carcinoma in situ.**

chromonychia: color changes in the nail unit.

clubbing: a raising of the nail bed resulting in a club appearance of the end of the finger caused by fibrovascular hyperplasia of the nail unit; a sign of lung disease.

digital fibrokeratoma: a benign tumor of fibrous tissue origin occurring on the tips of the fingers.

Dupuytren contracture: inflammatory process of the palmar fascia, occasionally extending into the fingers, in which severe contractures and nodular proliferation (skin dimples) may result. There are three phases: proliferative (nodular), involutional, and resolved. In the resolved state, the remaining constricting tissue is referred to as bands. Also called **palmar fibromatosis.**

epidermoid cyst: benign cyst composed of epidermal fragments that have been pushed to the deeper layers by minor trauma; also called **inclusion cyst.**

keratosis: premalignant lesions seen in sun-exposed, fair-skinned individuals causing skin atrophy and telangiectasias. If allowed to progress, it may become squamous cell carcinoma.

leukonychia: whitening of the nail plate.

macronychia: an unusually large or wide nail.

micronychia: small, short, or narrow nail.

onychalgia: nail unit pain.

onychia: inflammation of the nail plate.

onychogryphosis: nail plate hypertrophy that is horn-like resulting from trauma; also called **onychogryposis** and **ram's horn deformity.**

onycholysis: distal separation of the nail plate from the underlying nail bed.

onychomadesis: proximal separation of the nail plate from the nail matrix.

onychomycosis: fungal infection of the nail unit.

onychophagia: nail biting.

onychoptosis: loss of the nail plate.

onychorrhexis: spontaneous longitudinal splitting of the nail plate.

pincer deformity or **trumpet nail deformity:** a pathologic curling of the nail plate and nail bed with ingrowing of the nail plate into the nail folds and progressive pinching off of the soft tissue of the distal fingertips, which results in pain and deformity.

pitted nail: surface pits of nails less than 1 mm in diameter; may be a sign of psoriasis.

pterygium: scarring of the eponychial fold and the nail fold to the nail bed in nail trauma leading to functional and esthetic deformities such as absence of nail growth or splitting of the nail. This has also been associated with nail bed ischemia and collagen vascular disease.

racket nail: thumbnail shorter than it is wide. Usually, the distal ends of the fingers are also short.

reedy nail: fingernail marked by longitudinal furrows.

sclerodactyly: a scleroderma in which the fingers become thin and shiny with sclerotic skin at the tip, which is due to subcutaneous and intracutaneous calcinosis and diffused fibrosis of the collagen.

scleroderma: an autoimmune disease that causes the skin of the hands to become thin, tense, and shiny; IP joint stiffness, distal ischemic ulceration, and auto-amputation are common.

spoon nail: a central depression of the nail with raised sides.

subungual exostosis: a bone spur emanating from the distal phalanx dorsally under the nail bed, causing pressure pain, necrosis, and possible infection of the nail bed. Also called **Dupuytren exostosis.**

subungual hematoma: usually posttraumatic with nail bed laceration under an intact nail. A collection of blood under the nail plate.

turtle-back nail: a distorted fingernail, being more convex than normal.

unguis incarnatus: ingrown nail.

watch crystal nail: a nail as broad as it is long and convex lengthwise and crosswise; seen in pulmonary osteoarthropathy.

Other Specific Terms

aponeurotic fibroma: fibrous lesions of the hands commonly seen in childhood and adolescence. They are benign, but can be locally aggressive.

Bouchard node: thick nodular swelling caused by bone spurs in the PIP joints, not necessarily associated with systemic arthritis.

carpal bossing: prominence seen particularly at the dorsal index CMC joint; may be painful but usually causes no symptoms.

cheirospasm: spasms of the muscles of the hand; also called **writers cramps.**

flexor origin syndrome: tendonitis of pronator teres and wrist and finger flexor muscle origin on medial epicondyle of elbow; also called **medial epicondylitis** and **golfer's elbow.**

ganglion: a clear, viscid, fluid-filled sac found near the wrist joints or fingers, arising from capsuloligamentous structures; rarely associated with other diseases; most commonly found on dorsum of wrist.

glomus tumor: small vascular lesion that is usually very painful and associated with hypersensitivity to pressure or temperature; usually in fingertip.

hamartoma: unusual tumors of the peripheral nerves most commonly involving the median nerve of the hand. It starts as a slowly progressive swelling in the distal forearm of the palm; common symptoms of nerve compression may be present.

hand-foot syndrome: swelling in hands and feet as seen in sickle cell disease.

Heberden node: a thick nodular swelling caused by bone spurs in the DIP joints; not necessarily associated with systemic arthritis.

inclusion cyst: a noninfectious process following healing of laceration or puncture wound; germinal matrix of dermal growth, causing mass composed of desquamated dermal cells.

Luck classification of Dupuytren disease divided into three phases: proliferative phase, involutional phase, and residual phase, based on the histologic behavior of Dupuytren fibroblast.

mucous cyst: a misnomer; this is a ganglion of the DIP joint, which makes a cyst under the skin in the eponychial area.

nodular fasciitis: an uncommon reactive lesion that may simulate a sarcoma usually seen on the volar surface of the forearm, usually a rapidly growing small nodule. This has been confused with fibrosarcoma or myxoid liposarcoma leading to overtreatment.

overlap syndrome: seen in scleroderma patients with associated findings characteristic of lupus, dermatomyositis, or rheumatoid arthritis.

Preiser disease: spontaneous loss of blood supply and collapse of scaphoid, usually seen in young adults.

Raynaud disease: a condition characteristic of color changes in the tip of the fingers either blanching or cyanosis in both hands and may not be involved with vasospastic disease and not lead to ulceration of the fingertips.

Raynaud phenomenon: a clinical sign describing intermittent color changes that occur after exposure to cold or stress. A condition characteristic of color changes in the tip of the fingers either blanching or cyanosis in both hands; may not be involved with vasospastic disease and not lead to ulceration of the fingertips.

stenosing tenosynovitis: a bulbous swelling of the tendon, causing the tendon to catch as it passes through the pulley (the thick fibrous tunnel that holds the tendon in place); sometimes caused by rheumatoid arthritis; also called **trigger fingers** and **snapping tendons.**

Infections

The hand has many structures that are vulnerable to infections. When edema and swelling place pressure on muscles,tendons, blood vessels, and nerves, function is disrupted and compartmental ischemia could result. Adhesions or fibrosis following infection may reduce hand function temporarily or permanently. Terms related to infections are the following.

barber's interdigital pilonidal sinus: a foreign body granuloma usually caused by a reaction to hair implanted in the intradigital skin of the hand; first described in barbers; also called **interdigital pilonidal sinus.**

collar-button abscess: a digital webspace infection usually in the subdermal fatty layers. Drainage is usually required; also called **shirt-stud abscess.**

dactylitis: nonsuppurative insidious chronic infections of the hands and fingers commonly seen in syphilis and tuberculosis.

deep space infection: refers to infection of the thenar or midpalmar spaces; also called **palmar space infection.**

ecthyma contagiosum: a chronic infection causing large tumorlike lesions in immunodeficient host; believed to be contracted from exposure to sheep and goats.

eponychia: a nail-fold infection involving the entire eponychial fold and lateral nail fold. These are relatively rare.

fasciitis: a rapidly advancing necrotizing infection affecting the skin and subcutaneous tissue sparing the underlying muscle associated with high morbidity and mortality, seen commonly in group A *streptococcus* infections.

felon: a subcutaneous abscess involving the tissue of the distal fingertip. These may be under great pressure and require drainage, usually through a midlateral approach.

Hansen disease: commonly involves the hands; caused by *Mycobacterium leprae*. Peripheral neuropathy predominates with intrinsic atrophy and clawing. Later, soft tissue necrosis can result in actual loss of digits. Also called **leprosy**.

herpetic whitlow: a fascicular outbreak with an erythematous rim seen usually in fingertips of health care workers. These are commonly misdiagnosed and mistakenly drained. Supportive treatment is the mainstay. These are usually self-limited.

hockey-stick incisions: incisions placed at the lateral and distal aspects of the finger to facilitate drainage of felons (abscesses) of the fingertips.

horseshoe abscess: in those hands in which thenar and hypothenar spaces are interconnected, an abscess may spread to both sides of the hand in the shape of a horseshoe. Palmar space infection usually results from a penetrating wound. The deep spaces of the hand may fill with purulent material. Drainage is the key.

interdigital granuloma: small pyogenic granulomas found in the hand of cow milkers resulting from penetration of bovine hairs into the skin of the hand causing a foreign body reaction.

Kanavel sign: for pyogenic flexor tenosynovitis; there is a flexed position of the finger, symmetrical enlargement of the finger, excessive tenderness over the course of the tendon sheath, and extreme pain on passive extension of the digit.

Meleney infection: life- or limb-threatening infection with anaerobic bacteria or microaerophilic streptococcus. Amputation is usually required to save the patient's life; also called **gas gangrene**.

paronychia: infection in the soft tissue folds around the nail that usually results from injection of *Staphylococcus aureus* by a sliver of nail tissue, a manicure instrument, or a tooth. Drainage is mandatory.

pyogenic flexor tenosynovitis: a closed space infection of the flexor tendon sheath of the fingers and thumb generally caused by *Staphylococcus aureus*, *Streptococcus*, or *Pasteurella* presented with Kanavel signs, which are semiflexed position of the fingers, symmetrical enlargement of the whole digit, excessive tenderness limited to the flexor tendon sheath, and excruciating pain on passively extending the finger.

pyogenic granuloma: an exophytic friable growth over the surface of the skin. These are usually caused by *Staphylococcus aureus* and will require complete excision to effect a cure.

shooter's abscess: infections caused by parenteral drug abuse involving accessible sites on the hand and forearm. These appear as raised ulcers with cellulitis.

subungual abscess: a collection of pus under the nail plate or over the nail bed.

tenosynovitis: inflammation of the tendon sheath. Causes are multifactorial and include overuse, rheumatoid arthritis, infection, and nonspecific onset.

verruca vulgaris: a viral wart involving the nail or skin tissue. A carbon dioxide laser is usually curative.

Surgery of the Hand and Wrist

Surgical procedures of the hand and wrist are more commonly described anatomically than by eponyms. All terms, including eponyms, are listed according to the goals of the surgical procedure.

Arthrodeses of the Fingers

chevron a.: a rigid stable construction for IP joint fusion; a precise, chevron-shaped fitting of the bone cuts of the joint to be fused with resection of the joint surface.

Goldfarb and Stern a.: thumb CMC arthrodesis.

Haddad and Riordan a.: method of arthrodesis of wrist.

interphalangeal a.: cup and cone technique useful for MCP or IP fusion, allows for fine adjustment of angles and rotatory alignment after joint surfaces have been prepared.

Moberg dowel graft: for an IP arthrodesis in which there has been bone loss or nonunion. A finger joint fusion using a small, squared, bone peg.

Potenza a.: a finger joint fusion using bone peg taken from the adjacent phalanx or metacarpal.

trapeziometacarpal fusion: for advanced trapeziometacarpal disease in the thumb in young, active patients.

Arthrodeses of the Wrist

intercarpal a.: for wrist instability or collapse patterns, Kienböck disease, rheumatoid arthritis, localized degenerative changes in the carpus. These include triscaphe (scaphotrapeziotrapezoid), scaphocapitate, capitolunate, scapholunate, lunatotriquetral capitohamate (four-poster fusion). Moberg dowel grafts are useful in securing these fusions.

radiocarpal a.: commonly a total wrist fusion with or without autogenous graft. Useful for (1) a heavy laborer with posttraumatic arthritis, (2) failed RC arthroplasty, (3) rheumatoid arthritis, (4) tetraplegia with deformity of the wrist, and (5) tendon transfer surgery to stabilize the wrist.

radioulnar a.: for the creation of a one-bone forearm for advanced disease of the distal radioulnar joint.

scapholunate advanced collapse (SLAC) procedure: for the common combination of radioscaphoid and MC arthritis often seen in chronic nonunions of the scaphoid; a MC arthrodesis with excision of scaphoid.

total wrist a.: fusion of the distal radius and proximal and distal carpal rows. Useful salvage procedure for severe carpal arthritis.

triscaphe a.: of the scaphotrapeziotrapezoid articulation. Useful for localized arthritis and for rotatory subluxation of the scaphoid.

Arthrodeses of the Wrist (Eponyms)

Abbott a.: using only cortical bone grafts; also called **Abbott-Saunders-Bost a.**

Brockman-Nissen a.: intraarticular wrist fusion.

Carroll a.: rabbit ear–shaped bone graft fusion.

Feldon 2-pin wrist a.: a technique for fusing the wrist in rheumatoid patients using two thin Steinmann pins inserted through the second and third webspaces between the metacarpal bones across the carpus and the intramedullary canal of the radius.

Gill-Stein a.: extraarticular fusion using the dorsal distal radius as the graft; also called **radiocarpal a.**

Haddad-Riordan a.: intraarticular fusion using iliac crest bone graft.

Johnson and Alexander p.: for thumb arthritis, truncated cone arthrodesis of first metatarsophalangeal joint.

Liebolt a.: fusion using chips of bone graft.

Nalebuff a.: fusion that includes use of a Steinmann pin.

Seddon a.: intraarticular fusion involving resection of the distal ulna.

Smith-Petersen a.: fusion that includes resection of the distal ulna.

Wickstrom a.: fusion of the wrist using bone graft inserted into both the radius and carpus.

Arthroplasties

An arthroplasty is the reconstruction of joints to restore motion and stability. It involves the MCP, CMC, and PIP joints of the fingers and wrist, often with implants. The hand specialist frequently treats joint destruction commonly found in rheumatoid arthritis.

An implant arthroplasty involves a prosthetic replacement of joints by metallic or silicone-rubber parts, usually for arthritic conditions or traumatic ankylosis. Swanson silicone-rubber arthroplasty is a popular choice. (**Volz prosthesis, Steffe prosthesis, Swanson prosthesis.**)

anchovy procedure (Carroll p.): rolled PL graft placed into the space that remains after trapezium excision for pantrapezial arthritis.

Blatt capsulodesis: dynamic rotatory subluxation of the scaphoid. A proximally based flap of dorsal wrist capsule is attached to the distal pole of the scaphoid; this will prevent downward movement of the distal pole during radial deviation of the wrist; also called **dorsal capsulodesis.**

Broadbent and Woolf p.: four-flap Z-plasty in adducted thumb.

Brunelli and Brunelli p.: carpal ligament reconstruction, for scapholunate injury.

Burton and Pellegrini p.: tendon interposition arthroplasty with ligament reconstruction.

capsulectomy: PIP joint flexion contractures unresponsive to conservative treatment; proximal release of the joint capsule (volar plate) will improve movement.

Carroll a.: an interposition rolled tendon (palmaris longus) used as a spacer when the trapezium is removed for pantrapezial arthritis; also called **Froimson a.**

Curtis p.: capsulotomy of PIP joint.

Darrach resection: resection of the distal 1 to 1.5 cm of distal ulna at the wrist. Once considered as the standard procedure for the treatment of a myriad of distal radioulnar joint problems; now useful primarily in older adults and for severe rheumatoid arthritis. Also called **Albright and Chase p.**

dorsal capsulectomy: the removal of the dorsal joint capsule; for example, in the treatment of distal radial ulnar joint fracture.

Eaton volar plate a.: a chronic subluxation of the PIP joint after a displaced large volar lip fracture of the proximal end of the middle phalanx, greater than 50% of the articular surface. If left untreated, a chronic subluxation results. The volar plate is then advanced into the fracture site and tightened to prevent subluxation.

Eaton p.: for thumb metacarpal-carpal arthritis, tendon interposition arthroplasty with ligament reconstruction.

flexible hinge implant: a design for silastic implant arthroplasty developed by Swanson used in MP and PIP arthroplasties.

Fowler metacarpophalangeal a.: for arthritis of the MCP joint. The metacarpal is cut in the form of a chevron at the base of the proximal phalanx and then cut into a V shape, with an interposition of extensor tendon fusion.

hemiresection interposition arthroplasty: for distal radioulnar joint arthritis, resection of the articular surface of the distal ulna and interposition of a rolled tendon graft. Also called **Bowers arthroplasty.**

matched ulnar resection: popularized by Watson; resection of the articular surface of the distal ulna to match the shape of the radial styloid notch. This is useful for the treatment of distal radioulnar joint instability and arthritis.

Neibauer prosthesis: silicone hinge joints with built-in ties; useful in MCP joint arthroplasty.

perichondral autografts: use of osteocartilaginous grafts (from ribs) to resurface the injured articular surface of a small joint in the hand.

proximal row carpectomy: a salvage procedure whereby the scaphoid, lunate, and triquetrum are excised. This is useful in treating advanced arthritis involving the RC joint of wrist where motion is still desired by the patient.

radial styloidectomy: excision of the tip of the radial styloid; useful in isolated radioscaphoid arthritis or as part of the scapholunate advanced collapse wrist reconstruction.

Stefee thumb a.: a cemented metal polyethylene prosthesis useful in thumb MCP arthroplasty.

Suave Kapanje p.: fusion of the articular surface of the distal radioulnar joint with proximal resection of a distal ulnar segment of approximately 1.5 cm to facilitate motion. Also called **Lauenstein p.**

suspensionplasty p.: for advanced trapeziometacarpal arthritis, removal of the trapezium, and placement of half of the flexor carpi radialis as an anchor to the metacarpal and as a spacer. An improvement on the classic anchovy procedure. Also called **ligament reconstruction tendon interposition (LRTI) p.** and **Burton p.**

Swanson a.: complete array of silicone implants for all digital articula, joints, carpal bones, total wrist arthroplasty, distal ulna, and proximal radius. This is most useful in rheumatoid arthritis for the reconstruction of MCP joints. Its use in the carpus had to be discontinued because of concerns regarding silicone synovitis.

Swanson prosthesis (silicone): most useful for MCP and PIP arthroplasty in rheumatoid arthritis. In selected situations, a total wrist arthroplasty is useful (i.e., in bilateral involvement). Carpal silicone arthroplasty is now falling out of favor because of silicone synovitis.

trapezial hemiarthroplasty: resection of the distal half of the trapezium, sparing the scaphotrapezial joint; useful for trapeziometacarpal arthritis.

Tupper a.: in MCP joint arthritis, the volar plate may be used as an interpositional material after excision arthroplasty.

Vainio metaphalangeal interposition: MCP joint resectional arthroplasty with interposition of the extensor tendon and collateral ligaments.

Voltz a.: a metal-polyethylene cemented total wrist arthroplasty useful in selected cases of end-stage degenerative or rheumatoid arthritis.

Zancholli capsuloplasty: a volar plate advancement of the MCP joint of the thumb to treat congenital hyperextension.

Zancholli-Lasso p.: transfer of the flexor digitorum sublimus tendon to the lateral band or the A2 pulley to prevent metaphalangeal hyperextension and clawing; found in low ulnar nerve palsy.

Zancholli static-lock p.: a volar plate advancement (plication) for the treatment of metaphalangeal hyperextension; seen in claw deformities in low ulnar nerve palsy.

Neurologic Procedures

Boyes p.: repair of deep branch of ulnar nerve; tendon transfers for radial nerve palsy; tendon transfers to restore thumb adduction.

cable nerve grafts: a method of uniting strands of nerve graft and interposing them into a gap to repair a polyfascicular nerve discontinuity (of historic interest).

epineural repair: repair of lacerated nerve segments by repairing the epineurium. This is useful in digital nerves or in oligofascicular proximal nerves.

epineurotomy: the opening of the epineurium during a neurolysis procedure. This can be useful in certain cases of chronic nerve compression.

funiculectomy: for chronic end neuromas; peeling back the epineurium and resecting nerve fascicles, with reclosure and ligation of the epineurium. May aid in the treatment of end neuromas.

group fascicular repair: a perineural repair; useful in treating laceration of mixed motor and sensory nerves. Presumably, exact anatomic reapproximation will facilitate maximal functional return.

hemi-pulp flap: neurosensory free flaps from the great or second toe indicated for large single pulp defect. This is indicated when sensory function is essential for proper hand function and protection. This is best indicated for thumb reconstruction.

hetero-digital flaps: a cross-finger flap of dorsal skin to cover a significant palmar surface defect in an adjacent defect. Digital island transfer of pedicle flaps that are lifted with its neurovascular bundle and transferred to a defect on an adjacent digit.

internal neurolysis: presumably, internal dissection of intraneural scarring will facilitate return of nerve function. Originally thought to be useful in the treatment of carpal tunnel syndrome but now found to be harmful in many cases. This technique, however, is useful in the removal of intraneural neurilemmoma.

medial epicondylectomy: one method to decompress the ulnar nerve in the cubital tunnel by removing its bony floor, the medial epicondyle of the distal humerus.

Moberg p.: for tetraplegia; to restore the ability of key pinch in group II or III level tetraplegia. This includes CMC thumb arthrodesis, extensor pollicis longus tenodesis, and FPL tenodesis or transfer. Also called **key pinch p.**

neurectomy: the resection of a portion of nerve of an end neuroma (and presumed buried in bone or muscle).

neurotization: in patients with a profound brachial plexus injury with a flare anesthetic arm, the use of a live intercostal nerve grafted to a distal neural segment of the brachial plexus has restored some upper extremity function in select patients.

Trauma Procedures

Belsky-Eaton p.: pinning of proximal phalangeal fracture

Bentzon p.: attempt to convert a painful scaphoid nonunion to a painless pseudarthrosis by soft tissue (capsular flap) interposition; of historic interest.

Bevin Auriglass p.: a digital web-deepening procedure for the correction of burn syndactyly.

Buchler p.: open reduction and fixation of a Rolando base of thumb metacarpal fracture.

Chung p.: volar plate fixation of distal radial fracture.

Cooney p.: open repair of triangular fibrous cartilage complex for class 1D injury.

Culp p.: open repair of triangular fibrous cartilage complex class 1C injury

distal finger amputation revision: procedure performed following traumatic amputation involving the distal phalanx (fingertip) by the following techniques: healing by secondary intention, reamputation, V-Y flap (Kutler or Atasoy), volar flap advancement (Moberg), Bipedicle dorsal flap, crossfinger flap, and thenar flap.

Eaton and Littler p.: for recurrent dislocation of thumb CMC joint, ligament reconstruction; also called **trapeziometacarpal ligament reconstruction.**

Eaton and Malerich p.: open reduction of PIP joint fracture-dislocation.

Fernandez p.: grafting for scaphoid nonunion; also called **opening-wedge free graft**.

finger flaps: to preserve sensation.

    Atosoy p.: volar single V-Y advancement.

    cross-finger flap: a section of skin with its blood supply intact from a neighboring finger used to cover open area.

    Kutler p.: lateral double V-Y advancement.

    thenar flap: one raised from the thumb side of the base of the palm.

    Wolfe graft: free skin (pinch) graft; a section of full-thickness skin placed on the open area.

Fisk-Fernandez volar wedge: anterior cortical cancellous bone graft for the correction of scaphoid nonunion or malunion.

Gibraiel flap: a form of rotational skin flap using moving skin from the lateral aspect of the digit to the flexor surface with little or no movement of the pivot point.

Glickel p.: closed reduction and percutaneous pinning of distal radial fracture; graft reconstructions of chronic thumb ulnar collateral ligament injuries.

Herbert screw osteosynthesis: the use of a dumbbell-shaped bone screw with variable pitch to affect rigid compressive internal fixation of a scaphoid fracture or nonunion. This can be used with or without bone graft.

Kapandji fixation: for distal radius fracture; use of two K-wires inserted at 90 degrees at fracture site lateral and posterior and then angled 45 degrees anteriorly.

Kaplan p.: open reduction of finger MCP dislocation.

Kawai and Yamamoto p.: for scaphoid nonunion, vascularized bone graft.

Kirschner (K) wire fixation: small threaded or non-threaded wires are used to transfix fractures or to produce traction with the use of an external appliance.

Lamey and Fernandez p.: for distal ulnar pseudarthrosis, distal radial-ulnar joint arthrodesis

metacarpal lengthening: useful for irretrievable thumb amputation at the MCP joint level; metacarpal osteotomy, application of a distraction device, slow distraction, and later bone grafting will partially restore length of the thumb ray. Secondary first web deepening may be required. Also called **Matevp p.**

Russe bone graft: for scaphoid nonunion fracture; cortical cancellous graft placed by a volar approach through a longitudinal trough in the volar surface of the scaphoid that will enhance bony union.

Microvascular Procedures

anastomosis: term used for the direct repair of nerves and blood vessels.

back wall first technique: a microsurgical procedure in which the vessel wall away from the surgeon is sutured first, most useful in vessels of approximately equal size when one or both of the presenting ends cannot be rotated within a double clamp.

Chinese flap (radial forearm flap): a radial forearm rotation flap based on the radial artery to repair radial and hand defects.

cross-arm flaps: random flaps using tissue from random pedicle flap using tissue from the patient's upper arm to cover a large defect on the patient's contralateral hand.

denervation: the accidental or intentional removal of sensory or motor nerve input to a distal site in the hand or arm.

dorsalis pedis flap: a microvascular free flap using the dorsalis pedis artery of the foot as the donor artery used to cover small defects in the upper extremity.

fibrin clot glue: a method of augmenting nerve apposition by using fibrin clot glue to cement the suture line.

flipping technique: used in microsurgery repairing a small vessel that is freely mobile. One can flip the vessel to repair the back wall. Used in vein grafting and free-tissue transfer technique.

four-flap Z-plasty: a double Z-plasty used commonly in the reconstruction of the first webspace.

free flaps: a method of free tissue transfer using skin, muscle, bone, or all three. Tissue is transferred using its vascular pedicle and microsurgical anastomotic technique.

interposition graft: generally used for either nerve or vascular (vein) grafts to bridge a gap for direct microanastomosis of nerves and vessels.

laser Doppler fluxometry: this evaluates cutaneous microvascular perfusion. This evaluates the motion of the red blood cells in the area directly beneath the probe.

lateral arm flap: a free flap based on the posterior radial collateral artery; useful for covering large, full-thickness defects in the dorsum of the hand.

no reflow phenomenon: a microvascular anastomosis with arterial anastomosis. Disruption of the neurovascular tree may result in no venous return into the field.

sympathectomy: a method to improve peripheral blood flow by ablating the central or peripheral sympathetic innervation to arteries in treatment of chronic regional pain syndrome by surgery.

toe-thumb transfer: complete transfer of a toe with its full complement of neurovascular, tendinous, and bone structures to the hand to add to a digit or thumb on a posttraumatic or congenitally deficient hand.

wraparound procedure: the medial aspect of the great toe with its neurovascular bundles is removed from the toe and wrapped around a free bone graft at the tip of an amputation stump. This is then reattached using microvascular techniques. The donor site is secondarily grafted to close its defect.

Congenital Deformity Repairs

Barsky macrodactyly reduction: (1) filleting out of the distal phalanx, then placing all distal structures on to the end of the middle phalanx (this will shorten the macrodactylous digit); (2) hemiresection of the middle phalanx and DIP joint fusion.

Bayne and Klug p.: centralization of hand with transfer of flexor carpi ulnaris.

Bilhaut-Cloquet p.: for Wassel II thumb duplication (bifid thumb). The narrow half of each thumb tip is united with the other, discarding the central units and allowing the thumb to become one phalanx.

Bonola p.: a dorsally based closing wedge osteotomy of the distal phalanx to correct a Kirner deformity.

Bracket resection: epiphyseal resection of the apex of a delta phalanx accompanied by fat grafting.

Buck-Gramcko p.: centralization of hand lengthening brachymetacarpia in hypoplastic hand; pollicization of another finger.

Carstan reverse wedge osteotomy: for the treatment of a delta phalanx; a central wedge is reversed and turned 180 degrees to straighten a digit.

callotasis: technique of one-stage bone lengthening by placement of an external fixator on both sides of osteotomy and stretching the bone out to lengthen short digits. Also called **distraction lengthening.**

Cronin technique: a technique for separating syndactylized digit using a combination of palmar and dorsal triangular flaps.

House p.: for thumb-in-palm deformity, contracture release; for flexion and key pinch capacity, reconstruction of index finger

Kessler p.: for partial thumb amputations or other defects, metacarpal lengthening.

Krukenberg p.: in the congenital absence of a hand, the radius and ulna are surgically separated and covered with soft tissue so that the two bones will act as a claw.

Manske and McCarroll opponensplasty: for congenital radial dysplasia, abductor digiti minimi opponensplasties.

physiolysis: the selective obliteration of the growth plate and area of uneven bone growth such as seen in Madelung deformity. This is frequently accompanied by fat grafting to inhibit further bone growth.

radialization, centralization: an attempt to rebalance the hand and wrist on to the distal forearm in radial clubbed hand.

Skin, Nails, and Fascia Procedures

advancement flaps: flaps cut either from the volar pad or from the radial and ulnar pad of the distal fingertip for the reconstruction of fingertip injuries with skin and subcutaneous loss; also called **V-Y flaps** and **Kleinert-Atosoy.**

axial cutaneous flaps: free or island flap on a subscapular artery pedicle for medium-sized defect coverage in the hand; also called **scapular flap.**

axial flag flaps: a rotational skin flap based on a dorsal digital artery used for digital skin and subcutaneous defects.

axial pattern skin flap: a long skin flap possible because of an underlying vascular supply running along its long axis underneath.

Bednar and Lane p.: advancement of skin to cover base of a finger nail.

cocked-half flap: reconstruction of a thumb amputation at the MCP joint level with a local skin graft, iliac crest graft, and skin graft; also called **Gillies flap.**

composite nail bed flap: a full-thickness nail bed graft from a toe to cover a defect in a finger nail bed.

cross-finger flap: the dorsal skin of one digit is flapped over itself to create coverage for a volar skin defect of an adjacent digit.

cryotherapy: a method of using extreme cold to freeze skin lesions such as actinic keratosis.

escharotomy: in the management of deep thermal burns, burned and contracted skin is incised to decompress deeper tissues and prevent further necrosis.

fasciectomy: generic term used to describe excision of the palmar fascia, usually when involved in Dupuytren disease.

fasciotomy: (1) opening of muscle compartments and decompressing intrinsic muscle spaces in compartment syndrome; spaces to be decompressed are interosseus muscles (through dorsal incisions or volar thenar and hypothenar compartments); (2) incision into a Dupuytren central cord to release contracture; this is useful in older and debilitated patients, but contracture recurrence is common.

flag flap: a rotational pedicle flap harvested on the dorsum of the finger and used to cover defects on adjacent fingers or over the MCP joint. The same can be performed as a volar flap as well.

Macindo procedure: a form of palmar fasciectomy for Dupuytren contracture when the palmar skin is left open to granulate.

marsupialization: a technique used to expose the germinal matrix of a nail in patients with chronic paronychia in which a crescent of the eponychial fold is removed to uncover chronic fungal infection.

Moberg flap: useful in thumb tip reconstruction; the volar half of the thumb soft tissue is elevated with its neurovascular structures, and by flexing the IP joint of the thumb, the flap is then stretched over the thumb tip.

neurovascular island transfer: a method of transferring sensibility to an important part of the hand such as the thumb tip from a less important part of the hand, whereby a portion of skin is left connected to its neurovascular structures and passed subcutaneously to a different part of the hand.

onychectomy: removal of a fingernail.

onychotomy: the method of cutting into a nail, usually to remove a mass under the nail.

pedicle flap: a procedure that permits an island of skin and subcutaneous tissue to be transferred from one place to another on its own vascular supply, using multiple operative stages.

pedicle grafts: a term used for pedicle flaps but also includes *pedicle bone grafts*. *Island pedicle grafts* and *neurovascular pedicle grafts* are pedicle, skin, or subcutaneous tissue containing blood and nerve supply, thus providing sensation for the skin graft.

thenar flap: for fingertip coverage, an H-flap is raised on the thenar eminence and the digit tip is flexed down to it. By 10 to 14 days, the flap provides a good skin and soft tissue coverage to the distal digit tip. However, digital stiffness is common.

Muscle Transfers and Procedures for the Hand

There are two types of tendon procedures: (1) restoration of tendon function by direct repair of a tendon, its advancement, or its transfer, and (2) freeing of tendon from scar tissue, restrictive bands, or abnormal lining tissues. In some cases muscle attachments are transferred or used as a cover fro soft tissue defects.

Bateman p.: indicated in axillary and suprascapular nerve palsy, which involves an acromial fragment to the humerus to facilitate shoulder abduction.

Chen p.: posterior interosseous muscle flap.

deltoid flap: a muscular-free flap using the deltoid to cover small to moderate deficits in the upper extremity.

Hammond p.: multiple muscle transfers for reconstruction of the paralyzed shoulder in brachial plexus injuries. Transfer of the posterior third of the deltoid to the lateral aspect of the clavicle and from the tendinous origins of the long head of the triceps and the short head of the biceps to the lateral aspect of the acromion to aid in shoulder abduction. Transfer of the latissimus dorsi to teres major tendons.

House reconstruction: complete array of reconstructions to facilitate hand function in patients with varying degrees of quadriplegia (tetraplegia) depending on the level of the lesion in the cervical spine.

Steindler flexorplasty: in brachial plexus injury causing paralysis of elbow flexion (biceps and brachialis) with sparing of distal forearm musculature, the flexor pronator mass with the medial epicondyle of the distal humerus is transferred anteriorly and proximally on the humerus to effect elbow flexion.

Tendon Suture Repair Techniques

Numerous techniques and types of sutures are used in repairing tendons. A tendon repair is any reapproximation of a partially or completely severed tendon. The specific technique is directed at gaining maximal strength with minimal scarring.

Becker p.: multiple cross-stitching technique for approximation of fresh tendon edges.
Bunnell opponensplasty: the use of the flexor digitorum sublimis IV as a donor motor for thumb opposition, using the pulley in the region of the flexor carpi ulnaris and the pisiform.
Kleinert p.: modification of Bunnell technique, burying suture knot at tendon edge.
modified Kessler suture: a direct end-to-end grafting suture for flexor tendon lacerations, especially in zone II. These are usually augmented with epitendinous sutures.
Pulver-Taft weave: the strongest method of reattaching two tendons where space is not at a premium. It involves weaving tendon ends in and out of each other.
Tsuge: multiple cross-stitching technique for tendon reapproximation.
Verdan suture: multiple cross-stitching technique for tendon reapproximation.

Other specific techniques include **four-strand cruciate p., Tajima p., Halsted p., Salvage p.,** and **Silfverskiöld p.**

Tendon Grafts and Transfers

A tendon transfer is the relocation of a tendon from one place to another. The tendon retains attachment to its muscle. By contrast, free tendon graft requires complete excision of a tendon and its repositioning in a new location. Tendon transfers may be static or dynamic.

Tendon transfers are commonly required to replace or assist voluntary muscle function that is lost because of nerve injury, nerve disease, or direct and indirect sequelae of trauma to the muscle. Substantial numbers of transfers are used in central nervous system paralyses such as those caused by strokes and polio. Transfers are listed by categories that define function.

Aichef technique: a method of central slip reconstruction in Boutonnière deformity by designing a tendon flap using the central half of the lateral bands and bringing them toward the midline to recreate a central slip in which the central slip has been irreparably damaged by trauma.
Brand p.: hand web deepening with sliding flap; ring finger sublimis tendon used as motor; transfer of extensor carpi radialis longus or brevis tendon; transfer of sublimis tendon.
Brent-Moberg tenodesis: thumb flexor tenodesis to restore key pinch in quadriplegics. A technique using flexor or extensor tendon graft to restore and treat functions in ulnar nerve palsy.
Burkhalter p.: transfer of extensor indicis proprius tendon.
Burkhalter transfer: threading digital flexors through the proximal phalanx to facilitate MCP flexion in low ulnar nerve palsy with claw deformities.
Camitz p.: the palmaris longus, with its distal attachment tubularized, is passed under the thenar eminence and attached to the radial aspect of the base of the proximal phalanx of the thumb to act as an opponensplasty. This is useful in chronic carpal tunnel syndrome.
central slip repair and reconstruction: procedure designed to repair the common extensor insertion into the proximal dorsal end of the middle phalanx, thus restoring active PIP extension.
Clark pectoralis major transfer: transfer of the sternocostal portion of the pectoralis major muscle for the restoration of elbow flexion in brachial plexus injury.
crossed intrinsic transfer: in rheumatoid arthritis, with ulnar deviation of the digits at the metaphalangeal joint, a conjoined ulnar intrinsic tendon is

released from one digit and placed into the radial conjoined intrinsic tendon of the adjacent digit on its ulnar side.

dynamic tendon transfer: one that brings about motion by direct action of muscle contraction.

finger extension p.: Boyes procedure.

finger flexion p.: for flexion of the MCP joint (intrinsic transfer); **Boyes, Fowler, Bunnell, Stiles-Bunnell, Riordan,** and **Pulver-Taft procedures,** and **Brand I** and **Brand II procedures.**

flexor pronator slide: release of the flexor pronator muscle group origin allowing the muscle to slide distally. This helps correct wrist and digital flexion deformity and forearm pronation deformity in cerebral palsy.

flexor tenolysis: method used to free flexor tendon from its surrounding scars approximately 4 months after flexor tendon repair with secondary tendon adherence.

Fowler tenodesis: static tendon grafts originating in the extensor retinaculum, passing volarly to the deep transverse metacarpal ligament, and inserting it into the radial lateral bands. A procedure to prevent hyperextension of the MCP joint as seen in the claw deformity of low ulnar nerve palsy.

Green transfer: flexor carpi ulnaris to extensor carpi radialis brevis transfer to correct a wrist flexion deformity in cerebral palsy. Overcorrection is common.

Groves and Goldner transfer: transfer of flexor carpi ulnaris combined with sublimis tendon.

Huber transfer: a procedure designed to restore thumb opposition based on a transfer into the thenar eminence of the abductor digiti minimi, that is, a neurovascular pedicle.

Hui-Linscheid p.: a tenodesis procedure designed to reconstruct the volar ulnar carpal ligament using a strip of flexor carpi ulnaris tendon particularly useful in primary ulnar-carpal instability or secondary distal radial ulnar joint instability.

Jones transfer: in radial nerve palsy, tendon transfer designed to restore thumb, digital, and wrist extension.

Lasso p.: flexor digitorum superficialis in a tenodesis mode to flex the MCP joint used commonly in tetraplegia and patients with hyperextension deformities of the MCP joint and with hyperextension of the PIP joint.

Lennox Fritschi technique: a palmaris longus motored four-tail transfer used in ulnar palsy to correct claw deformities to promote MCP flexion and PIP extension.

Littler-Eaton ligament reconstruction: method of stabilizing the base of the thumb metacarpal in stage I basal joint arthritis by using local tendon graft reconstruction.

Littler boutonnière reconstruction: includes dorsal transposition of the lateral bands and repair of the central SLIP to the base of the middle phalanx.

Mennen opponensplasty: the extensor pollicis longus is passed through the interosseous membrane to the volar aspect of the forearm and backed out along the thenar eminence to the dorsal surface of the MCP joint, thus creating opponens function.

opponensplasty: the use of any of the intrinsic or extrinsic muscle tendon units to restore thumb opposition (i.e., in median nerve palsy); also called **Brand, Burkhalter, Groves, Goldner, Riordan, Phalen-Miller, Littler, Huber,** and **Fowler procedures.**

Parke tenodesis: static tenodesis using wrist extensors as grafts to treat claw deformities to promote MP flexion.

Ranney technique: an extensor digiti minimi transfer to the neck of the fifth metacarpal to restore the transverse metacarpal arch in ulnar nerve palsy.

Riordan technique: a flexor carpi radialis transfer using a free graft passing from the flexor to the extensor side of the forearm, radial lateral bands of the fingers involved in claw deformity in low ulnar nerve palsy.

static tendon transfer: transfer of a free tendon graft attached to two or more bony locations, such that the active movement of one joint will cause the passive movement of some other joint. For example, a tendon appropriately inserted proximal to the wrist and in the fingers will cause flexion of the fingers if the wrist is extended.

tendolysis: a tendon release. It describes two different types of procedures: (1) one in which the tendon is freed from scar tissue or entrapment so that it may move properly, and (2) tenosynovectomy, whereby all or part of the sheath of a functioning tendon is excised. Also called **tenolysis.**

tendon advancement: done when the damage segment of a tendon is so near its insertion that a direct tendon-to-bone rather than tendon-to-tendon repair is necessary. One such technique is the **Wagner advancement** of the profundus tendon.

tenodesis: the fixation of a tendon onto two bony locations to keep a joint from flexing or extending beyond a selected range. This procedure lends itself to prevention of hyperextension of the MCP joints in ulnar claw deformity. Two commonly done are the Fowler and Riordan procedures.

tenorrhaphy: the repair of a lacerated tendon, either immediate or delayed.

tenotomy: a procedure in which a tendon, either flexor or extensor, is sectioned purposely to correct a deformity to bring back the position or function of the hand or wrist.

thumb abduction p.: pulling thumb away from the side of the hand; also called **Boyes p.**

thumb adduction p.: pulling the thumb to side of index finger; also called **Boyes p., Bunnell p., Edgarton-Grand p.,** and **Royle-Thompson p.**

wrist extension p.: Boyes p. using pronator teres to the extensor carpi radialis brevis muscle.

Tenosynovectomy

Tenosynovectomy refers to the excision of thickened tendon sheath and other tissue surrounding a tendon, commonly seen in infection, chemical irritation, and rheumatoid arthritis (synovectomy). It also refers to the following procedures in hand surgery.

abductor pollicis longus release: a release of the fibrous canal surrounding the abductor pollicis longus at the wrist for symptoms of de Quervain syndrome (pain on abduction of the thumb). Also called **de Quervain release.**

Howard p.: freeing of adherent flexor tendon.

tenosynovectomy: a procedure whereby the tenosynovium surrounding the tendon sheaths are removed such as in rheumatoid arthritis to prevent tendon rupture or to treat tendon entrapment.

tenovaginotomy: procedure designed to release stenosing tenosynovitis by incising a retinaculum or flexor pulley.

trigger finger release: a release of fibrous covering of tendon (pulley) at the base of the finger to prevent a tendon with nodular changes from snapping with motion of the finger. Also called **snapping tendon release.**

Other Tendon Procedures

boutonnière reconstruction: a classic extensor tendon reconstruction for boutonnière deformity, designed to restore active extension of the PIP joint and to prevent its flexion posturing. This procedure is fraught with difficulty, and prognosis is guarded; also called **Littler, Matev,** and **Fowler procedures.**

Hunter rod: a silicone-rubber tendon spacer or rod that is used to form a new synovium-filled channel. It is removed during a second-stage procedure, and a tendon graft is threaded through. Useful as a two-stage procedure when the tendon bed is extremely scarred and a direct tendon graft is impossible. Also called **passive tendon implant.**

Kortzeborn p.: a lengthening of the extensor tendons of the thumb and formation of a fascial attachment of the thumb to the ulnar side of the hand to relieve ape hand deformity.

swan-neck revision: surgery designed to eliminate a swan-neck deformity in the fingers by revision of tendons; also called **Swanson revision** and **Littler modified tendon revision.**

Other Hand and Wrist Procedures

Agee p.: single-incision endoscopic carpal tunnel release.

Almquist p.: carpal ligament reconstruction.

Beckenbaugh p.: correction of hyperextension deformity of PIP joint.

Beskin p.: proximal phalangeal osteotomy.

Brand p.: hand web deepening with sliding flap; ring finger sublimis tendon used as motor; transfer of extensor carpi radialis longus or brevis tendon; transfer of sublimis tendon.

Broadbent and Woolf p.: four-flap Z-plasty in adducted thumb

Broudy and Smith p.: rotational osteotomy of first metacarpal.

Broudy and Smith p.: rotational osteotomy of first metacarpal.

capsular release: an incision of a joint capsule done to regain lost motion caused by contractures; also called **capsulectomy.**

capsulodesis: in hand surgery, the capsule, which may include the dorsal or volar plate, may be tightened to help hold an affected joint in a position that can no longer be held voluntarily. This is done often for nerve injuries and is commonly called the **Zancolli** procedure (for clawhand deformity); also called **volar capsular reefing** and **Blatt dorsal capsulodesis.**

carbon implant: a new form of resurfacing arthroplasty for the MCP and PIP joints used commonly in osteoarthritis; also called **pyrocarbon implant.**

carpal tunnel release: a division of the strong ligamentous band (transverse carpal ligament) that covers the median nerve and flexor tendons of the finger and thumb. This is usually done to relieve pressure on the median nerve that may result from arthritis, trauma, or unknown causes. A *tenosynovectomy*, if necessary, may be done through the same incision.

carpectomy: the removal of the proximal row of carpal bones, usually indicated in some forms of arthritis or severe spastic contractures.

Chow p: two-incision carpal tunnel release.

Chun and Palmer p.: an ulnar shortening osteotomy

Cowen and Loftus p.: metacarpal lengthening with distraction.

dermodesis: the removal of a segment of skin and then closure of the skin margins to shorten skin and restrict motion of a joint. It is frequently done in conjunction with a *Zancolli* capsulodesis for ulnar clawhand.

Dupuytren contracture release: named after a French surgeon, this surgical procedure is the excision of the contracted fibrotic bands of the palmar fascia. However, the skin is often adherent and recurrent deformity is a problem. Specific techniques for resection of these bands are:

Luck p.: percutaneous transection of fibrotic bands without removal of tissue.

McCash p.: transverse skin incision with transection of bands and then passive stretch dressing applied, leaving the wounds open.

fishmouth incision: a wraparound incision over the distal end of the finger to facilitate drainage.

Foucher technique: a procedure for internal fixation of metacarpal neck fractures using multiple prebent Kirschner wires in a wire-stacking technique.

ganglionectomy: the excision of a ganglion, which usually occurs on the dorsum of the wrist or the base of the fingers.

Hammond procedure: multiple muscle transfers for reconstruction of the paralyzed shoulder in brachial plexus injuries. Transfer of the posterior third of the deltoid to the lateral aspect of the clavicle, and from the tendinous origins of the long head of the triceps and the short head of the biceps, to the lateral aspect of the acromion, to aid in shoulder abduction. Transfer of the latissimus dorsi to teres major tendons.

Illarramendi and De Carlit p.: radial decompression for loss of blood supply to the lunate bone.

infiltration technique: a method of axillary block for regional anesthesia in upper extremity surgery. The anesthetic is injected around the axillary artery inside the sheath of the neurovascular bundle spreading local anesthetic around the brachial plexus.

interscalene block: a brachial plexus block using a needle in the interscalene space to numb the brachial plexus to effect regional anesthetic commonly used in shoulder surgery.

island flaps: either pedicle or free flaps of small amounts of tissue either skin, bone, muscle, or a combination of both for the reconstruction of small area defects.

joint leveling procedures with ulnar lengthening and radial shortening: used to restore the anatomic relationship between the distal radius and ulna (generally, the ulnar variance seen on the contralateral normal side).

Kanaya procedure: for limited pronation and supination of the wrist caused by distal radial ulnar joint disorders; interposition of vascularized fascia-fat graft with corrective osteotomy of the radius.

kite flap: an island pedicle of flap proximally based on the first dorsal metacarpal artery designed on the radial side of the distal portion of the second metacarpal and MCP joint; used to reconstruct defects on the dorsum of the hand usually on the radial side.

latissimus dorsi flap: a form of myocutaneous pedicle or free flap in which blood supply derives from the thoracodorsal artery and is used to cover large soft tissue defects.

mallet finger revision: designed to regain active extension of the DIP joints of the finger.

Fowler release: technique used at the PIP joint for a mallet finger.

palmar advancement flaps: a proximally based flap used to cover distal soft tissue defects; most commonly used in the thumbs. Also called **Moberg flap.**

palmar fasciectomy, fasciotomy: the release, with or without resection of tissues, of shortened, thickened, and contracted fasciae in the palm or finger in flexion deformities resulting from Dupuytren contracture.

phalangectomy: the excision of a part or all of a phalanx because of trauma or arthritis. Rarely performed in the hand; more commonly done in the foot.

pollicization: any operation replacing a congenitally or traumatically missing thumb by reconstruction of the index, long, ring, or little finger such that it acts or functions as a thumb; also called **Buck-Gramko p., Riordan p., Littler p., Gillies p.,** and **Verdan p.**

random pattern flaps: skin flaps that are generally quadrilateral in shape and are raised by incising three of the four sides and depends on the minute vessels of the subdermal and subcutaneous plexus.

RASL p.: acronym referring to the *reduction association of the scapholunate* joint. This consists of an open reduction of the scapholunate articulation, repair of the ligamentous remnants, and protection of the repair by internally blocking the scapholunate joint with a transverse Herbert screw for a year to provide intercarpal fibrosis.

ray amputation: a procedure to remove a metacarpal and all phalangeal segments of a finger distal to that metacarpal.

regional flaps: those derived from tissues not immediately adjacent to the primary defect but in its vicinity. They can be random or axial pattern flaps depending on their blood supply.

replantation: a microsurgical procedure that requires the reattachment of nerves, veins, and arteries to attempt restoration of function to a freshly severed part such as a finger.

revision polydactyly: polydactyly usually affects the thumb and little finger. Revision requires reattachment of specific tendons or ligaments; also called **Marks and Bayne p.**

saphenous flap: a myocutaneous flap based on the saphenous artery and nerve. This is used to cover small- to medium-sized defects.

synovectomy: removal of synovium in joints. The procedure is done frequently for rheumatoid arthritis.

tendinocutaneous flaps: vascularized tendon graft that can be transferred with a dorsalis pedis or radial forearm flap. This is indicated for one-stage reconstruction of degloving injury to the dorsum of the hand with loss of skin and extensor tendons for example.

Tikhor-Linberg p.: an alternative to the arm amputation of well-localized tumors around the shoulder, which represents a resection of the shoulder girdle with preservation of the arm.

transposition flaps: skin flaps used to cover small deficits. These may be axial pattern or random pattern.

trapeziectomy: removal of the trapezium bone in the treatment of basal joint arthritis, which may be done alone or in concert with an interposition arthroplasty.

ulnar forearm flap: a fascial cutaneous flap that is based on the ulnar artery and is harvested from the ulnar aspect of the forearm; used to cover deficits of the ulnar side of the hand or used as a free flap for distal defect.

wafer p.: for ulnar plus wrist; resection of the distal 2 to 3 mm of the ulnar head, leaving the styloid intact.

Approaches

Wrist

dorsal a.: on the back side of the wrist, this approach is used for tendon transfers, fusions, and ganglionectomies.

Henry a.: for volar forearm.

lateral a.: used on the radial side of the wrist for tendon transfers, radial styloidectomy, and visualization of the navicular bone.

medial a.: an approach to the ulnar side of the wrist used for some tendon transfers and for the Darrach procedure; also called **Smith-Petersen a.**

volar a.: approach from the palmar aspect of the wrist, used for carpal tunnel releases, tendon explorations, and some bony procedures.

Hand

Surgical approaches are too numerous and complicated to describe here. Refer to Canale ST, Beaty J, 2013.

The Foot and Ankle

The human foot is a marvelous anatomic structure that provides a stable base to support large amounts of weight, and shifts in any direction to maintain structural support. The bones of the foot are arranged to both balance body weight and negotiate irregular terrain. The average person will walk an estimated 20,000 to 46,000 miles in a lifetime, and, for that reason, may seek the expertise of an orthopaedic foot and ankle specialist or a podiatrist.

The **orthopaedic surgeon** is a board-certified, medical school graduate who treats many major problems related to the foot and ankle such as congenital deformities, traumatic injuries, degenerative conditions, athletic injuries, and deformities. The orthopaedic foot and ankle specialist provides surgical and nonsurgical care. Problems of the feet are so numerous and treatment has become so complex that foot and ankle care has become a subspecialty of orthopaedics. The American Orthopaedic Foot and Ankle Society and the American Academy of Orthopaedic Surgeons have been directly responsible for establishing a subspecialty devoted to injuries, diseases, and surgery of the foot and ankle. This subspecialization is now a part of many residency training programs.

The **podiatrist,** a doctor of podiatric medicine, is a graduate of a 4-year, doctoral-level program in podiatry. After residency, he or she becomes board certified in foot and ankle surgery and primary care in podiatric medicine. The podiatrist is devoted to diagnosing and treating diseases and disorders of the human foot, including biomechanics applied to orthotics and prosthetics, instructing patients in proper shoe fit and providing general foot care. The practice encompasses nonsurgical and surgical treatment

The **pedorthist,** a board-certified specialist in special footwear modifications and orthoses, provides services such as footwear modifications and filling prescriptions for special lines of shoes, customized inserts, and numerous foot support orthotics in the treatment of a variety of conditions.

In larger institutions, the orthopaedist may work in association with a podiatrist and pedorthist in the care of patients with ankle- and foot-related problems. A team approach provides the advantage of comprehensive, convenient, coordinated foot and ankle care. This team includes the orthopaedist, podiatrist, pedorthist, orthotist, and physical therapist. These specialists work independently, but may also make up the orthopaedic foot and ankle service team. For that reason, we have included many terms specific to podiatry along with the generally interchangeable terms of anatomy, diseases, and surgery of the foot and ankle.

Anatomy

The human foot is composed of 26 bones plus a varying number of ossicles or sesamoid bones and is divided into three functional units: the hindfoot (talus and calcaneus), midfoot (cuneiforms, cuboid, and navicular), and forefoot (metatarsals and phalanges). The joints between the calcaneus, talus, navicular, and cuboid bones permit most of the motion in turning the foot inward (inversion) or outward (eversion).

The bones of the midfoot and hindfoot are part of the longitudinal arch. The arch's function is to smoothly transmit weight from the hindfoot to the forefoot during gait, and to negotiate irregular terrain. During gait, the foot experiences forces that can be as much as two to four times the body weight. The joints between all of the bones of the arch work together to remain flexible and absorb shock when the heel strikes the ground. The joints remain flexible as weight is transferred through the midfoot to allow the foot to conform to the terrain. The joints tighten and the arch becomes fixed as body weight shifts to the forefoot so that the foot becomes a rigid lever to propel the body forward. Coordinated muscle forces control the transition from flexible to rigid and back to flexible.

During a step on a normal foot, the focus of force on the foot starts at the heel, travels toward the forefoot along the lateral border of the foot, and then travels medially across the ball of the foot to finish at the hallux (great toe). The mechanical complexities of the foot make it fascinating to study. Figures 11-1 to 11-4 will assist in understanding these structures. Injuries around the ankle joint receive the most attention and are discussed in Chapter 1.

Bones of the Ankle and Foot

accessory navicular: an "extra" bone or ossicle on the medial side of the navicular, present in up to 14% of the population. It is actually a tertiary center of ossification, and its interface with the navicular bone can be a source of pain. Also called **os tibiale externum.**

calcaneus: the heel bone; largest of the bones of the foot, articulates with the talus and cuboid. The combining form is *calcaneo,* for example, calcaneofibular ligament, or calcaneocuboid joint.

cuboid: cube-shaped bone on the lateral side of the foot, just distal to the calcaneus and articulating with the bases of the fourth and fifth metatarsals.

cuneiforms: three wedge-shaped bones lying just proximal to the first three metatarsals and distal to the navicular bone. They form the transverse arch. From medial to lateral, they are called the first, second, and third cuneiforms or the medial (middle and lateral cuneiforms).

FIG 11-1 Bones of right foot viewed from above. Tarsal bones consist of cuneiforms, navicular, talus, cuboid, and calcaneus. *(From Anthony C, Kolthoff N:* Textbook of anatomy and physiology, *ed 9, St Louis, 1975, Mosby.)*

distal interphalangeal (DIP) joint: the joint between the middle phalanx and distal phalanx of one of the lesser toes.

forefoot: portion of foot containing metatarsals, phalanges, and sesamoids.

The Foot and Ankle   **345**

Flexor digitorum longus tendons

Flexor digitorum brevis tendons

Adductor hallucis muscle (transverse head)

Flexor hallucis longus tendon

Lateral plantar nerve (deep branch)

Dorsal pedis artery

Plantar arch

Abductor hallucis muscle

Adductor hallucis muscle (oblique head)

Flexor hallucis brevis muscle

Peroneus longus tendon

Medial plantar artery

Flexor digitorum longus tendon

Flexor digitorum accessorius muscle

Medial plantar nerve

Lateral plantar nerve

Lateral plantar artery

Abductor digiti minimi muscle

Abductor hallucis muscle

Flexor digitorum brevis muscle

Calcaneal branch

FIG 11-2 The arteries and nerves of the plantar surface of the foot. *(Figure taken from* Textbook of Human Anatomy *copyright United Kingdom, 1976, W.J. Hamilton. Reproduced by permission of Macmillan Publishers, Ltd.)*

FIG 11-3 Muscles of sole. **A,** First layer. **B,** Second layer. **C,** Third and fourth layers. *(Figure taken from* Textbook of Human Anatomy *copyright United Kingdom, 1976, W.J. Hamilton. Reproduced by permission of Macmillan Publishers, Ltd.)*

hallux (pl. halluces): the great toe.
hindfoot: calcaneal (heel bone) and talar (ankle bone) portion of the foot; also called **rear foot.**
interphalangeal (IP) joint: the joint between the proximal phalanx and distal phalanx of the great toe.

lateral column: main weight-bearing structures of the outer side of the foot including the calcaneus, cuboid, and fourth and fifth metatarsals.
malleolus: the prominence of bone on either side of the ankle. The medial and lateral malleoli come from the

C

FIG 11-3, cont'd

tibia and fibula, respectively. The posterior malleolus is deep to the Achilles tendon and is a part of the tibia.

medial column: main weight-bearing structure including the talus, navicular, cuneiforms, and the first through third metatarsals.

metatarsals: the five long bones of the foot between the tarsals and the phalanges.

midfoot: portion of foot containing the navicular, three cuneiforms, and cuboid.

midtarsal joint: comprises the talonavicular and calcaneocuboid articulations and permits adduction-abduction and inversion-eversion motions of the forefoot; also called **transverse tarsal joint** and **Chopart joint.**

navicular: tarsal bone on medial side of foot that articulates proximally with head of talus and distally with three cuneiforms. Formerly called the **scaphoid.**

os: bone; also used in conjunction with a whole bone such as the calcis (calcaneus). However, *os* usually refers to small ossicles (small bones) or anatomic variants:

os intercuneiforme: between the medial and intermediate cuneiform.

os intermetatarseum: between the proximal fourth and fifth metatarsal.

os peroneum: in the peroneal tendon plantar and lateral to the cuboid.

os sustentaculum: the medial junction between the talus and calcaneus.

os talocalcaneus: the large accessory bone bridging the lateral talus and calcaneus.

ossa tarsi: the seven proximal bones of the foot connecting the tibia and fibula to the five metatarsals. The combining form *tarso* is used often, for example, tarsometatarsal joints and ligaments; also called **tarsus, bony tarsus,** and **tarsus osseous.**

os tibiale externum: medial navicular of foot; also called **accessory navicular.**

os trigonum: posterior to talus; can be easily confused with a fracture of the posterior lateral tubercle of the talus; also called **Bardeleben bone.**

os vesalianum: directly proximal to the fifth metatarsal.

phalanx: the toe; more specifically, the two bones of the great toe and three bones of each of the four small toes. It is not uncommon for the fourth or fifth toe to have the middle and distal phalanges fused and to have two phalanges only.

proximal interphalangeal (PIP) joint: the joint between the proximal and middle phalanx of one of the lesser toes.

sesamoid: two seed-shaped bones in the flexor hallucis brevis tendon located beneath the first metatarsal head, helping to plantar flex the great toe and protect the flexor hallucis tendon, which is situated between them.

FIG 11-4 A, Retinacular and synovial sheaths of ankle region, medial view. **B,** Retinacular and synovial sheaths of ankle region, lateral view. *(Figure taken from* Textbook of Human Anatomy *copyright United Kingdom, 1976, W.J. Hamilton. Reproduced by permission of Macmillan Publishers, Ltd.)*

subtalar joint: the main shock absorber for the foot; this joint comprises the talocalcaneal articulation and permits complex movement of the hindfoot in all three planes simultaneously.

sustentaculum tali: a bony projection of the medial calcaneus that supports the talus.

talocalcaneal bar: a tarsal coalition that denotes a bony or fibrocartilaginous bridge between the talus and the calcaneus.

talus: large bone beneath tibia that helps make up one third of the ankle joint, permitting the foot to go up or down. The talocalcaneal (subtalar joint) below the ankle joint allows the heel to turn in and out. The talonavicular ligaments originate from the talus; also called **astragalus**. The spring ligament (the inferior calcaneonavicular ligament) extends from the sustentaculum of the calcaneus to the navicular and supports the head of the talus.

tarsal coalition: an abnormal bony, fibrocartilaginous, or fibrous bridge between the tarsal bones. It is present at birth, but does not manifest itself until after bony maturity.

tarsometatarsal joint: this joint comprises the tarsal and metatarsal articulations and is also called **Lisfranc joint**.

Muscles and Tendons

abductor hallucis: short muscle on medial side that pulls the great toe away from other toes and supports medial longitudinal arch.

Achilles tendon: the long tendon of the calf composed of the gastrocnemius, soleus, and plantaris muscles and inserting into the calcaneus; also called **heel cord** and **tendocalcaneus**.

adductor hallucis: short muscle that attaches to base of great toe, pulls it toward the second toe, and prevents spreading of the metatarsal bones.

anterior tibial tendon (tibialis anterior): long tendon of the anterior leg; inserts into the medial cuneiform and first metatarsal; helps to dorsiflex the foot.

extensor digitorum longus and brevis: long tendon from the leg and short tendon from foot, respectively; pulls the lesser toes up in dorsiflexion (extension) and stabilizes the lesser metatarsophalangeal joints. There is no brevis tendon to the fifth toe.

extensor hallucis longus and brevis: long tendon from the leg and short tendon from foot, respectively; pulls the great toe up in dorsiflexion (extension) and stabilizes the first metatarsophalangeal joint.

flexor digitorum longus and brevis: long tendon from the leg and short muscle and tendon from the foot, respectively; insert into the distal and middle phalanges, respectively; plantar flexes the toes at all three joints.

flexor hallucis longus and brevis: long tendon from the leg and short muscle from the foot, respectively; insert into distal and proximal phalanges of the great toe, respectively; function to flex the great toe and support the medial longitudinal arch of foot; may have a role in equilibrium.

interosseous muscles: the group of small muscles between the metatarsals that attach to the extensor tendons over the toes; extend the interphalangeal joints and flex the metatarsophalangeal joints.

intrinsic muscles: similar to the hand, the intrinsic muscles arise from the metatarsals. The intrinsic muscles include:
- abductor hallucis
- abductor digiti minimi
- adductor hallucis
- dorsal and plantar interosseous
- extensor digitorum brevis
- extensor hallucis brevis
- flexor digitorum brevis
- flexor digiti minimi
- flexor hallucis brevis
- lumbricals
- quadratus plantae

peroneus brevis tendon: arises from the leg and courses along the posterior fibula; inserts onto the dorsolateral base of the fifth metatarsal; functions to evert the hindfoot.

peroneus longus tendon: arises from the leg and courses along the posterior fibula; turns medially at the cuboid to cross the foot and insert onto the plantar base of the first metatarsal; functions to plantar flex the first metatarsal, stabilize the arch, and everts the hindfoot.

peroneus tertius: arises from the leg and courses along the anterior fibula; inserts onto the dorsolateral base of the fifth metatarsal; functions to dorsiflex and evert the foot.

peroneus quartus: arises from the leg and courses along the posterior fibula; inserts onto the lateral calcaneus, cuboid, or base of the fifth metatarsal. It is not commonly present.

posterior tibial tendon: tendon of the tibialis posterior muscle; passes along the medial malleolus and inserts diffusely into the navicular, medial cuneiform, and plantar aspect of the midfoot; functions to invert and plantarflex the foot, assist the gastrocsoleus complex, and stabilize the longitudinal arch; also called **tibialis posterior.**

quadratus plantae: muscle arising from the plantar surface of the calcaneus; functions to assist toe flexion and stabilize the longitudinal arch.

Ligaments

Ligaments are typically named for the bones connected by ligament and include the following:

collateral l.: of the phalangeal and metatarsophalangeal joints.

bifurcate l.: originates from the anterior process of the calcaneus and has two branches; one inserting onto the cuboid and the second inserting onto the navicular.

deltoid l.: broad, triangular ligament on the medial side of the ankle that connects the medial malleolus to the talus and calcaneus.

lateral collateral ligaments: three ligaments that stabilize the lateral ankle; **anterior talofibular l., calcaneofibular l.,** and the **posterior talofibular l.**

Lisfranc l.: a ligament that connects the plantar surface of the medial cuneiform and plantar surface of the second metatarsal.

long plantar l.: connects the proximal plantar aspect of the calcaneus to the cuboid.

short plantar l.: connects the distal plantar aspect of the calcaneus and cuboid lies deep to the long plantar ligament.

spring l.: very strong and key ligament of the arch; connects the sustentaculum tali of the calcaneus to the plantar navicular; provides plantar support to the head of the talus; also called **plantar calcaneonavicular l.**

tarsal ligaments
    deep transverse metatarsal l.
    dorsal and plantar cuneocuboid l.
    dorsal and plantar cuneonavicular l.
    dorsal and plantar intercuneiform l.
    dorsal and plantar metatarsal l.
    dorsal and plantar tarsometatarsal l.
    talocalcaneal l.
    talonavicular l.

The Nail

eponychium: the epidermal layer covering the nail root; also called **cuticle.**

hyponychium: the thickened epidermis underneath the free distal edge of the nail plate.

lunula: half-moon-shaped, lighter area at the proximal base of the nail next to the root.

nail matrix: the proximal portion of nail bed from which growth chiefly proceeds; also, the tissue on which the deep aspect of the nail rests; also called **matrix unguis** and **nail bed.**

nail plate: hard portion of epidermis on dorsal side of hallux and phalanges from which the nails grow; also called **unguis.**

Miscellaneous Foot Terms

1–2 intermetatarsal angle: formed at the intersection of lines drawn along the longitudinal axes of the first and second metatarsals on an anteroposterior x-ray of the foot; used to assess **metatarsus primus varus** when evaluating a **bunion** or **hallux valgus.**

1–5 intermetatarsal angle: formed at the intersection of lines drawn along the longitudinal axes of the first and fifth metatarsals on an anteroposterior x-ray of the foot; used to assess **splayfoot.**

angle of Gissane: formed at the intersection of lines drawn along the margins of the posterior facet of the calcaneus and the anterior body of the calcaneus on a lateral x-ray of the foot; used to assess alignment of a calcaneus fracture.

ankle mortise: a rectangular cavity formed by the tibia and fibula; a joint space to receive the talus.

anterior talo-first metatarsal a.: formed at the intersection of lines drawn along the longitudinal axes of the first metatarsal and talus on an anteroposterior x-ray of the foot; used to assess forefoot adduction and abduction.

Bohler a.: formed at the intersection of lines drawn from the posterosuperior process of the calcaneus tuberosity to the anterior margin of the posterior facet; and from the anterior process of the calcaneus to the anterior margin of the posterior facet on a lateral x-ray of the foot; used to assess the amount of depression of the posterior facet of the calcaneus in a calcaneus fracture.

distal metatarsal articular a.: formed at the intersection of a line formed by connecting the medial and lateral margins of the first metatarsal head articular surface, and a line perpendicular to the longitudinal axis of the proximal phalanx on an anteroposterior x-ray of the foot; used to evaluate **bunion** or **hallux valgus**.

fat pad: thick fibrous collection of fat on the plantar surface of the foot.

Feiss line: a line drawn from the tip of the medial malleolus to plantar aspect of the first metatarsophalangeal joint during clinical examination; used to assess arch height.

Gschwind classification: for cerebral palsy, 4 group classification of foot pronation deformities.

Haglund process: enlargement of the posterosuperior process of the calcaneus; usually congenital.

hallux valgus a.: formed at intersection of lines drawn along longitudinal axes of proximal phalanx of the hallux and the first metatarsal on an anteroposterior x-ray of the foot; used to assess **bunion** or **hallux valgus**.

interdigital space: the area between the adjacent metatarsals and phalanges.

Meary a.: measured between lines drawn along the longitudinal axes of the talus and the first metatarsal on an anteroposterior x-ray of the foot; used to assess pes planus and pes cavus; also called **lateral talo-first metatarsal a.**

Meyer line: a line drawn through the longitudinal axis of the big toe to midpoint of heel during clinical examination; used to assess foot position while walking.

parallel pitch lines: two lines drawn on a lateral x-ray of the heel to assess prominence of the posterior superior process of the calcaneus; also called **Haglund deformity**.

plantar fascia: dense fascia of the plantar aspect of foot arising from calcaneus and inserting into base of proximal phalanges; also called **plantar aponeurosis**.

ray: complex of the metatarsals and phalanges that, on anteroposterior radiographs, appear as five rays.

sinus tarsi: small channel between the midanterior lateral calcaneus and talus; also called **tarsal sinus**.

talocalcaneal a.: measured between lines drawn along the longitudinal axis of the talus and the plantar cortex of the calcaneus on a lateral x-ray of the foot; used to assess talocalcaneal alignment in both **pes planovalgus (flatfoot)** and **pes cavovarus**.

tarsal tunnel: a fibroosseous tunnel along the medial aspect of the tarsal bones that contains the flexor tendons and the branches of the posterior tibial arteries and nerves.

Arteries, Veins, Nerves

Baxter n.: first branch of the lateral plantar nerve. It is a motor branch to the abductor digiti quinti muscle.

calcaneal branch of the posterior tibial a. and n.: supplies the heel (os calcis, calcaneus).

digital a. and n.: terminal arteries and nerves that travel together on the sides of the toes in the interdigital spaces.

dorsalis pedis a.: branch from the anterior tibial artery, going into the dorsum of the foot.

malleolar a.: anterior, medial, and lateral branches supply the medial and lateral malleolus.

plantar a.: supplies the plantar surface of the foot on medial and lateral side; also called **deep branch posterior tibial a.**

plantar arch: medial plantar artery that transverses the foot to anastomose with lateral plantar artery.

medial and lateral plantar nerves: branches of the posterior tibial nerve. Provide sensation to the medial and lateral portions of the plantar side of foot, respectively, and motor branches to intrinsic muscles of foot.

posterior tibial artery, nerve, and vein: travel through a fascial tunnel on the inner ankle (tarsal tunnel) and branch to supply the plantar aspect of the foot and toes.

Diseases and Conditions of the Foot and Ankle

The pathologic and neuromusculoskeletal changes that take place in the foot can be the result of multiple entities. For example, excessive weight, overuse, improper shoe fit, and similar causes can place stress and strain on the feet. Simple effects on the foot can relate to dermal abrasions, blisters, ulcers, fissures, bunions, corns, calluses, fungi, and other infections. The more severe problems involve peripheral vascular (ischemia) diseases, metabolic disorders (diabetes, gout), musculoskeletal changes (bunion and hammer toe deformities), and trauma (fractures, dislocations). All of these may cause or contribute to disability and inability to function. Diseases and conditions of the foot are listed alphabetically for reference. Systemic diseases are listed in Chapter 2.

Achilles tendonitis: dysfunction of the Achilles tendon caused by inflammation of the surrounding tissue (peritendinitis) or degeneration of the tendon tissue itself (tendinosis). **Retrocalcaneal bursitis** refers to inflammation of the bursal sac between the calcaneus and Achilles tendon.

ainhum: a rare condition of unknown cause, seen primarily in African-Americans wherein there is a constricting ring around a digit causing a very slow spontaneous lysis or autoamputation, usually of the fourth or fifth toe, but sometimes other toes; also called **dactylolysis spontanea.**

anonychia: absence of toenails.

athlete's foot: fungal infection of skin on the plantar surface of the feet and between the toes and nails caused by one of the dermatophyte species (*Trichophyton* or *Epidermophyton*); disease consists of scaling, fissures, maceration, and eroded areas between the toes; also called **tinea pedis** and **dermatomycosis pedis.**

Baxter nerve syndrome: compression of the first branch of the lateral plantar nerve by the plantar fascia and is implicated in heel pain syndrome.

blue foot syndrome: bluish discoloration of the feet most commonly caused by vascular disturbances.

bunion: joint deformity and enlargement of bone at the base of the metatarsophalangeal joint of the big toe with malposition of the first metatarsal, and overgrowth of bone at the first metatarsal head. This deformity, called **hallux valgus,** may or may not affect the position of the great toe. If the great toe is affected, then one of the following designations would be given: **hallux abductus** with bunion, **hallux adductus** with bunion, and **hallux abductovalgus** with bunion.

dorsal bunion: overgrowth of bone (exostosis) on the dorsal surface of the first metatarsal head or a dorsal malposition of the first metatarsal.

bunionette: similar to the bunion deformity but affecting the fifth metatarsal, causing the metatarsal head to be prominent laterally; also called **tailor's bunion.**

bursitis: inflammation of a fluid-filled sac that is normally present around a bony prominence to cushion it.

calcaneal spur syndrome: a spur-shaped bony growth at the origin of the flexor digitorum brevis, quadratus plantae, and abductor hallucis on the inferior calcaneus. It can cause pain on the bottom of the heel.

callosity: hard, thickened skin on the bottom of the foot like a clavus; also called **tyloma, keratoma, callus (pl. calluses).**

Charcot foot: an acquired foot deformity caused by multiple neuropathic fractures most often seen in diabetic patients; also called **Charcot arthropathy** and **neuropathic foot.**

Eichenholtz Classification for Foot Charcot Arthropathy
Development: bone fragmentation.
Coalescence: absorption of small bone fragments, fusion of joints.
Remodeling: healing and new bone formation.

Charcot-Marie-Tooth disease: in the foot, a spontaneous deterioration of the neuromuscular complex affects the peroneal nerve, causing cavus foot and ankle weakness.

checkrein deformity: fixed, flexion deformity of the hallux resulting from tethering of the flexor hallucis longus tendon after a lower limb fracture.

Clanton and McGarvey classification: for ankle ligament injury and treatment.

clavus: any corn or hyperkeratotic tissue involving a toe; a reaction of skin to intermittent chronic pressure, producing extra layers of hard skin; caused by restrictive footwear or by abnormal position or motion of the toes.

clavus: soft skin thickening between the toes, usually between the fourth and fifth toes; also called **soft callus, heloma molle, soft corn,** and **clavus mollis**.

clawtoes: fixed hyperextension of the metatarsophalangeal joints associated with flexion of the proximal and distal interphalangeal joints, producing a clawlike appearance; also called **claw toe deformity**.

clubfoot: congenital foot deformity resulting in the appearance of a golf club. The components include forefoot adduction with flexion and varus of the talus neck, ankle equinus, and heel varus. The result is that the foot turns in with the sole of the foot and the heel pulled medially.

Pirani Classification for Clubfoot Deformity
Each component is assigned a score of 0, 0.5, or 1, depending on severity.
The hindfoot contracture score is composed of findings of a posterior crease, an empty heel, and rigid equinus.
The midfoot contracture score is composed of findings of a medial crease, curvature of the lateral border, and the position of the head of the talus.

coalition: an abnormal fibrous, cartilaginous, or bony bridge between two bones. Most commonly occurs between the calcaneus and navicular (calcaneonavicular) or the talus and calcaneus (talocalcaneal or subtalar). Also called **congenital bars**.

congenital rocker-bottom flatfoot: condition present at birth; abnormal equinus position of talus with valgus position of the heel, resulting in a foot that looks like a rocker and has a prominence below the medial ankle; also called **congenital vertical talus** and **congenital convex pes valgus**.

curly toe: a bilateral congenital deformity in which one or more toes, usually the fourth toe, is supinated, medially deviated, and in plantar flexion.

dactylitis: infarcts in the small bones of the foot caused by sickle cell disease.

diabetic foot disease: general term applied to a variety of foot conditions that are associated with diabetes. This can include ulcers, peripheral vascular changes, peripheral neuropathy, joint destruction, and osteomyelitis.

Diabetic Foot Infection Classification
This classification is based on perfusion, extent (size), depth (tissue loss), infection, and sensation (neuropathy) (PEDIS) and is referred to as **PEDIS grade**.
Grade 1 uninfected: Wound lacking purulence or any manifestations of inflammation (erythema, pain, tenderness, warmth, or induration).
Grade 2 mild: Presence of two or more manifestations of inflammation, cellulitis or erythema extending 2 cm or less around the ulcer, with infection limited to the skin or superficial subcutaneous tissues. No other local complications or systemic illness.
Grade 3 moderate: Infection (as in grade 2) in a patient who is systemically well and metabolically stable but that has one or more of the following characteristics: cellulitis extending 2 cm, lymphangitic streaking, spread beneath the superficial fascia, deep-tissue abscess, gangrene, and involvement of muscle, tendon, joint, or bone.
Grade 4 severe: Infection in a patient with systemic toxicity or metabolic instability (e.g., fever, chills, tachycardia, hypotension, confusion, vomiting, leukocytosis, acidosis, severe hyperglycemia, or azotemia).

dorsiflexed metatarsal: a metatarsal that is deformed or malpositioned so that its head is higher than the adjacent metatarsal heads, resulting in increased plantar pressure over the adjacent metatarsal heads with limitation of motion of the involved metatarsophalangeal joint.

drop foot: paralysis or weakness of the dorsiflexor muscles of the anterior compartment of the leg innervated by the peroneal nerves, causing the foot and toes to drag when walking; also called **foot drop** and **peroneal nerve palsy**.

Dupuytren fibromatosis: plantar fibromas of the plantar fascia of the foot; present as solitary or multiple nodules occurring most often along the medial border of the plantar fascia.

Egyptian foot: a foot with a long first ray.

equinus: abnormal position of plantar flexion and used in combining form with other words to denote the anatomic location; ankle equinus, forefoot equinus, metatarsus equinus.

exostosis: in children, a bony growth protruding from the surface of bone formed by endochondral ossification. It ceases to grow when growth plate closes; also called **osteochondroma** and **osteocartilaginous exostosis**.

flail foot: a foot with poor neuromuscular function and control.

flatfoot: a foot with a depressed longitudinal arch. This term covers a wide range of conditions. In most cases, a flatfoot is due to imbalances of the muscles and ligaments that control the arch and is referred to as a **flexible flatfoot**. If musculoskeletal changes occur during adult life or if there is an injury, the term **acquired flatfoot** might be used. Many individuals with flatfeet go through life with no functional interferences.

Johnson Classification of Adult Acquired Flatfoot Associated with Posterior Tibial Tendon Insufficiency
Used for treatment planning:
Stage I comprises tenosynovitis without deformity.
Stage IIA comprises a flexible flatfoot with hindfoot valgus and a normal forefoot.
Stage IIB comprises a flexible flatfoot with hindfoot valgus and forefoot abduction with more than 40% of the talar head uncovered by the navicular.
Stage III comprises a rigid flatfoot deformity.
Stage IV is the same as Stage III with the addition of valgus instability of the tibiotalar joint.

foot cramps: an involuntary action involving a muscle-tendon reflex contraction, stretching the tendon, which sends nerve messages to the spinal cord, which in turn stimulates the muscle even more, producing a painful cramp. This can be related to abnormal levels of minerals (calcium, potassium, and magnesium), a decrease in blood supply to the muscle, a pinched nerve, holding the foot in pronation for a length of time, or a problem with the muscle itself.

forefoot equinus: describes a high-arched foot characterized by excessive plantar flexion of forefoot in relation to hindfoot.

forefoot valgus: describes pronated position of forefoot with respect to the hindfoot.

forefoot varus: describes supinated position of forefoot with respect to hindfoot.

ganglion: a benign soft tissue cystic mass filled with clear fluid, usually coming from a joint or a tendon sheath, usually in the midfoot or hindfoot.

gastrocnemius equinus: a tightness or contracture of the gastrocnemius muscle that restricts ankle dorsiflexion when the knee is fully extended; also called **Silverskold test**.

gout: a metabolic disorder wherein deposits of uric acid crystals form in the joints, the kidneys, and especially the great toe, causing pain and inflammation. Aspiration of joint fluid can help differentiate gout from an infection.

Greek foot: a foot with a short first ray.

Haglund deformity: prominent posterosuperior aspect of the calcaneus; also called **retrocalcaneal exostosis** or a "pump bump."

Haglund syndrome: pain on the superior and lateral side of the heel usually associated with a callus of the skin, bony prominence (**Haglund deformity**), and retrocalcaneal bursitis. A variety of conditions and shoe types can contribute to this condition; also called **retrocalcaneal exostosis.**

hallux abductus: great toe pointing toward second toe (transverse plane deformity).

hallux adductus: great toe pointing toward midline of body (transverse plane deformity).

hallux elevatus: fixed dorsiflexed position of entire first ray.

hallux extensus: fixed dorsiflexed position of the great toe.

hallux flexus: fixed flexion position of great toe at the metatarsophalangeal joint.

hallux malleus: hammer toe deformity of the great toe; fixed flexion position of great toe at the interphalangeal joint.

hallux rigidus: painful, stiff metatarsophalangeal joint; caused by arthritic changes.

hallux valgus: great toe pointing toward second toe, often rotated in frontal plane so that the nail plate is facing away from second toe.

hallux valgus interphalangeus: a hallux valgus deformity caused by deformity of the proximal or distal phalanx.

hallux varus: great toe pointing toward midline of body, often rotated in frontal plane so that the nail plate is facing second toe.

hammer toes: combined distal interphalangeal extension, proximal interphalangeal flexion, and metatarsophalangeal extension deformity of one or more lesser toes.

hard corn: a particularly hard, thickened area of skin over the dorsum of the toe; also called **heloma durum, clavus durum,** and **hard clavus.**

heel pain syndrome: a common orthopaedic problem of the foot characterized by plantar fascial inflammation, entrapment neuropathy, heel spur, or a painful heel pad caused by excessive loading on heel strike; also called **heel spur syndrome, plantar fasciitis,** and **calcodynia.**

heel spur: osteophyte that protrudes from the plantar or posterior aspect of the calcaneus causing pain; also called **calcaneal spur.**

Scranton and McDermott Classification of Ankle Osteophytes
Grade I: synovial impingement with osteophytes 3 mm or smaller on the tibial side of the ankle joint.
Grade II: an osteochondral reaction exostosis with osteophytes larger than 3 mm on the tibial side of the ankle joint.
Grade III: severe exostoses with or without fragmentation on both sides of the ankle joint.
Grade IV: same as Grade III with the addition of degenerative osteoarthritis of the ankle joint surfaces.

hindfoot equinus: characterized by plantar flexion of the calcaneus with a decrease of calcaneal inclination angle (low-arched, flatfoot, rocker-bottom foot).

ingrown nail: condition of the nail growing into the skin distally; also called **unguis incarnatus** and **onychocryptosis.**

intractable plantar keratosis (IPK): well-defined callous tissue with a central core located beneath a metatarsal head and usually the result of abnormal plantar pressure over a bony prominence.

lobster foot: congenital cleft secondary to the lack of the central three rays and middle and lateral cuneiforms producing a lobster claw appearance.

macrodactyly: enlargement of a toe or toes.

Madura foot: a severe deep fungal infection of the foot.

mallet toes: fixed flexion of the distal interphalangeal joint of the second to fifth toes, such that the toenails are pointing into the ground when walking.

malum deformans: a deep foot ulcer commonly associated with diabetes mellitus or other neuropathic conditions.

metatarsal cuneiform exostosis: an overgrowth of bone usually involving the dorsal surface of the first metatarsal base and first cuneiform.

metatarsalgia: pain in the plantar aspect of the metatarsal head area caused by a variety of disorders.

metatarsus abductus: turning out of the forefoot (metatarsals); also called **m. valgus.**

metatarsus adductocavus: forefoot turned inward in association with a high arch, usually seen in clubfoot deformity that includes heel varus (talipes equinovarus).

metatarsus adductus: turning in of the forefoot (metatarsals); also called **m. varus.**

metatarsus atavicus: abnormal shortness of the first metatarsal bone.

metatarsus equinus: very plantar flexed metatarsals.

metatarsus latus: broad foot caused by spreading of the metatarsals; widened forefoot, splay foot.

metatarsus primus varus: refers to medial deviation of the first metatarsal with splaying between first and second metatarsals; can be the cause of a bunion deformity.

Morton foot: short first metatarsal and long second metatarsal that causes changes in the weight-bearing pattern of the foot.

Morton neuroma: nerve compression syndrome of the interdigital nerve that most commonly occurs in the third web space; also called **interdigital neuroma.**

Morton syndrome: short, hypermobile first ray resulting in plantar pressure at second metatarsal.

neuropathic fracture: fracture or fractures secondary to loss of protective sensation; also called **Charcot fracture.**

nonplantigrade foot: foot alignment with a portion of the weight-bearing sole not in alignment with the floor.

onychauxis: overgrowth and thickening of a nail plate with fragmentation and discoloration of the nail, most frequently the great toenail; also called **onychogryphosis.**

onychocryptosis: condition of nail growing into the skin distally; also called **ingrown nail** and **unguis incarnatus.**

onychomycosis: fungal infection of the nail plate.

osteochondrosis: bone and cartilage disorder believed to be due to disruption of the blood supply to a growth center of a bone. These have been given eponyms after the persons who first reported them:

    Köhler disease: osteochondrosis of the navicular bone

    Freiberg infraction: osteochondrosis of the metatarsal head

    Sever disease: osteochondrosis of the calcaneus apophysis

overlapping toe: a toe that overlaps an adjacent toe; commonly affecting the second toe, which overlaps the great toe.

pachyonychia: extreme thickening of the toenails; usually congenital, the nails are more solid and regular than in onychogryphosis.

paronychia: an inflammation of the soft tissues around the nail plate, secondary to infection or trauma.

peroneal spastic flatfoot: flatfoot deformity associated with spasm of the peroneal muscles.

Persian slipper foot: the clinical appearance of the paralytic form of vertical talus in which the lateral column of the foot has an abducted plantar contour and the medial longitudinal column is elongated and convex. The lateral toes are elevated and clawed, which is the basis for the term.

pes: generally speaking, the term *pes* (foot) is used as a prefix to denote an acquired deformity of the foot, The terms *pes* and *talipes* are generally interchangeable.

   pes cavus: high arches in midfoot.

   pes planus: lowering of the longitudinal arch; flatfoot. There are two basic categories:

      flexible pes planus: flatfoot with general laxity in which the foot appears normal when not bearing weight but flattens with weight-bearing.

      rigid pes planus: nonflexible flatfoot that is present whether bearing weight or not.

pigeon toe: term that is often applied to any intoeing gait.

plantar fasciitis: inflammation in a band of tissue that runs from the heel to the bones in the ball of the foot that makes walking quite painful; caused by improper shoe fit, excess weight, uneven terrain, and Achilles tendon tightening.

plantar flexed metatarsal: a metatarsal that is malpositioned so that its head is lower than the adjacent metatarsal heads.

plantar wart: an epidermal growth affecting the plantar surface of the foot caused by a papillomavirus; also called **verruca vulgaris.**

plantigrade foot: foot alignment with the weight-bearing sole in alignment with the floor.

podagra: although it literally means "pain in the foot," this term is usually used for a painful attack of gout in the great toe.

polydactyly: congenital deformity resulting in extra digits of the toes.

polysyndactyly: condition in which more than two toes are joined together.

posterior tibial tendon insufficiency: weakness, degeneration, or rupture of the posterior tibial tendon associated with acquired flatfoot.

prehallux: accessory navicular; also called **os tibiale externum.**

pronation: a combination of motions, including abduction and eversion of the foot, that produces a relaxing of the arch for heel strike.

pump bumps: a thickening of skin forming a callus in the back of the heel above the calcaneus as a result of tight-fitting shoes and a **Haglund deformity.**

rheumatoid nodule: synovial mass associated with rheumatoid arthritis, which can form on the weight-bearing surface of the foot.

rocker-bottom foot: deformity of the foot such that the arch is disrupted and resembles a rocking chair rocker bottom.

sinus tarsi syndrome: inflammation of tissues in the canal between talus and calcaneus causing lateral foot pain with walking.

skew foot: a complex deformity involving adduction and supination of the forefoot (metatarsus adductovarus) and hindfoot valgus; also called **z-foot.**

splay foot: abnormally wide forefoot caused by abnormally wide intermetatarsal angles.

squatter's talus: a dorsal articular facet on the talar neck found in cultures that are accustomed to squatting.

stiff ray: immobility of all joints of any toe or toes.

subungual exostosis: a benign osteocartilaginous spur that grows from the distal phalanx under the nail bed.

supination: a combination of motions including adduction and inversion of the foot that produces a stiffening of the arch for push-off. This motion is normal during gait; however, excessive supination can lead to pathologic changes of the foot such as stiff cavus foot.

syndactyly: congenital anomaly of the foot (or hand) marked by a complete webbing between the toes; may involve two or more toes; may contain bone or merely soft tissue.

tailor's bunion: a pronounced prominence on lateral side of fifth metatarsal head. The term is derived from the historical cross-legged sitting behavior of tailors.

talipes: generally speaking, the term *talipes,* meaning ankle and foot, is used as a prefix to denote an affection of the foot, for example, *talipes equinovarus* (clubfoot).

talipes calcaneocavus: high-arched foot with fixed dorsiflexion; also called **pes c.**

talipes calcaneus: abnormally dorsiflexed hindfoot, with increased dorsiflexion of the calcaneus; also called **cavus foot** and **pes c.**

talipes calcaneovalgus: abnormally dorsiflexed hindfoot with turning out of the heel; also called **pes c.**

talipes calcaneovarus: abnormally dorsiflexed hindfoot with turning in of the heel; also called **pes c.**

talipes cavovalgus: high arch and turning out of the heel; also called **pes c.**

talipes cavovarus: high arch associated with turning in of the foot; also called **pes c.**

talipes equinovalgus: plantar flexion and turning out of the calcaneus; also called **pes e.**

talipes equinovarus: turning of the heel inward with increased plantar flexion. More precisely, a clubfoot, often having the components of talipes equinovarus with metatarsus adductus; also called **clubfoot** and **pes e.**

talipes planovalgus: depression of the longitudinal arch associated with heel valgus; also called **pes planovalgus.**

talipes planus: depression of the longitudinal arch; no specified heel valgus is implied by this term; also called **pes planus** and **flatfoot.** A *flexible pes planus* is flatfoot with general laxity but no other specific disease process.

ulcer: a breakdown in the skin secondary to neuropathic or ischemic conditions; also called **neuropathic u.** and **ischemic u.**

There are two classification systems for ulcers:

Wagner Classification Foot Ulcers
Grade 0: no open lesions
Grade 1: superficial ulcer
Grade 2: deep ulcer
Grade 3: localized osteomyelitis or abscess
Grade 4: forefoot gangrene
Grade 5: gangrene of entire foot

Depth-Ischemia Classification Foot Ulcers
Depth
Grade 0: at-risk foot, no ulcer
Grade 1: superficial ulcer, no infection
Grade 2: deep ulceration
Grade 3: extensive ulceration with exposed bone and deep infection
Ischemia
Grade A: not ischemic
Grade B: ischemia without gangrene
Grade C: partial forefoot gangrene
Grade D: complete forefoot gangrene

vertical talus: a spectrum of conditions in which the talus is oriented in a plantar-flexed and medially directed position resulting in a flatfoot with heel valgus and a rocker-bottom or convex sole. In the more severe congenital form, congenital rigid flatfoot, it is usually associated with a neurologic disorder such as arthrogryposis or myelomeningocele; also called **congenital convex pes valgus.**

Surgery

Descriptions of Procedures

Akin p.: for hallux valgus or deformed great toe; an osteotomy of the proximal phalanx of the great toe.

Aly p.: correction of valgus malunion of extraarticular calcaneal fracture.

Anderson p.: for lateral ankle instability, use of plantaris tendon for lateral ligament reconstruction.

Anderson and Fowler p.: for pes planus; an opening wedge osteotomy of the distal lateral calcaneus with tibial bone graft, closing wedge osteotomy of the medial cuneiform, and capsulotomy of the talonavicular joint.

arthroplasty: any type of procedure to reconstruct a joint, typically in the setting of degenerative or inflammatory arthritis.

arthroereisis: realignment of a joint by limiting certain movements or positions. Most commonly used in the treatment of pediatric painful flexible flatfoot deformity.

Austin p.: for hallux valgus; an osteotomy in the form of a chevron or V cut made in the distal aspect of the first metatarsal; also called **chevron procedure**.

avulsion of nail plate: a nonpermanent removal of the nail plate, either partial or complete, without disrupting the matrix cells that produce the nail plate.

Baker p.: for Achilles tendon tightness; relaxation of proximal tendon with a rectangular sliding slot incision.

Baker and Hill p.: for dynamic foot varus deformity caused by cerebral palsy; transposition of posterior tibial tendon anterior to medial malleolus.

Banks p.: for nonunion medial malleolus; resection of nonunion, addition of locally obtained tibial cancellous bone, and screw fixation.

Barr p.: for paralytic clubfoot; transfer of the posterior tibial tendon to the third cuneiform or metatarsal.

Barr-Record p.: for clubfeet; subcutaneous plantar fasciotomy and tendon Achilles lengthening done as separate procedures, with tibiotalar fusion.

Bartlett p.: for ingrown toenail; excision of wedge of skin with no excision of nail.

Batchelor-Brown p.: for flat feet; fusion of the subtalar joint with a fibular bone graft.

Benirschke and Sangeorzan p.: open reduction of calcaneal fracture.

Berkowitz p.: salvage of failed total ankle arthroplasty.

Berman and Gartland p.: for metatarsus adductus; dome-shaped osteotomy of all five proximal metatarsals.

Berkowitz p.: salvage of failed total ankle arthroplasty.

Bircher-Weber p.: for ankle fracture malunion with syndesmosis diastasis; osteotomy and corrective fibular lengthening with screw and plate fixation.

Bose p.: for ingrown toenail; excision of wedge of skin without excision of nail.

Bosworth p.: for repair of old rupture of Achilles tendon; fashioning direct tendon graft from median raphe (central portion of tendon).

Boyd amputation: an amputation at the ankle with tibial calcaneal fusion.

Braham and Pankovich p.: direct repair of neglected ruptures of Achilles tendon.

Brahms p.: for mallet toe; transfer of flexor digitorum profundus to dorsum of proximal phalanx.

Braly et al. p.: lateral decompression of malunited calcaneal fracture.

Bridle p.: for foot paralysis; posterior tibialis tendon transfer through interosseous membrane to dorsum of foot, and dual anastomosis to anterior tibialis and anteriorly transposed peroneus longus.

Brockman p.: for clubfoot; a soft tissue release of the medial capsule of the foot as well as a release of the posterior tibial tendon.

Broström p.: anatomic repair of lateral collateral ligaments for chronic lateral ankle instability; the **Gould modification** incorporates the extensor retinaculum with the repair.

Bugg-Boyd p.: for repair of old Achilles tendon rupture; use of fascia lata graft.

bunionectomy: for simple bunion or bunion associated with hallux valgus; a general class of many different operations that are designed to correct bunion deformity.

Butler p.: arthroplasty of fifth metatarsophalangeal joint

Campbell p.: for drop foot or talipes equinus; creates a posterior bone block to prevent plantar flexion.

Carr p.: subtalar distraction bone block arthrodesis; distraction arthrodesis for calcaneal malunion.

Carroll p.: two-incision technique for clubfoot correction.

Carstam and Eiken p.: opening-wedge osteotomy of distal phalanx.

Carstam and Theander p.: a reverse wedge osteotomy of the distal phalanx.

Carter and Ezaki p.: dome osteotomy and excision of Vickers ligament.

cheilectomy: for hallux rigidus; removal of an exostosis usually on the dorsal surface of the distal first metatarsal.

chevron osteotomy: for hallux valgus; an osteotomy in the form of a chevron or V cut made in the distal first metatarsal; also called **Austin p.**

Chopart amputation: of the forefoot through the talonavicular and calcaneocuboid joint.

Chrisman-Snook p.: reconstruction of the lateral ankle ligaments using peroneus brevis tendon; also called **modified Elmslie procedure**.

Cincinnati incision: an incision to correct clubfoot.

Clare p.: correction of calcaneal malunion through extensile lateral approach.

Clayton p.: for deformity of toes in rheumatoid arthritis; resection of proximal phalanx and entire metatarsal heads of all toes.

closing abductory wedge osteotomy (CAWO): for hallux valgus; proximal metatarsal laterally based wedge osteotomy to bring first metatarsal closer to second metatarsal.

Cole p.: for cavus foot deformity; an anterior tarsal wedge osteotomy with fusion.

Coleman p.: for talipes valgus; soft tissue and tendon release associated with a subtalar fusion.

condylectomy: for painful callus; removal of a condyle from a metatarsal or phalanx.

cone arthrodesis: for fusion of the first metatarsophalangeal joint; the metatarsal head is shaped into a cone, and a matching, concave cone is cut into the proximal phalanx at a proper angle to accept the metatarsal head for fusion; also called **Wilson p.** and **Johnson and Barington p.**

cotting: for ingrown nail; excision of a nail.

Clare p.: correction of calcaneal malunion through extensile lateral approach.

Cracchiolo p.: for deformity of toes in rheumatoid arthritis; silastic implant arthroplasty for metapharangeal joints of all toes.

Crawford p.: uses Cincinnati incision for clubfoot.

crescentic osteotomy: for hallux valgus; a dome-shaped or crescentic osteotomy at the base of the first metatarsal to reduce the metatarsus primus varus.

cylindrical osteotomy: to shorten long bones; removal of a cylinder of bone.

Deland p.: deltoid ligament reconstruction with peroneus longus tendon autograft.

Dennyson and Fulford p.: for hindfoot valgus deformity, subtalar arthrodesis.

Dias and Giegerich p.: for triplane fracture of ankle; open reduction with screw fixation when required.

Dickson-Diveley p.: for clawing of the big toe; the interphalangeal joint is fused, and the extensor hallucis longus is transferred to the flexor hallucis longus.

digital prosthesis: excision of interphalangeal joint with insertion of prosthetic device in that space.

Dillwyn-Evans p.: for severe resistant clubfoot deformity; Achilles and posterior tibial tendon, talonavicular joint capsulectomy, and fusion of the calcaneocuboid joint.

distal interphalangeal (DIP) fusion: for mallet toes; removal of the DIP joint and then fusion.

dorsal-V osteotomy: for plantar callosity; an osteotomy at the neck of a lesser metatarsal to allow the metatarsal to assume a slightly higher position.

dorsal wedge osteotomy: for plantar callosity; a dorsally-based wedge osteotomy at the base of a metatarsal to allow the metatarsal to move to a higher position.

Drennan p.: for ankle flexion weakness; posterior transfer of anterior tibial tendon.

Dunn-Brittain p.: for paralytic clubfeet; a method of triple arthrodesis excising most of the head of the talus.

Dunn-Brittain triple arthrodesis: removal of entire navicular bone.

Durham p.: for flatfoot; closing wedge osteotomy and fusion of cuneiform-navicular joint.

DuVries arthroplasty: for fixed hammer toes and mallet toes; resection of the head of the proximal phalanx (hammer toe) or middle phalanx (mallet toe).

DuVries plantar condylectomy: for plantar callosities; resection of plantar condyles from the lesser metatarsals.

DuVries p.: (1) for chronic instability of deltoid ligament of ankle; cross-shaped imbrication of deltoid ligament; (2) for hallux valgus; a modified McBride bunion procedure with vertical medial capsular imbrication and suturing of lateral capsule to second metatarsal head.

Dwyer p.: lateral closing wedge osteotomy of the calcaneus; associated with soft tissue release for clubfeet and other disorders.

Ellis Jones p.: for subluxing peroneal tendon; reconstruction of retinaculum using portion of Achilles tendon.

Elmslie p.: for lateral ankle instability; peroneal tendon used in ligament reconstruction.

Elmslie-Cholmely p.: double wedge osteotomy for high-arched feet.

Essex-Lopresti p.: for fractured calcaneus; use of a Steinmann pin or other metal pin to help achieve and hold fracture reduction.

Evans p.: (1) for lateral collateral ligament instability of ankle; use of peroneus brevis tendon; (2) for severe flatfoot deformity; distal lateral opening wedge osteotomy of the calcaneus.

exostectomy: removal of any excess prominences of bone.

Eylon p.: tibiocalcaneal arthrodesis with thin-wire external fixation.

Eyring and Guthrie p.: lateral repair of chronic ankle instability.

Farmer p.: for hallux varus; soft tissue repair with the use of a skin flap.

Fowler p.: (1) for metatarsus varus with severe cavus deformity; plantar fascia and muscle release associated with an opening wedge osteotomy of the first cuneiform; (2) for deformity of toes in rheumatoid arthritis; resection of proximal phalanx and varying portions of metatarsal heads of all toes; (3) for ingrown toenail; excision of entire nail.

Freid-Green p.: for paralysis of posterior tibial muscle; transfer of the peroneus longus, flexor digitorum longus, flexor hallucis longus, or extensor hallucis longus to posterior tibial tendon.

Frey p.: proximal phalangeal osteotomy

Frost p.: for ingrown nail; a skin flap is made over the lateral nail bed, with removal of the nail and bed followed by closure of flap.

Fulford p.: for spastic valgus deformity of foot; peroneus brevis elongation.

Gaenslen split-heel p.: a split incision approach for osteomyelitis of the calcaneus.

Gallie p.: for malunion calcaneus; subtalar arthrodesis using a tibial bone graft.

Garceau p.: for clubfeet; anterior tibial tendon transfer.

Garceau-Brahms p.: for paralytic clubfeet; transection of the motor branches of the plantar nerve.

Gelman p.: for clubfeet; identical to the McCauley procedure, except that the inferior calcaneonavicular ligament is not incised.

Giannestras p.: for plantar callosity; proximal shortening of metatarsal.

Gill p.: for drop foot; wedge of bone taken from the superoposterior calcaneus with insertion of that block into the posterior tibiotalar joint.

Girdlestone p.: for flexible hammer toe deformities; transfer of the long flexors of the involved toe(s) to the extensor hood mechanism (top of toe).

Gould p.: for pes cavus caused by tight plantar fascia; a double plantar fasciotomy through a lateral heel approach proximally and a distal medial approach.

Greene p.: one-stage release of circumferential constricting band; open ankle synovectomy in hemophilia; posterior tibial tendon transfer to dorsum of foot.

Grice p.: for congenital talipes valgus; a soft tissue medial and lateral foot release procedure.

Grice-Green p.: (1) for talipes valgus; tibial bone graft to subtalar joint; (2) for paralysis of gastrocsoleus; transfer of peroneus longus, peroneus brevis, and posterior tibial tendon.

Haddad p.: use of extensor digitorum brevis transfer for crossover toe deformity.

Hark p.: for congenital talipes valgus; multiple extensor and flexor Z-tendon lengthenings with bony repositioning.

Harris-Beath p.: for flat feet; talonavicular and subtalar arthrodesis.

Hauser p.: (1) for hallux valgus; excision of the medial exostosis and transfer of the adductor tendon from the proximal phalanx to the distal metatarsal; (2) for tight heel cord; division of proximal posterior and distal medial two-thirds of the Achilles tendon.

Heifetz p.: for ingrown nail; excision of affected ingrown side of nail and nail bed.

hemiphalangectomy: for shortening or straightening of a toe; resection of a portion of the phalanx.

Herndon-Heyman p.: for congenital talipes valgus; medial and lateral foot release with tendon lengthening.

Heyman p.: for clubfeet; soft tissue release for clubfoot, including deltoid ligament.

Hibbs p.: for claw toes and cavus feet; plantar fascia release with transfer of the extensor digitorum longus to the third cuneiform.

Hirose and Johnson p.: for correction of compensatory forefoot varus in a flatfoot deformity; an opening-wedge medial cuneiform osteotomy.

Hiroshima p.: for spastic equinus and equinovarus deformity; anterior transfer of long toe flexors.

Hoffer p.: for spastic inversion of foot; transfer of anterior tibial tendon to cuboid.

Hoffman-Clayton p.: resection of metatarsal head; resection of metatarsal heads and bases of proximal phalanges for cock-up deformities of toes as seen in rheumatoid arthritis.

Hoke p.: (1) triple arthrodesis done with reshaping of the head of the talus; (2) for flat feet; navicular bone and two medial cuneiforms are fused.

Hoke-Kite p.: for calcaneocavovarus deformity; excision and fusion with some shortening of talonavicular joint and a posterior closing wedge fusion of the talocalcaneal joint.

Hueter-Mayo p.: for simple bunion deformity; resection of prominent portion of first metatarsal.

Ingram p.: for congenital talipes valgus; Z-plasty lengthening of peroneus brevis tendon, medial release, reduction of navicular bone, and anterior tibial tendon transfer.

intermediate phalangectomy: for hammer toe deformity; excision of the middle phalanx.

Jahss p.: for cavus foot with clawtoes; excision of metatarsotarsal joint with dorsal wedge closed to reduce cavus and with adequate bone excision to relax plantar fascia.

Jansey p.: for ingrown toenail; excision of wedge of skin without excision of nail.

Japas p.: for high-arched feet; a combination of plantar fascia release and dorsal wedge osteotomy of the tarsal bones.

Johnson and Spiegl p.: for hallux varus; fusion of interphalangeal joint great toe and transfer of extensor hallucis longus to lateral proximal phalanx.

Jones p.: (1) for cock-up deformity of great toe; transfer of the extensor hallucis longus to the distal first metatarsal; currently done with a distal interphalangeal joint fusion; (2) for ankle instability; repair of the fibular collateral ligament using the peroneus brevis muscle.

Joplin p.: for splay foot deformity; transfer of fifth toe flexor to first metatarsal.

Juliano p.: for hallux varus; extensor hallucis brevis tenodesis.

Juvara p.: for hallux valgus; an oblique osteotomy at the proximal portion of the metatarsal to correct an abnormal transverse or sagittal plane deformity.

Karlsson p.: for lateral ankle ligament instability; reconstruction using original ligament; also called **Brostrum procedure.**

Kashiwagi p.: for malunion calcaneus fracture; lateral subtalar and calcaneocuboid joint fusion.

Kates-Kessel-Kay p.: for deformity of toes in rheumatoid arthritis; resection of metatarsal head only.

Kaufer p.: for spastic inversion of foot; transfer of posterior tibial tendon to peroneus brevis.

Keller p.: for hallux rigidus or hallux valgus; resection of the base of the proximal phalanx of the great toe.

Kendrick p.: for metatarsus adductus; soft tissue release for all tarsal metatarsal joints.

Kessel-Bonney p.: for lack of great toe extension; a closing wedge osteotomy of proximal phalanx. Also called **Moberg p.**

Kidner p.: for an accessory navicular bone; removal of the accessory navicular bone with or without transfer of the posterior tibial tendon under the navicular bone.

Kiehn-Earle-DesPrez p.: for plantar ulcer; closure of ulcer and transfer of extensor digitorum longus to distal metatarsal shaft.

Koman p.: for hindfoot valgus; medial displacement calcaneal osteotomy.

Kumar p.: arthrodesis of the first metatarsophalangeal joint.

Lambrinudi p.: a triple arthrodesis done by resection of the head and inferior portion of the talus.

Lange p.: for metatarsus varus; simple oblique osteotomy of the second, third, and fourth metatarsals; lateral closing wedge osteotomy of the first metatarsal at the base.

Lapidus p.: for hallux valgus; arthrodesis of the first metatarsocuneiform joint and a distal soft tissue procedure.

Larmon p.: for rheumatoid foot deformity; arthroplasty by resection of medial metatarsal head and proximal phalanx of great toe and resection of plantar part of metatarsal head of lesser toes.

Lichtblau osteotomy: for persistent clubfoot deformity in adults; medial soft tissue release, closing wedge osteotomy of the cuboid, and opening wedge osteotomy of the medial cuneiform.

Liebolt p.: for paralytic equinus foot; a two-stage procedure involving a Hoke triple arthrodesis followed by an ankle fusion.

Lindholm p.: for repair of ruptured Achilles tendon; fashioning of fascial flaps from superior tendon.

Lipscomb p.: for deformity of toes in rheumatoid arthritis; resection of proximal phalanx and plantar metatarsal head of all toes.

Lisfranc amputation: amputation through the tarsometatarsal joint.

Lloyd-Roberts p.: for clubfoot deformity in early childhood; soft tissue release.

Lowman p.: for flatfeet; transfer of the anterior tibialis with navicular cuneiform fusion.

Ludloff p.: for hallux valgus; an oblique osteotomy of the first metatarsal from proximal dorsal to distal plantar.

Lynn p.: for repair of Achilles tendon rupture; use of fanned out portion of plantaris tendon to cover direct repair.

Ma-Griffith p.: for Achilles tendon rupture; percutaneous technique of suture repair.

Majestro-Ruda-Frost p.: for spastic posterior tibial tendon; intramuscular lengthening.

malleolar osteotomy: a procedure or approach that provides access to the ankle joint in fracture reductions or in excising abnormal bone or cartilage.

Mammon p.: first metatarsal osteotomy and bone graft for a dorsal bunion.

Mann p.: for hallux valgus; a modified McBride bunion procedure with a vertical medial capsular imbrication and suturing of lateral capsule to second metatarsal head; also called **DuVries p.**

matricectomy: for toenail deformity or chronic disease; excision of all or a part of the nail plate and its germinal matrix to eliminate growth of the nail.

Mau p.: for hallux valgus; an oblique osteotomy of the first metatarsal from proximal plantar to distal dorsal.

Mayer p.: for deformity caused by poliomyelitis; transfer of peroneal tendon.

Mayo p.: (1) for bunion exostosis of first metatarsal head without significant angular deformity; excision exostosis; (2) for first metatarsophalangeal joint arthritis; oblique excision of the first metatarsal head.

McBride p.: for hallux valgus; excision of the medial exostosis, medial capsular reefing, fibular sesamoidectomy, and transfer of the adductor hallucis tendon into the distal first metatarsal.

McCauley p.: very extensive medial release of multiple joint capsules, tendon sheaths, and abductor hallucis and, if needed, posterior capsulotomy later.

McElvenny p.: (1) excision of a plantar nerve neuroma; (2) for hallux varus; lateral capsular reefing procedure associated with use of the extensor hallucis brevis tendon for repair.

McKeever p.: for hallux valgus or rigidus; fusion of the first metatarsophalangeal joint; also called **arthrodesis.**

McReynolds p.: for fractured calcaneus; open reduction and fixation with staples using a medial approach.

Meisenbach p.: for callosity on plantar aspect of foot; dorsal displacement of metatarsal head(s).

metatarsal head resection with prosthesis: removal of the metatarsal head to create an artificial joint with a silastic implant.

metaphyseal osteotomy: osteotomy through the neck or base of the metatarsal.

Miller p.: (1) for severe flatfoot deformity; naviculo-cuneiform-metatarsal fusion; (2) for hallux varus; repositioning of stump of adductor hallucis and transfer of abductor hallucis to lateral proximal phalanx.

Mitchell p.: for hallux valgus; a distal metatarsal osteotomy with a step cut and shifting of the metatarsal head laterally with excision of exostosis and medial capsular reefing.

Naughton-Dunn p.: for severe foot deformity; a triple arthrodesis with wedge resection.

neurectomy: excision of a portion of or an entire nerve.

Ober p.: for paralytic clubfeet; a method of transfer of the posterior tibial tendon to the third cuneiform or metatarsal.

onychotomy: incision into the nail bed.

opening abductory wedge osteotomy (OAWO): for hallux valgus; osteotomy of the first metatarsal base with use of bone graft to open the wedge and bring the first metatarsal closer to the second.

opening wedge osteotomy: a cut through bone followed by distracting the bone on one side to "open" the cut. Used for changing the angle of a bone.

Osmone-Clarke p.: for talipes valgus; soft tissue release of the medial and lateral foot with peroneus brevis tendon transfer.

osteotripsy: for callosities; may be any percutaneous reduction of a bony prominence.

panmetatarsal head resection: usually for severe arthritic deformity; resection of all of the metatarsal heads.

pantalar fusion: for instability of the hindfoot; fusion of the tibiotalar, subtalar, calcaneocuboid, and talonavicular joints.

partial ostectomy: to relieve pressure on the skin; removal of bony prominence.

Peabody p.: (1) for metatarsus varus; resection of the proximal portion of the second, third, and fourth metatarsals, with osteotomy of the fifth and capsular release of the first tarsometatarsal joint; (2) for paralysis of gastrocsoleus complex; transfer of anterior tibial tendon to the calcaneus.

Perry p.: for talipes equinovarus; split transfer of anterior tibialis to proximal third metatarsal, and flexor hallucis longus to dorsum of fourth metatarsal.

phenolization: for nail deformity in which a permanent elimination of a part or all of nail plate is desired. Phenol is applied to the nail matrix after the nail plate is removed to destroy any further nail growth.

Pierrot-Murphy p.: for ankle dorsiflexion weakness; transfer of Achilles tendon anteriorly on calcaneus.

proximal interphalangeal (PIP) fusion: operation commonly done for clawtoes or hammer toes; removal of the proximal interphalangeal joint and then fusion.

Pridie-Koutsogiannis p.: for flexible flatfoot with excessive heel valgus; medial displacement osteotomy of calcaneus.

Putti-Mayer p.: for treatment of polio foot deformity; transfer of posterior tibial tendon.

Quenu p.: for ingrown toenail; excision of nail bed germinal matrix through skin flap incision, leaving distal nail intact. Also called **Fowler p.** and **Zadik p.**

Reverdin-Green p.: for hallux valgus; a closing wedge osteotomy of the first metatarsal head.

Richardson p.: for malunited calcaneal fracture; posterior subtalar fusion using iliac bone graft as necessary.

Rose p.: for ingrown nail; removal of the ellipse of soft tissue to ingrown portion of nail.

Ruiz-Mora p.: proximal phalangectomy of the fifth toe for cock-up (or curly toe) deformity.

Samilson p.: for calcaneocavus foot; a crescentic osteotomy of the calcaneus.

scarf p.: for hallux valgus; a midshaft osteotomy to correct metatarsus primus varus.

shock wave therapy: the use of either low-energy or high-energy shock waves, like those used to break up kidney stones, to treat chronic inflammatory conditions of the Achilles tendon or plantar fascia.

Siffert-Foster-Nachamie p.: for paralytic clubfeet; triple arthrodesis.

Silver p.: excision of medial first metatarsal exostosis with lateral capsular release and medial capsular imbrication.

simple, effective, rapid, and inexpensive (SERI) p.: for hallux valgus; a distal metatarsal neck osteotomy through a minimal incision, stabilized with a longitudinal K-wire.

Staples-Black-Broström p.: for acute, severe ankle sprain; method of repair of lateral collateral ligaments.

Steindler matricectomy: for nail deformity; removal of a part of the nail matrix to eliminate one border of the nail plate.

Steindler p.: plantar release of the proximal muscles and fascia of the foot for high-arched feet.

step down osteotomy: for abnormally long lesser metatarsal; an osteotomy to shorten the bone.

Stone p.: for hallux rigidus; resection of the dorsal first metatarsal exostosis.

Strayer p.: for tight heel cord; gastrocnemius lengthening leaving soleus intact.

subtalar arthrodesis: for arthritis and other conditions of the talocalcaneal joint; fusion of the talus to the calcaneus.

subtalar arthroereisis: for severe flatfoot with calcaneal valgus; insertion of a metallic or ceramic spacer into the subtalar joint.

Suppan p.: for nail deformity; this is a name applied to a variety of procedures to eliminate all or a part of the nail matrix.

Syme amputation: an ankle disarticulation with preservation of the heel pad for weight-bearing.

syndactylization: a soft tissue procedure in which two adjacent toes are intentionally joined together.

talectomy: excision of the talus for severe soft tissue contractures.

tendon Achilles lengthening (TAL): a variety of procedures used to lengthen a tight or spastic Achilles tendon.

Thomas p.: for malunion calcaneus; subtalar arthrodesis using an iliac crest graft.

Tohen p.: for spastic equinovarus deformity of foot; transfer of conjoined extensor hallucis longus and anterior tibial tendon to second or fifth metatarsal.

transmetatarsal amputation: an amputation through the midportion of the metatarsals.

triple arthrodesis: for arthritis or unstable deformity of the hindfoot. Comprises fusion of the calcaneus to the cuboid, navicular to the talus, and talus to the calcaneus.

Turco p.: for clubfeet; soft tissue release of the posteromedial capsule as well as Achilles tendon lengthening.

Vulpius-Compere p.: for Achilles tendon tightness; proximal inverted V-shaped lengthening.

V-Y plasty: for clawtoes; transection of skin in V-shaped incision with closure in the shape of a Y.

Warner-Farber p.: for trimalleolar fractures with large posterior fragment; detachment of the fibula from tibia to get screw fixation of posterior fragment.

Watson-Cheyne p.: for ingrown toenail; excision of vertical wedge avoiding bone; also called **Burghard p., O'Donoghue p.,** and **Mongensen p.**

Watson-Jones p.: for lateral ankle instability; use of peroneus brevis tendon in reconstruction of lateral ligament.

Weil p.: for an unstable lesser metatarsophalangeal joint or for a plantar callosity or metatarsalgia caused by a long metatarsal; a distal oblique metatarsal shortening osteotomy.

Westin p.: for paralytic talipes calcaneus; a tenodesis of the Achilles tendon to the fibula.

White slide p.: for Achilles tendon tightening in spastic hemiplegia; anterior fibers of the Achilles tendon are cut distally, and medial fibers are cut proximally. The foot is then dorsiflexed, producing the slide.

Whitman talectomy p.: talectomy for calcaneovalgus foot.

Whitman-Thompson p.: for talipes calcaneus or talipes calcaneovalgus; complete excision of the talus.

Wilson p.: for hallux valgus; an oblique osteotomy of the first metatarsal neck area.

Wilson and Jacob p.: for tibial plateau fracture; use of patella and its cartilage surface for joint replacement graft.

Winograd p.: for an ingrown nail; excision of an ingrown portion of toenail, with curettage of the nail bed.

Wolf p.: for plantar callosity; proximal shortening of the metatarsal.

Wu p.: (1) for hallux valgus; an oblique osteotomy of the metatarsal neck with lateral and plantar displacement; (2) for hallux rigidus; first metatarsophalangeal joint fusion.

Young p.: anterior tibialis transfer for flatfoot.

Z-plasty: for tight heel cord; complete Z-shaped cut and repair in a lengthened position.

Zadik p.: for ingrown nail; excision of the entire nail.

Ankle Prostheses

The forces acting on the ankle are biplanar, yet by design, the prosthetics are monoplanar. With the highly active forces that exist across the ankle joint, there are fewer occasions for replacement of that joint. Prosthetic fixation is not as secure for these lower-limb joint replacements, with loosening a continuing problem. A historical list of prostheses is in previous editions.

Ankle and Foot Approaches

anterior a.: for tendon repairs, transfers, and some ankle fusions; also called **Kochler a.** and **Ollier a.**

Bassett et al. a.: approach to posteromedial ankle through posterior tibial tendon sheath.

Campbell a.: a posterior approach, for ankle arthrodesis; a posterior lateral approach to the elbow.

Cincinnati a.: incision for clubfoot.

Henry a.: direct lateral approach to the fibula.

Kocher a.: curved L to calcaneus; lateral to tarsus and ankle.

lateral and posterolateral a.: for repair of fractures, ligamentous injuries, and some tendon transfers; also called **Kocher a.** and **Gatellier and Chastang a.**

medial and posteromedial a.: for ankle fractures, tendon transfers, and correction of clubfeet; also called **Broomhead a., Colonna and Ralston a., Koenig and Schaefer a.,** and **Garceau a.**

Physical Medicine and Rehabilitation: Physical Therapy and Occupational Therapy

Physical Medicine and Rehabilitation

Physical medicine and rehabilitation (PM&R), also called physiatry, is a medical specialty based on the fundamentals of neuromuscular physiology, exercise physiology, and functional anatomy. Physiatry aims to enhance and restore functional ability and quality of life to those with physical impairments or disabilities.

The **physiatrist** is the physician specializing in PM&R and certified by the American Board of Physical Medicine and Rehabilitation after completing a residency and other requirements. In some distinct centers for rehabilitation, a physiatrist is the medical director of the unit. However, some units are organized on a programmatic basis and have a group of other medical specialists overseeing individual programs, for example, a rheumatologist with the arthritis program, a neurologist with the neuromuscular disease program, and an orthopaedist with the musculoskeletal program. The **physical therapist** is a health care professional who has completed a Doctor of Physical Therapy (DPT) degree, Master of Physical Therapy (MPT) degree, or Master of Science in Physical Therapy (MSPT) degree.

These education programs are accredited by the Commission on Accreditation in Physical Therapy Education. Board-certified physical therapy specialties are in the following areas: cardiopulmonary, neurologic, clinical electrophysiologic, orthopaedic, pediatric, geriatric, and sports physical therapy.

In a hospital setting, the physiatrist may direct a rehabilitation team that may include the occupational therapist, speech therapist, rehabilitation nurse, social worker, and psychologist. Additional members might include a vocational counselor, special educator, prosthetist and orthotist, and numerous medical specialists depending on patient needs. The physical therapist assistant is a skilled technical health worker who, under the supervision of a physical therapist, assists in the patient's treatment program.

The goal of the rehabilitation team is to enhance each patient's physical capabilities by using the team members' individual professional skills, expertise, and knowledge to evaluate, plan, and implement treatment interventions tailored to the needs of the patient. In this patient-centered approach, the patient and family participate in setting realistic goals to be achieved during the rehabilitation process.

In association with orthopaedic surgery, the rehabilitation team works closely with and is considered an integral part of the orthopaedic rehabilitation program. The physical therapist consults with the orthopaedist and other primary care physicians in the evaluation and treatment of patients and establishes the treatment plan.

Services are provided for preoperative and postoperative care of the surgical patient after restorative surgery, trauma, or correction of congenital anomalies. In addition, treatments include the prevention of pulmonary complications after surgery. Strengthening and range of motion (ROM) exercises are designed for patients with ligamentous tears and fractures. Amputees fitted with prostheses are instructed in their use and maintenance. The patient with a spinal cord injury is taught **activities of daily living (ADLs),** gait with braces, the use of assistive devices, and exercises to improve function. Specialized rehabilitation centers are designed to most effectively address these patients' needs.

Physical therapist services provide identification, prevention, remediation, and rehabilitation of patients with acute or prolonged physical dysfunction. Such intervention encompasses examination and analysis, therapeutic application of physical and chemical agents, exercises, and education to promote functional independence.

Physical therapy treatments may include the evaluation and treatment of abnormal gait patterns resulting from pathologic conditions, such as muscle weakness, paralysis, or biomechanical defects. Patients may also be referred for rehabilitative services for treatment of neuromuscular diseases (e.g. stroke, or spinal cord injuries), musculoskeletal impairments (e.g., arthritis), temporomandibular joint syndrome, and chronic pain. The goal is to decrease pain, increase function, and prevent deformity.

Physical Therapy Services

Physical therapists practice in a variety of settings: acute care hospitals, rehabilitation centers, skilled nursing facilities, convalescent homes, home health, schools, industry, sports clinics, pediatric facilities, and private practice.

The following is a quick reference to typical services (although not all inclusive) that are routinely provided by the physical therapist.

Physical Therapy Evaluation (General)	
strength	coordination
functional ability	sensation
range of motion	ambulatory status
cognitive status	

Physical Therapy Evaluation (Specific)	
manual muscle testing	posture
cardiopulmonary function	muscle tone
electroneurophysiology	skin integrity
neurodevelopmental	neonatal
isokinetic	thermography
gait mechanics	functional capacity evaluation

Physical Therapy Treatment Techniques
Therapeutic Exercise
passive range of motion
active-assistive range of motion
active range of motion
resistive (isometric, isotonic, concentric, eccentric, isokinetic) exercises
work hardening
coordination exercises
Specific Techniques
proprioceptive neuromuscular facilitation (PNF)
Bobath (neurodevelopmental)
Rood
Brunstrom
plyometrics
Muscle Reeducation
brushing
icing
tapping
quick stretch
neurodevelopmental training
Manual Therapy
cross-friction massage
manual lymph drainage
stretching soft tissue mobilization
joint mobilization
myofascial release
craniosacral therapy
McKenzie technique
muscle energy technique
pelvic floor therapy
Mobility
bed (bedbound patient)
transfer techniques
wheelchair mobility and safety
ambulation—parallel bars, walker, crutches, cane, prosthetic, orthotic
Hydrotherapy
cold/ice
heat (moist)

whirlpool (for increasing circulation, decreasing pain, debriding open wounds)

therapy pool (for gravity-free exercise and ambulation)

paraffin

Physical Modalities

electrical stimulation

functional electrical stimulation (FES)

diathermy

transcutaneous electrical nerve stimulation (TENS)

ultrasound

infrared

ultraviolet

laser

kinesio taping

McConnell taping

Cardiac Care

cardiac rehabilitation

cardiac stress testing

Pulmonary

bronchial drainage

breathing exercises

chest physical therapy: percussion, vibration, postural drainage

incentive spirometry

Pediatric

neurodevelopmental

scoliosis care (education and exercise, preoperative and postoperative care)

musculoskeletal

Intermittent Compression

edema control

Traction

cervical

pelvic

extremity

Patient Education (an essential element of every treatment plan)

Consultation Services

Consultative services are available for patients with special or extraordinary needs that require the recommendations of a multidisciplinary group.

Physical Therapy Modalities

balneotherapy: medical use of spa pools and mineral baths particularly for arthritis therapy.

cervical traction: a means of separating the cervical vertebrae 1 to 2 mm to help relieve painful neck conditions or cervical radiculopathies; may be intermittent or continuous.

contrast baths: alternately exposing affected limb to warm and cool water for specified periods. This is a means of reducing swelling, diminishing pain, and improving joint ROM.

cryotherapy: use of low temperatures to decrease inflammation, decrease pain and spasm, promote vasoconstriction.

diathermy: electromagnetic waves with a specific wavelength (shortwave diathermy, microwave diathermy) used as a means of producing heat deep inside tissues.

electrical stimulation:

    alternating current: sinusoidal or faradic; stimulates normally innervated muscles to relieve pain and relax muscle spasm.

    galvanic: direct current used to stimulate denervated muscles and for ion transfer (iontophoresis).

    high-voltage pulsed galvanic: to relieve pain and relax muscle spasm. Stimulates normally innervated muscles.

    iontophoresis: the use of direct current to drive water-soluble ions through the skin. Dexamethasone and lidocaine (Xylocaine) are commonly used to treat acute and subacute localized inflammation and pain.

    microamperage electrical nerve stimulation (MENS): microamperage current that is below patient's threshold; to relieve pain.

    transcutaneous electrical nerve stimulation (TENS): self-contained, modulated galvanic current (low voltage) that seems to block painful afferent nerve impulses. Helps to control pain so patient may exercise.

fluidotherapy: the use of forced warm air through a container holding fine cellulose particles to provide dry heat and exercise to upper and lower extremities. Both the temperature and the particle agitation can be controlled for edema and desensitization of hypersensitive area.

hot packs: silicone gel, clay, or other material in bags that can be heated to provide superficial heat for tissues.

Hubbard tank: a large full-body water tank used to assist in ROM and endurance exercise.

hydrostatic bed: essentially a waterbed that supports the patient for specific therapies.

hydrotherapy treatments: as commonly used today, immersion of affected limbs (sometimes including the trunk) in a tank of water at a specified temperature. The water may be moving (whirlpool), which is one means of debriding tissue. There are also tanks in which patients may sit (Lo-Boy) and in which they may be almost totally immersed (Hubbard tank). In a pool, the buoyancy of water can assist patients with partially paralyzed legs to walk. Some therapists refer to the **Archimedes principle** because the buoyancy in the water supports the weight, eliminates shock, and decreases the concern for need of balance.

interferential current: application of two medium-frequency alternating currents that interfere with each other. Used for pain control and muscle stimulation.

intermittent compression: a boot or sleeve that encloses the leg or arm and is alternately pressurized with air and then deflated. The inflate-deflate action provides a pumping effect that reduces disabling edema. It is often prescribed for breast cancer patients after a mastectomy and for lymphedema that may result.

paraffin bath: a combination of wax and mineral oil at 126° F used as a means of heating the hands or feet.

phonophoresis: the use of ultrasound to drive molecules of medications through the skin to the underlying tissues.

rest, ice, compression, and elevation (RICE): for the initial treatment of an injury; the treatment of choice for acute musculoskeletal injuries that include sprains, strains, and hematomas.

traction: for low back pain; application of pelvic belt with caudad pull, which may be continuous or use greater force intermittently.

ultrasound: ultra-high-frequency sound waves that mechanically vibrate soft tissue. Secondary deep heat may develop according to method of application.

whirlpool: a form of hydrotherapy using fast moving water that is usually heated.

Physical Therapy Procedures

acupressure: sustained deep pressure over muscular trigger points.

aerobic exercises: exercises in which oxygen is inhaled at a rate sufficient for a continuous process of energy production for muscle contraction; the goal is to increase endurance required for long-distance running or after cardiac complications.

agility training: to improve balance and coordination; trains in the ability to make rapid changes in movement and direction.

anaerobic exercises: exercises in which the expenditure of energy is at a faster rate than that for which the muscles can function without a period of recovery before there is further exertion.

aquatic exercise: exercise performed in a pool or large hydrotherapy tank that uses the buoyancy of water.

closed chain exercise: exercise that occurs when the distal segment of an extremity is fixed, such as performing a squat, in which the foot is in contact with the ground. Motion can take place in all planes. Also called **closed kinetic chain exercise.**

Codman exercises: exercises for a stiff shoulder in which the patient is bent over at the waist (90 degrees) and the hand hangs like a pendulum toward the floor. A weight may be placed in the hand and the arm is then moved through various arcs to increase the ROM in that shoulder.

concentric contraction: muscle shortening with part moving in direction of muscle pull; also called **positive work.**

cross-training: a complex training regimen in which two or more sports or activities are combined into either a solitary or a cyclical program to exercise different muscle groups and to provide variety and protection from repetitive use syndromes.

DeLorme exercises: originally established on the basis of the 10 repetition maximum, which is the maximal amount of resistance a muscle can lift through full ROM exercises 10 times; the term is frequently interchanged with *progressive resistive exercises*, which are designed to build strength and increase endurance through graduated resistance for a prescribed number of repetitions.

eccentric contraction: muscle lengthening during contraction; strengthening exercises in which the external force overcomes the actively contracting muscle, forcing the muscle to lengthen. Also called **negative work.**

effleurage: a method of massage that uses a flowing motion with the hands over a tight muscle to relieve tightness.

endurance training: high-repetition exercise designed to give maximum endurance for repeated muscle contraction.

gait training: the use of parallel bars, crutches, walkers, and canes with specific instructions to the patient. Weight-bearing may be described as *non–weight-bearing, partial weight-bearing,* or *full weight-bearing*. Ambulation with crutches is often described as *three-point gait,* and with walker, *four-point gait.*

isokinetic exercises: constant velocity; strengthening exercises requiring special equipment in which there is an accommodating resistance, resulting in a maximal force against the contracting muscle throughout its full ROM. Can be used for the spine as well as the upper and lower extremities.

isometric exercises: muscle contraction without joint movement in which the resistance may be provided by a fixed object (wall, stabilized bar) or the antagonistic muscle group (flexors versus extensors); a muscle-strengthening exercise that does not impel muscle to work through its ROM; also called **constant angle exercise** and **static exercise.**

isotonic exercises: muscle contraction with movement of the joint through a specified ROM against a fixed amount of resistance; also called **constant force exercise.**

joint manipulation: any skilled manual technique applied to a joint that moves one particular surface in relation to another.

joint mobilization: skilled passive movements applied to joint surfaces to restore joint play and ROM or to treat pain.

joint play: involuntary movements of joint surfaces allowed by capsular elasticity that allow for normal, pain-free voluntary motion; also called **accessory movement.**

lumbar stabilization: exercise program to stabilize the torso by developing the corset muscles of the lumbar spine, particularly the abdominal muscles.

manual lymphatic drainage: a specialized form of manual therapy that mobilizes protein-rich fluid toward intact lymphatics to reduce edema

manual therapy: any treatment in which hands are used to manipulate, massage, or mobilize a part of the body.

McConnell taping: the technique of specific taping to correct abnormal tilt, glide, and rotation of the patella in patients with patellofemoral disorders.

McKenzie extension exercises: exercises performed to decrease the compression on the intervertebral disk.

muscle energy technique: manual technique that uses active contraction of a patient's muscle to correct joint dysfunction.

myofascial release: manual therapy technique that applies prolonged stretching to release restrictions in the muscle-fascia system.

open chain exercises: exercise that occurs when the distal segment of an extremity is free, such as performing a seated knee extension exercise. Non–weight-bearing and usually in one plane of motion; also called **open kinetic chain exercises.**

pétrissage: a massage maneuver similar to kneading.

prehensile: the use of the thumb opposing the hand to grasp an object. The term *prehensile* implies function in which the thumb can be placed in opposition to the object. An atavistic hand lacks that capacity.

pulley exercises: a rope-on-pulley system used to increase ROM of a joint or strengthen muscles; resistance can be applied by another limb or by weights.

range of motion (ROM) exercises: designed to maintain or increase the amount of movement in a joint. They may be one of the following:

   passive ROM exercise: force is applied to bring about motion in a joint or joints by either a therapist or the patient, without any muscle function in these joints.

active-assistive ROM exercise: exercise performed by the patient but requiring assistance from a therapist, another extremity, or a mechanical device because of muscle weakness or pain.

active ROM exercise: exercise performed by patient without assistance or resistance; the therapist is only an instructor-observer.

resistive exercise table: commonly used for lower extremity problems, such as after knee surgery; resistance can be applied by weights (NK table in some locales) or by a graded hydraulic system.

spray and stretch: use of a vapocoolant, such as Fluori-Methane or ice, for treatment of trigger points in muscles. The vapocoolant is sprayed over a stretched muscle to increase ROM.

strength training: exercise directed to achieve the maximum capacity of a muscle to pull in a single effort.

Swiss ball exercises: use of an inflatable gymnastic ball with various movements for mobility, strength, balance, coordination, and stabilization of the spine and the extremities.

tapotement: a method of massage that involves percussion such as used in chest therapy.

therapeutic massage: soft tissue manipulation using techniques such as friction, stroking, and kneading to reduce muscle spasm and edema, stimulate circulation, and encourage relaxation. Also used to stretch scar tissue.

Williams exercises: for patients with low back pain; exercises are performed to open the lumbar intervertebral foramina and decrease the compression on the facet joints by flexing the lumbosacral spine, thereby stretching the extensors of the back and strengthening the abdominal muscles. Also called **flexion exercises.**

Tests and Measurements*

Given that the circulation is intact, the major parameters in assessing the function of a limb are ROM, sensation, and strength. These can be tested directly by the application of forces to the muscle through the ROM of individual joint and stimuli to the skin. Muscle testing can be supplemented by electrodiagnostic modalities such as electromyography. In muscle testing, strength is graded by the following scale as assessed directly by the examiner. ROM is measured with a goniometer, an instrument that measures joint motion in degrees.

Key to Manual Muscle Evaluation			
% of Normal Strength	Numerical Score	Letter Score	Muscle Strength Criteria
100%	5	N	Normal: Complete ROM against gravity with full resistance
75%	4	G	Good: Complete ROM against gravity with some resistance
50%	3	F	Fair: Complete ROM against gravity
25%	2	P	Poor: Complete ROM with gravity eliminated
10%	1	T	Trace: Evidence of contractility
0	0	0	Zero: No evidence of contractility (no palpable muscle contractility)
		S	Spasm*
		C	Contracture*

ROM, Range of motion.
*If spasm or contracture exists, place S or C after the grade of a movement incomplete for this reason.
From Daniels L, Worthingham C: Muscle testing: techniques of manual examination by comparison, ed 4, Philadelphia, 1980, WB Saunders.

dynamometer: an instrument to measure muscle strength and its effects from exercise, such as a handgrip d. that can be adjusted to test strength in different positions of grasp; or from a bicycle d. that measures muscular, respiratory, and metabolic effects of exercise, recording directly from a pressure gauge; also called **ergometer.**

computerized isokinetic dynamometer: an apparatus that can be used to test and record the maximal strength of a muscle as it acts on a joint through a full ROM. The recording is used to evaluate the progress of a patient's condition during recovery or to confirm the existence and extent of injury.

---
*For more specific information on various tests and examinations, an excellent source is American Orthopaedic Association, 1985.

Institute of Sports Medicine and Athletic Trauma (ISMAT) muscle testing: manual assessment of muscle strength with a small, force-measuring device held by the examiner.

osteokinetic movement: movement that occurs between two bones such as rotation, swing, or spin.

Sensory Testing

heat and cold testing: self-explanatory.

pinprick test: a gross test to check two variables: (1) the actual ability to feel a pinprick and (2) the ability to determine the difference between sharp and dull.

pressure testing: involves sensation produced by touch to a localized area using an instrument that indicates the pressure needed to produce sensation.

proprioceptive testing: tests the ability to sense the position of a body part with the eyes closed.

tendon reflex examination: graded from 0 to 4 and varies widely in meaning from examiner to examiner; the test is performed by striking the tendon briskly and watching muscle reaction.

two-point discrimination: ability to perceive difference between one or two points of touch at the fingertips or elsewhere; this test of fine sensation is measured in centimeters or millimeters.

vibrator sense examination: tests the patient's ability to feel vibrations with use of a tuning fork.

Electrical Testing

electromyography (EMG): evaluation of physiological state of the muscle by direct insertion of a small needle-electrode into a muscle fiber. Muscular activity is analyzed during the insertion, resting state, and active recruitment (contractile activity) of muscle fibers. EMG machine can convert small electrical activities of the muscle fibers to a wave form and sound that can be analyzed for abnormalities. Disorders affecting the nerve, muscle, or neuromuscular junction will eventually cause changes in the wave pattern of the muscle. Other disorders commonly evaluated with this study include entrapment syndromes and other neuropathic and muscle disorders.

conduction time: the measurement of time required for the nerve to transmit impulse. The conduction time is increased in neurologic disorders, such as vitamin B_1 deficiency and carpal tunnel syndrome caused by local nerve compression or disorders of myelin or axons.

nerve conduction study: a diagnostic test often performed in conjunction with the EMG. This is a test of the integrity of peripheral nerves that involves stimulating peripheral nerve in point A and picking up response at point B. Usually the conduction velocity and response (amplitude) of the nerve is recorded as a wave form and analyzed. Useful in the diagnosis of nerve entrapment syndrome and polyneuropathies.

Occupational Therapy

Occupational therapists are skilled clinicians in the art of maximizing patient functional outcomes in a variety of settings. Through functional client-based treatment, occupational therapists enable patients to restore, reinforce, and enhance performance; facilitate new adaptation and learning; diminish or correct abnormalities; and promote and maintain health. By looking at the client holistically, as well as outside factors such as environment, therapists endeavor to apply the skills and modifications needed to complete everyday activities of living.

The occupational therapist, registered/licensed (OTR/L) is a health professional who has been educated in a baccalaureate, master's, or doctoral curriculum accredited jointly by the Committee on Allied Health Education, American Medical Association, and the American Occupational Therapy Association's (AOTA) Accreditation Council for Occupational Therapy Education (ACOTE). In all educational programs, OTR/Ls must have completed clinical placements (field work) under supervision in settings ranging from hospitals and school systems to private clinics. They have passed the National Board for Certification in Occupational Therapy to become registered OTR/Ls and hold state licensure for practice, and have completed clinical placements under supervision in settings ranging from hospitals and school systems to private clinics. A certified occupational therapy assistant has satisfactorily completed an occupational therapy assistant curriculum approved by ACOTE and has passed a national certification examination to become certified and works under the supervision of an OTR/L.

Occupational therapists can specialize in specific practice areas by receiving further training, certification, and education. Those holding the title of *certified hand therapist* have been trained extensively in hand and upper extremity rehabilitation and have passed a comprehensive examination. Other specialties can include gerontology, mental health, pediatrics, and physical rehabilitation.

As of 2005, all graduating occupational therapists are required to possess a master's degree or higher for entry into the field. Having a master's degree as a minimum educational requirement allows clinicians to further venture into evidence-based practice wherein research provides rationale and helps to guide and justify treatment choices. Within the last decade, occupational therapists have pushed this imperative practice to the forefront of clinical application. As quantity and quality of research improve, therapists will be able to continue to align occupational therapy practice with that of other medical arenas.

Specific Occupational Therapist Interventions

Specific occupational therapy interventions include but are not limited to the following:

- education and training in ADLs
- administering and interpreting such tests as manual muscle and ROM
- design, fabrication, and application of splints and other orthoses
- developing perceptual-motor skills and sensory integrative functioning
- restoration of hand functioning decreased by a disease process, after surgery, or by a traumatic event
- instruction in work simplification, energy conservation, and use of proper body mechanics during activity for work, leisure, and daily living
- guidance in the selection and use of adaptive equipment
- therapeutic activities to enhance functional performance
- prevocational evaluation and training and physical capacity evaluation
- consultation concerning adaptation to home or work environments

Occupational Therapy Assessment

Services are provided to all age groups in a variety of settings, including hospitals, hand clinics, rehabilitation facilities, sheltered workshops, schools, extended care facilities, private homes, community agency clinics, and industrial settings.

Orthopaedists most frequently refer patients to occupational therapy for treatments of amputation, arthritis, soft tissue trauma, fractures, total joint replacement, sports injury, osteoporosis, elbow and shoulder arthroplasty, spinal cord injury, and chronic pain. One fourth of AOTA's more than 40,000 members work with orthopaedic patients.

Before intervention is provided, each potential patient's or client's case is screened to determine the need for occupational therapy. This is followed by evaluation, which consists of obtaining and interpreting data necessary for treatment, including that needed to plan for and document the evaluation process and treatment results. The occupational therapy evaluation includes assessment of functional abilities and deficits as related to the client's needs.

Specific Evaluations, Tests, and Devices

Specific evaluations, tests, and devices used in the assessment process include but are not limited to the following:

Baltimore therapeutic equipment (BTE) work simulator: a device used for evaluation and work hardening as well as regaining specific movement via attachments.
bulb dynamometer: a soft, cylindrical, rubber-filled squeeze bulb that measures gross isometric grasp and pinch, calibrated in pounds per square inch, measuring force in pounds by multiplying the reading by four.
Crawford small parts dexterity test: for fine eye-hand coordination and manipulation of small hand tools.
functional capacities assessment: a performance evaluation that determines a person's ability to perform physical work.
Jamar dynamometer: measures gross isometric grip strength in five positions and records in either pounds or kilograms.

Jebsen-Taylor hand function test: consisting of seven subtests to measure major aspects of hand function related to ADLs.

Martin vigorimeter: to test handgrip strength.

Minnesota rate of manipulation test: measures gross coordination and dexterity.

O'Connor finger dexterity test: designed to measure fine motor ability.

Pennsylvania bimanual work sample: measures finger dexterity of both hands, gross movements of both arms, eye-hand coordination, ability to use both hands simultaneously.

pinch: two-point, three-point, and lateral and pinch strength is tested with pinch gauge recorded in pounds or kilograms.

Purdue pegboard: measures gross movements of arm, hand, and fingers and fingertip dexterity.

Semmes-Weinstein monofilament: a series of monofilaments with different ratings to determine amount of sensory loss; also called **VonFrey hair test.**

Smith physical capacities evaluation (PCE): objective test to measure ability of individual to perform selected aspects of occupations.

two-point discrimination: most commonly measured with the Disk-Criminator or Boley gauge.

Valpar component work sample series: standardized test consisting of 16 work samples designed to measure 17 work behaviors by task analysis; developed for workers with industrial injuries.

volumeter set: accurately measures hand and distal forearm edema for objective monitoring of edema-reducing treatment modalities with water displacement.

Occupational Therapy Interventions

Occupational therapists are known for providing intervention that takes personal factors into account for each person. This client-centered approach allows clinicians to creatively target specific needs to further patient outcomes. This is especially important with patients who have a multitude of problems in different areas such as an orthopaedic patient who may have residual deficits from a neurologic event. Treatment refers to the use of specific activities or methods to promote, improve, or restore the performance of necessary functions, compensate for dysfunction, or minimize debilitation.

The therapist plans for and documents treatment performance to show progression as well as where more intervention is needed. The following are categories of necessary functional activities treated in occupational therapy for orthopaedic problems:*

activities of daily living (ADLs) and instrumental activities of daily living (IADLs): components of everyday activity, including self-care, work, and play or leisure activities. These may also be referred to as *life skills* or *life tasks* and consist of the following:

bathing: ability to obtain and use supplies and soap, rinse and dry all body parts, maintain bathing position, transfer to and from bathing position, use adapted bathing equipment such as bath mitt, tub bench, grab bars, scrub brush, and so forth.

dressing: ability to select appropriate clothing; obtain clothing from storage area; dress and undress in sequential fashion; fasten and unfasten clothes and shoes; and don and doff appliances, for example, glasses, prostheses, or orthoses.

feeding and eating: ability to set up food, use appropriate regular or adapted utensils and tableware, and bring food or drink from table to mouth.

communication device use: ability to use equipment or systems to enhance or provide communication, such as writing equipment, telephones, computers, communication boards, call lights, emergency systems, braille writers, augmentative communication systems, and computers.

functional mobility: ability to move from one position or one place to another as in bed mobility, wheelchair mobility, transfers (bed, chair, tub, toilet, car), and functional ambulation with or without adaptive aids, driving, or use of public transportation.

personal hygiene and grooming: ability to obtain and use supplies to shave, apply and remove cosmetics, wash, comb, style, and brush hair, care for nails, care for skin, and apply deodorant.

---

*Definitions taken from Roley SS, DeLany JV, Barrows CJ, et al: Occupational therapy practice framework: domain & process, 2nd edition, *Am J Occup Ther* 62(6):625-683, 2008. doi:10.5014/ajot.62.6.625

toilet hygiene: ability to obtain and use supplies, clean self, and transfer to and from and maintain toileting position on bedpan, toilet, or commode.

current life activities: activities that include home, work, and play.

cognitive skills: necessary mental processes, including orientation, conceptualization and comprehension (concentration, attention span, memory), and cognitive integration (applying diverse knowledge to environmental situations, including ability to generalize and problem solve).

employment seeking and acquisition: vocational exploration, job acquisition, and timely and effective job performance.

home: includes home management tasks such as clothing care, cleaning, meal preparation and cleanup, household maintenance, care of others, and safety procedures. The latter is important in preventing falls in areas such as bathroom, kitchen, and stairs.

play or leisure: choosing and engaging in activities for amusement, relaxation, spontaneous enjoyment, or self-expression.

prevention and minimization of debilitation: refers to programs for persons with predisposition to disability, as well as for those who have already incurred a disability, and includes the following:

energy conservation: activity restriction, work simplification, time management, or organization of the environment to minimize energy output.

joint protection: procedures to minimize stress on joints, including use of proper body mechanics, avoidance of static or deforming postures, and avoidance of excess weight-bearing.

positioning: placement of body part in alignment to promote optimal functioning; or position of tasks and objects in a position to maximize performance.

sensorimotor skills: consist of performance patterns of sensory and motor behavior prerequisite to self-care, work, and play and leisure performance, such as:
- ROM
- gross and fine coordination
- muscle control
- coordination
- dexterity
- strength and endurance
- sensory awareness, including
  - tactile awareness
  - stereognosis
  - kinesthesia
  - proprioceptive awareness

therapeutic modifications: design or restructuring of the physical environment to assist self-care, work, and play and leisure performance through selecting, obtaining, fitting, and fabricating equipment, as well as instructing client, family, and staff in its proper use and care, including making minor repairs and modifications for correct fit, position, or use. Some categories of therapeutic adaptation are:

orthotics, splints, or slings: to relieve pain, maintain joint alignment, protect joint integrity, improve function, or decrease deformity.

dynamic splints: an orthotic device that achieves its effects by movement and force generated by the patient's own musculature or external forces such as springs and rubber bands (Fig. 12-1).

functional fracture bracing using thermoplastics: proximal or distal to fracture, fracture alignment and stability when motion occurs.

static splints: an orthotic device that immobilizes all involved joints and surrounding musculature for protection and healing purposes (see Fig. 12-1).

FIG 12-1 Dynamic splint for patient with high radial nerve lesion. *(From Amanda Calhoon, Shady Grove Center for Sports Medicine, Rockville, MD.)*

static progressive splints: provide a low-load stretch; as a patient progresses, the splint can be advanced to provide more of a challenge to further advance movement and overall ROM.

prosthetics: in this context, an artificial device used to replace a missing body part such as a limb, tooth, eye, or heart valve. Occupational therapists play a key role with said clients in adaptation and functional integration of prosthetic.

assistive and adaptive equipment: additions or devices that assist in performance or in structural or positional changes, such as installing ramps and bars, changing furniture heights, adjusting traffic patterns, and modifying wheelchairs. Some typical adaptive equipment examples for orthopaedics are reachers, sock aids, raised toilet seats, leg-lifter straps, and walker adaptations (platforms and walker bags).

The Research Enterprise

Orthopaedic research encompasses a wide range of clinical, basic science, and epidemiologic investigation on the embryology, growth, development, and remodeling of the musculoskeletal system and of its response to disease and treatment. The single clinician-scientist working alone in a laboratory is becoming increasingly rare; most research efforts of recent years are interdisciplinary and take the form of teams of clinicians, basic scientists, engineers, epidemiologists, statisticians, and laboratory technicians.

A relatively small amount of the effort and time involved in biomedical research is taken up in actually performing the experiment and analyzing the results. Considerable effort is taken in the process of developing the research proposal, through which the investigators request permission or funds to conduct a study, and in reporting the results to the general scientific community.

The Research Proposal

Research proposals are submitted to internal, institutional bodies; to not-for-profit foundations; to corporations for extramural research; or to government agencies for extramural research; often in response to a **request for applications (RFA)** announced by the agency. By far the largest sources of orthopaedic research funding in the United States is the **National Institutes of Health (NIH)**, an agency of the Department of Health and Human Services consisting of 19 separate institutes (e.g., the **National Institute of Arthritis and Musculoskeletal and Skin Diseases [NIAMS]**).

There are many avenues for research proposals for the different stages of career. Grants are available for training and initiation of early research proposals from government grants such as NIH and the Department of Defense. Also orthopaedic foundations such as the Orthopaedic Research and Education Foundation and the Arthritis Foundation have small and large grants for new and established investigators.

The objective of the research proposal is to demonstrate to the reviewers that the proposed studies are necessary, reasonable, and feasible. The research proposal and the process of evaluating it differ between funding mechanisms and agencies, but most follow this general outline:

- The investigators list **specific aims** for the proposed research, overall questions for which the research program is designed to provide general answers.
- The investigators propose a testable **hypothesis** or **hypotheses** associated with the specific aims, to which the proposed work will be addressed.
- The **background and significance** of the research question is reviewed; what is known in the field, and what is controversial, are established and delineated.
- The **materials and methods** of the proposed studies are outlined, as is a **plan for data analysis**.

Preliminary data (either supporting the proposed hypotheses, or demonstrating the ability to perform the proposed experiments) and a **sample size analysis** are presented.

Finally, a research budget is proposed, with provisions for both direct costs (those actually involved in performing the study, including supplies, equipment, personnel, etc.) and **indirect costs** (usually a percentage of the direct costs used for institutional overhead [keeping the lights on]).

Review processes differ between applications and institutions, but generally this task is given to a board of anonymous **peer reviewers** (scientists working in the same or closely related field). Many times, comments of the reviewers are forwarded to the investigators (in the case of the NIH, taking the form of the infamous **pink sheets,** which long ago stopped being pink), in the interests of improving the proposal for subsequent submissions. Often the task of evaluating a proposal is kept institutionally separate from the actual funding decisions. As a result, at times a research proposal may be approved but not funded.

Provisions for adequate protection and humane use of subjects must be addressed (in the case of human patients, by the **institutional review board [IRB]**; in the case of other animals by the **institutional animal care and use committee [IACUC]**). Local, institutional committees are also charged with reviewing the proposed use of radioisotopes, toxic material, or recombinant DNA; the concerns of these bodies must be addressed before the study is allowed to begin.

Reporting the Results

Usually the first step in reporting results to the scientific community takes the form of **abstracts** (poster presentations, or short podium presentations) at regional, national, or international meetings, such as those of the American Academy of Orthopaedic Surgeons, the Orthopaedic Research Society, or the American Society for Bone and Mineral Research. Some of these venues provide anonymous peer reviews but with limited feedback to the investigators in the form of comments (in most cases, the investigators are told that the submitted abstract is either accepted or rejected, with no further comment). Published abstracts, with improved Internet applications, are becoming more available to those members of the community who do not personally attend the meetings, but these reports tend to be short, preliminary, and terse. The advantage of these venues is their relative speed and the opportunity for feedback from peers at the actual meeting.

Full **reports of original research,** to be published in journals (such as *Bone, Journal of Biomechanics, Journal of Orthopaedic Research, Journal of Bone and Mineral Research*), the next step in the process, are fully analyzed and interpreted by the investigators. These are submitted to the editors of the journals, who then forward the manuscripts (often with authors and institutions redacted) to anonymous peer reviewers. Detailed feedback is provided to the investigators regarding methods and interpretations; often several iterations of the process are required before a paper is accepted for publication.

Review papers, often invited papers in journals by recognized leaders in a particular field, are designed to summarize the current state of the art and historical perspectives on a topic from many sources but generally do not include new data.

General Research Terminology

The following terms are likely to be found in many areas of research. They have been divided into statistics, biomechanics, techniques in measurements, and orthopaedic cell and tissue biology (general, cartilage, and bone).

Statistics and Epidemiology

accuracy: the property of a measurement denoting its proximity to some gold-standard true value. A measurement may be accurate without being precise (e.g., giving a wide range of test results, centered about the true value).

alpha value: the benchmark value that, *a priori*, is established to determine statistical significance. The alpha value is compared to the *p* value given by the data. If p is ≤ 0.05 α, then statistical significance has been established. In most cases, α = 0.05.

analysis of variance (ANOVA): a method for evaluating differences in a continuous variable between multiple groups. The ANOVA may be further classified as to the number of grouping types being considered:

one-way ANOVA: considers only one categorical variable, which may itself have many possible values (e.g., gender, ethnicity, disease status). When the number of groups is two (e.g., male/female, young/old, diseased/not diseased), the one-way ANOVA reduces to a *t* test.

two-way ANOVA: (and more complex versions, involving three, four, or more ways) considers simultaneously the effect of two or more categorical variables (e.g., the effect of gender and ethnicity on patient height would be properly addressed using a two-way ANOVA), along with the **interaction** between the variables.

Bayesian statistics: (after Rev. Thomas Bayes, 1702–1761, British cleric) a family of statistical techniques in which the interpretation of the results of an experiment includes an evaluation of the results of similar, previous experiments to establish statistical significance. Used in some applications of evidence-based medicine.

categorical variable: a parameter characterized by having a limited number of possible values (e.g., male/female, old/middle-aged/young, right/left) (cf. *continuous variable*).

chi-square analysis (χ^2): a test for determining whether the proportions of data described by two or more categorical variables is random (e.g., 51% of the people with a particular disease are men. Is the disease gender-related?).

confidence interval (CI): an estimate of the range in which a particular percentage of values (usually 95%) may be found.

continuous variable: a parameter characterized by having an infinite number of possible values (e.g., height, weight, blood pressure, age) (cf. *categorical variable*).

correlation: the strength of the relationship between two continuous variables, with no assumption as to which of the variables may be causative (cf. **regression analysis**). The method gives a *p* value and an **r value.** The range of r values is between −1.000 (perfect negative relationship) and 1.000 (perfect positive relationship), with a value of 0.000 denoting no statistical relationship.

Fisher exact test: (after Sir R.A. Fisher, 1890–1962, British statistician and agronomist) a test for determining whether the proportions of data described by two or more categorical variables is random. It is similar in concept to the χ^2 analysis but is more appropriate in cases in which the number of observations is small.

input variable: the parameters that are varied experimentally (cf. output variable); also called **predictor variable, independent variable,** and **the X-axis.**

logistic regression: a special form of regression, in which the dependent variable is a categorical (usually binary) parameter. It is often used in outcomes research and epidemiology, in which the output variables are parameters such as diseased/not diseased, healed/not healed, and so forth.

nonparametric test: a distribution-free method (usually rank-ordered) of dealing with nonnormally distributed data (e.g., a Spearman rank-order test in place of a Pearson product-moment correlation; a Wilcoxon signed-rank test in place of a paired *t* test; a Kruskal-Wallis statistic in place of a one-way ANOVA).

normal distribution: a continuous parameter characterized by a frequency distribution that is Gaussian, that is, bell-shaped, symmetrical, with a maximum number of values at the average, 68% of the values found within one standard deviation of the mean, and 95% of the values found within 1.96 standard deviations of the mean. A normal distribution of the data is a basic assumption of a parametric test; if the data are decidedly nonnormal, then nonparametric tests should be used.

odds ratio (OR): the effect of a risk factor in increasing or decreasing the probability of an outcome, often determined by a logistic regression. By convention, if OR > 1, the outcome is more probable with addition of the risk factor (e.g., body mass index as a risk factor and osteoarthritis as the outcome); if OR < 1, the outcome is less probable with addition of the risk factor (e.g., regular exercise as the risk factor, and heart disease as the outcome).

output variable: the variables that are measured to represent the response to changes in the input variable(s) (cf. input variable); also called **dependent variable** and **the Y-axis**.

***p* value:** the probability that a finding of a difference between groups, or of a correlation between parameters, is due to chance alone.

parametric test: statistical methods, such as linear regressions, ANOVAs, and *t* tests, which are based on estimates of the mean and variance of a population and which inherently assume a normal distribution of these values (Table 13-1).

***post-hoc* tests:** when an ANOVA provides evidence of a statistically significant effect of a particular parameter with three or more possible values (e.g., ethnicity, old/middle-aged/young), these tests are used in place of multiple *t* tests to determine which groups are different from which other ones. For instance, blood pressure may be significantly higher in a group of older patients than in the corresponding group of young patients, but neither may be significantly different from the values found in the middle-aged groups. Several methods are in common use, including the Tukey, Student-Newman-Kuels, Fisher least-squared difference, Duncan, and Bonferroni tests when making all pair-wise comparisons; Dunnett's test when comparing test groups with a single control group, or McNemar's test as a nonparametric, pair-wise test. Also called **multiple comparison test**.

power: the probability that a finding of no difference between groups, or of no correlation between variables, is in fact true; alternatively, the probability of being able to statistically discern a significant difference between groups, or a correlation between variables, should one exist, given the existing sample size and variance. Generally, the minimum power for a definitive finding of no difference or no correlation is 0.80.

precision: the property of a measurement denoting its repeatability. A measurement may be precise without being accurate (e.g., tightly clustered about a value that is not correct).

pseudoreplication: statistical situation that occurs when more than one measurement is taken from a single individual. Such measurements cannot be considered as independent of one another. Special statistical tests are used in these cases, for example, the paired *t* test, the repeated-measures ANOVA, and the mixed-model ANOVA.

regression: a method of comparing two or more continuous variables, in which the relationship between the variables (usually in a linear form) is specifically described in terms of one or more independent, or causative variables, and a single dependent, or output variable. The method gives the geometric equation of the relationship (in the linear form, dependent variable = a **constant** + [a **slope** × independent variable]), a ***p* value** for both the constant (determining whether the constant is significantly different from zero) and for the slope (determining whether the slope is significantly different from zero), and an **r^2** value, which is often interpreted as denoting the percentage of the variability in the data that is explained by the regression equation. The square root of the r^2 value is exactly the r value that would be obtained if a simple correlation between the variables were calculated.

sample size: in general, the sample size for a study, at best determined before the study is initiated, depends on:
- the variability of the measurements:
  - measurement accuracy and precision (which may be estimated by the standard error). The more accurate and precise the measurement, the smaller the sample size required.
  - variability within the population (which may be estimated by the standard deviation). The smaller the population variability, the smaller the sample size required.
- the nature of the question to be addressed:
  - for comparisons of data between categories (e.g., male vs. female, diseased vs. nondiseased), the difference between means of categories (quantified as the *effect size,* the difference between means,

TABLE 13-1 Basic Parametric Statistical Techniques

	Input Variable	
Output variable	**Continuous**	**Categorical**
Continuous	Regression, Correlation	ANOVA t test
Categorical	Logistic, Regression	Chi-square, Fisher exact test

ANOVA, *Analysis of variance.*

divided by the standard deviation). The larger the effect size, the smaller the sample size required.
- for comparisons of continuous variables (e.g., age vs. blood pressure), the slope of the relationship between predictor and outcome variables, in a regression. The further the slope is from 0, the smaller the sample size required.
- the chance of being wrong that the investigator is willing to accept (the alpha value, and the power). The higher the chance of being wrong the investigator is willing to accept, the smaller the sample size required.

standard deviation (SD): a measure of the variability of a parameter in a population, equal to the positive square root of the variance. By definition, in a normally distributed population, 95% of the values of the parameter will be found within 1.96 standard deviations of the mean. Unlike standard error, the standard deviation is relatively insensitive to the sample size. It is always larger than the standard error.

standard error (SE): a measure of the reliability of the mean of a parameter. By definition, if samples are taken of a normally distributed population, 95% of the time, the true mean will fall within 1.96 standard errors of the sample mean. The standard deviation is quite sensitive to the sample size; as the sample size approaches a census of the target population, the standard error by its very definition approaches zero. The standard error may be estimated as (the standard deviation) / (the square root of the sample size). Also called **standard estimate of the mean (SEM).**

statistical errors: these are generally divided into two types:
  type I error: in which a correlation between continuous variables or a difference between groups is asserted when such correlations or differences do not in fact exist. The probability of making a type I error is α.
  type II error: in which a finding of no correlation between continuous variables, or no differences between groups is asserted, when such correlations or differences do in fact exist. The probability of making a type II error is 1-power, or β.

t test: a method for evaluating differences in a continuous variable between two groups. As such, it comprises a special case of the **one-way ANOVA.** Also called **Student's t test.**

variance (s²): a measure of the spread of the data. The formula for this measure is:

$$s^2 = \left(\left(\sum x^2\right) - \left(\left[\sum x^2\right]/n\right)\right)/(n-1),$$

where $\sum x^2$ is the sum of all the squared values, $(\sum x^2)$ is the square of the summed values, and n is the number of observations.

Evaluating Clinical Tests

Assuming that there is some readily available gold standard of disease status, clinical tests may be evaluated using the terms found in Table 13-2.

Population Indices on the Columns

sensitivity: a/a + c (the part of the first column that is true).
specificity/selectivity: d/b + d (the part of the second column that is true).

Individual Indices on the Rows

positive predictive value: a/a + b (the part of the first row that is true).
negative predictive value: d/c + d (the part of the second row that is true).

Therefore, for example, if {Low Test Result} = Diseased, and {High Test Result} = Not diseased, then

- make a test more sensitive (move the cutoff to the right in the previous example; Fig. 13-1), and you will correctly classify more of the diseased population (more true positives). You will also falsely classify more of the nondiseased population as diseased (more false positives).

TABLE 13-2 Evaluating Clinical Tests

		True Disease Status	
Test Result	Positive	Negative	Negative
Positive	a	b	a + b
Negative	c	d	c + d
Totals	a + c	b + d	a + b + c + d

FIG 13-1 A comparison of the terms *sensitive* and *selective*, for a test in which a low value implies disease and a high value implies no disease.

- make a test more specific or selective (move the cutoff to the left in the previous example), and you will correctly classify more of the nondiseased population (more true negatives). You will also falsely clear more of the diseased population (more false negatives).

Study Design

Studies may be classified as a series of binary descriptors:

experimental/interventional: the investigator actively does something to change a risk factor (e.g., drug/placebo tests) compared with **observational/effectiveness,** in which the investigator takes no active role in the status of a risk factor.
prospective: the risk factor may or may not have occurred at the time of the study, but the outcome has not compared with **retrospective,** in which both the risk factor and the outcome have occurred at the time of the study.
descriptive: in which the outcomes are qualitatively reported compared with **analytic,** in which the outcomes are subjected to quantification and numerical analysis.

Study Groups

target population: the group to whom the results of the study will be inferred (e.g., all mammals, all people, all young people).
sample population: the specific part of the target population that the investigator has the ability to measure.
disease incidence: new cases per population at risk per time. This may be estimated with a *cohort* study, in which a group of subjects are followed, with multiple observations, over a defined period.
disease prevalence: cases per population at risk at one point in time (generally given as a percentage). This may be estimated with a *cross-sectional* study, in which all observations are made, once per subject, at a defined time (e.g., next Thursday, or at first presentation).

Biomechanics

The field of biomechanics is concerned with the application of physical and engineering principles to issues of biologic interest.

acceleration: change in velocity per unit of time.
  angular acceleration (degrees, or radians/time^2): change in rotational velocity per time.
  linear acceleration (distance/time^2): change in velocity in a straight line/time.
adaptation: biologically mediated changes in mechanical properties of tissues associated with the mechanical milieu of the tissues.
anisotropy: the quality, usually of a material, of having varying mechanical properties (e.g., strength, stiffness) depending on the direction of applied forces (e.g., reflected in the grain in a piece of wood).
bending: deformation of a structure in response to a load applied to an unsupported portion of the structure.
bending moment: the product of force applied and the distance from the point of application to the point of interest; also called **torque** and **newton meter (N-m).**
brittle: characterized by having a relatively small deformation before failure (e.g., glass) (cf. *plastic* or *ductic*).
center of mass: the point about which the mass of the object can be balanced; also called **center of gravity.**
centroid: the geometric center of a body. In an object of constant thickness, made of a homogeneous material, the centroid and the center of mass are at the same point.

coefficient of friction: ratio of tangential force to the interbody compressive force required to initiate motion between bodies.

compliance: deformation per load (inverse of stiffness).

compression: tending to push objects together. By convention, compressive forces or motions are considered to be negative in sign.

couple: a pair of equal and opposite parallel forces acting on a body and separated by some distance.

creep: deformation with time under a constant load (cf. *stress relaxation*).

degrees of freedom: the number of independent variables in a coordinate system required to completely define the position of an object in space.

displacement: a measurement of change in position in response to force; expressed in units of volume such as fluid displacement.

dynamic load: load that varies over time (cf. *stress relaxation*).

elastic: tending to return to original dimensions after the deforming force has been removed. By this definition, rubber bands might be considered elastic (nonlinearly elastic), but so might concrete (linearly elastic).

elongation: deformation caused by a tensile load, a measure of ductility.

Energy measures: the ability to do work, or the work added to a system by a force or a deformation; examples are **newton meters** and **joules.**

equilibrium: the state of not accelerating, in which the sum of all forces acting on a body is zero.

factor of safety: ratio of structural or materials strength of a body to its load (structure) or stress (materials) encountered in normal service.

fatigue: failure or damage as a result of the cyclic application of multiple submonotonic-failure loads.

fatigue limit: the cyclic load a material or structure can endure indefinitely without damage; also called **endurance limit.**

finite element analysis (FE, FEA): a method of stress analysis, usually done on a computer. The geometry of the structure of interest is divided into regularly shaped elements, each with multiple nodes. The material of each element is defined in terms of its modulus and Poisson ratio. Loading conditions (nodes of application and direction of loads) and constraints (limits on node motion) are defined. Changes in node-to-node distance are then calculated; from these can be calculated local stresses and strains. Also called **finite element modeling (FEM).**

free-body diagram (FBD): analytical technique in which a body and all the forces acting on it, and their points of application, are delineated. In its simplest form, an assumption is made of no net motion (equilibrium), although dynamic FBDs are also used.

helical axis of motion: a unique axis in space that completely defines a three-dimensional motion between two rigid bodies, analogous to instantaneous axis of rotation for planar motion.

hysteresis: consequence of cycling of a nonlinearly elastic material, or of postyield, prefailure cycling of a linearly elastic material or structure, in which the stress-strain or force-deformation curves for increasing and decreasing deformations are not superimposed. The area of the stress-strain curve between the increasing and decreasing legs of the test represent the energy lost in the maneuver (Fig. 13-2).

impulse (units: N-s): a measure of impact properties.

inertia (units: kg): the property of a body that imparts **mass;** the tendency of a body at rest to remain at rest and of a body in motion to remain in motion.

instantaneous axis of rotation: when one body rotates about another, the distance from each point in the moving body to a single point in the stationary body remains constant. In more complex kinematics, the position of this point in the stationary body itself moves. The instantaneous axis of rotation is a

FIG 13-2 Energy loss (energy, or work = force × distance), caused by hysteresis in one cycle.

line perpendicular to the plane of motion and passing through this point.

isotropy: the quality, usually of a material, of having constant mechanical properties (e.g., strength, stiffness) regardless of the direction of applied forces.

kinematics: the study of motion, without respect to energy input or output.

kinesiology: the study of motion and of the forces that produce it.

kinetic energy (KE) (= 0.5 × mass × velocity^2): the energy possessed by a body in motion.

kinetics: the study of energy relationships with respect to motion.

load (= mass × acceleration): force applied to an object.

lubrication: any of a number of means towards reducing friction between surfaces (e.g., joint surfaces).

    boundary lubrication: characterized by a thin layer (down to a single molecule thick) of fluid between surfaces.

    film lubrication: in this type of lubrication, the opposing surfaces are kept completely apart by a thick layer of fluid.

    elastohydrodynamic lubrication: lubrication that occurs when the bearing surfaces are relatively compliant and deform away from their opposing surface by the action of the lubricant.

    squeeze film lubrication: characterized by a pressurized layer of fluid between surfaces.

    hydrodynamic lubrication: in a relatively thicker layer of lubricant, hydrodynamic lubrication is created when the friction between lubricant molecules (related to the viscosity) acts to drag fluid into the space between surfaces. Generally, most applicable during rapid joint movement.

    weeping lubrication: lubrication caused by the extrusion of fluid from the matrix of the surfaces.

moment of inertia (MOI): one of several measurements of the distribution of material around an arbitrary plane or axis; in general, proportional to the structure's resistance to bending about that axis. Where m = the mass of a particle in the body, A = the area of that particle, x = the distance from that particle to the plane, and r = the distance from that particle to the axis.

    area MOI: second moment of the area: $(I = \Sigma Ax^2)$, units in m^4; essentially the mass moment of inertia of a material whose density is 1 kg/m^2, but useful as a generalization or first approximation in which the density variability within the body is negligible or unknown.

    mass MOI: $(I = \Sigma mx^2)$, units in kg•m^2.

    polar MOI: $(I = \Sigma mr^2$, or $I = \Sigma Ar^2)$, units in kg•m^2 or m^4, respectively; useful in the special case of torsion about an axis.

momentum: a characteristic of a moving body, related to its ability to maintain its motion.

    linear momentum (units N•s): the tendency of a moving body to pursue a straight path at a constant velocity.

    angular momentum (mass moment of inertia × angular velocity, units N •m •s, or Planck): the tendency of a spinning body to continue spinning at a constant angular velocity.

normal (not the statistical definition): perpendicular to a surface.

plastic deformation: characterized by having a relatively large deformation before failure (e.g., a willow stick) (cf. *brittle*). Also called **ductile deformation.**

Poisson ratio (v, no units): ratio of lateral deformation to axial deformation (e.g., barreling in a compression test, necking in a tensile test).

potential energy (PE): the capacity of a body at rest to do work (e.g., by virtue of its height, PE = mass × acceleration because of gravity × height).

rheology: the study of fluid flow.

scalar: a parameter having only a quantity, with no directional information (cf. *vector*).

shear: a force or deformation oriented parallel to a surface.

stiffness: units differ, depending on the application; force/deformation, a structural property.

strain: strictly speaking, strain (deformation/original dimension) has no units. However, it is often expressed in microstrain (με), where 1 με = a deformation/original dimension ratio of 1×10^{-6}. 10,0000.25 με = 1% deformation.

strength: maximum load (structure) or stress (materials) before yield or failure, depending on the specific application, occurs.

stress relaxation: viscoelastic decrease in load with time under constant deformation (cf. *creep*).

stress-strain curve: all mechanical tests, especially of objects of biologic origin, are tests of structure (e.g., whole-bone tests, tests of individual trabeculae), and most result in the development of a force (Y-axis) deformation (X-axis) curve. Under certain conditions (e.g., milled specimens, continuum assumptions, or simplified geometry), a useful fiction is that of the material (or materials) test, in which the units are theoretically controlled for specimen size and shape (Fig. 13-3).

energy to yield: energy put into the system (can be measured as the area under the stress-strain curve) from the beginning of the test to the yield point, or to the failure point, respectively. Also called **energy to failure, work to yield,** and **work to failure.**

failure point: point of maximum stress. Stress at the failure point is the **ultimate strength (Pa)** of the material. For some materials, plastic deformation can continue past the failure point.

linear elastic region: region in which the increase in stress is directly proportional to the increase in strain.

modulus (Pa): material stiffness, defined as change in stress/change in strain.

plastic region: region between yield and failure; also called **postyield region.**

toe region: nonlinear region at the beginning of the test. Generally considered as an artifact of the testing machine-specimen gripping apparatus.

yield point: point at which the strain begins to increase disproportionately to the increase in stress, in comparison to the ratio suggested by the modulus. Stress at the yield point is the yield strength of the material; associated with the onset of permanent damage and deformation.

tangent-delta (Tan-δ; units radians): in an oscillatory viscoelastic test, a measure of the phase angle between an applied stress or strain and the resulting strain or stress, respectively (Fig. 13-4).

tension: tending to pull objects apart; by convention, tensile forces or motions are considered to be positive in sign.

tribology: the study of friction, lubrication, and wear; also called **tiotribology.**

vector: a parameter having both a quantity and a direction (cf. *scalar*).

viscoelasticity: a materials or structural property, characterized by demonstrating a change in mechanical properties as a function of the speed of load application.

viscosity (units pascal-second, or kg/sm): a measure of the resistance of a fluid to flow.

wear: loss of surface material, associated with relative motion of interacting surfaces.

abrasive wear: wear caused by contact between a relatively soft and a relatively hard material, resulting in a cutting of the softer material.

adhesive wear: wear caused by formation of a temporary junction between one surface and another, pulling out fragments of the weaker material.

weight: (units N) mass times the local gravitational pull (on Earth, 9.81 m/s^2).

work: force times displacement (units Nm).

FIG 13-3 A classical stress-strain curve of a linearly elastic-plastic material, with the important components marked.

FIG 13-4 An example of the results of a dynamic mechanical analysis, with time on the horizontal axis. Delta (δ) represents the phase-angle difference (the lag) between the applied stress and the resulting strain.

Measurements and Techniques

computed tomography (CT): two- and three-dimensional imaging modality in which multiple x-ray absorption profiles are taken as the x-ray source and collection device are rotated about the patient or specimen. These are then constructed into two- and three-dimensional images by computer postprocessing. Also called **computer-assisted tomography (CAT).**

   quantitative CT (QCT): computed tomography in which the patient or specimen is imaged along with a set of solid or fluid calibration controls.

   micro CT: extremely high-resolution (on the order of μm), small-specimen CT.

cytomorphology: the study of the structure of cells.

dual-energy x-ray absorptiometry (DXA, DEXA): two-dimensional imaging modality in which two simultaneous single-energy x-ray sources are passed over the patient or specimen. With appropriate computerized postprocessing, the resulting image can for instance give a measure of bone density that is independent of the overlying soft tissue densities.

electrophoresis and blotting: any of a number of techniques for separating molecules by their electric charge, in which the unseparated mixture is placed in a gel substrate and subjected to an electric field. The individual molecules then migrate until they reach their isoelectric point, at which point a combination of the molecular size and charge prevents further motion within the gel. The pattern of molecules is then transferred (blotted) by contact to nitrocellulose or nylon sheets.

   Western blot: a method of measuring protein presence. A solution of many proteins is fractionated and transferred. The sheet is then exposed to an antibody specific to the protein in question, which is then imaged with autoradiography (a radiolabeled protein or antibody, exposed to photographic or radiographic film) or by stain-linked second antibodies.

   Northern blot: a method of measuring gene expression. Single-stranded RNA is fractionated and transferred, and the sheet is exposed (hybridized) to a radiolabeled DNA probe, which, if the strands are complementary, stick together. The sheet is then washed and exposed to photographic or radiographic film. Areas in which hybridization has occurred, that is, in which the RNA is complementary to the probe, appear dark.

   Southern blot: a method of measuring gene presence. Double-stranded DNA is fractionated and transferred, and the sheet is exposed to a radiolabeled DNA probe. The sheet is then washed and exposed to photographic or radiographic film. Bands that contain DNA that is complementary to the probe appear dark.

   There is no Eastern blot.

enzyme-linked immunosorbent assay (ELISA): a competitive binding assay using an immunoglobulin attached to an enzyme-generated chromophoric substance that, when the complex attaches to a specific antigen, will reveal and quantitate (when read by a photosensor) the amount of antigen present.

flow cytometry: device and techniques for sorting particles (usually cells) by differential fluorescence. Particles in a suspension are stained with a fluorescent dye. The particles are then run past a laser fluorescent excitatory and emission detector in single file.

force plate: a device used in kinetics and kinematics, generally consisting of a flat plate with multiple piezoelectric sensors underneath. The forces imparted by interaction between the test subject and the plate (for instance, while running across the plate) can then be measured, as a function of time, in the X (in the direction of motion), Y (in the lateromedial direction), and Z (normal to the plate) directions.

high-performance liquid chromatography (HPLC): a means of making rapid separation of solutes with the use of small-bead ion-exchange or gel-filtration columns under high pressure; also called **high-pressure liquid chromatography.**

in vitro: (in glass) (also, **ex vivo**) analysis of a process that takes place outside the living body (e.g., cell culture, dissection), often written in italics.

in vivo: (in the live) analysis of a process within a living animal, often written in italics.

magnetic resonance imaging (MRI): two- and three-dimensional imaging modality, based on the magnetic spin characteristics of molecules (for the most part, water) within a tissue.

mechanical testing: devices and techniques for applying controlled loads or deformations to structures and materials and for measuring resulting deformations or loads, respectively.

microarray: a glass or nylon substrate, to which has been adhered nucleic acid probes for known genes or gene products in spots of 200-μm diameter or less. When an unknown sample in solution is placed in contact with this chip and subjected to standard hybridization techniques (miniaturized), the state of expression of thousands of genes can be determined simultaneously and quickly; also called **genome chip.**

microscopy: devices and techniques for preparing specimens, magnifying images, and measuring features on the resulting images.

    backscatter electron microscopy (BSE): scanning electron microscopy in which the energy of the resulting photons is analyzed for characteristics of the elements present within the sample.

    bright-field microscopy: classical laboratory unit, in which a light is passed through a condenser, then transmitted through a thinly sliced specimen (embedded in wax [paraffin] or plastic [commonly polymethylmethacrylate]), then through an objective lens, and finally through an ocular lens to the user or to a camera. With oil immersion lenses, resolution of 0.2 μm is possible.

    confocal scanning microscopy (CSM): computerized bright-field microscopy (usually used in conjunction with fluorescence), in which the focus point is altered automatically during the imaging process, resulting in a longer depth of field.

    dark-field microscopy: a means of imaging living microscopy, in which the light source is directed parallel to the microscope slide, and the scattered light is collected by the lenses.

    differential interference contrast (DIC) microscopy: a means of imaging living cells, in which the brightness of the image is proportional to the gradient in refraction index of the material; also called **Nomarski microscopy.**

    fluorescence microscopy: bright field microscopy, in which a fluorescent dye (one which absorbs light at one frequency, causing it to emit light at a different frequency) is applied to tissues being studied. Two filters are used, one which limits the light entering the specimen to the **excitation frequency,** and one that limits the light after it passes through the specimen to the **emission frequency.**

Fourier transform infrared spectroscopy and microscopy (FTIR): a means of imaging material based on the reflection and analysis of infrared portion of the spectrum.

histomorphometry: any of a number of methods, both manual and automated, for measuring the size and shape of objects as they appear on a histologic section.

microradiography: high-resolution (<1 μm) x-ray imaging of thin specimens, imaged with bright-field microscopy.

phase contrast microscopy: a means of imaging living cells, complementary to differential interference contrast, in which the brightness of the image is proportional to the refractive index of the material.

polarized light microscopy: bright-field microscopy, in which two polarizing filters are placed in the light path, one above and one the specimen. Often used to determine the general direction of populations of collagen molecules.

Raman spectroscopy and microscopy: a means of imaging material based on the Raman effect, in which a certain number of photons directed at a surface are reflected inelastically, that is, a loss of energy is recorded, generally as a function of the molecular bond length and vibration status.

scanning electron microscopy (SEM): in this imaging modality, the surface of a structure is bombarded at a discrete point in a raster pattern by an electron beam, and the electrons that are scattered by this interaction are counted by a detector. The brightness of the corresponding point on an imaging device (usually a cathode-ray tube) is set proportionally to the number of electrons counted. The electron beam on both the specimen and on the imaging device are then moved, and the process is repeated.

transmission electron microscopy (TEM): the principles of TEM are not unlike those of bright-field microscopy; the illumination source used is the accelerated electron, the specimens are much thinner, and the resolution is improved to the angstrom range.

microsphere: small glass or polystyrene beads, injected intravenously or intraarterially for studies involving vascularization and local ischemia.

motion analysis: any of a number of techniques for quantifying kinematics and kinetics, usually involving light or radiographic imaging, as well as measurements of joint angles **(goniometry),** force plate analysis and electrical evidence of muscle activity **(electromyography [EMG]).**

photogrammetry: technique for motion analysis, in which two or more images are taken with the image collection devices at known positions. The relative positions of known points that are present on both images can then be calculated. **Radio-photogrammetry** is photogrammetry accomplished with x-ray equipment.

polymerase chain reaction: a method for amplifying selected DNA (for instance, from a particular gene of interest) to measurable amounts from small samples by repeated gentle heating (to separate DNA strands), cooling (annealing) with hybridization with known DNA primers, and polymerization with the four DNA bases in the presence of a DNA polymerase. A reverse polymerase chain reaction can measure the presence of mRNA in the cell.

radioactive tracers: a variety of compounds are used in orthopaedic research to follow specific biologic activity. The most common tracers used are:

^{45}Ca	^{67}Ga
^{3}H (tritium)	^{99m}Tc
^{51}Cr	^{85}Sr
$^{35}SO_4$	

real-time polymerase chain reaction (qPCR): uses the method of polymerase chain reaction to quantitatively amplify and measure a targeted DNA or reverse transcribed RNA sequence. A **reverse transcriptase polymerase chain reaction (RT PCR)** is used to determine the presence of a specific mRNA. The DNA sequence is then multiplied and measured with a fluorescent DNA dye. This allows for determining the quantity of mRNA in the sample. This method can also quantify the absolute or relative amount of DNA of a specific gene and is carried out in a thermal cycler that uses fluorescent dyes that bind the DNA and then can be detected and quantified by a computer in real time.

stress-generated potentials (SGP): any electrical potential (voltage) produced by mechanical deformation.

> **Piezoelectric potential:** a potential that is developed on the molecular surface of a material when that material is deformed.
>
> **streaming potential (zeta):** a potential that is created by the passage of charged ions in fluids passing by fixed surface charges.

strain gauge (or gage): a device for measuring deformation. Designs and construction differ between applications, but generally these consist of a miniature conductor printed on a thin piece of plastic, which is then glued to the structure of interest. As the structure is deformed, there is a change in the resistance of the conductor, which can then be amplified and calibrated through a **Wheatstone bridge** circuit, and converted into units of strain.

transgenic animals: animals in which particular genes have been added to **(knockins)** or removed from **(knockouts)** the germ line.

Units of Measurement

The basic International System (SI) units for length, mass, time, and temperature are, respectively, the meter, gram, second, and degree Celsius (centigrade), and are listed in Table 13-3, along with their English system equivalents. The dalton is used as a measure of molecular mass. Force and pressure are derived quantities.

The triple point of water is 0.01° C (that point at which water may exist as a gas, liquid, and solid in thermodynamic equilibrium at standard atmospheric pressure); –273.16° C (0 Kelvin) is defined as absolute zero, and water boils at standard atmospheric pressure at 100° C.

One **hertz (Hz)** is defined as one cycle per second.

TABLE 13-3 SI Units of Measurement

Magnitude	Length	Mass	Time	Force	Pressure
10^{-15}	Femtometer, fm	Femtogram, fg	Femtosecond, fs		
10^{-12}	Picometer, pm	Picogram, pg	Picosecond, ps		
10^{-10}	Angström, A				
10^{-9}	Nanometer, nm	Nanogram, ng	Nanosecond, ns		
10^{-6}	Micron, micrometer, μm	Microgram, μg	Microsecond, μs		
10^{-3}	Millimeter, mm	Milligram, mg	Millisecond, ms		
10^{-2}	Centimeter, cm				
10^{0}	Meter, m (39.37 inches)	Gram, g (0.0352 ounces); *Dalton*, Da (¹⁄₁₂ the mass of a C_{12} atom)	Second, s	Newton, N (1 kg accelerated 1 m/s²; 0.225 lb on Earth)	Pascal, Pa(1 N/m²); 1.45 × 10⁻⁴ lb/square inch
10^{3}	Kilometer, km	Kilogram, kg; Kilodalton, kD		Kilonewton, kN	Kilopascal, KPa
10^{6}					Megapascal, MPa
10^{9}					Gigapascal, GPa
10^{12}					Terapascal, TPa

SI, *Système International.*

Orthopaedic Cell and Tissue Biology

General

adipogenesis: the process of producing adipose, or fatty tissue.

agarose: purified plant protein gel, used in electrophoresis as the matrix through which the molecules travel.

angiogenesis: the process of creating new blood vessels.

apoptosis: programmed cell death, in which the cell and nucleus are systematically condensed and fragmented in a well-defined series of molecular events (cf. *necrosis,* in which the cells swell and burst).

biglycan: core protein with two glycosaminoglycan chains.

caspase: any of a group of cysteine proteases, crucial for apoptosis.

cathepsin: any of a number of lysosomal enzymes that can degrade the components of the extracellular matrix.

cell components: substructures within the cell. The ones most commonly described in orthopaedic research include:
 centriole
 endoplasmic reticulum
 filaments
 Golgi apparatus
 lysosome
 microsome
 microtubule
 mitochondria
 nucleolus
 nucleus
 plasma (or cell) membrane
 polyribosome
 ribosome
 vesicle

cell cycle: referring to several sequential phases in a cell's life, centered around cell proliferation. Most cells proceed slowly through the cycle or remove themselves from the cycle to enter the G_0 phase at some stage of their lives.

 G_0 phase: nonproliferative, resting (only in terms of cell division).

 G_1: the interval between the end of mitosis and the beginning of DNA synthesis.

 S (synthesis): DNA synthesis stage.

 G_2: the interval between the end of DNA synthesis and the beginning of cell division.

FIG 13-5 Cell cycle.

M (mitosis): active mitosis and cell division (Fig. 13-5).
chemokine: a type of cytokine that has the ability to induce directed cell migration (chemotaxis) in nearby responsive cells; the affected cells will migrate.
circadian: pertaining to a 24-hour biologic cycle.
collagen: any of at least 18 forms of extracellular proteins, which account for at least 30% of the protein in the mammalian body. It consists of a structure of small amino acids (glycine 35%, alanine 11%) and permanently kinked amino acids (proline 12–25%, hydroxyproline 9%), in which every third protein is glycine, in a pattern glycine-X-proline, glycine-proline-X, or glycine-X-hydroxyproline. The mixture of the amino acid X determines the collagen type. Usually seen as a stable triple helix, held together with hydrogen bonds, and a few covalent crosslinks. Major types found in the mammalian body include:
Type I: bone, skin, cornea, sclera, tendon, ligament
Type II: cartilage, intervertebral disk, vitreous humor
Type III: skin, blood vessels, repair tissue
Type IV, VI: basement membrane
Type X: growth plate, repair tissue, embryonic tissue
cyclooxygenase: a common enzyme in the synthesis pathway of prostaglandins, prostacyclines, and thromboxanes from arachidonic acid.
cytokine: one of many small molecules that typically signal adjoining or nearby cells to produce specific chemicals. Cytokines may be proteins, peptides, or glycoproteins produced cells located throughout the body. This is in contrast to many hormones that arise from glands. Examples are the interleukins and tumor necrosis factor alpha.
decorin: small proteoglycan, thought to modulate collagen fibril assembly and cross-linking in bone.
defensins: a group of short, naturally produced antimicrobial proteins important in naturally occurring bacterial contamination such as in and around the gums.
deoxyribonucleic acid (DNA): is the molecule that contains the genetic information for all living cells and is found in the nucleus. DNA is made up of four types of nucleotides: adenine (A), guanine (G), cytosine (C), and thymine (T). It is the combination of these four nucleotides that make up the genetic sequence found in chromosomes. DNA is found in a double strand forms a double-helix structure and the **human genome** consists about three billion nucleotides. It is DNA that contains the **genetic code** for mRNA transcription leading to translation into proteins. Changes to the nucleotides in the coding region of genes in DNA can result in mutations and altering the function of translated protein. Many diseases can be traced to a single nucleotide change (SNP) in the DNA sequence of a gene.
epigenetics: changes in genetic expression caused by changes outside of the DNA genetic code. This includes DNA methylation and histone modification.
fibromodulin: noncollagenous protein found in articular cartilage, associated with fibril assembly, and found in greater abundance away from the chondrocytes.
gene expression: messenger RNA production, which is necessary but not sufficient for protein production.
genotype: genetic make up of an individual. This is in contrast to phenotype which is the appearance of an individual based on their genetic inheritance.
interleukins: a family of cytokines that were initially described in leukocytes. The term *interleukin* derives from (*inter-*), "as a means of communication," and (*-leukin*) "deriving from the fact that many of these proteins are produced by leukocytes and act on leukocytes." It has now been shown to be expressed in most cells in the body. Interleukins have been shown to promote inflammation, matrix remodeling, and autoimmunity in connective tissues.
ischemia: local decrease in oxygen tension, often resulting from damage to blood supply.

lysosomal protease: degradative enzymes found in lysosomes, generally active at acid pH, may be associated with extracellular matrix breakdown.

messenger ribonucleic acid (mRNA): is made of long chains of nucleic acid from transcription of DNA. mRNA is involved in the translation process of making proteins, by binding to ribosomes and coding for the specific protein sequences. mRNA is found as a single strand molecule as opposed to the double strand of DNA.

metalloproteinases: protein-cleaving enzymes that often have an association with a Zn ion; also called **metalloproteases** and **matrix metalloprotease (MMP)**. Some of the major musculoskeletal MMPs include:
   collagenases: (MMP I and MMP XIII).
   gelatinase: (MMP II, which cleaves specific collagens, fibronectin, and proteoglycans).
   stromelysin: (MMP III, which cleaves core protein and, thereby, aggrecan from hyaluronic acid).

microRNAs (miRNA): small, short, noncoding RNA molecules (~22 nucleotides long) and involved in the regulation of genes after translation to messenger RNA. They function by binding complementary sequences of their target mRNAs resulting in silencing them so they can not be used in protein translation. Each miRNA can silence many gene targets. The miRNA's themselves are found in the noncoding regions in the chromosome and hold the potential to be used as drugs to silence genes.

mitogen-activated protein kinase (MAP) kinase: serine/threonine-specific protein kinase cascade that responds to extracellular stimuli to regulate gene expression, mitosis, differentiation, and cell survival and apoptosis, and that are well conserved across species.

neuropeptides: neuroactive peptides, 2–40 amino acids long, which can act as hormones, neurotransmitters, or neuromodulators (e.g., substance P, luteinizing hormone releasing hormone, somatostatin).

nondisjuction: failure of a chromosome or chromosomes to separate normally during meiosis, resulting in germ cells (sperm or ovum) lacking in a chromosome or with an extra chromosome.

phenotype: the appearance of an individual based on their genetic inheritance. This is in contrast to genotype, which is the DNA-based inheritance of the individual.

proteomics: the identification and characterization of gene protein products.

reactive oxygen species: highly transient and chemically reactive species of oxygen atom; includes oxygen ions, free radicals, and peroxides. Important in some cell-signaling mechanisms, increased levels can result in significant damage to subcellular structures (oxidative stress).

small interfering RNA (siRNA): a method by which genes can be selectively turned off in cell culture or in live animals without resort to transgenic methods, by hybridizing small complementary strands of RNA to messenger RNA. This blocks the ability of the RNA to transcribe a protein.

single nucleotide polymorphism (SNP): a single nucleotide (A, G, T, or C) that changes the genetic coding of DNA. This often results in altered production of a specific protein.

stem cell: pluripotential cell; a subset of these, **Mesenchymal stem cells** can differentiate into osteocytes, chondrocytes, or adipocytes.

tissue inhibitor of metalloproteinases (TIMP): a specific protein that inhibits matrix metalloprotease.

transforming growth factor (TGF): a family of cytokines associated with growth and development, which includes the bone morphogenic proteins.

tumor necrosis factor–alpha (TNF-α): an inflammatory cytokine that is involved in systemic inflammation. It is largely produced by macrophages, but can also be made by synoviocytes, chondrocytes and osteoblasts. The primary role of TNF-α is to stimulate proinflammatory genes that are involved in cell signaling and matrix remodeling in cartilage and bone.

Cartilage

ADAMTS: proteases characterized by *a d*isintegrin-like *a*nd *m*etalloprotease domain (reprolysin-type) with *t*hrombo*s*pondin type I motifs; ADAMTS 4 and ADAMTS 5 are also called *aggrecanase 1* and *2*, respectively.

aggrecanases: proteolytic enzymes that belong to the ADAMs (a disintegrin and metalloprotease) family of proteases. They have been shown to degrade large proteoglycans such as aggrecan. Two forms of aggrecanase have been shown to be made in humans: ADAMTS4 (aggrecanase-1) and ADAMTS5 (aggrecanse-2).

cartilage: smooth, relatively low-cellularity tissue, consisting of chondrocytes in lacunae, and a large amount of extracellular matrix composed of water, collagen, and proteoglycans.

> **calcified cartilage:** forming the thin layer of cartilage between the hyaline articular cartilage and the subchondral bone.
>
> **elastic cartilage:** found in the ligamentum nuchae, epiglottis, external ear. Yellow, flexible.
>
> **fibrocartilage:** found in intervertebral disks, symphyses, and repair tissue of damaged hyaline cartilage. Histologically shows a herringbone fiber pattern.
>
> **hyaline cartilage:** found at the articular surface of joints, tracheal rings, at the distal end of ribs. Blue-white, shiny, smooth.
>
> **physeal cartilage:** forming the growth plate of endochondral ossification. Appears much like hyaline cartilage, and in some species (e.g., reptiles) the two are often coincident.

Hierarchy of Cartilage Structure

aggrecan: large matrix molecule composed of a hyaluronic acid backbone with numerous proteoglycan chains covalently attached via link proteins.

cartilage oligomeric protein (COMP): a large non-collagenous matrix glycoprotein that consists of five identical glycoprotein subunits which contain epidermal growth factor and thrombospodin-related regions. COMP also binds to other matrix proteins such as collagen by divalent cations. COMP has been proposed to be a marker of cartilage turnover.

chondrocyte: the major type of cell found in cartilage. Generally encased in a cartilage **lacuna**.

chondroitin sulfate: a sulfated sugar with 40 to 60 repeating units of N-acetylgalactosamine and glucuronic acid, part of the glycosaminoglycan seen in cartilage.

core protein: the central protein of the proteoglycan subunit, to which the glycosaminoglycans are associated.

fibril: several strands of tropocollagen held together with crosslinks.

fiber: an assembly of several fibrils.

glucosamine: one of the components of glycosaminoglycan; a glucose with a nitrogen-containing group.

glycosaminoglycan (GAG): linear carboxylated and sulfated sugar polymers, covalently attached to a small peptide.

hyaluronic acid: nonsulfated glycosaminoglycan of glucuronic acid and N-acetylglucosamine that makes up the backbone of the aggrecan molecule in cartilage.

keratin sulfate: a glycosaminoglycan with 5 to 20 repeating units of galactose and N-acetylglucosamine.

link protein: a 44- to 55-kD protein that associates the core protein to the hyaluronic acid chain.

lubricin: a large protein product from the *PRG4* gene that has been shown to be present in many connective tissues such as ligament, bone, tendon, skin and cartilage. It has been shown to be present in synovial fluid and in the surface layer (superficial zone) of articular cartilage. It is believed that it plays a role in joint lubrication, synovial homeostasis, and as a low-friction interface for tendons as well as the heart covering.

perichondrium: the fibrous tissue on the outside (non-articular) border of cartilage or continuous with periosteum in the case of a physis.

proteoglycan: a polymer consisting of a core protein associated with multiple glycosaminoglycans; also called **mucopolysaccharide.**

procollagen: triple-helical form of collagen immediately after extracellular polymerization of intracellularly-produced **tropocollagen α-chains** into **procollagen** and subsequent cleavage of terminal peptides.

tidemark: border in articular cartilage between calcified and uncalcified cartilage layers.

Bone

alkaline phosphatase: a serum marker for bone formation.

bone morphogenic protein (BMP): a family of at least 18 proteins involved in the stimulation of bone formation, part of the transforming growth factor superfamily.

Bone Cells

osteoblast: cells of mesenchymal origin, capable of laying down bone matrix (**osteoid,** which is mostly collagen), which then calcifies extracellularly.

osteoclast: multinucleate cells of monocyte origin, whose major role is in the removal of bone.

osteocyte: osteoblasts encased in **lacunae,** which communicate (quite possibly, information about mechanical strain) with one another and with bone lining cells, via cell processes encased in **canaliculi** or tunnels within the bone matrix.

Bone Lining Cell

basic multicellular unit (BMU): the combination of osteoclasts and osteoblasts, working in concert in the remodeling of bone.

calbindin: a protein involved in cytoplasmic transport of calcium; also called **calcium binding protein.**

calcitonin: a short-chain protein hormone that is involved in bone accretion. The activity of this hormone can reduce the level of serum calcium by its effect on new bone formation.

calcium hydroxyapatite: $Ca_{10}(PO_4)_6(OH)_2$, the major mineral form found in bone.

cancellous bone: thresholds differ between authors, but generally bone with a porosity of more than 40%, usually found toward the ends of long bones and in the body of vertebrae; also called **trabecular bone.**

cement line: the outer edge of a basic multicellular unit (BMU), which stains dark under toluidine blue, representing the furthest extent of osteoclastic activity during the remodeling process that resulted in the BMU; also called **reversal line.**

compact bone: thresholds differ between authors, but generally bone with a porosity of less than 40% is usually found in the diaphysis and metaphysis of long bones, and in the shells of vertebrae; also called **cortical bone.**

diaphysis: the tubular, central section of a long bone.

endochondral ossification: process of bone development in which bone replaces a cartilage anlage. Usually characterized by the presence of a physis (e.g., most long bones, vertebrae).

epiphysis: the portion of a long bone between the physis and the end of the structure.

Haversian system: (after Clopton Havers, 17th-century British microscopist) a secondary osteon with its associated canal.

Hueter-Volkmann law: physiologic compressive forces stimulate accelerated growth of articular, epiphyseal, or physeal cartilage.

Howship lacuna: (after John Howship, 19th-century British surgeon) the surface (or, in some definitions, the space bordered by the surface) of bone after osteoclastic activity has begun and before osteoblastic refilling as begun. Characterized by scalloped edges, in which individual osteoclasts have been actively resorbing bone. Often, osteoclasts are present at these surfaces.

intramembranous ossification: process by which bone is formed without a preexisting cartilage anlage, for example, most of the bones of the skull, and the increase in width of long bone diaphyses.

lamellar bone: bone that is laid down in orderly sheets, in which the collagen fibers are parallel to one another.

leptin: a hormone made by fat tissue that acts on brain to regulate food intake and body weight. Mice with a homozygous mutation (ob/ob) eat voraciously, are massively obese, and have increased bone mass, suggesting a relationship between obesity and bone. Recently, elevated levels of leptin have been associated with obesity and osteoarthritis.

matrix vesicle: extracellular depot of enzymes near osteoblasts that are involved in the initiation of bone mineral formation.

metaphysis: the cone-shaped portion of a long bone between the physis and the diaphysis.

modeling: placement of bone material where there was none earlier; does not require osteoclastic activity.

osteon: circumferential pattern of lamellar bone around an Haversian canal containing blood vessels.

  primary osteon: osteon that is laid down de novo, without previous osteoclastic activity (thus, no cement line), usually as a result of periosteal expansion.

  secondary osteon: osteon that is the result of remodeling (osteoclastic and subsequent osteoblastic activity, thus, a cement line is present).

osteocalcin: the most abundant noncollagenous protein in bone, important in the mineralization of new bone and as a chemoattractant for bone cells.

osteopontin: noncollagenous bone matrix protein, possibly involved in cell attachment to the matrix and in force transduction.

osteonectin: noncollagenous bone matrix protein involved in mineralization, binding of growth factors, regulation of bone formation, and matrix control of metastasis; also called **secreted protein, acidic, rich in cysteine (SPARC).**

osteoprotegerin (OPG): a protein inhibitor of osteoclastogenesis.

parathyroid hormone (PTH): polypeptide hormone involved in elevation of serum calcium, bone resorption, and renal calcium retention.

periosteum: the fibrous tissue covering on the nonarticular, nonligament-tendon attachment surfaces of a bone.

physis: the growth plate, a highly organized cartilaginous structure in which most long bone growth occurs.

plexiform bone: lamellar bone, often seen in ungulates, formed by filling in a surface trabecular network.

receptor activator of nuclear factor kappa B (RANK) and **receptor activator of nuclear factor kappa B ligand (RANKL):** osteoclast precursors expressing RANK on their cell surfaces interact with osteoblasts or with stromal cells expressing RANKL on their cell surfaces, an important step in osteoclastogenesis and in bone resorption.

remodeling: removal and replacement of bone material; requires osteoclastic as well as osteoblastic activity.

sclerostin: a secreted glycoprotein produced by the osteocyte. It has antianabolic effects on bone formation. Sclerostin exerts its effects by interfering with Wnt signaling, which plays a key role in the regulation of bone formation. Sclerostin may also promote the apoptosis of osteoblasts, further inhibiting bone growth.

vitamin D: alternatively considered a vitamin or a hormone, it is produced in the skin on exposure to ultraviolet light and altered in the kidney and liver. It acts by affecting the intestinal absorption of calcium, renal retention of calcium, and the remodeling process at the bone surface. Related terms include **1,25-dihydrocholecalciferol, 1,25-dihydroxyvitamin D3, 25-hydroxycholecalciferol,** and **24,25-dihydroxycholecalciferol.**

Wolff's law: (after Julius Wolff, 19th-century German surgeon and pathologist) the clinical observation that bone will model and remodel in response to and in the direction of the forces acting on it.

woven bone: bone that is placed in a relatively disorganized fashion, with no clear order under polarized light microscopy; generally laid down quickly, as in the early stages of fracture repair (callus) or in rapid growth phases of ungulates, and replaced later with **lamellar** bone.

Appendix: Orthopaedic Abbreviations

The Joint Commission on Accreditation of Healthcare Organizations (JCAHO) has directed that each hospital establish a standard list of abbreviations and acronyms that are known by all specialties. Listed here are those approved by the JCAHO, and include many more that are used by orthopaedic physicians to expediently document patient records in a clinical situation. These additional abbreviations and acronyms are included as a compendium for recognition as a reference only.

Care must be taken when using abbreviations. In some cases, a single abbreviation may refer to several words. For example, the abbreviation *quad* could refer to *quadrilateral* (hip), *quadriceps* (musculature), and *quadriplegic* (paralysis). The context of the material determines which word is used. Use of capitalization of abbreviations varies widely. Professional organizations are included and listed separately.

AA: active-assisted (range of motion)
AAA: abdominal aortic aneurysm
AAI: ankle-arm index
AAL or ant ax line: anterior axillary line
AAROM: active assisted range of motion
ab: antibody
abd: abdomen; abdominal (pad)
ABD: abduction
abd poll: abductor pollicis
ABI: ankle-brachial index
ac: before meals
AC: acromioclavicular (joint)
ACL: acromioclavicular ligament (shoulder)
ACL: anterior cruciate ligament (knee)
ACLS: advanced cardiac life support
acid PO₄: acid phosphatase
ACS: acetabular cup system
AD: assistive devices
ADD: adduction
add poll: adductor pollicis
ADL: activity of daily living
ad lib: as desired
adm: admission
ADQ/ADM: abductor digiti quinti (or minimi)
AE: above elbow
AF: atrial fibrillation; also called **a-fib**
AFO: ankle-foot orthosis s
AG: antigravity
AGE: angle of greatest extension
AGF: angle of greatest flexion
AIDS: acquired immunodeficiency syndrome
AIIS: anterior inferior iliac spine
AJ: ankle jerks
AK: above knee
AKA: above-knee amputation
Alb: albumin
ALPSA: anterior labrum periosteum shoulder arthroscopic lesion
ALRI: anterolateral rotatory instability (knee)
ALS: amyotrophic lateral sclerosis; anterolateral sclerosis
ALT: same as serum glutamic pyruvic transaminase (SGPT)
AMI: acute myocardial infarction

AML: anatomic medullary locking (total hip replacement)
amp: ampule
ANA: antinuclear antibody (for lupus erythematosus)
Anes: anesthesia
ANF: antinuclear factor
ANOVA: analysis of variance
ANS: autonomic nervous system
AO: Arbeitsgemeinschaft für Osteosynthesaefragen
AP: anteroposterior (view)
APB: abductor pollicis brevis
APC: anteroposterior compression (pelvic fracture)
APL: abductor pollicis longus
aq, aqu: aqueous; water solution
ARDS: acute respiratory distress syndrome
ARIF: arthroscopically assisted reduction and internal fixation
AROM: active range of motion
AS: arteriosclerosis; aortic stenosis
ASAP: as soon as possible
ASD: atrial septal defect
ASI: acromial spur index
ASIS: anterosuperior iliac spine
ATLS: advanced trauma life support (courses)
AV: arteriovenous; atrioventricular
AVF: arteriovenous fistula
AVM: arteriovenous malformation
BB to MM: belly button to medial malleolus (examination)
BE: below elbow
BFO: balanced forearm orthosis
bid: twice a day (ii)
BJ: biceps jerks
BK: below knee
BKA: below knee amputation
BMD: bone mineral densitometry
BMI: body mass index
BMP: bone morphogenic protein
BP: blood pressure
Bx: biopsy
C: centigrade
C/E angle: center edge angle
c/o: complaint of
C-1 through C-7: cervical vertebrae or nerve roots
C3-4 through C6-7: intervertebral disk spaces between cervical vertebrae
C7-T1: intervertebral disk space between seventh cervical and first thoracic vertebra
C8: eighth cervical nerve root
Ca: calcium, carcinoma
CABG: coronary artery bypass graft
CAD: coronary artery disease
CAD-CAM: computer-assisted design–computer-assisted manufacturing
CA lig: coracoacromial ligament
CAM: controlled ankle motion
CAMBA: calcaneal axis first metatarsal base angle
CAOS: computer-assisted orthopaedic surgery
CASH: cruciform anterior spinal hyperextension orthosis
CAT-CAM: contour-adducted trochanteric–controlled alignment method
CBC: complete blood count
cath: catheterization
CC: chief complaint
CCU: coronary care unit
CCK: constrained condylar knee
CFS: cerebrospinal fluid
CG: contact guarding
CHF: congestive heart failure
CID: carpal instability dissociative
CIND: carpal instability, nondissociative
CK: creatine kinase (enzyme)
CLIP: capitolunate instability pattern
CMC: carpometacarpal
CMF: chondromyxoid fibroma
CNS: central nervous system
CPM: continuous passive motion
co: complaint of
CO: certified orthotist
COMP: cartilage oligometric protein (research)
CP: cerebral palsy
CP: certified prosthetist
CPA: condylar-plateau angle
Cpd: compound
CPO: certified prosthetist and orthotist
CPPD: calcium pyrophosphate deposition (disease)
CPR: cardiopulmonary resuscitation
CPRS: chronic regional pain syndrome
CPT: current procedural terminology
CREST: calcinosis, Raynaud, esophageal, sclerodactyly, telangiectasia

CRMO: chronic recurrent multifocal osteomyelitis
CROW: Charcot restraint orthotic walker
CRP: cross-reactive protein
CRT: cathode-ray tube
CSF: cerebrospinal fluid; colony stimulating factor
C-spine: cervical spine
CSVL: central sacral vertical line
CT: computed tomography; also called **computed axial tomography (CAT)**
CTO: cervicothoracic orthosis
CTR: carpal tunnel release
CTS: carpal tunnel syndrome
CTSO: cervical thoracolumbosacral orthosis
CV: cardiovascular
CVA: cerebrovascular accident (stroke)
cva: costovertebral angle
CX: culture
CXR: chest x-ray examination
D1, D2, etc.: dorsal vertebrae 1, 2, etc.
Da: Dalton (research)
DANA: designed after natural anatomy (prosthesis)
DBS: Denis Browne splint
dc, D/C: discontinue
DC: dorsal capsulodesis
DCP: dynamic compression plate
DDH: developmental dysplasia of the hip
decub: decubitus position; lying down
dev: deviation
DEXA/DXA: dual energy x-ray absorptiometry
DIE: died in emergency room
dig: digitorum
DIP: distal interphalangeal
DIPJ: distal interphalangeal joint
disch: discharge
DISH: diffuse idiopathic skeletal hyperostosis
DISI: dorsal intercalated segment instability
Disl: dislocation
Distal/3 or D/3: distal third
DJD: degenerative joint disease
DKB: deep knee bends
DM: diabetes mellitus
DMARD: disease modifying antirheumatic drug
DNA: deoxyribonucleic acid
DNR: do not resuscitate
DO: doctor of osteopathy
DOA: date of admission; dead on arrival

DOE: date of examination
DOMS: delayed-onset muscle soreness
DP: distal phalanx
DPP: dorsalis pedis pulse
DPA: dual photon absorptiometry
DPC: distal palmar crease
DPD: dual photon densitometry
dr: dram (4 ml)
DRUJ: distal radioulnar joint
DSA: digital subtraction angiography
D-spine: dorsal spine; thoracic spine
DTR: deep tendon reflex
DVT: deep vein thrombosis
Dx or diag: diagnosis
Dz: disease
EBL: estimated blood loss
EBV: Epstein-Barr virus
ECF: extended care facility
ECG, EKG: electrocardiograph (or electrocardiogram)
ECRB: extensor carpi radialis brevis
ECRL: extensor carpi radialis longus
ECU: extensor carpi ulnaris
ED: elbow disarticulation; emergency department
EDB: extensor digitorum brevis
EDC: estimated date of confinement
EDC: extensor digitorum communis
EDL: extensor digitorum longus
EDQ/EDM: extensor digiti quinti (or minimi)
EDS: Ehlers-Danlos syndrome
EEG: electroencephalograph(gram)
EIP: extensor indicis proprius
EJ: elbow jerks
ELISA: enzyme-linked immunosorbent assay
ELPS: excessive lateral pressure syndrome
EMG: electromyography
EOM: extraocular movement
EPB: extensor pollicis brevis
EPL: extensor pollicis longus
EPP: end-plate potential (depolarization of muscle)
ERE: external rotation in extension
ERF: external rotation in flexion
ESIN: elastic stable intramedullary nailing
ESO: electrospinal orthosis
ESR: erythrocyte sedimentation rate
ETOH: alcohol
expir: expiration

EXT: extremities
F: Fahrenheit
FA: false aneurysm
FABER: flexion in abduction and external rotation
FADIR: flexion in adduction and internal rotation
FB: foreign body
FCR: flexor carpi radialis
FCU: flexor carpi ulnaris
FDI: first dorsal interosseous (hand or foot)
FDL: flexor digitorum longus
FDP: flexor digitorum profundus
FDQB: flexor digiti quinti brevis
FDS: flexor digitorum sublimis (or superficialis)
FES: functional electrical stimulation
FF: further flexion
FFC: fixed flexion contracture
FFP: fresh frozen plasma
FH: family history
fl: fluid
FPB: flexor pollicis brevis
FPL: flexor pollicis longus
FQF: four-quadrant fusion
FRA: femoral ring allograft
Fx or fract: fracture
FRAX: fracture risk assessment tool
FTA: femorotibial angle
FUO: fever of undetermined origin
FWB: full weight-bearing
G or gm: gram (15 grain)
GAG: glycosaminoglycans
GB: gallbladder
GCS: Glasgow Coma Score
Gd-DTPA: gadopentetate dimeglumine
GHL: glenohumeral ligament
GI: gastrointestinal
Gla: γ-carboxyglutamic acid
Glut: gluteal
GMFCS: gross motor function classification system
Gpa: gigapascal
gr: grain (60 milligram)
gt: drop
gtt: drops (0.05 ml)
GU: genitourinary
H&P: history and physical (examination)
H: per hypodermic
H/H: hemoglobin and hematocrit

HA: hallux abductus
HAGL: humeral avulsion of glenohumeral ligament
Hct: hematocrit
HCTU: home cervical traction unit
HD: heloma durum (hard corn)
HD: hip disarticulation
HEENT: head, ears, eyes, nose, throat (examination)
Hg: mercury
Hgb: hemoglobin
HIV (HTLV): human immunodeficiency virus
HLAM: hemilaminectomy
HM: heloma molle (soft corn)
HNP: herniated nucleus pulposus
HP: hot packs
HPI: history of present illness
HPLC: high-performance (pressure) liquid chromatography
hs: at bedtime
HT: hammertoe
HT: Hubbard tank
HV: hallux valgus
Hx: history
Hz: hertz
I&D: incision and drainage
I&O: intake and output
ICS: intercostals space (ribs)
ICT: intermittent cervical traction
IDK: internal derangement of the knee
IHW: inner heel wedge
IM: intramuscular; intramedullary (rod)
IMF: intramedullary fixation
Inf: inferior
INFH: ischemic necrosis of femoral head
IP: interphalangeal (joint)
IPJ: interphalangeal joint
IPK: intractable plantar keratosis
IPOP: immediate postoperative prosthesis
IPSF: immediate postsurgical fitting
IRE: internal rotation in extension
IRF: internal rotation in flexion
IS: interspace
ISIS: integrated shape imaging system
ITB: iliotibial band
ITT: internal tibial torsion; iliotibial torsion
IV: intravenous
IV: intravenous (injection)

IVP: intravenous pyelogram
Jct: junction
JRA: juvenile rheumatoid arthritis
K: potassium
Kg: kilogram (1000 gram)
KJ: knee jerks
KMFTR: Kotz modular femur and tibia resection (system)
Kp: Kilopond
KUB: kidney, ureter, and bladder view of abdomen
KVO: keep view open (for intravenous fluids)
L: liter
L&W: living and well
L1-L5: lumbar vertebrae
LAC: long-arm cast
LAD: ligamentous anterior dislocation
LAM: laminectomy
LAMI: laminotomy
LANC: long-arm navicular cast
LAS: long-arm splint
LASER: light amplification by stimulated emission of radiation (lower case in context)
lat: lateral
lat men: lateral meniscus or meniscectomy
LBP: low back pain
LBQC: large-based quad cane
LC/DCP: limited-contact dynamic-compression (plate)
LCP: Legg-Calvé-Perthes (disease)
LCS mb: low-contact stress meniscal bearing
LCS rp: low-contact stress rotating patella
LE: lupus erythematosus (also called **systemic lupus erythematosus [SLE]**); lower extremity
LFA: low-friction arthroplasty
LHD: left-hand dominant
LIFO: locked intramedullary fracture osteosynthesis
lig: ligature; ligament
Liq: liquid
LISS: less invasive spine surgery
LLC: long-leg cast
LLD: leg-length discrepancy
LLE: left lower extremity
LLL: left lower limb
LLQ: left lower quadrant
LLS: long-leg splint
LLWC: long-leg walking cast

LOM: limitation of motion
LP: lumbar puncture
LS: lumbosacral (spine)
LSK: liver, spleen, and kidneys
LS: lumbosacral
L-spine: lumbar spine
LSS: lumbosacral spine
LUE: left upper extremity
LUL: left upper limb
LUQ: left upper quadrant
MAC: monitored anesthesia care
MACS: MAST-associated compartment syndrome
MAL: midaxillary line
MARS: modular acetabulum reconstruction system
MAST: medical antishock trousers
MC: metacarpal; midcarpal
MCI: midcarpal instability (volar, palmar, extrinsic)
MCL: midclavicular line
MCP: metacarpophalangeal (joint)
MD: muscular dystrophy
Med: medial or medical
MED: multiple epiphyseal dysplasia
med: medicine
med men: medial meniscus or meniscectomy
MENS: microamperage electrical nerve stimulation
MESS: mangled extremity severity score
mg: milligram (1/60 grain); myasthenia gravis
MHW: medial heel wedge
MI: myocardial infarction
Middle/3 or M/3: middle third
MIO: minimally invasive osteosynthesis
MIS: minimally invasive surgery
M/L: medial lateral (narrow M/L)
MLD: median lethal dose (radiation)
ml: milliliter
mm: millimeter
mm: muscles; mucous membrane
MMT: manual muscle testing
MOI: moment of inertia
MP: middle phalanx or metaphalangeal (joint)
MPC: midpalmar crease
MPV: metatarsus primus varus
MRA: magnetic resonance angiography
MRI: magnetic resonance imaging
MRSA: methicillin resistant *Staphylococcus aureus*
MS: multiple sclerosis

MSD: microsurgical discectomy
MSL: midsternal line
MT: muscle testing
MTA: metatarsus adductus
MT bar: metatarsal bar
MTJ: midtarsal joint
MTP: metatarsophalangeal (joint)
MTV: metatarsus varus
MUA: manipulation under anesthesia
MVA: motor vehicle accident
mx: management
NaCl: sodium chloride
NB: note well
NCV: nerve conduction velocity
Neg: negative
NISSA: nerve, ischemia, soft tissue, skeletal injury, shock, age (prediction for amputation)
NKA: no known allergies
NMR: nuclear magnetic resonance
NOS: not otherwise specified
NPO: nil per os (nothing per mouth)
NSAID: nonsteroidal antiinflammatory drug
NSNA: normal shape, normal alignment
NV: neurovascular
NWB: non–weight-bearing
O$_2$: oxygen
OA: osteoarthritis
OAWO: opening abductory wedge osteotomy
obl: oblique
OCD: osteochondritis dissecans
OD: oculus dexter (right eye); overdose
ODQ/ODM: opponens digiti quinti (or minimi)
OI: osteogenesis imperfecta
OP: opponens pollicis
OPD: outpatient department
OR: operating room; open reduction
ORIF: open reduction/internal fixation
ORTHO: orthopaedic
os: small bones
OS: oculus sinister (left eye); also abbreviated OL
OT: occupational therapy
OU: both eyes
OWO: open wedge osteotomy
oz: ounce (8 dram, 30 ml)
P&A: percussion and auscultation

1/2P: hemiparesis
P: passive
PA: pascal (expressed as Newtons/square meter)
PA: psoriatic arthritis
PA: posteroanterior
PAD: peripheral arterial disease
PAL: posterior axillary line
PAO: peripheral arterial occlusion
Path: pathology
PB: paraffin baths
PB: peroneus brevis
pc: after meals
PCA: patient-controlled anesthesia
PCA: porous-coated arthroplasties
PCA: porous-coated anatomic (total hip replacement)
PCE (Smith): physical capacities evaluation
PCP: primary care provider
PE, Px: physical examination
PE: pulmonary embolism
PEMF: pulsating electromagnetic fields
PEMF: pulsed electromagnetic fields
PERRLA: pupils equal, round, regular to light accommodation
PF plantar flexion
PFC: pelvic flexion contracture
PFFD: proximal femoral focal deficiency
Ph: phosphorus
PH: past history
phal: phalanx or phalanges
PHT: pseudohypothyroidism
PI: present illness
PID: pelvic inflammatory disease
PIP: proximal interphalangeal (joint); PIPJ
PL: palmaris longus
PLIF: posterior lumbar interbody fusion; posterolateral interbody fusion
PLRI: posterolateral rotary instability
PMA: progressive muscle atrophy
PMD: progressive muscular dystrophy
PMHx, PMH: past medical history
PMMA: polymethylmethacrylate
PMRI: posteromedial rotary instability
PNF: proprioceptive neuromuscular facilitation
PNS: peripheral nervous system
PO: per oral

POC: plan of care
polio: poliomyelitis
Post: posterior
Post-op: postoperatively
pp: postprandial (after meals)
PP: proximal phalanx
PPD: purified protein derivative (tuberculosis test)
PPM: parts per million
PPO: passive prehension orthosis
PQ: pronator quadratus
PR: pelvic rock
pre-op: preoperatively
prep: preparation
PRE: progressive resistive exercises
PRN: as often as necessary; ad lib
prog: prognosis
prox/3 or P/3: proximal third
PSI: predictive salvage index
PSIS: posterosuperior iliac spine
PSS: progressive system scoliosis
pt: patient
PT: physical therapy
PT: pronator teres
PTA: prior to admission
PTB: patella tendon bearing; pretibial bearing (socket type)
PTB: patellar tendon bearing (cast, orthosis, prosthesis)
PTBS: patellar tendon bearing suspension
PTB-SC: patellar tendon-bearing-supracondylar
PTB-SP: patellar tendon-bearing-suprapatellar
PTH: parathyroid hormone
PTP: posterior tibial pulse
PTT: patellar tendon transfer; partial prothrombin time
PVC: premature ventricular contraction
PVD: peripheral vascular disease
PVS: peripheral vascular system
PW: plantar wart
PWB: partial weight-bearing
q: every
q3h: every 3 hours
qam: every morning
QCT: quantitative computed tomography
qd: every day
qh: every hour
qid: four times a day (iiii)
qod: every other day
qoh: every other hour
qs: as much as suffices; quantity sufficient
QSAC: quadrant-sparing acetabular component
qt: quart (32 oz, 0.946 liter)
quad: quadriceps; quadrilateral; quadriplegic
quant: quantity
R: roentgen unit, x-ray examination
Ra: radium
RA: rheumatoid arthritis
rad: radiology, radiation absorbed dose
RC: radiocarpal (joint)
rem: roentgen-equivalent-man
RF: rheumatoid factor
RGO: reciprocating gait orthosis
Rh–: rh negative
Rh+: rh positive
RHD: right-hand dominant
Rheum: rheumatology
RICE: rest, ice, compression, elevation
RLE: right lower extremity
RLL: right lower limb
RLQ: right lower quadrant
RM: repetition maximum
R/O: rule out
ROM: range of motion
ROS, SR: review of systems
RR: recovery room; relative risk
RRE: round, regular, and equal
RSD: reflex sympathetic dystrophy
RTC: return to clinic
RUE: right upper extremity
RUL: right upper limb; right upper lobe
RUQ: right upper quadrant
RV: return visit
S1-S5: sacral vertebrae
SAC: short-arm cast
SACH: solid ankle cushioned heel
SAFE: stationary ankle flexible endoskeletal (foot)
SANC: short-arm navicular cast
SAPHO: synovitis-acne-pustulosis-hyperostosis-osteomyelitis syndrome
SAS: short-arm splint
SBQC: small base quad cane
SC: sternoclavicular (joint)

SCFE: slipped capital femoral epiphysis
SCSI: subaxial cervical spinal injury
SCIWORA: spinal cord injury without radiographic abnormality
SCSP: supracondylar-suprapatellar
SD: shoulder disarticulation
SD: standard deviation
SDD: sterile dry dressing
SDR: surgical dressing room
SE: standard estimate
SEM: standard estimate of the mean
Sed Rate: erythrocyte sedimentation rate
Segs: segmented white cells
SEM: scanning electron microscopy
SERI: simple, effective, rapid, and inexpensive (foot procedure)
SGOT: serum glutamic oxalacetic transferase
SGP: stress-generated potentials
SGPT: serum glutamic pyruvic transferase
SH: social history
SI: Système International d'Unités (Fr.); International System of Units (extension of metric system)
SI: sacroiliac (joint)
SICS: subaxial injury classification scale
Sig: let it be labeled; directions
SIS: Standard International System
SL: serious list
SLAP: superior labrum anterior to posterior (shoulder lesion)
SLC: short-leg cast
SLE: systemic lupus erythematosus
SLR: straight leg raise
SLS: short-leg splint
SMA: spinal muscular atrophy
SMPS: sympathetic maintained pain syndrome
SNF: skilled nursing facility
SNP: single nucleotide polymorphisms
SOAP: subjective, objective, assessment, plan—a problem-oriented medical record-keeping system
sol, soln: solution
SOMI: sternal-occiput-mandibular immobilization (orthosis)
SOS: if necessary, repeat once if need exists
SP: suprapatellar
SPECT: single-photon-emission computed tomography
SPGR: spoiled grass (image)

SSEP: somatosensory-evoked potentials (research)
SSI: segmental spinal instrumentation
staph: *Staphylococcus* or implies *S. aureus* species
STAT: immediately
STEN: stored energy
STIR: short tau inversion recovery
STJ: subtalar joint
strep: *Streptococcus*
STSG: split-thickness skin graft
SUFE: slipped upper femoral epiphysis
Sub-Q, SQ, SC: subcutaneous (under the skin)
sup: superior
surg: surgical; surgery
SWASH: sitting, walking, and standing hip (orthosis)
SWD: shortwave diathermy
sympt or Sx: symptoms
Sz: seizure
T: temperature
T1-T12: thoracic vertebrae
tabs: tablets
TAL: tendon Achilles lengthening
TAMBA: talar axis first metatarsal base angle
TARA: total articular replacement arthroplasty
TB: tuberculosis
TEM: transmission electron microscopy
TENS: transcutaneous electrical nerve stimulation
TEV: talipes equinovarus
TFCC: triangular fibrocartilage complex
TFD: target-film distance
TG: tendon graft
TH: transhumeral (amputation)
THA: total hip arthroplasty
THF: triquetrohamate fusion
THR: total hip replacement
TIA: transient ischemic attack
tid: three times a day (iii)
TIMP: tissue inhibitor of metalloproteinase
TJ: triceps jerks
TJR: total joint replacement
TKA: total knee arthroplasty
TKR: total knee replacement
TLIF: transforaminal lumbar interbody fusion
TLR: triquetrohamate ligament reconstruction
TLSO: thoracic lumbosacral orthosis
TMJ(s): temporomandibular joint (syndrome)
TMT: talometatarsal (angle)

Tomo: tomogram
TPC: thenar palmar crease
TPN: total parenteral nutrition (intramuscular, intravenous, subcutaneous, intramedullary)
TPR: temperature, pulse, respiration
TR: transradial (amputation)
TSD: target-scan distance
T-spine: thoracic spine
TSS: toxic shock syndrome
TT: tendon transfer
TT: tilt table
TTAP: threaded titanium acetabular prosthesis
Tx: traction; treatment, transfusion
UCL: ulnar collateral ligament
UE: upper extremity
UHMWPE: ultrahigh molecular weight polyethylene
UN: ulnar nerve (finger spreader)
URI: upper respiratory (tract) infection
US: ultrasound
ut dict: as directed
UTI: urinary tract infection
UV: ultraviolet (light)
VATER: vertebral, and tracheoesophageal, esophageal, radial, and renal
VC: volar capsulodesis
VDDR: vitamin D–dependent rickets
VDRR: vitamin D–resistant rickets
VISI: volar intercalated segment instability
VS: vertical shear (pelvic fractures)
VSL: very serious list
VTED: venous thromboembolic disease
VWF: vibratory white finger (Raynaud phenomenon)
WBC: white blood cell count
WC: wheelchair
WD: wrist disarticulation
WD, WN: well developed, well nourished
WEST: work evaluation systems technology
WFE or Wms flex ex: Williams flexion exercises
WNL: within normal limits
WPB: whirlpool bath
Wt: weight
XIP: x-ray in plaster (examination)
XLIF: extreme lateral interbody fusion
XMATCH: cross match
XOP: x-ray out of plaster (examination)
>: greater than
<: less than
1°: primary
2°: secondary
3°: tertiary

Professional Organizations

AAOP: American Academy of Orthotists and Prosthetists
AAOS: American Academy of Orthopaedic Surgeons
AATB: American Association of Tissue Banks
ABOS: American Board of Orthopaedic Surgery
AF: Arthritis Foundation
AOA: American Orthopaedic Association
AOFAS: American Orthopaedic Foot and Ankle Society
AOPA: American Orthotics and Prosthetics Association
AORI: Anderson Orthopaedic Research Institute
APRL: Army Prosthetic Research Lab
ARCO: Association Research Circulation Osseous
ASBMR: American Society for Bone and Mineral Research
ASES: American Shoulder and Elbow Surgeons
ASIA: American Spinal Injury Association
ASIF: Association for the Study of Internal Fixation
DEA: Drug Enforcement Agency
DoD: Department of Defense (research)
FAAOS: Fellow, American Academy of Orthopaedic Surgeons
HHS: Department of Health and Human Services
HMO: Health Maintenance Organization
ICRC: International Committee of the Red Cross
IRE: Institutional Review Board
ISMAT: Institute of Sports Medicine and Athletic Training
JCAH: Joint Commission on Accreditation of Hospitals
JCAHO: Joint Commission on Accredited Health Organizations
MEDLARS: Medical Literature Analysis Retrieval System
MRE: Medical Research Council
MTS: Musculoskeletal Tumor Society

NIAMS: National Institute of Arthritis and Musculoskeletal and Skin Diseases
NIH: National Institutes of Health
OREF: Orthopaedic Research and Education Foundation
OSHA: Occupational Safety and Health Administration
OTA: Orthopaedic Trauma Association
SI: Système International, System of Units (extension of metric system)
TASTM: The American Society for Testing Metals (and Alloys)
WHO: World Health Organization

Appendix: Anatomic Positions and Directions

In orthopaedics, anatomic positions and directions are routinely used to provide an accurate description of specific anatomic locations. These basic directions may be compared to looking at a map to determine the longitude and latitude of an area. Humans are three-dimensional subjects with points of reference made in the orthograde (upright) position. The surface locations and anatomic planes are described as follows.

Surface Location

The location of a structure is described in reference to a standing person facing the examiner with outstretched hands in a palms-up position. The basic directional terms are:

anterior (ventral): forward or front surface (Fig. B-1)
inferior: lower area, below, toward the tail end
lateral: sides, away from midline
medial: middle, toward the midline
posterior (dorsal): back surface
superior: upper area, above, toward the head

These reference points may be combined to give a more precise location to a specific region on a surface or in structures deep within the body, for example, the exposed hip in a surgical procedure. When these terms are compounded and hyphen omitted, the combining forms may be:

anteroinferior: front and below
anterolateral: front and to outer side
anteromedial: front and to inner side
anteroposterior: front and toward back
anterosuperior: front and above

These can be used in combination with locations in reverse order, such as:

posteroinferior: back to below
posterolateral: back to outer side
posteromedial: back to inner side
posterosuperior: back to front toward head

In some cases, dorsal (back) may be used for posterior (e.g., dorsolateral).

Anatomic Planes

The term *plane* comes from the Latin word *planus*, meaning a flat, level surface. There are three directions of planes, all in reference to a standing person facing the examiner: vertical anterior to posterior (sagittal), vertical side to side (coronal or longitudinal), and horizontal (transverse).

anteroposterior planes
    median (midsagittal) plane: vertical plane directly through the midline of the body, transecting the nose, navel, and spine, and dividing the body into left and right halves.
    median or sagittal plane: any of the anteroposterior planes through the midaxis, dividing the body in half; the term sometimes implies the median plane only. If the word *sagittal* is used to denote

Fig B-1 Anterior view of human figure demonstrating meaning of terms used in describing the body. (From Anthony CP, Kolthoff N: *Textbook of anatomy and physiology*, ed 9, St Louis, 1975, Mosby.)

the median plane, then other sagittal planes are called *parasagittal planes.*

horizontal (transverse) plane: any of the horizontal planes across the body at right angles to coronal and sagittal planes parallel to baseline.

neutral plane: the plane of a structure around which bending occurs.

vertical side to side planes

coronal (frontal plane): a plane parallel with long axis of body at right angles to median sagittal plane going through coronal sutures of the skull (approximately center of body) and dividing body into front and back parts.

longitudinal: lengthwise and parallel with long axis of body or part; any of the vertical side to side planes. Coronal and longitudinal planes have been used interchangeably to describe each other. In this case, the context of the sentence will indicate the reference point of the plane.

Specific Locations

When describing limb anatomy, the nomenclature is very specific. The four appendages are correctly referred to as the *upper* and *lower limbs,* two *forelimbs,* and two *hind limbs.* The **thigh** indicates that portion above the knee and the **shank** the portion between the knee and ankle. The **calf** is the posterior aspect and the **shin** the anterior aspect of the leg. The sole (bottom) of the foot is called the **plantar surface,** and the top is the **dorsal surface.** The **brachium** refers to that portion of the arm above the elbow and below the shoulder. The **antebrachium** refers to the portion of the arm below the elbow but above the wrist. The **ventral side** of the hand is the palm or **volar surface,** with the opposite side being the **dorsum** or **dorsal surface.** The forearm is similarly divided into volar and dorsal aspects.

Joint Motions* (Fig. B-2)

Ranges of joint motion refer to the extent of movement within a given joint. Joint motion may be active, passive, or active assistive. The major joint areas involve the shoulder (glenoid), elbow (cubitus), hip (coxa) (Fig. B-3), and knee (genu).

All the hinge joints have motion described in terms of **flexion** and **extension.** Except for the ankle, the 0-degree position occurs when the limb is held out straight, and the degree of flexion is then stated in terms of degrees from the 0-degree extended position. The knee and elbow will occasionally extend beyond the

---

*Further information about the assessment and recording of joint motions is obtainable from American Academy of Orthopaedic Surgeons, 1985.

Fig B-2 A, Elbow. *Flexion:* 0 to 150 degrees. *Extension:* 150 degrees to 0 (from angle of greatest flexion to 0 position). *Hyperextension:* measured in degrees beyond the 0 starting point: This motion is not present in all individuals; when it is, it may vary from 5 to 15 degrees. **B,** Elbow and wrist, *Pronation:* 0 to 80 or 90 degrees. *Supination:* 0 to 80 or 90 degrees. *Total forearm motion:* 160 to 180 degrees. **C,** Wrist. *Flexion* (palmar flexion): 0 to about 80 degrees. *Extension* (dorsiflexion): 0 to about 70 degrees, **D,** Wrist. *Radial deviation:* 0 to 20 degrees. *Ulnar deviation:* 0 to 30 degrees. (From American Academy of Orthopaedic Surgeons: *Joint motion—method of measuring and recording,* Chicago, 1985, The Academy.)

0-degree limit, and this motion is expressed in degrees of **hyperextension.** The wrist has approximately 90 degrees of extension and 90 degrees of flexion (dorsiflexion and palmar flexion).

The Neutral Zone Method is used for measuring joint motion. The anatomic position of the joint defines the starting position at zero, and motion is measured in degrees of a circle. Other measured motions include:

circumduction: a maneuver or movement of a ball-and-socket joint in a circular motion; for example, the shoulder can circumduct 180 degrees with six movements possible.
flexion: to bend from the joint as in flexion movements of the spine at the waist (anterior or lateral). In the foot or hand is expressed as:

dorsiflexion: the toe-up motion of the ankle expressed in degrees from the 0-degree position of the foot at rest on the ground in standing position.
plantar flexion: the toe-down motion of the foot at the ankle expressed in degrees from 0-degree position of the foot at rest on the ground in standing position.
palmar flexion: of the wrist with palm up in flexion.
extension: extending distally away from body as in the limbs, or bending back posteriorly as in the spine.
pronation: palm-down position of hand with elbow at a 90-degree angle, brought about by the motion of the radius around the ulna (posterior rotation). In the foot, the plantar surface is turned down.
supinate, supination: palm-up position of the hand with elbow flexed at a 90-degree angle, brought

THE HIP

Fig B-3 The hip. **A,** *Inward rotation:* measured by rotating leg outward. *Outward rotation:* measured by rotating leg inward. **B,** *Inward rotation (internal):* measured by rotating leg away from midline of trunk with thigh as the axis of rotation, thus producing inward rotation of the hip. *Outward rotation (external):* measured by rotating leg toward midline of trunk with thigh as the axis of rotation, thus producing outward rotation of the hip. **C,** *Abduction:* outward motion of the extremity is measured in degrees from 0 starting position. *Adduction:* to measure, examiner should elevate opposite extremity a few degrees to allow leg to pass under it. (From American Academy of Orthopaedic Surgeons: *Joint motion—method of measuring and recording,* Chicago, 1985, The Academy.)

about by motion of the radius around the ulna (anterior rotation). In the foot, the plantar surface is turned inward.

ulnar deviation: of the hand at the wrist such that the hand is directed in an ulnar direction; measured in degrees from 0 with hand in midline.

radial deviation: of the hand at the wrist such that the hand is directed radially; measured in degrees from 0 with hand in midline.

abduction: movement away from midline of body in frontal plane; applied to hip, shoulder, fingers, thumb, and foot. The midline reference point is a central line in the body for proximal joints and the central part of a limb for distal joints (Figs. B-4 and B-5).

adduction: movement toward the midline in frontal plane as in abduction. On verbal transcription in clinical notes the person dictating will sometimes say "a-b-duction" or "a-d-duction" to clarify distinction between *abd*uction and *add*uction (see Fig. B-4).

anteversion: to lean forward at an angle; in reference to the neck of humerus or femur, an anterior rotation.

anteroflexion: bending forward.

eversion: turning outward, when applied to the heel, describes the degree of motion of the heel pushed outward with ankle in neutral position; when applied to the foot, describes the combined motions of dorsiflexion, pronation, and abduction (Fig. B-6).

inversion: when applied to the heel, describes the degree of motion of the heel pushed inward with ankle in neutral position; when applied to the foot, describes the combined motions of plantar flexion, supination, and adduction (see Fig. B-6).

retroflexion: bending backward.

retroversion: turned toward the back; in reference to the neck of femur or humerus, a posterior rotation.

apposition: contact of two adjacent parts; bringing together as in a finger movement, the thumb to index finger.

opposition: applied mostly to the thumb but also to little finger; describes the motion required to bring about opposition, or the setting opposite, of thumb against little finger (pulp surfaces). For the thumb, opposition is the combined action of abduction, rotation, and flexion.

external rotation: in frontal plane is away from midline.

internal rotation: in a frontal plane is toward the midline.

valgus: turned outward; the distal part is bent away from the midline; for example, genu valgus (knock-kneed).

varus: turned inward; the distal part is toward the midline; for example, genu varus (bow-legged).

Anatomic Associated Terms

The following are other associated terms referring to directions of anatomy or physical signs.

Fig B-4 A, Nomenclature of fingers. To avoid mistakes, fingers and thumb are referred to by name rather than by number. **B,** Finger spread in abduction and adduction can be measured in centimeters or inches from the tip of index finger to tip of little finger. Individual fingers spread from tip to tip of indicated fingers. (From American Academy of Orthopaedic Surgeons: *Joint motion—method of measuring and recording,* Chicago, 1985, The Academy.)

a, an: no, not, against.
AAL: anterior axillary line.
ab: away from (abduct).
abducens: drawing away from median line of the body; also called **abductor m.**
ad: toward (adduct).
adjacent: close to, beside
AGE: angle of greatest extension.
AGF: angle of greatest flexion.
alignment: linear position of one part of an extremity compared with another; to bring into a straight line.
ambi: on both sides.
ambidextrous: using both right and left hands effectively.
amph-, amphi-: both ways, all around, both sides.
an-: not, against, without.

THE THUMB

Zero starting position

Abduction

Rotation

Flexion

Flexion to tip of little finger

or

Flexion to base of little finger

Fig B-5 Thumb opposition. The motion is a composite of three elements: abduction, rotation, and flexion. This motion is considered complete when tip, or pulp, of thumb touches tip of fifth finger or, according to some surgeons, when tip of thumb touches base of the fifth finger. (From American Academy of Orthopaedic Surgeons: *Joint motion—method of measuring and recording,* Chicago, 1985, The Academy.)

HIND PART OF THE FOOT

Inversion

Eversion

0° Neutral

0° Neutral

A

FORE PART OF THE FOOT

90°

90°

0°

0°

Inversion (supination, adduction, and plantar flexion)

Eversion (pronation, abduction, and dorsiflexion)

B

Fig B-6 A, Hindpart of the foot. *Inversion:* heel is grasped firmly in cup of examiner's hand. Passive motion is estimated in degrees, or percentages of motion, by turning heel inward. *Eversion:* motion is estimated by turning heel outward. **B,** Forepart of the foot. *Active inversion:* foot is directed medial. This motion includes supination, adduction, and some degree of plantar flexion; can be estimated in degrees or expressed in percentages as compared with the opposite foot. *Active eversion:* sole of foot is turned to face laterally. This motion includes pronation, abduction, and dorsiflexion. (From American Academy of Orthopaedic Surgeons: *Joint motion—method of measuring and recording,* Chicago, 1985, The Academy.)

anatomic axis: the true axis of an extremity measured by lines.
angle: the figure or space outlined by the diverging of two lines from a common point or by the meeting of two planes; a projecting or sharp corner.
angulation: deviation from the norm; sharp bend of a structure to form an angle.
aniso: unequal, asymmetrical, dissimilar.
annulus: any circular structure, ring-shaped.
ante-: forward, before.
antecedent: to precede, or go before.
anteflexion: to bend forward.
anterior: front view, ventral side, face surface, superior.

antero-: before, in front of.
anteversion: tipping forward.
anticus: foremost, in the front.
antimere: the right or left half of the body; a segment of an animal body formed by planes, cutting the axis of the body at right angles.

apex: top, tip, point of activity, summit, vertex (refers to C2).
apical: pertaining to apex; situated near point of reference.
apo-: away from.
asymmetric: lacking symmetry; uneven, as one limb to another.
axis: line of symmetry, rotation, or revolution; pivot dividing line; also second vertebra.
axis of rotation: circular arcs of limb segments that move in a line of right angles to the plane.
basal, basilar: base of a part.
bilateral: both sides.
cata-: prefix meaning down, against, or according to.
caudal, caudad: toward the lower end of the erect trunk or tail, inferior to or bottom point of reference.
centri-: center.
cephalic: toward the head; uppermost point of reference.
circumference: around, outer circular boundary.
circumflex: describes an arc of a circle; winding around.
co-, com-, con-: together, with.
concave: rounded, depressed surface.
contralateral: opposite side.
convex: rounded, elevated surface.
coronal: a plane dividing the body with front and back portions; in the direction of the coronal suture; a longitudinal plane passing through the body at right angles to the median plane.
craniad: toward the head.
curvilinear: curved away from straight line.
de-: away, from, down.
deep: depth from surface.
delta: triangle (deltoid).
dexter: right.
dia-: between, through, across, apart.
diffuse: widely distributed.
dis-: apart from.
distal: away from, furthest point of reference.
dorsal: back or posterior aspect.
ec-: out, out from.
ectopic: located away from normal position; out of place.
em-, en-: in, within.
endo-: within, in.
epi-: on, above, over.

eso-: in, inward, inside.
ex-, exo-: out, outside.
external: outside, describing walls, cavities, or hollow viscera.
extra-: beyond, outside, without.
facet: flat surface.
flexure: curved or bent.
fore: in front of, before.
fusiform: spindle-shaped, tapered.
geniculum: an abrupt bend or angle in a small structure (knee).
hyper-: over, above, excessive.
hypo-: under, below, deficient.
in-, ino-: into, within.
inferior: below point of reference, underneath.
infra: below or under.
in situ: in its natural place or position.
inter-: between.
intercalary: middle.
internal: inside; describing walls, cavities, or hollow viscera.
interspace: the space between two similar parts (e.g., the vertebrae, ribs).
interstitial: spaces within a structure.
intra-: within.
intro-: into, beginning.
ipsilateral: same side.
iso-: equal, symmetrical.
juxta-: prefix for close to, near, in apposition, side by side (e.g., juxtaposition).
lat, latero-, lateral: sides, right and left; away from median plane, outer surface.
latus: broad.
length: the linear distance between two joints. The International System unit of length is measured in meters.
levo: left.
linea aspera: linea (line) and aspera (rough).
linear: elongated, straight line.
longitudinal: lengthwise, parallel to the long axis of a part (coronal or frontal planes).
MAL: midaxillary line.
medi-, medial: middle or median plane, toward midline, inner surface, link making halves.
megalo-: large.
meso-: middle intermediate.

met-, meta-: beyond, from one place to another, point of change.
multiangular: many angles.
neutral axis: the longitudinal line of a structure around which torsion occurs; the longitudinal line in a long structure where normal axial stresses are zero when structure is subjected to bending.
oblique: slanting diagonal; inclined.
oblongata: oblong.
orthograde: upright position, as in a standing person.
palmar: side of hand surface, face up.
para-, par-: beyond, beside.
parallel: equal in lines or surface; in the same direction.
pars: a division or part; a particular part of a greater structure (e.g., pars interarticularis).
patent: open, unobstructed, apparent, evident.
peri-, peripheral: immediately around, sphere.
perpendicular: exactly upright; being at right angles to a given line or plane.
pivot: to turn as in a circular motion.
plantar: sole, bottom of the foot.
posterior, postero-, post-: after, behind, tail end, back, inferior to surface.
prone: face down (lying face down).
protract: pull forward.
proximal: close to nearest point of reference.
quadratus: four-sided.
re-: back, again.
recurvatum: bending backward; a flexure or hyperextension.
residual: left behind.
retract: pull back.
retrad: backward, toward back part.
retro-, retrograde, retroflex: bending backward, behind.
rotation: turning in a circular motion.
scalene: having unequal sides; said of a triangle (e.g., scalenus muscle).
scalenus: uneven.
sinister: left.
striate: having transverse lines (muscles).
sub-: under.
subjacent: lying underneath (sub-: under + -jacent: to lie).
summit: top.
super-, supra-: above, beyond, upon, over.
superficial: near the surface.
superior, sup.-: uppermost side, above point of reference, toward head (cephalic).
supine: lying on back, face up.
sym-, syn-: together.
symmetric: exhibiting symmetry, even, alike.
terminal: end.
trans-, transverse: through, across, horizontal.
ultra: beyond.
unilateral: one side.
ventral: belly side (abdomen), anterior, front, face up.
vertex: the top or summit, apex.
vertical: perpendicular to the plane of the horizon (vertex).
volar: underneath surface, palm or sole side up.

Appendix: Etymology of Orthopaedics

The word *etymology* comes from the Greek *etymos*, meaning genuine or true, plus *logos*, study of. Etymology is the study of the original meaning of words (*origo*, beginning).

Most of our medical terminology originated from Latin and Greek history and mythology, and was nonmedical in use. Scientific language was attributed to early physicians and writers such as Hypocrites, Aristotle, and Galen. Latin terms were introduced by Galen, a Greek physician who moved to Rome, and the Flemish anatomist, Vesralius. Celsus, Aretaeus, Pliny, and Chaucer were among many others who contributed to the scientific vocabulary. Students receiving a medical degree are required to take the Hippocratic Oath, named for the most famous Greek physician, Hippocrates of Cos. He was a contemporary of Socrates, and the oath set forth a basic ethical code for the medical profession.

Galen gave the first account of musculi by describing and naming more than 300. In 1543 BC, Vesalius abandoned the system of naming muscles and accurately numbered them. In the sixteenth century, Jacque Dubois renamed muscles after parts to which they were attached; for example, tibialis, peroneus, and others were named by shape (rhomboid), size (longus, brevis), substance (membranous), or from the number of heads (biceps, triceps). Borelli added to names the action of muscles (pulley, lever, wheel). In the eighteenth century, Winslow, Albinus, Cowper, Douglas, and Riolan named muscles as we know them today. Leonardo da Vinci lettered his illustrations and occasionally gave a muscle a special name.

Centuries later, scholars preferred using the languages of Latin and Greek in science over other languages for a number of reasons, mainly because of the ease in which words could be used interchangeably in combining forms based on roots, prefixes, and suffixes. Special rules applied to plurals of such words. Anglo-Saxon English has a limited capacity for compounding words and often requires numerous words to make a point. Therefore Latin and Greek were retained as the main structure of scientific language as we know it today. Scholars for generations have studied word origins and discovered full histories for most words, found mostly in the authoritative *Oxford English Dictionary*.

Anatomy is a descriptive science. Many words that are nonmedical in origin describe sizes and shapes (deltoid, lamboid, piriformis) or plants (sesamoid: sesame seed; nucleus: little nut; pisiform: pea-shaped) or are taken from living creatures (lupus: wolf; musculus: little mouse; cauda equina: horse's tail; lumbrical: worm). Often, the Greek and Latin words having the same meaning are very different; for example, clavicle (Latin, dim. of *clavis,* a key) and *cleido* (Greek, a fastener or key), are used in combining form (sternocleidomastoid).

Anglo-Saxon (A-S) English favors monosyllabic words such as hand, foot, back, leg, arm, and so forth, and is augmented by many words from other languages such as Latin (L), Greek (Gr), French (Fr), Italian (It), Spanish (Sp), Middle English (ME), German (Ger), and other nonclassical origins. Greek mythology also contributed to the linguistics in use today. Achilles, a hero who fought at Troy, was killed by an arrow that pierced the single vulnerable spot on his body; his heel. "Achilles heel" now refers to a vulnerable spot. Atlas, a giant in Greek mythology, was compelled to bear the weight of the heavens on his shoulders. Today, the name *Atlas* is used to describe geography and collections of maps. Chemical elements also derive their names from myths, such as helium, titanium, and mercury. The space age programs today also chose mythological names such as Gemini, Nike, Saturn, Apollo, and Zeus.

A knowledge of word derivation is the best way to accurately use words in their proper form. A brief description of the origin of orthopaedic and associated terminology is given here to assist in the understanding of this specialty.

a, an: (G) negative prefix before a word that signifies the thing named is deprived of its quality (e.g., anaerobic, anorexic); not, without.

abdomen: (L) belly, the area between the chest and pelvis.

abductors: (L) abducens, led away; *ab-* from *ducere,* to lead. Muscle on contraction pulls away from median plane of body or axial line of extremity.

accident: (L) from *accidens,* a happening; *accidere,* to happen; (G) *cado,* to fall. An unexpected happening.

acetabulum: (L) *acetum,* vinegar cup + *bulum,* little cup, dim. of *abrum,* a holder or receptacle. Cup-shaped depression of the ilium (true hip) for holding head of femur.

acromion: (G) *akron* or *akros,* summit, peak + *-omos,* shoulder; outermost tip of scapula.

acute: (L) *acutus,* sharp, from *acuere,* to sharpen (cf. *acus,* needle).

adductor: (L) *adductus,* to bring toward median plane of body vs. abductor.

Adeno: (G) prefix for gland.

adhesion: (L) *ad,* to bring in + *haerere,* to stick; *adhaesio,* stuck to.

adipose: (L) *adeps, adipis,* fat. Term used to describe tissue fat.

adjuvant: (L) adjuvans, aiding; that which assists to increase the action desired.

adventitia: (L) *adventicius. Ad,* to + *veniere,* to come. An adventitious bursa is one formed from surrounding tissues in an unusual situation (e.g., tailor's bursa, student's elbow). A tunica adventitia is applied to the outer covering of a structure or organ (artery).

agonist: (G) *agonistes,* a rival or combatant, a prime mover; a muscle concerned with carrying out a movement (contraction) versus antagonist (opposite).

ala, alar: (L) winglike structure; alar ligament of first cervical vertebra, and sacral ala, the lateral portion.

allograft: (G) *allos,* other + (L) *graphium,* grafting knife. To transplant tissue from same species.

ambidextrous: (L) ability to use both hands as if they were right hands; *ambi,* on both sides + *dexter,* right.

amphiarthrosis: (G) *amphi,* on both sides + *arthron,* a joint. Limited mobility with movement in all directions. Diarthrosis and synarthrosis refer to incomplete joints (intervertebral disks).

amputation: (L) *amputare,* to cut around + amputation, a pruning. Hippocrates recommended this operation at the joint.

analgesia: (G) *an,* not + *algos,* pain. Absence of pain.

anaphylaxis: (G) *ana,* up + phylaxis, *protection.*

anapophysis: (G) *ana,* back + *apophysis,* an offshoot; an accessory spinal process of a vertebra.

anastomosis: (G) an opening created by a natural, pathologic or surgical communication between two normally distinct spaces, organs or tubular structure.

anatomy: (G) *ana,* apart + *tome,* a cutting; *anatome,* dissection. Hippocrates (420 BC) used word for a branch of medical education. The oldest treatise known on anatomy is an Egyptian papyrus (1600 BC) on dissecting bodies for medical purposes. The science was based on dissection, from which it got its name.

anconeus: (G) *ancon,* a bend, especially the elbow (cf. *angle*).

anesthesia: (A-S) *an,* against + *aesthesis,* sensation. Partial or complete loss of sensation.

ankle: (A-S) from (L) *angulus,* an angle, corner, or bend; (G) bend.

ankylosis: (G) *ankyl,* stiff + *osis,* condition. An ancient term for stiffening of joints, loss of mobility.

annulus: (L) ring-shaped structure; annular fibrosis of intervertebral disks.

anomaly: (G) *anomalia, an,* against + *omaly,* ordinary. Abnormality or deviation from normal, whether in structure, form, location, or function.

antagonist: (G) anti- or *an,* against, opposite + *tagon,* a struggle; *agonistes,* a rival. A muscle that opposes the action of another muscle (agonist).

anterior: (L) *ante-*, before, more in front; from *anterus*, positive form of anterior. antero-(L) ante- before, more in front; prefix used in combining form.

aorta: (L from Gr *aorte*) the main trunk of the arterial system of the body.

anti-: (G) prefix meaning against.

apex: (L) tip.

aplasia: (G) *a*, against + *plasia*, to mold or form. A failure in tissue formation.

aponeurosis: (G) *apo*, away from + *neuron*, tendon. Before Aristotle (c. 350 BC) introduced the word *neura* for nerves, everything of a fibrous nature was called a neuron. Galen (c. 180 AD) was first to use the word aponeurosis to refer to the insertion of a muscle that was not by flesh fibers but terminated in the white sheath.

apophysis: (G) *apo*, from + *physis*, growth; offshoot. Outcropping, but not end of bone, but rather the outgrowth of bone without an independent center of ossification. A place for tendinous attachment.

appendages: (L) *appendere*, to hang to, an extremity (pl. appendices).

arachnoid: (G) *arachne*, spiderlike + *eidos*, form, shape; resembling a web; cerebellum and spinal cord covering.

arcuate: (L) *arcualis*, arch-shaped, bowed. Refers to arcuate line of rectus sheath and arcuate ligament of wrist.

artery: (G) *aer*, air + *terso*, to carry; arteries were believed to be air carriers in vessels. Later referred to arteries carrying blood.

arthritis: (G) *arthro*, joint + *-itis*, inflammation.

arthrodesis: (G) *arthro*, joint + *desis*, binding; fusion of a joint.

arthrology: (G) *arthro*, joint + *-ology*, treatise or discourse, the science of joints. Galen recorded two main orders of joints: diarthrosis (articulation with movement) and synarthrosis (articulation without movement). He then divided the diarthroses into enarthroses, arthrodies, and ginglymus. Synarthroses were divided into suture, symphysis, and gomphosis.

articulatio: (L) *articulus*, little joint, dim. of *artus*, fitted close. Artus was used for limbs, thus, *articulatus*, jointed. Galen, Pliny, and Celsus preferred the Latin *articulus* to the Greek *arthro*; however, both continue to be used.

artifact: (L) *ars*, art + *facere*, to make; anything artificially produced and not occurring naturally. A feature of a test that stimulates a pathologic condition or interference with correct results of the test.

aspera: (L) *asper*, rough. Linea aspera is a roughened ridge on the femur associated with insertion of the adductor group of muscles.

asthenia: (G) *asthenis*, without strength; loss of strength, myasthenia—loss of muscle strength.

ataxia: (G) lack of order; defective muscular coordination (esp.) that is manifested when voluntary muscular movements are attempted.

atlas: (G) from *atlao*, endure or sustain. Galen (c. 180 AD) called the atlas *protos spondylos*, the first cervical vertebra, and second vertebra, epistropheus, to rotate on. The term was later changed to refer to the axis.

atrophy: (G) *atrophia*, a wasting; *a*, lacking + *trophia*, nourishment. A decrease in size of an organ or tissue, commonly a muscle.

autogenous: (G) *autos*, self + *genous*, to produce; self-produced or originating within the body.

autonomic: (G, A-S) *auto*, self + *nomos*, law; functioning independently.

auxe: (G) enlargement, increase; auxetic, to promote proliferation of leukocytes and other cells.

avulsion: (L) *avulsio*, to separate by force. From (G) *ab*, away from + (L) *vellere*, to pull.

axilla: (L) armpit. Uncertain origin, but thought to be a compound word from *axis alae*, meaning axle of a wing, where arm revolves at this point.

axis: (L) a line, real or imaginary, that runs through center of a body; or a pivot, about which a part revolves.

bacterium (pl. bacteria): (G) *bakterion*, rod; rod-shaped, one-celled organism.

biceps: (L) *bi*, two + *ceps*, head; caput; bicipital, having two heads. Refers to the biceps brachii and biceps femora muscle groups.

bifida: *bi*, two + *findere*, to cleave; having two parts (e.g., spina bifida).

biopsy: (G) *bio*, life + *op*, vision. Excision of living tissue for microscopic examination.

blasts: (G) suffix meaning *germ*; used in reference to cells that make other cells, such as the osteoblasts, bone-making cells.

bone: (A-S) from (L) *os* and (G) *osteon*.

boss: (Fr) *boce*, a swelling; a rounded eminence (e.g., carpal bossing). *Bosselated* refers to having many small prominences.

brachium: (L) arm, from (G) *brakhion*, shorter; *brachy*, short. Brachialis muscle of upper arm.

brevis: (L) short. Refers to short flexor of fingers (flexor digitorum brevis).

brisement: (Fr) crushing as in breaking by force; pronounced breez-mon.

bruise: (Fr) *bruiser*, to break. Broken vessel.

bruit: (Fr) noise; pronounced broo-ee.

bunion: (G) bunion, bugnone, a lump; bouvos, a hill or eminence; (L) *bunia*, enlargement.

bursa: (G) *bursula*, a pouch or sac, a purse; (L) pouch, wine skin. A sac between tendons, tendon and bone, muscle and bone that acts as a gliding surface at pressure points where friction can occur. Named in association with their anatomic location.

cadaver (pl. cadavera): (L) *cadere*, to fall, die.

calcar: (L) a spur, calcarine, spur-shaped; small spiny projection of bone.

calcaneus: (L) *calx*, a heel; *os calcis*, heel bone.

calcification: (L) *calx*, lime + *facere*, to make.

calcium: (L) *calx*, lime.

calisthenics: (G) *kalos*, beautiful + *sthenos*, strength.

callus: (G) *kalon*, callositas, dry wood; (L) *callum*, hard skin; (A-S) callus, new bone formation at site of fracture.

callous: hard, thickened skin (e.g., the foot).

canal: (L) *canalis*, channel. Conduit for vessels, nerves.

canaliculi: tunnels within bone matrix

cancellous: (L) *cancelli*, lattice work. A resemblance of cancellous tissue in bone to lattice work.

capitate: (L) *caput*, head-shaped; having a rounded extremity. Refers to small bone on distal row of hand; triquetrocapitate is the ligament.

capitellum: (L) *capitella*, small head. Knoblike protrusion of lateral condyle of the distal humerus.

capsule: (L) dim. of *capsa*, capsula, a little box; from *capio*, I receive.

caput: (L) a head; (G) *capitulum*, a little head. Modified to -ceps, as in biceps and triceps.

carotid: (G) *karos*, deep sleep; refers to main arteries of head and neck.

carpus: (L) *carpus, carpi*, wrist; (G) *karpos, karphyos*, dry bits of wood.

cartilage: (L) cartilage, gristle; (G) chondro.

cauda: (L) a tail, from *cadere*, to fall. Hence, cauda (tail) equine (horse), termination of the spinal cord, was believed to resemble a plaited horse's tail.

cell: (L) *cella*, a chamber.

cervical: (L) cervico, cervicalis; pertaining to the neck.

cheiro: (G) *chiro*, hand; (L) manus, to grasp.

chirurgery: (G) hand + work; one who works with his hands, a chirurgeon.

chondral: (G) from *chondros*, cartilage or gristle; (L) cartilage, gristle.

chronic: (G) *chronos*, time; of long duration.

cicatrix: (L) a scar left by a healed wound; to heal by scar tissue.

circulation: (L) *circulatio*, movement in a circular course.

claudication: (L) *claudicare*, to limp or be lame; disturbance of circulation.

clavicle: (L) *claviculum*, dim. of *clavis*, a key, probably related to *claudere*, to shut or close; (G) *cleido-* as in sternocleidomastoid. In both Latin and Greek, its use meant a key, bolt, fastener. The collar bone was likened to a key because it locks the shoulder girdle to the breast bone, and because of its shape.

clinic: (G) *klinikos*, to recline, a bed.

clonus: (G) *klonos*, turmoil; convulsing movements of epileptics. Now refers to spasm in which rigidity and relaxation alternate.

coccyx: (G) cuckoo's beak, from *kokkyx, coccygeus*, a cuckoo. Coccyx, tip of spine.

collagen: (G) *kolla*, glue + *gennan*, to produce; a glue-like substance that holds connective tissues together. Colloid, kollodes, glutinous.

collateral: (L) *con*, together + *lateralis*, latus, side; secondary accessory.

comitans: (L) companion. *Comes* (sing.), *cometes* (pl.); a blood vessel that accompanies a nerve trunk.

communis: (L) common, a vessel; that supplies several branches of the hand.

comminuted: (L) *com*, together + *minuere*, to crumble. To break into pieces, crushed.

concussion: (L) *concussus*, a shaking, from *concutio*, shake violently. An old term for *thunder*.

condyle: (G) *kondylos*, knuckle, knob; projections at the end of bones.

conjoined: (Fr) to meet, touch, overlap; refers to the aponeurotic tendon.

contusion: (L) *contusio*, a bruise; from *contundere: con*, together + *tundere*, to break.

coracoid: (G) *korax*, a crow + *oeides*, shape; (L) *corvus*. Anything hooked or pointed like a raven's beak. Variant of coronoid.

corpus: (L) *corporis*, body; (G) *somatos, soma*.

corpuscle: (L) *corpusculum*, small, rounded body; former term for blood cell.

cortex: (L) *corticis*, rind; outer hard layer of compact bone.

cortical: (L) cortex, a rind, outer layer.

costo-: (L) costa, from *costarum*, ribs. Refers to costovertebral cartilage.

coxa: (L) kaksha, the hip bone.

cranium: (L) skull.

crepitus: (G) *krepis*, a little noise, creaking; from *crepitare*, to crackle.

cribriform: (L) *cribrum*, a sieve + *forma*, form, sieve-like; anything perforated with holes (e.g., cribriform plate of ethmoid bone).

cricoid: (G) *krikos*, a ring + *oeides*, shape. Refers to cricoid cartilage shaped like a signet ring.

cruciate: (L) crux, shaped like a cross; refers to the two intraarticular ligaments of the knee joint that cross and give strong support to the knee.

cubitus: (L) elbow, from *cubo*, lying down (cf. decubitus). Cuboid is cube-shaped; (G) kyboides, cube.

cuneiform: (L) *cuneus*, a wedge + *forma*, shape. Anything wedge-shaped.

curettage: (Fr) curette, a cleanser; scraping out a cavity. Also called *debridement*.

cutaneous: (L) *cutis*, skin.

cuticle: (L) cuticula, little skin. The epidermis of the skin.

cyto-: (G) kytos, prefix denoting cell.

dactylos: (G) a digit, of the fingers or toes.

debridement: (Fr) de + bridle; thus, unbridling. Originally, to cut away as restricting bands, and later to include tissue.

decubitus: (L) lying down; position of lying down, decubitus ulcer may occur.

dehiscence: (L) *dehiscere*, to gape; to burst open, as in a wound.

deltoid: (G) *delta* (fourth letter of Greek alphabet); triangular-shaped.

dermas: (L) skin; *cutis vera*, true skin; corium, integumentary.

dermatome: (G) *dermu*, skin + *tome*, incision. Refers to dermatome distribution of spinal cord segments and nerve distribution.

desmoid: (G) from *desmos*, band, a ligament.

desiccant: (L) to dry up, as in a wound; desiccans (e.g., osteochondritis desiccans).

dexterity: (L) means right or to the right; dexter, right.

diagnosis: (G) *dia*, through + *gnosis*, knowledge; to discern.

diaphragm: (G) *dia*, through + *phragm*, a partition, wall. Any partition of the body; more specifically, the abdominal diaphragm.

diaphysis: (G) *dia*, through + *physis*, growth. To grow through, produce. Refers to center of ossification for shaft of long bones situated between growing regions at end of bone (epiphysis, metaphysis).

diarthrosis: (G) a joint, a movable articulation; freely movable hinge joint.

diastase: (G) *dia*, through + *stase*, to stand. A standing apart, separation. Now refers to complete separation of bone.

diathermy: (G) *dia*, through + *therme*, heat.

digitorum: (L) digitus, fingers or toes.

diplegia: (G) *di*, two + *plegia*, stroke; paralysis affecting one side only.

disk: (L) *discus*, plate; flat, round, platelike structure (intervertebral d.).

disease: (Fr) *desaise; des*, from + *aise*, depart from normal.

dislocation: (L) *dis*, apart + *locus* or *locare*, to place; dislocatio. Refers to separation of bone at joint area; formerly called a *subluxation*.

doctor: (L) from *docere*, to teach.

dorsum: (L) the back of a part.

dysfunction: (G) *dys*, difficult, painful + *functio* (L), a performance. Abnormal, impaired function.

dysplasia: (G) *dys*, bad + *plasien*, to form. Abnormal growth process.

dura: (L) hard. Refers to dura mater, the outermost and toughest of three membranes enclosing the spinal cord and brain. Syn. pia mater, soft.

dystrophy: (G) *dys*, bad, defective + *troph*, nourishment. Deficient by way of nutrition or metabolism; shortening of a muscle.

ebonation: (L) *e*, out + (A-S) *ban*, bone. Removal of bony fragments from a wound.

eburnate: (L) *eburnus, ivory;* refers to changes in bone density to an ivory-like structure in a process called *eburnation.*

ecchymosis: (G) *ek,* out + *chymos,* juice + *osis,* condition; *ecchy,* extravasation + *mosis,* to pour, shed. Extravasation of blood into tissue.

edema: (G) *oedema,* a swelling. Hippocrates referred to fluid buildup in tissue as oedematous, and the term continues to this day.

effusion: (L) escape of fluid.

elbow: (A-S) from *elboga; eln,* forearm + *boga,* bend. From *ell,* a measure of length used in early times from shoulder to fingers; *boga* was a bending or bow.

embolus: (G) plug.

enarthrosis: (G) *en,* in + *arthron,* joint; a ball-and-socket joint.

en bloc: (Fr) as a whole; in surgery to remove as a whole or a lump.

enchondroma: (G) *en,* within + *chondro,* cartilage + *oma,* tumor; tumor within cartilage.

endoskeleton: (G) *endo,* within + (A-S) *skeleton;* the bony and cartilaginous parts of the skeleton that develop from mesoderm and not ectoderm and that are buried within the soft parts.

endosteum: (G) *endo,* within; medullary cavity of bone.

ensiformus: (L) *ensis,* sword + *forma,* shape. Part of breastbone (xiphoid).

enthesis: (Gr) a putting in. The use of metallic or other inert substances to substitute for or replace lost tissue.

epicondyle: (G) *epi,* upon + *kondylos,* a knuckle, knob. Prominence on bone above or upon a condyle.

epidermis: (L) *epi,* upon + *dermis,* skin. Outer layer of skin.

epilepsy: (G) *epi,* upon + *lepsy,* falling sickness. Ancient term referring to infliction, seizures. The French terms are *petit mal* (short) and *grand mal* (large).

epimysium: (G) *epi,* upon + *mys,* muscle. The fibrous sheath enclosing a muscle.

epiphysis: (G) *epi,* upon + *physis,* outgrowth. Center of ossification where a part of the process ossifies separately before making an osseous union with the main portion of bone.

epithelium: (G) *epi,* upon + *thele,* nipple. Areas with nipplelike papillae. Term usually applied for the skin. The cognate word *endothelium* is usually applied to blood vessel inner lining and mesothelium to visceral lining such as the lung pleura and lining of the peritoneal cavity.

eponychium: (L) from *onyx,* nail; the structure from which the nail develops.

equilibrium: (L) *aequus,* equal + *libra,* balance. State of balance. Condition in which contending forces are equal.

equina: (L) from *equus,* horse; refers to equinovarus and valgus (a form of clubfoot).

erythema: (G) *erythros,* red + *ema,* condition. To redden, to blush.

erythropoietic: (G) *erythros,* red + *poietic,* suffix for making or producing.

ethmoid: (G) *ethmos,* a sieve + *oeides,* form, shape, resembles. Cribriform, sievelike. Perforations of the ethmoid plate.

etiology: (G) aetiology; refers to studying causes of disease.

eversion: (L) out + *ventere,* to turn the foot out at the ankle between the talus and calcaneus.

exacerbate: (L) *ex,* out + *acerbus,* harsh, bitter; from *exacerbare* and exasperate, an increase in symptoms, a flare-up, to make worse.

exostosis: (G) *ex,* out + *os,* bone + *osis,* condition. A bony outgrowth.

extrinsic: (L) *extrinsecus,* coming from; *extra,* outside + *secus,* otherwise.

euphoria: (A-S) *eu-,* well, good + *phoria,* being; a condition of good health.

fabella: (L) dim. of *faba,* a bean; a bean-shaped sesamoid fibrocartilage that may develop in the lateral head of the gastrocnemius muscle behind the knee joint.

facet: (Fr) *facette,* little face; refers to the small, smooth articular surface of bone as in facet joints of the spine.

falciform: (L) *falx,* sickle + *forma,* shape; triangular ligament of ischium (inguinal ligament).

falx: (L) sickle-shaped structure; denotes a ligamentous opening (e.g., conjoined tendon).

fascia: (L) a band, bandage. Anatomic fasciae denote sheathlike fibrous connective tissue that supports, separates, and covers muscles, joints, and other tissues of the body.

femur: (L) dim. of *ferendum,* bearing; bearing weight as in the thigh bone.

fenestra: (L) a window; to open or make a window; fenestrate, fenestration.

fiber: (L) *fibra,* threadlike; (G) fibrin, fibroid.

fibula: (L) a small clasp, or needlelike point, a broach, buckle; (G) anything pointed or piercing. Long, thin bone of lower limb behind the tibia.

fissure: (L) *fissura,* a cleft or groove; any groove in bone or fascia.

flap: (Dutch) *flappens,* to strike; named for a pedicle graft covering bone after resection.

flavum: term for *yellow;* refers to band of yellow elastic tissue of laminae of spine, called *yellow ligament* or *ligamentum flavum.*

flexor: (L) *flectere,* to bend; any muscle that flexes or bends a joint; flexion.

foramen: (L) *forare, foro,* to pierce; a natural opening or passageway in bone, fascia, vessels, or nerves; to pass through (e.g., obturator foramen).

fossa: (L) *fovea,* pit or hollow; (Fr) *fodere,* to dig. Any hollow depression in bone.

fracture: (L) *fractura,* a break; (Fr) *frangere,* to break.

ganglion: (G) *ganglia,* a knot, mass, tumor swelling.

gastrocnemius: (G) *gaster,* belly + *kneme,* leg. Refers to the large superficial calf muscle of the posterior lower limb.

gemellus: (L) for twin; one of two muscles inserted in the obturator internus tendon.

Genu-: (L) to bend. Geniculum referred to a knot or node. (G) *gony, gonu,* knee; genu recurvatum, valgus, and varus.

gladiolus: (L) dim. of *gladius,* a sword; main part of sternum.

glenoid: (G) *glene,* shallow socket + *oeides,* shape. Cup-shaped depression of scapula of shoulder.

glia: (G) glue; supporting tissue of spinal cord.

gluteal: (G) *gloutos,* a rump, buttock; any rounded eminence; gluteus maximus.

gout: (L) *gutta,* a drop, meaning poison falling drop by drop into a joint as a cause of pain and disease. Hippocrates described gout in the foot as *podagra.*

gracilis: (L) thin, lean, slender; a muscle of the thigh.

hallux: (G) *hallus, allomai,* to leap; (L) great toe, hallucis.

hamate: (L) *hamatus, hamatum,* hooklike process; hamate bone of wrist.

hamstring: (A-S) ham, back of thigh; flexor tendons behind knee that stand out like cords.

hang nail: (A-S) *angnaegl,* from *ange,* troublesome + *naeagl,* nail.

hemiplegia: (G) *hemi-,* half + *plege,* a stroke. Paralysis affecting one side of body.

histology: (G) *histos,* woven web + *logos,* a treatise; *histo* refers to any woven material, a web, and in Homer, the sail of a ship. The tissue structure of an organism or part.

humerus: (L) ossa humeri that involved the scapula, clavicle, and humerus. Later changed to mean only upper arm bone.

hyaline: (G) *hyalos,* glass; hyaloid, glasslike that denotes clear matrix (e.g., hyaline cartilage of joint surfaces).

hyoid: (G) U-shaped; from Greek letter upsilon.

idiopathic: (G) *idios,* own, peculiar to oneself + *pathos,* disease. Refers to a condition or disease state without known cause.

index: (L) from *dico,* to point out, a pointer; hence, the forefinger (pl. *indices*).

ilium: (L) flank, from ilia, soft parts, because the iliac bone supports the gut. It is the wide portion of bone of the pelvis.

incarnatus: to grow, as in to grow a fingernail or toenail.

infection: (L) *infectum,* from *inficere,* to taint or tinge; to alter by invasion of a pathogenic agent, to infect.

inflammation: (L) *inflammatic,* from *inflammare,* to burn, or flame within. In the eighteenth century, Sauvages introduced suffix *-itis* to refer to inflammation.

infrapatellar: (L) *infra-,* prefix for below, under + *patellar*; knee cap.

infraspinatus: (L) *infra-,* beneath + *spina,* thorn; beneath scapular spine.

innervation: (L) *in,* into + *nervus,* a nerve. Reciprocal innervation refers to muscles moving a joint.

innominate: (L) innominatus, from *in,* without + *nomen,* name. Given to three bones of the pelvis where compound bone was not named.

insertion: (L) *in,* into + *serere,* to plant. Place of attachment of muscle into bone which it moves.

in situ: (L) in position, in original place.

interossei: *inter,* between + *ossei,* bone; situated between bones, such as specific muscles of the hands and feet, muscles, ligaments, or vessels.

intramedullary: (L) within + *medullaris,* marrow. Within marrow cavity of bone.

intrinsic: (L) *intrinsecus,* situated inside; thus intrinsic muscles have their origin and insertion entirely within a structure and thereby are limited to it.

insertion: (L) *in,* into + *serere,* to plant. Place of attachment of a muscle into a bone that it moves.

interstitial: lying between; spaces within an organ or tissue.

in toto: (L) as a whole.

inversion: (L) *ventere,* to turn; to turn foot inward at the ankle.

in vitro: (L) in glass, as in a test tube.

in vivo: (L) in the living body or organism; a test performed on living organisms.

involucrum: from *volvere,* to wrap; a covering of newly formed bone enveloping the sequestrum in infection of bone.

ischemic: (G) *isch,* to keep back + *aemia,* blood. Deficiency of blood to a part, ischemia.

ischium: (G) *ischion,* hip, meaning strength; lowermost bone of innominate bones forming the bony pelvis, seat bone; (L) coxa.

joint: (L) *junctura, junctio,* from *jungere,* to join; the point of articulation between two bones.

juxtaposition: (L) near, close proximity + *positio,* place. Adjacent to or side by side.

kinematics: (G) *kinematos,* movement; relates to biomechanics and muscle movements.

knuckle: (Ger) *knokel;* (L) *articulus,* joint segment. Prominence of the distal heads of the metacarpals or dorsal aspect of any of the phalangeal joints.

kyphosis: (G) *kypho,* hump + *-osis,* condition. Convex prominence of spine.

lacuna: (L) a pit, hollow space; refers to microscopic resorption areas in bone, cartilage, or cementum. *Lacunula,* small or minute lacuna.

lamella: (L) a little plate, dim. of lamina; layer of bone or ground substance of osseous tissue situated in places within bone.

lamina: (L) flat plate; refers to flattened part of either side of the vertebral arch when used alone.

latissimus: (L) *latus,* broad; refers to latissimus dorsi back sheath muscle.

leio: (G) *leios,* smooth; prefix that refers to muscles.

lepto: (G) *leptos,* slender (e.g., *leptodactyly,* abnormally slim fingers).

levator: (L) *levo,* to lift, raise a part; refers to levator musculi.

ligamentum: (L) *ligare,* to tie, bind + *mentum,* a bandage. Fibrous band of tissue connecting articular ends of bone serving to bind them together to facilitate or limit motion, or to support viscera.

limbus: (L) edge, fibrocartilaginous rim of a joint; refers to glenoid (shoulder) and acetabulum (hip).

linea aspera: (L) *linea,* line + *aspera,* rough. Roughened ridge on femur for insertion of adductus group of muscles.

lipos: (G) *lipos,* fat; lipoid, resembling fat.

lordosis: (G) *lordo,* curved, to bend; an exaggeration of the normal forward convexity in the lumbar region of the spine.

lumbar: (L) *lumbus,* loin; refers to lumbar region.

lumbrical: (L) *lumbricus,* worm; refers to the four small, wormlike muscles of the palm of the hand and foot.

lunate: (L) *luna,* moon; crescent-shaped bone in wrist.

lunula: (L) dim. of *luna;* refers to half-moon-shaped white area at base of nail.

lupus: (L) wolf; named for gradual skin disease, lupus erythematosus.

luxation: (G) *luxatio,* dislocation, from *luxo,* to dislocate; subluxate is a partial dislocation.

lymph: (L) *lympha,* water; clear, transparent fluid found in lymphatic vessels.

magnum: (L) large or great; capitate bone, formerly called *os magnum,* the largest of carpal bones.

malacia: (G) *malakia,* softening; as of abnormal tissue softening.

malaise: (Fr) discomfort; indisposed, not well.

malleolus: (L) *malleus,* small hammer; refers to bony eminences on either side of the ankle. mandible; (L) *mandibula,* horseshoe-shaped bone of lower jaw.

manubrium: (L) a handle, from *manus,* hand + *hibrium* or *habeo,* to hold. Named for uppermost part of sternum (manubrium sterni) that is similar to the handle of a sword.

manus: (L) the hand; (G) *cheir.*

marrow: (A-S) *mearh,* unknown origin; (L) medulla. The spinal cord was formerly called the *spinal marrow* (fourteenth c.). Now, any soft central part of bone.

matrix: (L) *mater*, mother tissue; refers to intercellular substance of tissue, the formative portion of a structure.

maxilla: (L) upper jaw; paired bone with several processes.

mediastinum: (L) *medius*, middle + *stare*, to stand; taken from *per medium tensum*, that which is tight down the middle. (The term is applied to partitions and in no way is connected to the word *mediastinus* of Latin origin.)

medicine: (L) *medicina*, the art of healing; *medicor* meant to heal or cure. From thirteenth century, medicus applied to anyone associated with the art of healing in the care and treatment of patients.

medullary: (L) *medullaris*, marrow, from medius, middle (medio ossis); refers to the medullary cavity, medulla.

meninges: (G) *meninx*, a membrane; refers to membranes investing the spinal cord and brain.

-melia: (G) *melos*, limb; refers to absence of a limb (e.g., hemimelia).

meniscus: (G) *meniskos*, crescent-shaped, dim. of *mene*, moon; the medial and lateral crescent-shaped intraarticular fibrocartilage in the knee.

metabolic: (G) *metaballein*, to change; refers to metabolism.

metacarpus: (G) *meta*, beyond + *karpus*, wrist. Five bony rays distal to the wrist.

metaphysis: (G) *meta*, beyond + *physis*, growth. The line of junction of the epiphysis and the diaphysis.

metaplasia: (G) *meta*, beyond + *plasia*, to form. Virchow described connective tissue group changes into another tissue of the same group, such as cartilage into bone.

metatarsal: (G) *meta*, beyond + *tarsos*, ankle. Five bony rays distal to the tarsal bones of the foot.

mnemonic: (G) memory; a very old system for remembering, dating back to 477 BC.

monostotic: (G) *mon*, single + *osteon*, bone; refers to a single bone.

mucous: (L) *muco*, slimy exudate from membrane.

muscle: (L) little mouse, dim. of *mus*, mouse and (G) *myo*; probably derived from the way muscles move under the skin.

myo-: (G) muscle; prefix denoting relationship to muscle

myelos-: (G) marrow, the pith of plants; refers to the marrow cavity of the spinal cord.

navicular: (L) *navicula*, little boat, dim. of *navis*, a ship; boat-shaped structure hollowed out in form. Both navicular and scaphoid are used for the boat-shaped carpal and tarsal bones.

necrosis: (G) *nekrosis*, state of death; sequestrum of bone, sloughing of soft tissue. Insufficient blood supply to a part resulting in death of tissue.

nerve: (L) *nervus*, sinew and (G) *neuron*, sinew; refers to the nerve cells.

neurolemma: (G) *neuro*, nerve + *lemma*, sheath, husk. A thin membranous sheath covering a nerve fiber.

neuroma: (G) neuron, formerly any type of tumor composed of nerve cells.

nodule: (L) *nodulus*, a knot; refers to a small node or collection of cells.

nuchae: (L) nucha, back of neck; refers to neck area.

nucleus: (L) *nux*, nut, a little nut; the central part of a cell.

obturator: (L) *obturare/obturo*, to stop up, obstruct, or occlude; a membrane that covers an opening (e.g., obturator foramen).

occult: (L) from *occulere*, to hide or cover over; occultus, hidden, concealed.

odontoid: (G) *ondon*, tooth + *oid*, resembles; toothlike process of second cervical vertebra.

olecranon: (G) *olenes kranon, kranos*, helmet, olekranon, point of the elbow; elbow process at the proximal end of the ulna.

omo-: (G) *omos*, shoulder; prefix used in combining form (e.g., omovertebral).

omohyoid: (G) *omos*, shoulder + *hyoeides*, U-shaped. Shoulder muscle formerly called omohyoid because the muscle was attached to the scapula at one end and the hyoid bone at the other.

onco: (G) *onkos*, bulk, mass; prefix used in combining form (e.g., oncogene, a gene associated with tumors).

onychia: (G) *onychos, onyx*, nail; (L) *unguis*. Inflammation of nail bed.

opponens: (L) opposing; applied to the muscles of the hand and foot (e.g., thumb opposed to other digits).

organ: (G) *organon*, (L) *organum*, viscus, viscera.

orifice: (L) *orificium*, a natural opening.

orthopaedic: (G) *orthos*, straight + *paes*, a child. Literally means straightening of children. First introduced in 1741 by Nicholas Andry, French physician, who published the first book on orthopaedics. He proposed to prevent and correct deformities in children by exercise, diet, and mechanical means. His was the first work specifically devoted to the subject.

os: (L) *os, ossis*, bone; ossicle, ossiculum, small bone. (G) *oste*, allows for use in combining form.

ossification: (L) *os*, bone + *facere, to* make. Process of bone formation.

osteoblast: (G) *osteo*, bone + *blast*, a germ or sprout. A bone-producing cell.

osteoclast: (G) *osteo*, bone + *klasis*, to break up. Concerned with absorption and removal of unwanted tissue.

osteogenesis: (G) *osteo*, bone + *genesis*, origin. Bone production.

osteophyte: (G) *osseo*, bone + *phyte*, outgrowth; bony excrescence branched in shape.

pain: (L) *poena*, a fine, a penalty.

palmaris: (L) palm, hand; palmaris longus and brevis muscles of hand.

palpate: (L) *palpare, palpabilis*, to touch; perceptible by feel, touch.

palsy: (Fr) *paralysie*, (ME) *parlesie*; term *palsy* appeared in 1300.

paralysis: (G) *para*, besides + *lysis*, to loosen, *paralyein*, to disable. Disabling limb condition.

paraplegia: (G) *para*, besides + *plegia*, a stroke. Formerly meant stricken on one side, and now refers to paralysis of both limbs and maybe the trunk.

paratenon: *para*, around + *tenon*, tendon; fatty tissue surrounding tendon to fill in spaces.

paresis: (G) *parienai*, to let fall or pass; referred to muscle weakening and now includes partial paralysis.

pars: (L) a part of a larger structure; the pars interarticularis bridges the spine between articular facets.

paronychia: (G) *para*, besides + *nychia*, a nail. Refers to infection of marginal area of nail.

patella: (L) a saucer, small pan, dim. of *patera*, a round plate, and *patere*, to lie open or exposed; the kneecap.

patency: (L) *patens*, open, evident.

pathology: (G) *pathema*, disease + *logos*, word, reason. Study of the nature and cause of disease.

pectineus: (L) *pecten*, comb; muscle that flexes and adducts the thigh.

pectoralis: (L) from *pectus*, the breast; ancient term for an ornamental breast plate that was later included in medicine to mean the pectoralis major and minor muscles of the chest.

pedicle: (L) *pes, pedis*, foot, and *pediculus*, a little foot, stem; referred to stalks of plants originally, and later to structures of anatomy.

pelvis: (L) a basin, (G) tub or wooden bowl; any basin-shaped structure or cavity. Named for the large three innominate bones.

periosteum: (G) *peri*, around + *osteon*, bone. Hard protective fibrous membrane covering bone.

peritoneum: (G) *peri*, around + *teinein*, to stretch. Serous membrane that supports the abdominal cavity.

peroneal: (G) *perone*, pin, sewing needle, anything pointed for piercing; (L) fibula, brooch. Peroneal relates to the fibula; peroneus, perone, relates to one of three muscles of the leg causing motion of the foot.

pes: (L) *pedis*, a foot or footlike projection; applied to different structures such as pes cavus (hollow), pes planus (flat), pes anserinus (goose foot).

phalanges: (G) *phalanx*, a band of soldiers; (L) *internodia*, because joints of fingers and toes were called nodes in close knit row. Refers to the distal, medial, and proximal phalanges of the hands and feet; phalanx, line.

Phlebo-: (G) *phleps, phlebos*, vein; combining form for vein.

physician: (Fr) *physicien*; one who has successfully completed a prescribed course of studies in medicine.

physio: (G) prefix for nature.

physis: (G) *phyein*, to generate growth; portion of long bone involved in growth (e.g., diaphysis and epiphysis).

Pia: (L) soft, thin vascular membrane investing the brain and spinal cord; innermost of the three meninges (dura mater, pia mater, arachnoid).

pinna: a static, winglike projection.

piriformis: (L) pirun, a pear + *forma*, shape; piriformis muscle.

pisiform: (L) *pisum*, pea + *forma*, shape. Pea-shaped bone of wrist and smallest of carpal bones, proximal row, ulnar side.

placebo: (L) for shall please; an inactive agent designed to appear the same as an active therapeutic agent.

plantar: (L) *planta,* sole of foot, and (G) *platus, planus,* flat; from (L) *plantaris,* a sprout, twig, plant.

plaster: (G) *emplastron,* to form, mold. Hippocrates and Galen wrote extensively on the subject. Pliny described it in making casts. Originally, bandages were made of starch and paste, lime, and egg white. The gypsum variety was made in Paris, thus *plaster of Paris.*

-plasty: (G) suffix meaning to form or fashion.

pleura: (G) a rib. Now applied to serous membrane lining the chest wall.

plexus: (L) a braid, plait, entanglement; a complex, especially of blood and lymphatic vessels, and nerves (e.g., brachial plexus).

plica: (L) plicae, a fold; a fold, pleat, band or shelf of synovial membrane that projects into a joint cavity.

pollicis: (L) thumb, from *polleo,* strong; (pl. *pollices*); refers to the pollicis longus and brevis of the hand (formerly called *pollex*).

popliteal: (L) *poples,* the ham; ancient term from *plicare,* to fold. Refers to the popliteus muscle behind the knee between the hamstrings that flexes the leg and aids in rotation.

prima fasciae: (L) according to first appearance before final examination.

profundus: (L) deep seated; refers to source located deeper than indicated reference point (e.g., profundus tendon). Opposite of sublimis.

prognosis: (G) foreknowledge, prediction of course of disease and recovery.

pronator: (L) *pronatus,* prone (face down), from *pronare,* to bend forward and *pronus,* turned, inclined; pronator muscle that allows pronation. Vesalius used *pronum* and *supinum* to refer to muscles.

proprioceptive: (L) *proprius,* one's own, special + *capere,* to take, seize. A perception of sensations that creates awareness of what's going on within the body.

prosthesis: (G) prosthesis, an addition.

proximal: (L) nearest point of reference.

pseudo: (G): prefix for false, not true

psoas: (G) *psoa;* one of two muscles of the loins.

pubis: (L) grown up; anterior part of innominate bone, anterior pelvic bone.

pulse: (L) *pulsus,* beating; pulsate, *pulsare,* throb.

quadriceps: (L) *quadri,* four + *caput,* head. Four-headed as a quadriceps muscle.

rachio: (G) *rhachis,* spinal column; used in combining form.

radius: (L) a staff, rod, spoke of a wheel; (G) *radix,* a ray. The distal radius rotates around the distal ulna through a radius of 180 degrees.

ramus: (L) rami, branch; a branch of any given artery or nerve of the spine, extension.

ray: (L) radius; in orthopaedics, refers to the five rays of bones in the hands and feet.

rectus: (L) straight; refers to rectus abdominus muscle of the abdomen.

reflex: (L) *reflexus,* to bend back and (G) *reflectere,* to turn back; used to describe muscle movements of the body.

resection: (L) *resectio,* a cutting off; partial excision of a bone.

retinaculum: (L) halter, a tether, from *retinere,* to restrain; restraining fibers of fascia that hold a part in place (e.g., the patellar retinaculum, fibers that surround the knee cap and knee, and the flexor and extensor retinacula of the palm of the hand).

retroversion: (L) *retro,* back + *versio,* a turning.

rheumatoid: (G) *rheuma,* discharge + *eidos,* form, shape, resembling rheumatism.

rhexis: (G) a rupture of any organ, blood vessel or tissue.

rhomboids: (G) rhombus, kite-shaped; a four-sided figure with all sides equal. Refers to the rhomboid muscles, greater and lesser.

rickets: (A-S) to twist.

sacrum: (L) *sacer,* sacred, holy. In ancient times, the sacrum was used in sacrificial rites because it was the last bone to decay, and it was believed that the body would reform around it. Largest of vertebral bones, it protects and supports the lower organs.

sagittal: (L) *sagitta,* an arrow; the sagittal suture resembles an arrow. The sagittal plane is the medial vertical plane in line with the suture (i.e., the median plane of the body).

saphenous: (Arabic) *al safin,* hidden; saphenous vein or nerve in the lower limbs.

sarcolemma: (G) *sarx,* flesh + *lemma,* sheath. The delicate membranous sheath surrounding each individual muscle fiber.

sartorius: (L) *sartor,* a tailor; refers to a muscle whose action is to bring the leg into a flexed, adducted, and laterally rotated cross-legged sitting position habitually adopted by tailors.

scaleneus: (G) *scalenos,* uneven; refers to a triangle with unequal sides, and named for the neck muscle group of unequal length composed of the medius, minimus, and anterior m.

scaphoid: (G) *skaphe,* a small boat, and (L) *scapha,* skiff; scooped out, hence, boat-shaped bones in the hands and feet.

scapula: (L) *scapulae,* resembling a trough or digging tool and (G) *spathula,* broad implement, resembling a spade; the large, flat, triangular bone of the shoulder that articulates with the clavicle and humerus, shoulder blades.

sciatic: (L) *sciaticus,* and (G) *ischion,* a hip joint; refers to pain in the loins and hip, and is associated with the large sciatic nerve.

sclerosis: German in origin; meant degeneration of tissue. Later, referred to a hardening process.

scoliosis: (G) a curvature. In early times, meant anything bent or curved. Now refers specifically to a lateral curvature of the spine.

seizure: (Fr) *seiser,* a sudden attack of pain of certain symptoms of disease.

semilunar: (L) *semi,* half + *luna,* moon. The crescent-shaped lunate bone of carpus, lunate bone.

septum: (L) *saeptum,* a partition.

sequestrum: (L) *sequestrare,* to separate, set aside; fragment of necrosed bone that has detached from surrounding tissue.

serratus: (L) *serra,* a saw, serrated, having a sawtooth edge; serratus anterior muscles, anterior (chest) and posterior (back).

sesamoid: (G) *sesamon,* sesame plant + *-oid,* resembling. In Arabic, is *sem sem,* a sesame seed. Seed-shaped bones or fibrocartilage situated in tendons that move over a bony surface.

sinister: (L) to the left; left hand.

skeleton: (G) *skeletos,* a dried up body; the framework of the body consisting of 206 bones.

soleus: (L) *solea,* a flat fish; the flat, triangular-shaped muscle that inserts into the tendocalcaneus of the lower limbs.

spasm: (G) *spasmos,* convulsion, to draw out or pluck; refers to tonic or clonic muscle spasms.

spica: (L) ear of grain. Compares the overlapping of a cast to an ear of corn.

spina: (L) a thorn, (G) *spondylos*. In anatomy, thorn-like projections were called *spines* dating back to the fourteenth century; the vertebral column with its spinous processes.

spinalis: (L) a muscle attached to a spinal process of a vertebrae.

splay foot: (ME) *splayen,* to spread out + (A-S) *foot.* Flatfoot, pes planus.

splenius: flat muscle on either side of the back of the neck and upper thoracic region.

spondylo: (G) spine; prefix used in combining form to refer to the vertebrae; *spondylolisthesis,* to slip.

sprain: (L) *exprimere,* to press, squeeze, strain; (Fr) *espraindre,* to wring.

spur: (A-S) a pointed instrument. Refers to calcaneus of heel and femoral neck of femur (medial and underside where spurs are likely to occur).

stenosis: (G) *stenos,* narrow, a stricture; narrowing of a passageway.

sternum: (G) *sternon,* breast, chest + *steros,* hard, solid, and palpable. Thus the breastbone is composed of the manubrium (top portion), gladiolus (body), and ensiform or xiphoid process (lower portion).

stethoscope: (G) *stethos,* chest + *skopein,* to examine. Instrument used to mediate the sounds produced within the body.

styloid: (G) *stylos,* pillar and (L) *stilus,* any long, pointed instrument; the ulnar styloid is the large prominence of bone at the back of the wrist.

sublimis: (L) uplifted, up in the air; applied to physical position, such as sublimus tendon near the surface.

subclavian: (L) *sub,* under, below + *clavis,* key. Refers to muscle, artery, or vein under the clavicle (collar bone).

subscription: (L) *subscriptus,* written under.

sulcus: (L) groove; plural sulci. The sulci cutis are the ridges on the skin of the palmar surface of fingers that comprise the fingerprints.

superficialis: (L) superficial. Denotes an artery, vein, or nerve close to the surface.

supination: (L) *supinatio*, turning face upward; supinator muscle of forearm, or that of leg, turning leg or foot outward.

supraspinatus: (L) *supra*, above + *spinatus*, spines or thorn-shaped. Refers to the supraspinatus muscle above the spine of the scapula.

sural: (L) *sura*, calf; refers to calf muscle group, triceps surae (gastrocnemius, plantaris, and soleus muscles).

sustentaculum: (L) a supporting structure.; a process of the calcaneum that supports part of the astragalus.

surgeon: (G) from *chirurgeon, cheir*, meaning the hand + *ergon*, to work. One who works with the hands.

symphysis: (G) *syn*, together + *phyein*, to grow, growing together; a natural union. Refers to the symphysis pubis, two articular bones joined by fibrocartilage.

symptom: (G) *symptoma*, occurrence.

synarthrosis: (G) *syn*, together + *arthrosis*, a joint. An immovable joint.

syndesmosis: (G) *syn*, together + *desmos*, a band. A joint in which two bones are held together by ligaments.

syndrome: (G) concurrence, running together; clinical picture of a disease made by the presence of several typical signs and symptoms.

synergists: (G) *syn*, together + *ergon*, work, to cooperate. Refers to the smooth coordinated way in which muscles work together in the execution of movement, such as the synergist muscle group, organs, or parts acting in unison.

synostosis: (G) *syn*, together + *osteon*, bone. The union of two bones by osseous tissue such as the diaphysis and epiphysis of a long bone at the end of the growth period.

synovium: (G) *syn*, together + *oon*, egg, (L) ovum, egg white. Refers to the egg white appearance of fluid present in movable joints.

tabatiere anatomique: (Fr) anatomic snuff box; refers to space at the base of the thumb.

talipes: (L) *talipedare*, to be weak on the feet, to totter. Hence, talipes, club foot.

talus: (L) from Cicero, *ludere talis*, to play at dice, and *taxillus*, dice; bone resembling dice because dice were carved from the calcaneus of a horse. Talus, ankle bone.

tarsus: (G) from *tarsomai*, to become dry, tarsos; referred to anything flat or spread out. Thus applied to the flat part of the feet.

tectorial: (L) *tectum*, roof; pertains to a roof or covering.

tendon: (L) *tendere*, to stretch out; (Gr) *tenon*, a tightly stretched band; the elongated end of a muscle. Syn. sinew.

tensor: (L) *tendere*, tensum, to stretch; named for muscle that tenses or stretches and does not alter the direction of a part (e.g., tensor fascia).

teres: (L) from *terere*, to rub or grind smooth, well turned or rounded off; refers to the ligamentum teres, round ligament of the hip.

thecal: (G) sheath, capsule; relates to a tendon sheath, theca.

thenar: (G) from *theino*, to strike; referred to flat part of hand used to strike. Now refers to muscles of the palm divided into groups called thenar (major group) and hypothenar (lesser group).

thoraco: (G) thorax, chest, breast plate, stethos. In classical Greek, the thorax was armor (breastplate) to protect the chest and abdomen.

therapy: (G) *therapeia*, treatment, remedy, cure. First referred to the noun, *therapeutae*, healers, and later included treatment.

tibialis: (L) a pipe or flute, shin bone, variant of *tubia*, tube. In ancient times, musical instruments were made from shin bones of animals and objects of tubular form. Tibia, the larger anterior bone of the lower limb.

tonic: (G) *tonikos*, from *tonos*, tone; refers to muscular tension or contraction.

tourniquet: (Fr) *tournier*, to turn. Originally applied to a stick that turned to tighten a bandage or apply pressure over a large artery to stop blood flow.

trabecula: (L) little beam, dim. of *trabs, trapes*, timber; any large wooden beam, such as the rib of a boat or strands of supporting fibers. Refers to beamlike pattern or arrangement of bony lamellae in cancellous bone and muscle bundles raised up beneath ventricular endocardium of heart.

trapezoid: (L) an irregular, four-sided figure; referred to a four-sided geometrical figure with two sides parallel to two sides divergent. Named for a carpal wrist bone (os magnum), the muscle was also called *musculus cucullaris* because together with its fellow of the opposite side, it resembled a monk's cowl or hood.

trapezius: (L) the flat, triangular muscle covering the posterior surface of the neck and shoulders.

trauma: (G) *tro,* to wound or hurt + *ma,* results of action. Any wound or injury to the body by exterior forces inflicted or by physical agent.

triceps: (G) *tri,* three + (L) *tres,* three + *ceps,* head; a three-headed muscle with a single insertion (e.g., triceps brachii in the arm and triceps surae of the lower limb that combines the gastrocnemius and soleus muscles).

triquetrum: (L) *triquetrus,* having three corners; refers to the wedge-shaped cuneiform bone of the wrist.

trochanter: (G) *trochos,* a wheel or runner; two bony processes below the neck of the femur for muscle attachment. Galen applied term to greater and lesser trochanters and bony protuberance because of the way it moved in the act of running; a lever to turn the wheel.

trochlea: (L) *trochilsa,* a pulley and (G) *trochos,* a wheel; refers to trochlea of humerus, an articular cylinder around which the ulna moves, similar to a pulley, but cylinder does not turn. A structure having the function of a pulley, a ring through which a tendon or muscle projects.

tubercle: (L) *tuberculum,* a little swelling; in orthopaedics, bony prominences that provide ligamentous attachment.

tuberosity: (L) tuberosities, to roughen; any roughened areas of bone for muscle attachment (e.g., greater tuberosity of the humerus).

ulna: (L) from *ell,* a measure of length; (Gr) *olene,* the elbow. In earlier times, the word denoted the whole arm, and now refers to the inner and larger bone of the forearm and elbow opposite the thumb side.

unguis: (L) claw, talon, nail; the toe or fingernails under the nail bed.

uniceps: (L) *unus,* one + *ceps,* head. Having a single head or origin.

unilateral: (L) *unus,* one + *latus,* side; occurring on one side.

valgus: (L) bent outward, bow-legged; also, talipes valgus; hallux valgus, distal to a point outward, genu valgus.

varus: (L) bent, turned inward; talipes varus (foot), genu varum (knock-kneed).

vascular: (L) *vas,* a vessel or dish; hence, a vascular organ is one with a profuse blood supply.

vastus: (L) vast, wide and great; refers to the three large muscle groups of the thigh (v. lateralis, v. medialis, v. intermedius).

vena: (L) vein, vessel; refers to the vena cava, the large vein leading to the heart with an upper and lower distribution.

vertebrae: (L) joint, from *vertere,* to turn and *vertebratus,* jointed or articulated. Refers to the 33 bony segments of the spinal column.

viability: (L) *vita,* life + *habilis,* fit. The ability to live, grow, and develop.

vinculum: (L) a band, cord, or anything that binds; from *vincio,* I bind; ringlike ligaments of the wrists and ankles; blood vessel bridges to the flexor tendons (brevis and longus), vinculae.

viscera: (L) *vis,* strength, casing, cavity; internal organs enclosed in the abdominal cavity and thorax.

volar: (L) *vola,* palm of hand or sole, from vola manus, hollow of hand; (Gr) *ballo,* to hurl. Palma referred to outstretched open hand.

vulnerable: (L) *vulnerare,* to wound; easily wounded.

whitlow: (ME) *whitflawe,* white flow; suppurative inflammation at the end of a finger or toe, deep-seated or superficial. Paronychia, felon.

wound: (A-S) *wund*; trauma to tissue.

xiphoid: (Gr) *xiphos,* a sword + *oeides,* shape; sword-shaped bone of the inferior tip of the sternum to which ribs attach (ensiformis).

Bibliography

General

American Academy of Orthopaedic Surgeons: In Heck CV, editor: *Fifty Years of Progress (1922–1983)*, Chicago, 1983, The Academy.

American Medical Association: *International classification of diseases 9th revision clinical modification*, Dover, Del, 1997, American Medical Association.

American Medical Association: *Manual of style*, ed 8, Baltimore, 1989, Williams & Wilkins.

American Orthopaedic Association: History of orthopaedics, 1–8. In *Manual of orthopaedic surgery*, Chicago, 1985, AAOS.

Anthony C, Kolthoff N: *Textbook of anatomy and physiology*, ed 9, St Louis, 1975, The CV Mosby Co.

Brasher RH, Raney RB: *Handbook of orthopaedic surgery*, ed 10, St Louis, 1986, The CV Mosby Co.

Canale ST, Beaty JH: *Campbell's operative orthopaedics*, ed 12, St. Louis, 2012, Elsevier.

Carroll K, Edelstein J: *Prosthetics and patient management: a comprehensive clinical approach*, 2006, Slack Incorporated.

Chabner DE: *The language of medicine*, ed 8, St Louis, 2007, Saunders Elsevier.

Cozen L: *Office orthopaedics*, ed 4, Springfield, Ill, 1975, Charles C Thomas.

Cyriax J: *Textbook of orthopaedic medicine: diagnosis of soft tissue lesions*, vol 1, ed 8, Philadelphia, 1984, Bailliere Tindall.

Dorland's illustrated medical dictionary, ed 32, Philadelphia, 2011, Saunders.

Glanz WD, et al.: *Mosby's medical and nursing dictionary*, ed 2, St Louis, 1986, The CV Mosby Co.

Hilt NE, Cogburn SB: *Manual of orthopaedics*, St Louis, 1977, The CV Mosby Co.

Hoppenfeld S, Zeide MS: *The orthopaedic dictionary*, Philadelphia, 1994, JB Lippincott.

Miller MD, Thompson SR, Hart J: *Review of orthopaedics*, ed 6, Philadelphia, 2012, Elsevier.

Reider B: *The orthopaedic physical examination*, Chicago, 2005, Saunders.

Simpson JA, Weiner ESC: *The Oxford English dictionary*, ed 2, Oxford, 1989, Clarendon Press/Oxford University Press.

Smith DG, Michael JW, Bowker JH: *Atlas of amputations and limb deficiencies*, ed 3, Chicago, 2004, AAOS.

Soukhanov AH, Ellis K, Cook L, et al: *Webster's II new riverside university dictionary*, Rolling Meadows, IL, 1984, Riverside Publishing Company.

Stedman's medical dictionary, ed 28, Baltimore, 2005, Lippincott Williams & Wilkins.

Thomas CL: *Taber's cyclopedic medical dictionary*, ed 22, Philadelphia, 2013, FA Davis.

Turek SL: *Orthopaedics: principles and their applications*, vol 1, ed 4, Philadelphia, 1984, JB Lippincott.

Fractures

Allman FL: Fractures and ligamentous injuries of the clavicle and its articulation, *J Bone Joint Surg* 49A(4):774–784, 1967.

Anderson IF: Osteochondral fractures of the dome of the talus, *J Bone Joint Surg* 71A:1143–1152, 1989.

Anderson LD, D'Alonzo RT: Fractures of the odontoid process of the axis, *J Bone Joint Surg* 56A(8):1663–1674, 1974.

Arslan H, Kapukaya A, Kesemenli C, Subasi M, Kayikçi C: Floating knee in children, *J Pediatr Orthop* 23(4):458–463, 2003.

Ashurst APC: Classification and mechanism of fractures of the leg bones involving the ankle: based on a study of three hundred cases from the Episcopal Hospital, *Arch Surg* 4:51–129, 1922.

Badelon O, Bensahel H, Mazda K, Vie P: Lateral humeral condylar fractures in children: a report of 47 cases, *J Pediatr Orthop* 8(1):31–34, 1988.

Bado JL: The Monteggia lesion, *Clin Orthop Rel Res* 50:71–86, 1967.

Beaty JH, Kasser JR, editors: *Rockwood and Wilkins' fractures in children*, ed 6, Philadelphia, 2006, Lippincott Williams & Wilkins.

Beaulé PE, Dorey FJ, Matta JM: Letournel classification for acetabular fractures. Assessment of interobserver and intraobserver reliability, *J Bone Joint Surg Am* 85-A(9):1704–1709, 2003.

Boyd HR, Griffin LL: Classification and treatment of trochanteric fractures, *Arch Surg* 58:853–866, 1949.

Buckholtz RW: Pathomechanics of pelvic ring disruptions, *Adv Orthop Surg* 10:167, 1987.

Bucholtz RW, Heckman JD, Court-Brown CM, et al., editors: *Rockwood and Green's fractures in adults*, ed 7, Philadelphia, 2010, Wolters Kluwer Health/Lippincott Williams & Wilkins.

Cabenela ME, Morrey BF: Fractures of the proximal ulna and olecranon. In Morrey BF, editor: *The elbow and its disorders*, Philadelphia, 1993, WB Saunders.

Canale ST, Kelly FB Jr: Fractures of the neck of the talus: long-term evaluation of seventy-one cases, *J Bone Joint Surg Am* 60(2):143–156, 1978.

Chadwick CJ, Bentley G: The classification and prognosis of epiphyseal injuries, *Injury* 18:157–168, 1987.

Colonna PC: Fracture of the neck of the femur in children, *Am J Surg* 6:793–797, 1929.

Colton CL: Fractures of the olecranon in adults: classification and management, *Injury* 5:121–129, 1973.

Craig EV: Fractures of the clavicle. In Rockwood CA Jr, Matsen FA, editors: *The shoulder*, Philadelphia, 1990, WB Saunders, pp 367–412.

Crenshaw AH: Fractures of shoulder girdle, arm and forearm. In Crenshaw AH, editor: *Campbell's operative orthopaedics*, ed 8, St Louis, 1991, Mosby-Year Book.

DePalma AF: In Connelly JF, editor: *The management of fractures and dislocations: an atlas*, vols 1-2, ed 3, Philadelphia, 1981, WB Saunders.

Dias LS, Tachdjian MO: Physeal injuries of the ankle in children, *Clin Orthop Rel Res* 136:230–233, 1978.

Essex-Lopresti P: The mechanism reduction technique and results in fractures of the os calcis, *Br J Surg* 39:395–419, 1952.

Evans EM, Wales SS: Trochanteric fractures, *J Bone Joint Surg* 33B(2):192–204, 1951.

Ferkel RD, Cheng MS, Applegate GR: A new method of arthroscopic staging of osteochondral lesions of the talus. Presented at the American Academy of Orthopaedic Surgeons, Orlando, Fla, February 17, 1995.

Ferkel RD, Sgaglione NA, Del Pizzo W, et al.: Arthroscopic treatment of osteochondral lesions of the talus: technique and results, *Orthop Trans* 14:172–173, 1990.

Fielding JW, Magliato HJ: Subtrochanteric fractures, *Surg Gyn Obs* 122:555–560, 1966.

Filan SL, Herbert TJ: Herbert screw fixation of scaphoid fractures, *J Bone Joint Surg Br* (78):519–529, 1996.

Frykman G: Fracture of the distal radius including sequelae-shoulder-hand-finger syndrome disturbance in the distal radio-ulnar joint and impairment of nerve function: a clinical and experimental study, *Acta Orthop Scand* 108(suppl):1, 1967.

Garden RS: Malreduction and avascular necrosis in subcapital fractures of the femur, *J Bone Joint Surg* 53B(2):183–197, 1971.

Gartland JJ: Management of supracondylar fractures of the humerus in children, *Surg Gynecol Obstet* 109:145–154, 1959.

Gustilo RB: *The fracture classification manual*, St Louis, 1991, Mosby-Year Book, Inc.

Gustilo RB, Mendoza RM, Williams DN: Problems in the management of type III (severe) open fractures, *J Trauma* 24:742, 1986.

Gustilo RB, Merkow RL, Templeman D: The management of open fractures, *J Bone Joint Surg* 72A:299–304, 1990.

Hardcastle PH, Reschauer R, Kutscha-Lissberg E, Schoffmann W: Injuries to the tarsometatarsal joint: incidence classification and treatment, *J Bone Joint Surg* 64B(3): 349–356, 1982.

Hawkins LG: Fracture of the neck of the talus, *J Bone Joint Surg* 52A(5):991–1002, 1970.

Helfet DL, Howey T, Sanders R, et al.: Limb salvage versus amputation. Preliminary results of the mangled extremity severity score, *Clin Orthop Rel Res* 256:80–86, 1990.

Herbert TJ, Fisher WE: Management of the scaphoid fracture using a new bone screw, *J Bone Joint Surg* 66B:114–123, 1984.

Hohl M, Moore TM: Articular fractures of the proximal tibia. In Evarts M, editor: *Surgery of the musculoskeletal system*, ed 2, New York, 1990, Churchill Livingstone.

Hoppenfeld S, Zeide MS: *The orthopaedic dictionary*, Philadelphia, 1994, JB Lippincott.

Ideberg R: Fractures of the scapula involving the glenoid fossa. In *Surgery of the shoulder*, Toronto, 1984, BC Decker, pp 63–66.

Jensen JS: Classification of trochanteric fractures, *Acta Orthop Scand* 51:803–810, 1980.

Johansson JE, McBroom R, Barrington TW, Hunter GA: Fracture of the ipsilateral femur in patients with total hip replacement, *J Bone Joint Surg* 63A:1435–1442, 1981.

Judet R, Judet J, Letournel E: Fractures of the acetabulum: classification and surgical approaches for open reduction: preliminary report, *J Bone Joint Surg* 46A(8):1615–1646, 1964.

Kanis JA, Johnell O, Oden A, Johansson H, McCloskey E: Osteoporosis international, *Osteoporos Int* 19(4):385–397, 2011.

Key JA, Conwell HE: *Management of fractures, dislocations and sprains*, St Louis, 1951, CV Mosby.

Kilfoyle RM: Fractures of the medial condyle and epicondyle in children, *Clin Orthop Rel Res* 41:43–50, 1965.

Klafs CE, Arnheim DD: *Modern principles of athletic training*, ed 5, St Louis, 1981, The CV Mosby Co.

Krishnan KB, Khanna G, Clohisy D: Gene translocation in musculoskeletal neoplasms, *Clin Orthop Relat Res* 466(9): 2131–2146, 2008.

Kulund DN: *The injured athlete*, Philadelphia, 1982, JB Lippincott.

Kuhn JE: Shoulder injuries in athletes: a new classification system for shoulder instability, *Br J Sports Med* 44:341–346, 2010.

Kyle RF, Gustilo RB, Premer RF: Analysis of six hundred and twenty-two intertrochanteric hip fractures, *J Bone Joint Surg* 61A(2): 216–221, 1979.

Lauge-Hansen N: Fractures of the ankle. II. Combined experimental-surgical and experimental-roentgenologic investigations, *Arch Surg* 60:957–985, 1950.

Letts M, Vincent N, Gouw G: The "floating knee" in children, *J Bone Joint Surg* 68B:442–446, 1986.

Levine AM, Edwards CC: The management of traumatic spondylolisthesis of the axis, *J Bone Joint Surg* 67A(2):217–226, 1985.

Mallory TH, Kraus TJ, Vaughn BK: Intraoperative femoral fractures associated with cementless total hip arthroplasty, *Orthopaedics* 12(2):231–239, 1989.

Mason ML: Some observations on fractures of the head of the radius with a review of one hundred cases, *Br J Surg* 42:123–132, 1954.

Mast JW, Spiegel PG, Pappas JN: Fractures of the tibial pilon, *Clin Orthop Relat Res* 230:68–82, 1988.

Meyers MH, McKeever FM: Followup notes: fracture of the intercondylar eminence of the tibia, *J Bone Joint Surg* 52A(8):1677–1684, 1970.

Milch H: Fractures and fracture dislocations of the humeral condyles, *J Trauma* 4:592–607, 1964.

Mora Guix JM, Pedrós JS: Castaño Serrano A: Updated classification system for proximal humeral fractures, *Clin Med Res* 7(1–2):32–44, 2009.

Müller ME, Allgöwer M, Schnieder R: *Manual of internal fixation*, ed 3, Berlin, 1991, Springer-Verlag. 152–157.

Müller ME, Nazarian S, et al.: *The comprehensive classification of fractures of long bones*, Berlin, 1990, Springer-Verlag.

Neer CSI: Displaced proximal humeral fractures. Part I: classification and evaluation, *J Bone Joint Surg* 52A(6):1077–1089, 1970.

Neer CSI, Howrowitz BS: Fractures of the proximal humeral epiphyseal plate, *Clin Orthop Rel Res* 41:24–31, 1965.

Oestern HH, Tscherne H: Pathophysiology and classification of soft tissue injuries associated with fractures. In Tscherne H, Gotzen L, editors: *Fractures with soft tissue injuries*, Berlin, 1984, Springer-Verlag, pp 1–8.

Ogden JA: Skeletal growth mechanism injury patterns, *J Pediatr Orthop* 2:371–377, 1982.

Ogden JA, Tross RB, Murphy MJ: Fractures of the tibial tuberosity in adolescents, *J Bone Joint Surg* 62A(2):205–215, 1980.

Owen R, Goodfellow J, Bullough P: *Scientific foundations of orthopaedics and traumatology*, London, 1980, William Heinemann Medical Books, Ltd.

Pauwels F: *Der Schenkenholsbruck, em mechanisches Problem Grundlagen des Heilungsvorganges Prognose und kausale Therapie*, Beilageheft zur Zeitschrift fur Orthopaedische Chirurgie, Stuttgart, 1935, Ferdinand Enke.

Peterson L: *Sports injuries*, Chicago, 1986, Year Book Medical Publishing.

Pipkin G: Treatment of grade IV fracture-dislocation of the hip, *J Bone Joint Surg* 39A(5):1027–1042, 1957.

Poland J: *Traumatic separation of the epiphysis*, London, 1898, Smith, Elder and Company.

Riseborough EJ, Radin EL: Intercondylar T fracture of the humerus in the adult: a comparison of operative and non-operative treatment in twenty-nine cases, *J Bone Joint Surg* 51A(1):130–141, 1969.

Rockwood CA: Subluxations and dislocations about the shoulder. In *Fractures in adults*, Philadelphia, 1984, JB Lippincott, pp 1192–1198.

Rockwood CA, Green D, Buckholtz RW: *Fractures in adults*, vol 1–2, ed 3, Philadelphia, 1984, JB Lippincott.

Rockwood CA, Wilkins KE, King RE: *Fractures in children*, vol 3, Philadelphia, 1984, JB Lippincott.

Rowe CR, Lowell JD: Prognosis of fractures of the acetabulum, *J Bone Joint Surg* 43A:30–59, 1962.

Rüedi T, Allgöwer M: Fractures of the lower end of the tibia into the ankle joint, *Injury* 1:92, 1969.

Russell TA: Fractures of the hip and pelvis. In Crenshaw AH, editor: *Campbell's operative orthopaedics*, ed 8, St Louis, 1991, Mosby-Year Book.

Salter RB, Harris WR: Injuries involving the epiphyseal plate, *J Bone Joint Surg* 45A:587–622, 1963.

Samilson RL, Preito V: Dislocation arthropathy of the shoulder, *J Bone Joint Surg* 65A(4):456–460, 1983.

Schatzker J, McBroom R, Bruce D: The tibial plateau fracture: the Toronto experience 1968–1975, *Clin Orthop Rel Res* 138:94–104, 1979.

Schultz RJ: *The language of fractures*, Huntington, New York, 1976, RE Krieger.

Seinsheimer FI: Subtrochanteric fractures of the femur, *J Bone Joint Surg* 60A(3):300–306, 1978.

Seligson D, Pope M: *Concepts in external fixation*, New York, 1982, Grune & Stratton.

Stewart MJ, Milford LW: Fracture-dislocation of the hip: an end result study, *J Bone Joint Surg* 36A:315–342, 1954.

Thompson VP, Epstein HC: Traumatic dislocation of the hip: a survey of 204 cases covering a period of twenty-one years, *J Bone Joint Surg* 33A(3):746–778, 1951.

Tile M: Pelvic ring fractures should they be fixed, *J Bone Joint Surg* 70B:1–12, 1988.

Torode I, Zieg S: Pelvic fractures in children, *J Pediatr Orthop* 5:76, 1985.

Tronzo RG: Special considerations in management, *Orthop Clin North Am* 5(3):571–583, 1974.

Watson-Jones R: *Fractures and joint injuries*, Edinburgh, 1955, E and S Livingston.

Weber BG: Die Verletzungen des oberen Spurnggelenkes. In Bern, editor: *Aktuelle Probleme in der Chirurgie Verlag Han Huber*, 1966.

Winquist RA, Hansen ST: Comminuted fractures of the femoral shaft treated by intramedullary nailing, *Orthop Clin North Am* 11(3):633–647, 1980.

Young JW, Burgess AR, Brumback RJ, Poka A: Pelvic fractures: value of plain radiography in early assessment and management, *Radiology* 160:445–451, 1986.

Zickle RE: An intramedullary fixation device for the proximal part of the femur: nine years experience, *J Bone Joint Surg* 58A:866–872, 1976.

Zuix JM, Pedrós JS, Serrano AC: Updated classification system for proximal humeral fractures, *Clin Med Res* 7(1-2):32–44, 2009.

Diseases

Aegerter E, Kirkpatrick JA: *Orthopaedic diseases: physiology, pathology, radiology*, ed 4, Philadelphia, 1975, WB Saunders.

Albright JA, Brand RA: *Scientific basis of orthopaedics*, New York, 1979, Appleton-Century-Crofts.

Altman R, Alarcón G, Appelrouth D, et al.: The American College of Rheumatology criteria for the classification and reporting of osteoarthritis of the hand, *Arthritis Rheum* 33(11):1601–1610, 1990.

American Academy of Orthopaedic Surgeons and the International Society for the Study of the Lumbar Spine. In *Glossary on spinal terminology*, Chicago, 1980, The Academy, pp 675–680.

Babis GC, Sakellariou V, Parvizi J, Soucacos P: Osteonecrosis of the femoral head, *Orthopedics* 34(1):39–48, 2011. Available at http://www.healio.com/orthopedics/hip/journals/ortho/%7B71a60ea4-ff86-414f-9e2d-95f5bf60f447%7D/osteonecrosis-of-the-femoral-head.

Beighton Hypermobility Score, *Soulderdoc.co.uk*, 2014. Available at. http://www.shoulderdoc.co.uk/article.asp?article=645.

Bogumill GP, Schwamm HA: *Orthopaedic pathology: a synopsis with clinical and radiographic correlation*, Philadelphia, 1984, WB Saunders.

Dietz FR, Matthews KD: Update on genetic bases of disorders with orthopaedic manifestations, *J Bone Joint Surg* 78A:1583–1598, 1996.

Disease Database. Available from http://www.diseasesdatabase.com/content.asp.

Enneking WF: A system of staging musculoskeletal neoplasms, *Clin Orthop* 204:9–24, 1986.

Enzinger FM, Weiss SW: *Soft tissue tumors*, ed 2, St Louis, 1988, CV Mosby.

Fitzgerald RH, et al.: Orthopedic knowledge update, *American Academy of Orthopedic Surgeons*, Chicago, 1987.

Frantz CH, O'Rahilly R: Congenital limb deficiencies, *J Bone Joint Surg* 43(8):1202–1224, 1961.

Frassica FJ, Thompson RC: Evaluation diagnosis and classification of benign soft-tissue tumors, *J Bone Joint Surg* 78A:126–140, 1996.

Gartland JJ: *Fundamentals of orthopaedics*, ed 5, Philadelphia, 1991, WB Saunders.

Hall CB, Lambert CN, O'Rahilly R, Swinyard CA: Nomenclature for congenital skeletal limb deficiencies a revision of the Frantz and O'Rahilly classification, *Artificial Limbs* 2(1):24–35, 1966. Available at http://www.oandplibrary.org/al/1966_01_024.asp.

Hamada K, Yamanaka K, Uchiyama Y, Mikasa T, Mikasa M: A radiographic classification of massive rotator cuff tear arthritis, *Clin Orthop Relat Res* 469(9):2452–2460, 2011.

International Organization for Standardization: IOS 8548-1: *Prosthetics and orthotics-Limb deficiencies, Part 1: Method of describing limb deficiencies present at birth*, Geneva, Switzerland, 1989, International Organization for Standardization.

Jawad MU, Scully SP: Classifications in brief: Mirels' classification: metastatic disease in long bones and impending pathologic fracture, *Clin Orthop Relat Res* 468(10):2825–2827, 2010.

Levesque J: *A clinical guide to primary bone tumors*, Philadelphia, 1998, Lippincott, Williams & Wilkins.

Mercier LR: *Practical orthopaedics*, ed 5, St Louis, 2000, Mosby.

The Merck manual of diagnosis and therapy, ed 16, Rahway, NJ, Merck Research Laboratories.

Mirra JM: *Bone tumors: clinical, radiographic, and pathologic correlations*, ed 2, Philadelphia, 1989, WB Saunders.

Mourad LA: *Orthopaedic disorders*, St Louis, 1991, Mosby-Year Book.

Pappas AM: Congenital abnormalities of the femur and related lower extremity malformations: classification and treatment, *Pediatr Orthop* 3(1):45–60, 1983.

Praemer A, Furner S, Rice DP: *AAOS musculoskeletal conditions in the US*, Chicago, 1999, AAOS.

Röder C, Staub LP, Eichler P, et al.: Avoiding misclassification bias with the traditional Charnley classification: rationale for a fourth Charnley class BB, *J Orthop Res* 24:1803–1808, 2006, http://dx.doi.org/10.1002/jor.20224.

Salter RB: *Textbook of disorders and injuries of the musculoskeletal system*, ed 2, Baltimore, 1984, Williams & Wilkins.

Schajowicz F, Ackerman IV, Sissons HA: Histological typing of bone tumors. In *International classification of tumors*, vol 6, Geneva, 1972, World Health Organization.

Seddon HJ: A classification of nerve injuries, *Br Med J* 2(4260):237–239, 1942.

Steinberg ME, Hayken GD, Steinberg DR: A quantitative system for staging avascular necrosis, *J Bone Joint Surg* 77B:34–41, 1995.

Sunderland S: A classification of peripheral nerve injuries producing loss of function, *Brain* 74(4):491–516, 1951.

Imaging

Bansal A: The dripping candle wax sign, *Radiology* 246(2):638–640, 2008.

Camacho MA: The double posterior cruciate ligament sign, *Radiology* 233(2):503–504, 2004.

Carlson CL: The "J" sign, *Radiology* 232(3):725–726, 2004.

Donnelly EF: The Hawkins sign, *Radiology* 210(1):195–196, 1999.

Ewald FC: Knee Society total knee arthroplasty roentgenographic evaluation and scoring system, *Clin Orthop* 248:9–13, 1989.

Gor DM: The trough line sign, *Radiology* 224(2):485–486, 2002.

Goswami GK: The fat pad sign, *Radiology* 222(2):419–420, 2002.

Greulich WW, Pyle SI: *Atlas of the development of the hand and wrist*, ed 2, Stanford, Calif, 1959, Stanford University Press.

Hollar MA: The hair-on-end sign, *Radiology* 221(2):347–348, 2001.

Homma M, Kumar J: An early sign of avascular necrosis and late lateral growth arrest of the proximal femur in development dislocation of the hip: clinical case presentation Alfred I, *DuPont Institute*, 1996. Retrieved from http://gait.aidi.udel.edu/educate/avn.htm.

Johnson TS: The spur sign, *Radiology* 235:1023–1024, 2005.

Lesniak B, Jose J, Gupta A: Magnetic resonance imaging double popliteus tendon sign: a case report, *Sports Health* 3(4):390–392, 2011.

Ly JQ: The four-tendon sign, *Radiology* 247(1):291–292, 2008.

Papadopoulou P: The celery stalk sign, *Radiology* 245(3):916–917, 2007.

Persaud T: The polka-dot sign, *Radiology* 246(3):980–981, 2008.

Talangbayan LE: The inverted Napolean's hat sign, *Radiology* 243(2):603–604, 2007.

Tanner JM, et al.: *Assessment of skeletal maturity and prediction of adult height (TW2) method*, ed 2, London, 1983, Academic Press.

Todd TW: *Atlas of skeletal maturity*, St Louis, 1937, The CV Mosby Co.

Wakely SL: The posterior vertebral scalloping sign, *Radiology* 239(2):607–609, 2006.

Test, Signs, and Maneuvers

American Academy of Orthopaedic Surgeons: (1985): *Joint motion: method of measuring and recording*, ed 6, Chicago, 1985, The Academy.

Feller JA, Bartlett JR, Lang DM: Patellar resurfacing versus retention in total knee arthroplasty, *J Bone Joint Surg Br* 78(2):226–228, 1996.

Frankel HL, Coll JR, Charlifue SW, Whiteneck GG, Gardner BP, Jamous MA, Krishnan KR, Nuseibeh I, Savic G, Sett P: Long-term survival in spinal cord injury: a fifty year investigation, *Spinal Cord* 36(4):266–274, 1998.

Gerhardt JJ: *Measuring and recording of joint motion: instrumentation and techniques*, ed 2, Toronto, 1990, Hogrefe & Huber.

Hoppenfeld S: *Physical examination of the spine and extremities*, New York, 1976, Appleton-Century-Crofts.

Iankova A: The Glasgow coma scale: clinical application in emergency departments, *Emerg Nurse* 14(8):30–35, 2006.

Liang MH, Katz JN, Phillips C, et al.: The American Academy of Orthopaedic Surgeons Task Force on Outcome Studies: the total hip arthroplasty evaluation form of the American Academy of Orthopaedic Surgeons, *J Bone Joint Surg* 73:639–645, 1991.

Polly HF, Hunder GG: *Physical examination of the joints*, ed 2, Philadelphia, 1978, WB Saunders.

Reider B: *The orthopaedic physical examination*, ed 2, Philadelphia, 2005, WB Saunders.

Smits-Engelsman B, Klerks M, Kirby A: Beighton score: a valid measure for generalized hypermobility in children, *J Pediatr* 158(1):119–123, 2011.

Trumbly CM: *Physical disabilities*, ed 2, Baltimore, 1983, Williams & Wilkins.

Laboratory

Henry JB: *Clinical diagnostic management by laboratory methods*, ed 18, Philadelphia, 1991, WB Saunders.

Kjeldsberg CR, Knight JA: *Body fluids*, ed 2, Philadelphia, 1987, American Society of Clinical Pathologists.

Schumacher HR: Synovial fluid analysis and synovial biopsy. In Kelly WW, Harris ED, Ruddy S, Sledge CB, editors: *Textbook of rheumatology*, ed 3, Philadelphia, 1989, WB Saunders.

Casts, Splints, and Dressings

Crosby LA, Lewallen DG, editors: *American Academy of Orthopaedic Surgeons: Emergency care and transportation of the sick and injured*, ed 6, Chicago, 1997, The Academy.

Schmeisser GA: *A clinical manual of orthopedic traction techniques*, Philadelphia, 1963, WB Saunders.

Schneider RF: *Handbook for the orthopaedic assistant*, ed 2, St Louis, 1976, The CV Mosby Co.

Simon Koenigsknecht: SJ: *Emergency orthopaedics: the extremities*, ed 2, Norwalk, Conn, 1987, Appleton & Lange.

Prosthetics and Orthotics

American Academy of Orthopaedic Surgeons: *Atlas of limb prosthetics: surgical, prosthetic, and rehabilitation principles*, ed 2, St Louis, 1992, Mosby-Year Book.

American Academy of Orthopaedic Surgeons: *Atlas of orthotics*, ed 2, St Louis, 1985, CV Mosby Co.

American Academy of Orthopaedic Surgeons: *Atlas of orthotics, biomechanical principles and applications*, St Louis, 1975, Mosby.

Bunch WH, Keagy RD: *Principles of orthotic treatment*, St Louis, 1976, The CV Mosby Co.

Goldberg B, Hsu J: *Atlas of orthotics and assistive devices*, ed 3, St Louis, 1997, AAOS, Mosby.

Redford JB: *Orthotics etcetera*, ed 3, Baltimore, 1986, Williams & Wilkins.

Smith DG, Michael JW, Bowker JH: *Atlas of amputations and limb deficiencies: surgical prosthetic and rehabilitation principles*, Chicago, 2004, American Academy of Orthopaedic Surgeons.

Anatomy and Surgery

American Orthopaedic Association: *Manual of orthopaedic surgery*, Chicago, 1985, The Association.

Burchardt H: The biology of bone graft repair, *Clin Orthop* 174:28, 1983.

Casscells SW: *Arthroscopy: diagnostic and surgical practice*, Philadelphia, 1984, Lea & Febiger.

Crenshaw AH: *Campbell's operative orthopaedics*, vols 1-4, ed 10, St Louis, 2002, Mosby-Year Book, Inc.

Epps CH Jr: *Complications in orthopaedic surgery*, vols I and II, ed 3, Philadelphia, 1994, JB Lippincott.

Friedlaender GE: *Allografting*, St Louis, 1992, Mosby-Year Book.

Friedlaender GE: Immune responses to osteochondral allografts: current knowledge and future directions, *Clin Orthop* 174:58, 1983.

Haimovici H: *Vascular surgery: principles and techniques*, New York, 1984, Appleton-Century-Crofts.

Moore KL: *Clinically oriented anatomy*, ed 2, Baltimore, 1985, Williams & Wilkins.

Reckling F, Reckling JA, Mohn M: *Orthopaedic anatomy and surgical approaches*, St Louis, 1990, Mosby-Year Book.

Robertson PA: Prediction of amputation after severe lower limb trauma, *J Bone Joint Surg* 73A:639–645, 1991.

Rutherford RB, editor: *Vascular surgery*, ed 2, Philadelphia, 1984, WB Saunders.

Shahriaree H, editor: *O'Connor's textbook of arthroscopic surgery*, ed 2, Philadelphia, 1992, JB Lippincott.

Tomford WW, Friedlaender GE: Bone banking procedures, *Clin Orthop* 174:15, 1983.

Weiland AJ: Current concepts review: vascularized free bone transplants, *J Bone Joint Surg* 63A:166, 1981.

The Spine

Joaquim AF, Lawrence B, Daubs M, Brodke D, Patel AA: Evaluation of the subaxial injury classification system, *J Craniovertebr Junction Spine* 2(2):67–72, 2011.

Lee JY, Vaccaro AR, Lim MR, Oner FC, Hulbert RJ, Hedlund R, Fehlings MG, Arnold P, Harrop J, Bono CM, Anderson PA, Anderson DG, Harris MB, Brown AK, Stock GH, Baron EM: Thoracolumbar injury classification and severity score: a new paradigm for the treatment of thoracolumbar spine trauma, *J Orthop Sci* 10(6):671–675, 2005.

Lenke LG: Lenke classification system of adolescent idiopathic scoliosis: treatment recommendations, *Instr Course Lect* 54:537–542, 2005.

Mac-Thiong JM, Labelle H, Parent S, Hresko MT, Deviren V, Weidenbaum M, members of the Spinal Deformity Study Group: Reliability and development of a new classification of lumbosacral spondylolisthesis, *Scoliosis* 3:19, 2008.

Weinstein JN, Rydevik BL, Sonntag VKH, editors: *Essentials of the spine*, New York, 1995, Raven Press.

Wiltse LL: Classification terminology and measurements in spondylolisthesis, *Iowa Orthop J* 1:52–57, 1981.

Hand and Wrist

DiDio LJA: *Synopsis of anatomy*, St Louis, 1970, The CV Mosby Co.

Doyle JR, Blythe W: *American Academy of Orthopaedic Surgeons: symposium on tendon surgery in the hand*, St Louis, 1975, The CV Mosby Co.

Edmonson AS, Crenshaw AH, editors: *Campbell's operative orthopaedics* (vol 1), ed 9, St Louis, 1996, Mosby.

Green DP, editor: *Operative hand surgery*, New York, 1988, Churchill-Livingstone.

Lichtman DM: *The wrist and its disorders*, Philadelphia, 1988, WB Saunders.

Mackinnon SE, Dellon AL: *Surgery of the peripheral nerve*, New York, 1988, Thieme Medical Publishers.

Oneson SR, Scales LM, Timins ME, Erickson SJ, Chamoy L: MR imaging interpretation of the Palmer classification of triangular fibrocartilage complex lesions, *Radiographics* 16(1):97–106, 1996.

Scher RK, Daniel III CR: *Nails: therapy, diagnosis, surgery*, Philadelphia, 1990, WB Saunders.

Steichen JB, editor: *Comprehensive atlas of hand surgery*, Chicago, 1989, Year Book Medical Publishers.

Wolfe SW, Hotchkiss RN, Pederson WC, Kozin SH: *Green's operative hand surgery*, ed 6, Philadelphia, 2012, Elsevier.

Yen CH, Chan WL, Leung HB, Mak KH: Thumb polydactyly: clinical outcome after reconstruction, *J Orthop Surg (Hong Kong)* 14(3):295–302, 2006.

Foot and Ankle

Jahss MH: *Disorders of the foot*, vols. I and II. Philadelphia, 1982, WB Saunders.

Mann RA: *Surgery of the foot*, ed 5, St Louis, 1986, CV Mosby.

Coughlin MJ, Saltzman C, Anderson RB, editors: *Mann's surgery of the foot and ankle*, ed 9, Philadelphia, 2013, Saunders Elsevier.

Occupational Therapy and Physical Therapy

American Occupational Therapy Association Commission on Practice Uniform Reporting System Task Force: *Uniform terminology system for reporting occupational therapy services*, Rockville, Md, 1986, The Association.

Brotzman SB, Manske RC: *Clinical orthopaedic rehabilitation: an evidence-based approach*, ed 3, Philadelphia, 2012, Elsevier Mosby.

Kamenetz HL: *Dictionary of rehabilitation medicine*, New York, 1983, Springer.

Magee DJ: *Orthopaedic physical assessment*, ed 3, Philadelphia, 1997, WB Saunders.

Roley SS, DeLany JV, Barrows CJ, et al: Occupational therapy practice framework: domain & process, 2nd edition, *Am J Occup Ther* 62(6):625–683, 2008. doi:10.5014/ajot.62.6.625.

Research

Brighton CT, Black J, Pollack S: *Electrical properties of bone and cartilage*, New York, 1979, Grune & Stratton.

Frankel V: *Orthopedic biomechanics*, Philadelphia, 1970, Lea & Febiger.

Hoppenfeld S, deBoer P: *Surgical exposures in orthopaedics: the anatomic approach*, ed 3, Philadelphia, 2003, Lippincott, Williams & Wilkins.

O'Keefe RJ, Jacobs JJ, Chu CR, Einhorn TA: In *Orthopaedic basic science*, ed 4, Chicago, 2013, American Academy of Orthopaedic Surgeons, pp 43–53.

Poole AR: Cartilage in health and disease. In McCarthy D, Koopman W, editors: *Arthritis and allied conditions: a textbook in rheumatology*, ed 12, Philadelphia, 1992, Lea & Febiger, pp 279–333.

Suggested Readings

Journals and Tapes

AAOS Instructional Course Lectures (Park Ridge, Ill)
ACTA Chirurgiae Orthopaedicae et Traumatologiae Cechoslovaca (Praha)
ACTA Orthopaedica Scandinavica
Aktuelle Probleme in Chirurgie und Orthopadie (Bern)
Advances in Orthopaedic Surgery 1985 (Baltimore)
American Journal of Emergency Medicine (Philadelphia)
American Journal of Knee Surgery (Thorofare, NJ)
American Journal of Sports Medicine (Waltham, MA)
Archives of Orthopaedic and Traumatic Surgery (Berlin)
Archives of Physical Medicine and Rehabilitation (Chicago)
Archivio Putti di Chirurgia Degli Organi di Movimento (Firenze)
Arthritis and Rheumatism (Philadelphia)
Arthroscopy (New York)
Audio Digest Foundation (AAOS Ortho Tapes) (Chicago)
Beitrage zur Orthopadie und Traumatologie (Berlin)
Bone (New York)
Bone Marrow Transplant (United Kingdom)
Bone and Mineral (Amsterdam)
Buck CJ: *ICD-9-CM*, Vols 1 and 2, St Louis, 2006, Elsevier.
Bulletin of the Hospital for Joint Diseases Orthopaedic Institute (New York)
Chirurgia Degli Organi di Movimento (Bologna)
Chirurgia Narzadow Ruchu I Ortopedia Polska (Warszara)
Clinical Orthopaedics and Related Research (Philadelphia)
Clinics in Sports Medicine (Philadelphia)
Continuing Education in Orthopaedic Surgery (Recert) (AAOS) (Chicago)
Foot and Ankle (Baltimore)
Hand Clinics (Philadelphia)
Hip (Philadelphia)
Instructional Course Lectures; AAOS (Chicago)
International Orthopaedics (New York)
Italian Journal of Orthopaedics and Traumatology (Bologna)
Journal of the American Medical Association (Chicago)
Journal of the American Podiatric Medical Association (Bethesda, MD)
Journal of Arthroplasty (New Brunswick, NJ)
Journal of Bone and Joint Surgery, American Volume (Boston)
Journal of Bone and Joint Surgery, British Volume (London)
Journal of Bone and Mineral Research (New York)
Journal of Foot Surgery (Baltimore)
Journal of Hand Surgery (St Louis)
Journal of Hand Therapy (Philadelphia)
Journal of Orthopaedic Research (New York)
Journal of Orthopaedic and Sports Physical Therapy (Baltimore)
Journal of Orthopaedic Trauma (New York)
Journal of Pediatric Orthopaedics (New York)
Journal of Prosthetics and Orthotics (Alexandria, VA)
Journal of Rheumatology (Buffalo, NY)
Journal of Sports Medicine and Physical Fitness (Torino, Italy)
Journal of Trauma (Baltimore)
Magyar Traumatologia, Orthopaedia es Helyreallito Sebeszet (Budapest)
New England Journal of Medicine (Boston)
Nippon Seikeigeka Gakkai Zasshi (Journal of the Japanese Orthopaedic Association, Tokyo)
Orthopaedic Audio-Synopsis (AAOS) (Chicago)
Orthopaedic Clinical Update Monograph (AAOS) (Chicago)
Orthopade (Berlin)
Orthopaedic Nursing (Pitman, NJ) (NAON)
Orthopaedic Review (Lawrenceville, NJ)
Orthopaedic Survey (Chicago)
Orthopaedics (Thorofare, NJ)
Orthopedic Clinics of North America (Philadelphia)
Ortopediia Travmatologiia I Protezirovanie (Kharkov)
Pediatric Clinics of North America (Philadelphia)
Physical Therapy Journal (Alexandria)
Revue de Chirugie Orthopedique et Reparatrice de l'Appareil Moteur (Paris)
Skeletal Radiology (Berlin)
Spine (Hagerstown, MD)
Sports Medicine
Yearbook of Orthopaedic Trauma and Surgery (Chicago)
Yearbook of Orthopaedic and Traumatic Surgery (St Louis)
Yearbook of Orthopaedics (abstracts) (St Louis)
Yearbook of Sports Medicine (Chicago)
Yearbook of Sports Medicine (St Louis)
Zeitschrift fur Orthopadie und ihre Grenzgebiete (Stuttgart) Osteopathic Medicine

Index

A

Abbott
 approach, 275
 arthrodesis, 331
 method, 138
Abbott and Gill osteotomy, 214
Abbott and Lucas approach, 274
Abbott-Fisher-Lucas arthrodesis, 228
Abbott-Saunders-Bost arthrodesis, 331
Abdominal muscles, 288
Abdominal pads, 184
Abduction
 bar, 181
 external rotation test, 141
 injuries, 15
 orthoses, 198–199
 sign, 140
Abductor digiti minimi (ADM), 310
Abductor digiti quinti (ADQ), 310
Abductor hallucis, 349
Abductor lurch, 159
Abductor pollicis brevis (APB), 310
Abductor pollicis longus (APL), 310, 339
Ablate, 278
Ablative surgery, 278
Above elbow amputation, 190
Abrasion, 97
Abrasive wear, 385
Abscess, 97
Abstracts, 378
Acanthosis nigrican, 327
Acceleration, 382
Accessory bone, 307
Accessory ligament, 234, 312
Accessory movement, 369
Accessory navicular bone, 344, 347

Accommodative orthoses, 197
Accuracy, 378
Ace bandage, 184
Acetabular angle, 111
Acetabular coverage, 114
Acetabular depth, 114
Acetabular fracture, 10
 associated, 22–23
 elementary, 22
 Letournel and Judet classification for, 21–23
 Thompson and Epstein classification for, 30
Acetabular head quotient, 114
Acetabular index, 111
 angle, 112
Acetabular Classification for Congenital Deficiencies, 92t
Acetabular Labral Tear Classification, 91t
Acetabular line, 114
Acetabular notch, 254
Acetabular rim syndrome, 90
Acetabuloplasty, 259
Acetabulum, 254
 central fracture dislocation, 28
 deficiencies, 91–92
 Rowe and Lowell classification for, 28
Acheiria, 95, 320
Aichef technique, 337
Acheiropodia, 95
Achilles
 bulge sign, 154
 reflexes, 157
 squeeze test, 149
 tendon, 231–234, 262, 349
 tendonitis, 352
Achillobursitis, 69
Achillodynia, 69
Achondroplasia, 64–65

Page numbers followed by f and t indicate figures, tables respectively.

Achondroplastic dwarfism, 64–65
Achondroplastic stenosis, 294
Achterman and Kalamchi Classification for Fibular Hemimelia, 96t–97t
Acid-fast bacillus (AFB), 168–169
Acid phosphatase (AcP), 165
Acinetobacter baumannii, 169
AC joint, 240
　separation, 33
Acquired digital fibrokeratoma, 327
Acquired disease, 43
Acquired flatfoot, 354
Acquired thumb flexion contracture, 320
Acrocapitofemoral dysplasia, 84
Acrocephalosyndactylism, 59
Acrocyanosis, 77, 324
Acrofibrokeratomas, 327
Acrolentiginous melanoma, 327
Acromial angle, 111
Acromial profile, 119
Acromioclavicular separations, 28, 243
Acromioclavicular sprain, 35
Acromionectomy, 244
Acromion process, 241
Acromioplasty, 244
Acroosteolysis, 54
Acrosclerosis, 76
Acrosyndactyly, 320
Actinomyces, 169
Actinomycosis, 48
Activated partial thromboplastin time (APTT, PTT), 165
Active-assistive range of motion (ROM) exercise, 370
Active compression test, 140
Active glide test, 149
Active range of mostion (ROM) exercise, 370
Activities of daily living (ADLs), 365–366, 373–374
Acupressure, 368
Acute, 97
Acute calcific retropharyngeal tendonitis, 69
Acute calcific tendonitis, 69
Acute disease, 43
Acute osteomyelitis, 48
Acute postpartum scroiliitis, 292
Adactylia, 95
Adactyly, 320
Adamantinoma, 53
ADAMTS, 391
Adaptation, 382
Adaptic dressing, 183
Addison's keloid, 76
Addis test, 149
Adduction
　injuries, 15
　sign, 140
Adductor, 254
　hallucis, 349
　muscle, 261
　pollicis (AdP), 310
　tubercle, 261
　tuberosity, 261
Adenopathy, 97

Adhesions, 97
Adhesive
　bursitis, 72
　capsulitis, 72
　tape, 184
　wear, 225, 385
Adipogenesis, 389
Adipose tissue, 231
Adjustable Thomas splints, 185
Adjuvant therapy, 276
Adolescent scoliosis, 293
Adson
　maneuver, 136
　test, 136
Adult hypophosphatasia, 58
Adult scoliosis, 293
Advancement, 278
　flaps, 335
Adventitia, 235
Adventitious, 98
Aebi, Etter, and Cosica fixation, 301
Aerobic exercises, 368
Afebrile, 98
A-frame orthoses, 198
Agarose, 389
Agee procedure, 339
Aggravated, 98
Aggrecan, 392
Aggrecanases, 391–392
Aggressive fibromatosis, 54
Agility training, 368
Agonists, 231
-agra, 98
Ahlback changes, 119
Ainhum, 352
Air cast, 181
Air cast walker, 181
Airplane cast, 180
Airplane splint, 182, 201–202
Air pressure splints, 188
Air splint, 188
Aitken Classification for Longitudinal Deficiency of the Femur, Partial, 96t–97t
Akin procedure, 357
Alanine aminotransferase (ALT), 164–165
Ala of the ilium, 252
Alar dysgenesis, 291
Albee
　fixation, 302
　procedure, 306
Albers-Schönberg disease, 47, 59
Albert achillodynia, 69
Albright and Chase procedure, 332
Albright hereditary osteodystrophy, 83
Albright-McCune-Sternberg syndrome, 59
Albright syndrome, 59, 68
Albumin, 164
Alexander view, 108
-algia, 98
Algodystrophy, 54, 79
Alkaline phosphatase (ALP), 164–165, 392

Allen
  maneuver, 136
  test, 144
Allergenic arthritis, 70
Allergy, 98
Allis
  maneuver, 147
  sign, 147
  test, 151
Allman classification, 14
Anderson and d'Alonzo Classification, 14–15
Alloantibodies, 173
Allodynia, 81, 317
Allogenic, 216
Allograft, 216–217, 302–303
Almquist procedure, 339
Alpha angle, 111
Alpha-L-iduronidase, 67
Alpha value, 378
ALPSA lesion, 36
Alternating current, 367
Alumina, 225
Aluminum foam splint, 182
Aly procedure, 357
Ambling gait, 158
Amelia, 95, 320
American Academy of Orthopaedic Surgeons, 178, 378
American Academy of Orthotists and Prosthetists, 189
American Association of Blood Bank Standards, 171–172
American Association of Tissue Banks, 216–217
American Board for Certification, 189
American Joint Committee on Cancer (AJCC) Staging System, 50, 53
American Orthotics and Prosthetics Association (AOPA), 189
American Shoulder and Elbow Surgeons system, 159
American Society for Bone and Mineral Research, 378
American Society of Orthopaedic Professionals, 177–178
American Spinal Injury Association (ASIA) Impairment Scale, 159, 286, 297t
Aminoterminal propeptide (N-PCP), 168
Amniotic bands, 95, 320
Amoss sign, 138
Amputation, 277–278
  above elbow, 190
  defined, 277
  general, 277–278
Amputation neuroma, 80
Amspacher and Messenbaugh osteotomy, 214
Amspacher and Messenbaugh prostheses, 250
Amstutz and Wilson osteotomy, 214
Amyloid β-microglobulin, 58
Amyoplasia congenita, 62
Amyosthenia, 61
Amyotonia congenita, 62
Amyotrophic lateral sclerosis (ALS), 78
Anaerobic culture, 169
Anaerobic exercises, 368
Analgesia, 98
Analgia, 98

Analysis of variance (ANOVA), 379
Analytic, 382
Anastomosis, 98, 278, 334
Anatomic anterior cruciate ligament reconstruction, 267
Anatomic femoral axis, 115
Anatomic femorotibial angle (FTA), 111
Anatomic neck, 241
  fracture, 8
Anatomic planes, 405–406
Anatomic positions/directions
  anatomic planes, 405–406
  joint motions, 406–409
  location, 405–406
  terminology, 409–412
Anatomic snuff box, 313
Anchoring screws, 303
Anchovy procedure, 331
Anconeus, 247, 310
Anderson and Fowler procedure, 357
Anderson and Hutchins procedure, 272
Anderson Orthopaedic Research Institute Periprosthetic Bone Loss (AORI), 119
Anderson procedure, 272, 357
Andersson lesion, 294
André Thomas sign, 144
Andrews procedure, 267
Anesthesia, 98, 278
Aneurysm, 73
Aneurysmal bone cyst, 54
Aneurysmorrhaphy, 238
Angelman syndrome, 84
Anghelescu sign, 138
Angiogenesis, 389
Angiogram, 128–129
Angiography, 128–129
Angioplasty, 128
Angiosarcoma, 53–54
Angioscopy, 128
Angle of Gissane, 350
Angular acceleration, 382
Angular momentum, 384
Angular velocity, 384
Angulation, 6
  of fracture, 6
Anisospondyly, 291
Anisotropy, 382
Ankle, 343–364
  anatomy, 343–351
  arteries of, 266, 357
  bones of, 344–349
  components, 194–195
  conditions, 351–357
  diseases, 351–357
  dislocations of, 34
  fracture, 15, 17, 21, 31
  joint of, 199
  ligaments of, 350
  mortise of, 11, 350
  muscles of, 349–350
  nerves of, 357
  prostheses for, 364

Ankle *(Continued)*
   sprains of, 15
   stirrup, 181
   surgery, 357–364
   tendons of, 349–350
   veins of, 357
Ankle-arm index, 129
Ankle-brachial index (ABI), 129
Ankle clonus test, 155
Ankle corset, 206
Ankylodactylia, 72
Ankylosing spinal hyperostosis, 291
Ankylosing spondylitis, 76–77
Ankylosis, 70, 72–73
Annealing, 225
Annotated units
   length, 176
   other, 176
   volume, 176
   weight, 175–176
Annulus fibrosus, 287
Annulus fracture, 325
Anomaly, 98
Anonychia, 352
Ansa cervicalis, 286
Anserine bursa, 230
Anstrom suspension test, 138
Antagonists, 231
Antalgic gait, 159
Anteater nose sign, 116
Antebrachial cutaneous nerve, 314
Antecedent sign, 158
Antecurvatum, 6
Antefemoral cyst, 72
Anteflexion, 98
Anterior approach, 306, 364
   knee, 275
   leg, 275
Anterior axillary approach, 274
Anterior compartment, 74, 263
Anterior cruciate ligament, 263
   instability test, 149–150
   sprain, 35
Anterior dislocation, 34
Anterior displacement, 289
Anterior drawer sign, 152, 154
Anterior elbow approach, 274
Anterior forearm approach, 274
Anterior hiatal sign, 116
Anterior hip approach, 275
Anterior horns, 288
Anterior iliofemoral ligament, 255
Anterior inferior iliac spine, 252
Anterior interosseous nerve syndrome, 248, 318
Anterior lift-off test, 141
Anterior ligament
   longitudinal, 287
   sacroiliac, 253
Anterior shoulder dislocation, 33, 243
Anterior slide test, 140
Anterior spinal fusion, 301

Anterior spurring, 291
Anterior superior iliac spine, 252–253
Anterior talofibular ligaments, 350
Anterior talofibular sprain, 35
Anterior talo-first metatarsal angle, 350
Anterior thoracic nerve, 243
Anterior tibial
   artery, 265
   sign, 149
   spine, 261
   tendon, 349
   tubercle, 261
Anteroinferior glenohumeral ligament, 242
Anterolateral approach
   elbow, 274
   femur, 275
   hip, 275
   humerus, 274
   knee, 275
Anterolateral approach, 306
Anterolateral rotatory instability (ALRI), 93
Anteromedial approach
   elbow, 274
   humerus, 274
   knee, 275
Anteromedial cyst, 72
Anteromedial glenohumeral ligament, 242
Anteromedial shoulder, 274
Anterosuperior glenohumeral ligament, 242
Anteversion, 98, 114
Antibiotic beads, 279
Anticus reflex, 157
Anticus sign, 157
Anti–double-stranded (native) DNA, 165
Anti-HCV, 173
Anti-human immunodeficiency virus antibodies (anti-HIV), 173
Antinuclear antibody (ANA), 165–166
Antistreptolysin O titer (ASO), 166
Anvil test, 136, 147
AO, 219
AO/ASIF (Association for Osteosynthesis/Association for the Study of Internal Fixation)
   long bone fractures, 13–14
   soft tissue classification, 14
AO fixateur interne, 304
AO-Morscher plate, 222
AOPA, 196
Aortofemoral bypass (AFB), 238
Aortoiliac bypass, 238
Apert disease, 59
Apert syndrome, 320–321
Aphalangia, 321
Aphasia, 98
Apical lordotic view, 108
Apical view, 108
Apley grind test, 150
Apley scratch test, 141
Apley test, 150
Apodia, 95
Aponeurectomy, 231
Aponeurorrhaphy, 231, 235

Aponeurosis, 231, 310
　surgical procedures on, 231
Aponeurotic fibroma, 328
Aponeurotomy, 231
Apophyseal fractures, 4
Apophysis, 209
Apophysitis, 55
Apoplexy, 98
Apoptosis, 389
Apposition, 6
Apprehension test, 141, 143
Approximate, 279
Apraxia, 78
APRL voluntary-closing hand, 192
AP view, 108
Aquatic exercise, 368
Arachnodactyly, 95, 321
Arachnoid, 287
Arachnoiditis, 78
Arcade of Froshse, 249, 313, 318–319
Arcade of Struthers, 247, 249–250
Archer's shoulder, 36
Archimedes principle, 368
Arcuate ligament, 252, 263, 312
Area MOI, 384
Arizona universal leg support, 185
Arlet Ficat Marcus Classification for Femoral Head Osteonecrosis, 122t
Arm
　anatomy of, 246–250
　blood vessels of, 248
　bones of, 246–247
　cylinder cast, 179
　ligaments of, 249–250
　muscles of, 247
　nerves of, 248–249
　surgery of, 250–252
Arm pit, 241
Armstrong procedure, 244
Army Prosthetics Research Laboratory (APRL), 192
Arnold-Chiari syndrome, 299
Aronson and Prager prostheses, 250
Arrhythmia, 77
Arterial injury, 27
Arterial insufficiency, 73–74
Arterial occlusive disease, 74
Arteries, 235
　of Adamkiewicz, 288
　of ankle, 357
　anterior tibial, 265
Arteriogram, 107, 128–129
Arteriography, 128–129
Arterioles, 235
Arteriosclerosis, 74
Arteriovenous fistula (AVF), 74
Arteriovenous malformation (AVM), 74
Arteritis, 76
Arthralgia, 70
Arthrectomy, 229
　catheter, 238
Arthrempyesis, 70

Arthritis, 70
　allergenic, 70
　mutilans, 316–317
Arthrocace, 70
Arthrocele, 70
Arthrocentesis, 227
Arthrochalasis, 70
Arthrochondritis, 70
Arthroclisis, 227
Arthrodesis, 227–229, 362
　categories of, 228
　specific, 228–229
Arthrodial cartilage, 229
Arthrodysplasia, 70
Arthroendoscopy, 227–228
Arthroereisis, 227, 357
Arthrofibrosis, 321
Arthrogram, 107
Arthrography, 107
Arthrogryposis, 71, 321
Arthrogryposis multiplex congenita, 321
Arthro-(joints), 226–230
　anatomy of, 226–227
　arthrodesis, 228–229
　general surgery, 227–228
　types of, 227
Arthrokatadysis, 71, 90
Arthrokleisis, 71, 227
Arthrolith, 71
Arthrolysis, 227
Arthromeningitis, 71
Arthrometer test, 150
Arthroncus, 71
Arthroneuralgia, 71
Arthronosos, 71
Arthropathy, 71
Arthrophyte, 71
Arthroplasty, 227, 357
　for acromioclavicular separations, 243
　for anterior shoulder dislocations, 243
　for high-riding scapulae (Sprengel deformity), 243
　for posterior shoulder dislocations, 243
　for shoulder stabilization, 244
Arthropyosis, 71
Arthrorheumatism, 71
Arthro-root diseases, 70–71
Arthrosclerosis, 71
Arthroscopy, 227–228
Arthrosis, 44–45, 71
Arthrosteitis, 71
Arthrosynovitis, 71
Arthrotomy, 228
Arthroxerosis, 71
Arthroxesis, 228
Articular cartilage, 209, 229
　implant (ACI), 230
　transfer (ACT), 230
Articular fractures, 4
Articulating frame fixation, 224
Artifact, 158
Aseptic, 98, 279

Aseptic necrosis, 55
Ashhurst sign, 116
Ashurst classification, 15
　for ankle fracture, 15
ASIF, 219
Asnis procedure, 259
Asnis screw, 219
Aspartate aminotransferase (AST), 164
Aspergillus, 169
Asphyxia, 98
Aspiration, 98, 279
Assistive and adaptive equipment, 375
Assmann disease, 55, 59
Associated acetabular fracture, 22–23
Association Research Circulation Osseous Classification for Osteonecrosis (ARCO), 119t–120t
Asthenia, 98
Astragalus, 349
Asymmetry, 98
Asymptomatic, 98
Asynergia, 98
Atavistic epiphyseal, 212
Ataxia, 62, 98
Ataxic cerebral palsy (CP), 79
Ataxic gait, 159
Atheroma, 74
Atherosclerosis, 74
Athetoid cerebral palsy (CP), 79
Athetosis, 98
Athlete's foot, 352
Atlanta brace, 198
Atlas, 285
Atonia, 78, 98
Atony, 98
Atosoy procedure, 334
Atrophy, 77, 98
Attenuate, 279
Attenuation of tendons, 316
Attrition attenuation of tendons, 316
Atypical, 98
Austin procedure, 358
Autogenous, 216
Autogenous saphenous vein graft (ASVG), 238
Autograft, 216, 302
Autologous donor, 171
Autolyzed, antigen-extracted allogeneic (AAA) bone, 217
Autonomic dysreflexia, 78
Autonomic dystrophy, 318
Autonomic nervous system, 283
Autopsy, 279
Autosomal dominant hypophosphatemic rickets, 83
Autosomal inheritance, 100
Autosomes, 171
Avascular, 98
Avascular necrosis, 55
AV fistula, 74
Aviator's astragalus, 11
Avila approach, 274
Avulsion, 98
　fracture, 4
　of nail plate, 358

Axial compression test, 144
Axial flap
　cutaneous, 335
　flag, 335
　pattern skin, 335
Axilla, 241
Axillary artery, 242
Axillary block, 273
Axillary lateral view, 108
Axillary nerve, 243
Axillary sling, 205
Axillary vein, 242–243
Axillofemoral bypass (AxFem), 238–239
Axis, 285
　anatomic femoral, 115
　fracture, 23
Axolemma, 314
Axonotmesis, 78, 82t

B

B. H. Moore procedure, 245
Baastrup disease, 291, 298
Babinski-Fröhlich syndrome, 60
Babinski reflex, 155
Babinski sign, 155
Baciu and Filibiu arthrodesis, 228
Backfire fracture, 8
Background and significance, 377
Back-knee, 92
Backpack palsy, 36
Backscatter electron microscopy (BSE), 387
Back wall first technique, 334
Bacterial antigen assay, 169
Badelon Classification, 15
Badgley
　approach, 306
　arthrodesis, 228
　nail, 219
Bado Classification, 15
BAGHL, 36
Bailey and Dubow osteotomy, 214
Bailey approach, 306
Bailey-Dubow nail, 219
Bail knee lock, 199
Baker and Hill osteotomy, 214
Baker and Hill procedure, 358
Baker cyst, 92–93
Baker procedure, 271, 358
Balanced suspension, 185
Balkan frame, 187
Ball-and-socket joint, 227
Ball-and-socket osteotomy, 214
Balloon angioplasty, 239
Ballotable patella test, 150
Ballottement test, 144
Balneotherapy, 367
Baltimore therapeutic equipment (BTE) work simulator, 372
Bamboo spine, 116
Banana peel procedure, 272

Index 441

Bandage, 178
  Ace, 184
  adhesive, 184
Bankart
  fracture, 8
  fragment, 8
  lesion, 8
  procedure, 244
Bankhart lesion, 33
Banks approach, 276
Banks-Dervin rod, 304
Banks procedure, 358
Barber's intradigital pilonidal sinus, 329
Bardeleben bone, 347
Barlow splint, 199
Barlow test, 147
Barre-Lieou syndrome, 78–79
Barr procedure, 358
Barr-Record procedure, 358
Barsky macrodactyly reduction, 335
Bartlett procedure, 358
Barton fracture, 8, 325
Barton tongs, 185
Basal neck fracture, 10
Baseball elbow, 36
Baseball finger, 9, 36
Baseball splint, 182
Baseball throwers humerus, 36
Baseline radiograph, 106
Basicervical, 10
Basic hand splint, 200
Basic multicellular unit (BMU), 393
Basile screw, 219
Basilic vein, 248
Basketball foot, 36
Bassett et al. approach, 364
Batchelor-Brown procedure, 358
Batchelor plaster, 180
Bateman procedure, 244, 336
Bathing, 373
Baumann angle, 111
Baumgard and Schwartz prostheses, 250–251
Baxter and D'Astous procedure, 259
Baxter nerve, 351
Baxter nerve syndrome, 352
Bayesian statistics, 379
Bayne and Klug procedure, 335
Bayne classification, 321
Bayne Classification for Longitudinal Ulnar Deficiencies, 96t–97t
Bayne Classification for Radial Bone Deficiencies, 96t–97t
Bayonet position, 6
Bayonet sign, 150
Beaded, 225
Beak ligament, 312
Beak nail deformity, 327
Beal syndrome, 321
Beaufort seating orthoses, 205
Bechtol prosthesis, 246
Beckenbaugh procedure, 339
Becker locking grip hand, 192

Becker muscular dystrophy, 63
Becker procedure, 337
Bednar and Lane procedure, 335
Beefburger procedure, 272
Beevor sign, 155
Beggel-Hansen disease, 57
Behçet syndrome, 72
Beighton hyperlaxity score, 98
Beighton laxity score, 159
Bekhterev test, 138
Bell classification, 321
Bell-Dally dislocation, 33
Bell palsy, 81
Bellemore and Barrett osteotomy, 214
Belly press test, 141
Below elbow amputation, 190
Below-knee suspension, 194
Belsky-Eaton procedure, 333
Bench Burn disease, 138
Bench test, 138
Bending, 382
Bending moment, 382
Benediction attitude sign, 144
Benediction sign, 144
Benign, 98
Benign disease, 43
Benirschke and Sangeorzan procedure, 358
Bennett
  approach, 274
  dislocation, 327
  fracture, 9
  orthoses, 202
Benoit-Gerrard, 219
Bent finger, 321
Bentzon procedure, 333
Berkowitz procedure, 358
Berman and Gartland procedure, 358
Bernese osteotomy, 214–215
Bertol method, 120
Bertolotti syndrome, 291
Beskin procedure, 339
Betadine dressing, 183
Beta$_2$-microglobulin amyloidosis, 84
Bevin Aurglass procedure, 333
Biceps
  femoris, 261
  groove, 241
  muscle, 247
  reflexes, 157
  tuberosity, 247
Bicipital groove, 241
Bicipital tendonitis, 69
Bickel and Moe procedure, 271
Bicompartmental replacement, 271
Bicycle spoke injury, 36
Bier block, 273
Bifid thumb, 321
Bifurcate ligament, 350
Bifurcation, 98
Big femoral head (BFH), 225
Bigelow ligament, 255

442 Index

Bigelow reduction maneuver, 147
Biglycan, 389
BIL lesion, 36
Bilateral fixation, 224
Bilateral hip spica cast, 180
Bilhaut-Cloquet procedure, 335
Billet, 194
Bilobed pedicle, 273
Bimalleolar angle, 111
Bimalleolar ankle fracture, 11
Bimalleolar equivalent, 11
Biodegradable fixation, 219
Biomechanics, 382–385
Biopsy, 279
Bipartite, 98
Bipartite patella, 93
Bipolar hip replacement, 256
Birch Classification for Fibular Deficiencies, 96t–97t
Bircher, Weber procedure, 358
Bivalve cast, 181
Bizarre parosteal osteochondromatous proliferation (BPOP), 53
Black heel syndrome, 36
Blackburne-Peel ratio, 114
Black-dot heel, 36
Blade plate, 219
Blair arthrodesis, 228
Blair-Brown skin graft, 272
Blastomyces, 169
Blastomycosis, 48
Blatt capsulodesis, 331
Blatt dorsal capsulodesis, 339–340
Bleck procedure, 259
Blood bank
 immunologic tests, 173–174
 procedures, 171–172
 products, 172–173
 terminology, 171–172
Blood gases, 166
Blood urea nitrogen (BUN), 164
Blood vessels, 73–77
 of arm, 248
 arterial disorders, 73–76
 collagen vascular disorders, 76–77
 disorders, 77
 venous disorders, 73
Blount
 disease, 59
 displacement osteotomy, 214
 osteotomy, 214
 plate, 219
 prostheses, 251
 staple, 219
Blue foot syndrome, 352
Blue toe syndrome, 74
Blumensaat line, 114
Blundell Jones varus osteotomy, 214
Blunt dissection, 279
BMP 1 receptor type 1A (ACVR1), 57
Body casts, 179
Body jacket, 203

Boeck sarcoid, 59
Böhler
 angle, 111, 350–351
 nail, 219
 splint, 182
Böhler-Braun frame, 185
Bohlman pin, 219
Bohman procedure, 301
Bohn and Durbin classification for Epiphyseal Fractures, 15
Boitzy procedure, 261
Bollard, 219
Bone
 age, 120
 of ankle, 344–349
 arm, 246–247
 block, 218
 densitometry, 107
 diseases, 44–48
 infarct, 56
 island, 56
 loss, 27
 matrix, 210
 miscellaneous conditions, 54–59
 spur, 56–57, 326
 suture fixation, 213
 tumors, 49–53
Bone marrow, 210
 aspirate, 303
 biopsy, 163–164, 213
 pressure, 107
 transplant, 213
Bone morphogenic protein (BMP), 303, 392
Bone scan, 125–126
Bone scintigraphy, 125
Bone specific alkaline phosphatase (BAP, BSAP), 168
Bonola procedure, 335
Bony ankylosis, 72
Bony spurs, 295–296
Bony tarsus, 347
Booth test, 141
Boot-top fracture, 11
Borden and Gearen osteotomy, 214
Borden osteotomy, 214
Bose procedure, 358
Bossing, 98
Boston bivalve cast, 181
Boston brace, 203
Boston overlap brace (BOB), 203
Bosworth
 approach, 275
 arthrodesis, 228
 fixation, 302
 fracture, 11
 procedure, 244, 272, 358
 prostheses, 251
Bouchard node, 59, 328
Bouldering, 37
Bounce home test, 150
Boundary lubrication, 384
Boutonnière deformity, 316, 323, 327
Boutonnière reconstruction, 339

Bouvier manuever, 144
Bow, 6
Bowen disease, 327
Bowers arthroplasty, 332
Bowers hemiresection, 251
Bowing fracture, 6
Bowler's thumb, 36
Bowstring sign, 138
Bowstring test, 138
Boxer's elbow, 8
Boxer's fracture, 36
Boyd
  amputation, 358
  approach, 274
  side plate, 219
Boyd and Anderson prostheses, 251
Boyd and Griffin classification, 16
Boyd and McLeod prostheses, 251
Boyd and Sisk procedure, 244
Boyes procedure, 333, 338–339
Boyes test, 144
Bozan maneuver, 147
Bracelet test, 144
Brachial artery, 242, 248
Brachialgia statica paresthetica, 319
Brachialis muscle, 247
Brachial plexus, 243
Brachial vein, 248
Brachioradialis, 247, 310
Brachydactyly, 321
Bracket resection, 335
Brackett osteotomy, 214
Bradford frame, 187
Bradford procedure, 305
Brady and Jewett prostheses, 251
Bradycardia, 77
Bragard sign, 138
Braham and Pankovich procedure, 358
Brahms procedure, 358
Brailsford disease, 59
Braly et al. procedure, 358
Brand procedure, 337–339
Brattstrom procedure, 301
Braun procedure, 244
Braun skin graft, 273
Breaststroker's knee, 36
Brent-Moberg tenodesis, 337
Brendt and Harty Modified Classification, 16
Brett
  arthrodesis, 228
  osteotomy, 214
  procedure, 272
Brett and Campbell procedure, 271
Breuerton view, 108
Bridle procedure, 358
Bright-field microscopy, 387
Brisement, 244, 279
Bristow-Laterjet procedure, 244
Bristow procedure, 244
British test, 150
Brittain arthrodesis, 228

Brittain procedure, 244
Brittle, 382
Brittle bones, 46
Broaching, 279
Broadbent and Woolf procedure, 331, 339
Brockman-Nissen arthrodesis, 331
Brockman procedure, 358
Broden view, 108
Brodie abscess, 59
Brooker Classification for Heterotopic Ossification, 57t
Brooker-Willis nail, 219
Brooks and Jenkins fixation, 301
Brooks and Saddon procedure, 244
Broomhead approach, 364
Broom-stick cast, 180
Broström procedure, 358, 361
Broudy and Smith procedure, 339
Brown approach, 274
Brown procedure, 272
Brown-Séquard syndrome, 81
Brown tumor, 57
Brudzinski sign, 155
Bruit, 77, 98
Brunelli and Brunelli procedure, 331
Bryan and Morrey classification, 16
Bryan approach, 274
Bryant sign, 141
Bryant traction, 186
Buchler procedure, 333
Buchman disease, 55, 60
Bucholz and Ogden's Classification for Osteonecrosis, 120t
Bucket-handle fracture, 10
Bucket-handle tear, 92–93
Buck-Gramcko procedure, 335, 341
Buck traction, 186
Budin splint, 206
Buerger disease, 74, 324
Buford complex, 89
Bugg-Boyd procedure, 358
Bulb dynamometer, 372
Bulge sign, 150
Bumper fracture, 11
Bunion, 350–352
Bunionectomy, 358
Bunionette, 352
Bunkbed fracture, 11
Bunnell opponensplasty, 337
Bunnell procedure, 244, 338–339
Bura view, 109
Burghard procedure, 364
Burkhalter procedure, 337–338
Burkhalter transfer, 337
Burlap bone, 213
Burnham view, 109
Burns disease, 60
Burns test, 138
Burrows procedure, 244
Bursa-related diseases, 70
Bursa sac, 226
Bursectomy, 230
Bursitis, 70, 352

Bursocentesis, 230
Bursography, 107
Bursolith, 70
Bursopathy, 70
Bursoscopy, 230
Bursotomy, 230
Burst fracture, 9
Bursting fracture, 4
Burton and Pellegrini procedure, 331
Burton procedure, 332
Burton sign, 158
Butler procedure, 358
Butterfly fracture, 4

C

C bar, 202
Cable, 219
Cable nerve grafts, 333
Cable twister orthoses, 199
Cachexia, 98
Café-au-lait, 98, 158
Caffey disease, 58, 60
Cages, 256, 304
Caisson disease, 57
Calandriello procedure, 258
Calandruccio device, 219
Calandruccio nail, 219
Calbindin, 393
Calcaneal branch
 of the posterior tibial artery, 351
 of the posterior tibial nerve, 351
Calcaneal inclination angle, 113
Calcaneal spur, 355
 pad, 206
 syndrome, 352
Calcaneal tendon, 231–234
Calcaneofibular ligaments, 350
Calcaneofibular sprain, 35
Calcaneus bone, 344
Calcar, 252
Calcar femorale, 252
Calcific bursitis, 70
Calcific periarthritis, 84
Calcific tendonitis, 69
Calcification, 98, 209
Calcified cartilage, 229, 392
Calcinosis circumscripta, 76
Calcitonin, 167, 393
Calcium (Ca), 164, 210–211
 47, 125
 binding protein, 393
 hydroxyapatite, 393
Calcium pyrophosphate deposition disease (CPPD), 89
Calcodynia, 355
Caldwell and Durham procedure, 266, 271
Calf band, 199
Callahan and Scuderi approach, 274
Callahan approach, 275
Callahan procedure, 301
Callaway test, 141

Callosity, 98, 352
Callotasis, 213, 279, 335
Callus, 13, 98, 352
Cam impingement, 90
Cambium layer, 211–212
Camelback sign, 150
Camitz procedure, 337
Campanacci disease, 53, 90
Campanacci lesion, 46
Campanacci Radiographic Classification for Benign Bone
 Tumors, 120t
Campbell
 approach, 274, 364
 arthrodesis, 228
 procedure, 259, 267–268, 358
 prostheses, 251
Campbell and Akbarnia prostheses, 251
Campbell's Operative Orthopedics, 209
Camper chiasm, 311
Campomelia, 98
Camptocormia, 291
Camptodactyly, 321
Camurati-Engelmann Disease (CED), 60
Camurati-Engelmann dysplasia, 60
Canadian C-spine rule, 120
Canale procedure, 259
Canale view, 109
Canaliculi, 212, 393
Canaliculus, 211
Canal-to-calcar isthmus ratio, 114
Canale-Kelly Classification, 16
Cancellous
 bone, 211, 213, 393
 graft, 217
 screw, 219
Candida, 169
Canes, 183
Cannulated nail or screw, 219
Cantelli sign, 156
Capacitive coupling, 224
Capillaries, 235
Capital epiphysis, 254
Capitate, 307
Capitellar fracture, 16
Capitellocondylar prostheses, 251
Capitellum, 246
Capner procedure, 305
CAPP terminal device, 192
Capsotomy, 230
Capsular arthroplasty, 259
Capsular release, 339
Capsule, 226
Capsulectomy, 230, 331, 339
Capsulitis, 72
Capsulodesis, 230, 339–340
Capsuloplasty, 230
Capsulorrhaphy, 230
Capsulotomy, 230
Carbon implant, 340
Carboxyterminal propeptide (c-PCP, PICP), 168
Cardiovascular, 235

Carducci test, 144
Caries, 98
Caries sicca, 98
Carotid artery, 286
Carotid endarterectomy, 239
Carotid subclavian bypass, 239
Carotid tubercle, 285
Carpal
  bone, 307
  bossing, 328
  coalition, 321
  compression test, 144
  height ratio, 114
  instability, 327
Carpal instability dissociative (CID), 326
Carpal instability nondissociative (CIND), 326
Carpal pedal spasm, 323
Carpal tunnel, 313
  release, 340
  syndrome (CTS), 318
  view, 109
Carpectomy, 340
Carpus, 307
Carroll
  arthrodesis, 331
  arthroplasty, 332
  procedure, 272, 331, 358
Carr procedure, 358
Carrying angle, 111
Carstam and Eiken procedure, 358
Carstam and Theander procedure, 358
Carstan reverse wedge osteotomy, 335
Carter and Ezaki procedure, 358
Carter-Rowe view, 109
Cartilage, 226–227, 391–392
  arthrodial, 229
  bone, 211
  oligomeric protein (COMP), 392
  space narrowing, 295
  surgical procedures, 230
  tumors, 51–52
  types of, 229–230
Cartilage diseases
  chondro-root diseases, 64
  epiphyses abnormalities, 65–67
  miscellaneous, 64–65
  mucopolysaccharidoses, 67
Cartilage-hair hypoplasia, 65
Cartwheel fracture, 11
Caspase, 389
Cast
  accessories, 183
  air, 181
  airplane, 180
  arm cylinder, 179
  body, 179
  boot, 181
  brace, 2, 181
  burns, 181
  complications, 181–182
  components, 225

Cast (Continued)
  cutter, 178
  defined, 178
  devices applied to, 181
  frames, 184–187
  immobilization, 179–181
  limb, 179–180
  materials, 178–179
  orthosis, 181
  padding, 178
  protectors, 181
  shoe, 181
  sock, 195
  spica, 179
  suspensions, 184–187
  syndrome, 182
  terminology, 181
  tractions, 184–187
Castle and Schneider procedure, 259
CAT scan, 105, 125
Categorical variable, 379
Cathepsin, 389
Catheter, 106
Catheterization, 279
Cathode ray tube, 106
Caton-Deschamps ratio, 114
Catterall hip score, 120
Cauda equina syndrome, 287, 295
Causalgia, 79, 318
Cauterization, 279
Cautery, 279
Cave and Rowe procedure, 269
Cave approach, 275
Cavus foot, 357
C-clamp fixation, 224
Cedell fracture, 11
Celery stalk sign, 117
Cell components, 389
Cell cycle, 389–390
Cellular cartilage, 229
Cellulitis, 98
Cement line, 393
Cement-wedge sign, 117
Center edge (CE) angle, 111
Center of gravity, 382
Center of mass, 382
Centigray, 107
Central cord syndrome, 297
Central dislocation, 28, 34
Central fracture, 10, 28
Central nervous system, 283
Central polydactyly, 322
Central sacral line, 114
Central slip, 313, 337
Centralization, 335
Centroid, 382
Cephalic vein, 242, 248
Ceramic-ceramic bearing, 225
Cerebellar gait, 159
Cerebral palsy (CP), 79
Cerebral spinal fluid, 287

Cerebroside reticulocytosis, 60
Cerebrospinal fluid (CSF), 169
Cerebrovascular, 235
Cerebrovascular accident (CVA), 74–75
Certified orthotist (CO), 189
Certified prosthetist (CP), 189
Certified prosthetist-orthotist (CPO), 189
Cervical dislocation, 33–34
Cervical halter traction, 186
Cervical pedicle screws, 303
Cervical plexus, 286
Cervical rib, 291
Cervical spine, 284
   arteries and veins, 286
   bones and landmarks, 285–286
   fusion, 301–302
   injury, score system for, 16
   muscles, 286
   nerves, 286
Cervical traction, 367
Cervico-obturator line, 114
Cfba-1, 57
Chaddock reflex, 155
Chaddock sign, 155
Chadwick and Bentley Classification, 16–17
Chairback orthoses, 202
Chalk bones, 59
Chalk-stick fracture, 117
Chamberlain line, 114–115
Chamfer, 279
Chance fracture, 9–10
Chandler
   arthrodesis, 228
   procedure, 259, 271
Chapple test, 147
Chaput fracture, 11
Chaput tubercle, 261
Charcot
   arthropathy, 352
   disease, 78
   foot, 352
   fracture, 355
   joint disease, 81
Charcot-Marie-Tooth disease, 81, 319, 352
Charcot restraint orthotic walker (CROW), 197
Charleston bending brace, 203
Charley horse, 36, 63
Charnley
   arthrodesis, 228
   hip scale, 159
   screw, 219
   traction, 186
Charnley and Henderson arthrodesis, 228
Charnley Hip Arthroplasty Classification, 90t
Charnley-Müllerv approach, 275
Chauffeur's fracture, 8, 325
Chaves-Rapp procedure, 244
Checkrein deformity, 352
Check socket, 195
Cheilectomy, 358
Cheirospasm, 328

Chemokine, 390
Chemonucleolysis, 300
Chemosterilized grafts, 217
Chemotherapy, 276
Chen procedure, 336
Chest straps, 192
Chevron
   arthrodesis, 330
   osteotomy, 358
   procedure, 358
Chiasma tendinum, 311
Chicago test, 138
Chiene test, 147
Chilblains, 74
Childhood hypophosphatasia, 58
Children
   ankle fracture, 17
   epiphysis, 16–17, 27
   floating knee fracture, 23
   hip fracture, 17
   humeral physeal fracture, 25
   humerus, 19, 21, 24
   pelvic fracture, 30
   physis fracture, 29
   tibia, 24, 26, 31
Children's Amputee Prosthetic Program (CAPP), 189
Childress test, 150
Chinese flap, 334
Chin-on-chest deformity, 293
Chip fracture, 4
Chip graft, 218
Chisel fracture, 8
Chi-square analysis, 379
Cholesterol, 164
Chondralgia, 64
Chondrectomy, 230
Chondritis, 64
Chondroblastoma, 51
Chondroblasts, 231
Chondrocalcinosis, 316
Chondro-(cartilage)
   surgical procedures, 230
   types of, 229–230
Chondroclasts, 231
Chondrocyte, 231, 392
Chondrodiastasis, 230
Chondrodynia, 64
Chondrodysplasia, 64
Chondrodysplasia punctata, 64
Chondrodystrophia, 64
Chondrodystrophia fetalis, 64–65
Chondroepiphysitis, 64
Chondrofibroma, 53, 64
Chondroitin sulfate, 392
Chondrolipoangioma, 53, 64
Chondrolipoma, 53, 64
Chondrolysis, 64
Chondroma, 51
Chondromalacia, 64
Chondromalacia patellae, 92–93

Chondromatosis, 64
Chondrometaplasia, 64
Chondromyoma, 53, 64
Chondromyxoid fibroma, 51
Chondromyxoma, 64
Chondronecrosis, 64
Chondroosteodystrophy, 64, 67
Chondropathia tuberosa, 61
Chondropathology, 64
Chondropathy, 64
Chondrophyte, 64
Chondroplasty, 230
Chondroporosis, 64
Chondro-root diseases, 64
Chondrosarcoma, 51
Chondrosarcomatosis, 64
Chondrosteoma, 64
Chondrosternoplasty, 230
Chondrotomy, 230
Chondrum terminale, 285
Chop amputation, 278
Chopart, 193
   amputation, 358
   dislocations, 34
   joint, 347
Choppy sea sign, 117
Cho procedure, 267
Chordoma, 53
Chorea, 79
Chow procedure, 340
Chrisman-Snook procedure, 358
Chromonychia, 327
Chronic, 98
Chronic cervical sprain, 295–296
Chronic disease, 43
Chronic osteomyelitis, 48
Chronic recurrent multifocal osteomyelitis (CRMO), 48
Chronic regional pain syndrome (CRPS), 75, 318
Chronic sclerosing osteomyelitis of Garre, 48
Chuinard and Petersen arthrodesis, 228
Chun and Palmer procedure, 340
Chung procedure, 333
Chvostek sign, 157
Chvostek test, 157
Chvostek-Weiss sign, 157
Chylothorax, 98
Cicatrix, 98
Cierny-Mader Staging System, 120
Cincinnati approach, 364
Cincinnati incision, 358
Cinefluoroscopy, 125
Cineplastic amputation, 277
Cineradiography, 125
Cineroentgenogram, 125
Circadian, 390
Circular amputation, 277
Circular fixation, 224
Circumduction
   gait, 159
   manuever, 144
   test, 141

Clancy procedure, 267
Clanton and McGarvey classification, 352
Clare procedure, 358
Clark pectoralis major transfer, 337
Clasped thumb, 321
Claudication, 74
Clavicectomy, 244
Clavicle, 240–241
   fractures, 14, 24
   orthoses, 203
   straps, 183
Clavicotomy, 244
Clavus, 352–353
Clavus durum, 354
Clavus mollis, 353
Claw hand deformity, 319
Claw hand sign, 145
Claw toe deformity, 353
Claw-type basic frame, 187
Clay shoveler's fracture, 10
Clayton procedure, 359
Clear cell chondrosarcoma, 51
Clear cell sarcoma, 53
Cleavage fracture, 4
Cleeman sign, 149
Cleft, 60
Cleft hand, 321
Cleidocranial dysostosis, 57
Cleland ligament, 314
Clenched fist view, 109
Clinical pathology, 163
Clinical test evaluation, 381
Clinodactyly, 321
Clipping injury fracture, 11
Cloacae, 48
Clonus, 99
Closed amputation, 277
Closed biopsy, 279
Closed chain exercise, 368
Closed dislocation, 33
Closed fractures, 3
Closed integumentary injury, 14
Closed kinetic chain exercise, 368
Closed management, 1
Closed reduction, 213
Closed suction irrigation, 280
Closing abductory wedge osteotomy (CAWO), 359
Closing wedge cast, 181
Closing wedge osteotomy, 214
Cloth binder, 202
Clothespin graft, 218
Cloverleaf nail, 219
Cloward procedure, 301
Clubbing, 327–328
Clubfoot, 353, 357
Club foot orthose, 197
Cluneal nerve, 253
Coach's finger, 37
Coalition, 353
Coaptation splint, 182

Coast of Maine, 158
Coarse woven bone, 213
Cobb method, 120–121
Cobb syndrome, 293
Cobra plate, 220
Coccidioides, 169
Coccyalgia, 291
Coccydynia, 291
Coccygeal spine, 284
Coccygectomy procedure, 305
Coccygodynia, 291
Coccygotomy procedure, 305
Coccyodynia, 291
Coccyx, 287
Cocked-half flap, 335–336
Cock-up splint, 200
Codfish vertebrae, 117
Codivilla procedure, 269
Codman
 angle, 111
 approach, 274
 exercises, 368
 sign, 141
 triangle, 111
 tumor, 51
Coefficient of friction, 383
-coele, 99
Coffin-Lowry syndrome, 84
Cofield procedure, 244
Cognitive skills, 374
Cogwheel phenomenon, 158
Cogwheel sign, 158
Coleman lateral standing block test, 154
Coleman procedure, 359
Cole and Manske Classification for the First Distal Ray Absence with Ulnar Deficiency, 96t–97t
Cole osteotomy, 214
Cole procedure, 359
Collagen, 230–231, 390
Collagen oligomeric matrix protein (COMP), 89
Collagenases, 391
Collar and cuff, 181
Collar-button abscess, 329
Collateral circulation, 235–238
Collateral ligament, 234, 350
Colles fracture, 8
Colonna and Ralston approach, 364
Colonna capsular arthroplasty, 259
Colonna (Delbet) classification, 17
Colony count (CC), 169
Color Doppler, 129
Columnar zone, 212
Colton Classification, 17
Comatose, 99
Combined arch support, 206
Combined stenosis, 294
Commemorative sign, 158
Comminuted fracture, 4
Commission on Accreditation in Physical Therapy Education, 365
Commissural myelorrhaphy procedure, 305

Committee on the Hip, American Academy of Orthopaedic Surgeons, 91
Common digital arteries and nerves, 314
Common flora, 169
Common peroneal nerve, 266
Common tendon, 231
Communication device use, 373
Comolli sign, 141
Compact bone, 211, 393
Compartment syndrome, 74
Compensatory curve, 292–293
Compere and Thompson arthrodesis, 228
Complete aphalangia, 95
Complete dislocation, 33
Complete fracture, 4
Complete paraxial hemimelia, 95
Complete phocomelia, 95
Complex regional pain syndrome, 79, 317
Compliance, 383
Complicated dislocation, 33
Composite beam model, 256
Composite graft, 218
Composite nail bed flap, 336
Compound dislocation, 33
Compound lined pedicle, 273
Compound pedicle, 273
Compression, 383
 arthrodesis, 228
 dressing, 183
 fracture, 4, 9
 of nerve root, 295
Compressive neuropathy, 317
Computed axial tomography (CAT scan), 105, 125
Computed tomography (CT), 125, 386
Computed tomography (CT) angiography, 128–129
Computer-aided orthopaedic surgery (CAOS), 225
Computer-assisted design/computer-assisted manufacturing (CAD-CAM), 194
Computer assisted orthopaedic surgery (CAOS), 279
Computer-assisted tomography (CAT), 386
Computerized isokinetic dynamometer, 370
Concentric contraction, 368
Condensing osteitis of the clavicle, 57
Conduction time, 371
Condylar cuff, 194
Condylar fracture, 4, 8
Condylar-plateau angle (CPA), 111
Condyle, 211
Condylectomy, 213, 359
Condylotomy, 213
Cone arthrodesis, 359
Coned-down view, 109
Confidence interval (CI), 379
Confocal scanning microscopy (CSM), 387
Confrontational test, 145
Congenital, 99
Congenital bars, 353
Congenital convex pes valgus, 353, 357
Congenital disease, 43
Congenital dislocation, 33–34, 93
Congenital dysplasia of the hip (CDH), 34

Congenital hip
  disease, 91
  dislocation, 91
  dysplasia, 91
Congenital hypotonia, 62
Congenital myotonia, 62
Congenital pancytopenia, 100
Congenital pseudarthrosis, 57
Congenital rocker-bottom flatfoot, 353
Congenital scoliosis, 293
Congenital trigger thumb, 320–321
Congenital ulnar drift, 321
Congenital vertical talus, 353
Congestive heart failure, 78
Congruence angle, 111
Conjoined tendon, 231, 242
Connecting cartilage, 229
Connexin-32, 81
Connexus intertendineus, 311–312
Conoid ligament, 242
Conrad-Bugg trapping, 11
Consecutive dislocation, 33
Constant, 380
Constant angle exercise, 369
Constant force exercise, 369
Constitutional stenosis, 294
Constrained, 271
Constrained liner, 256
Constriction bands, 320
Constriction ring syndrome, 71
Constrictive edema, 182
Contagious disease, 43
Contamination, 27
Continuous passive motion (CPM), 186
Continuous variable, 379
Contour adducted trochanteric controlledalignment method (CAT-CAM), 194
Contractions, 99
Contracture, 99
Contralateral sign, 155
Contralateral straight leg raising test, 138
Contrast, 106
  baths, 367
  radiography, 106
  study, 106
Contrecoup, 99
Control belt, 195
Control cables, 191
Control orthoses, 203
Controlled ankle motion (CAM) walkers, 181, 206
Contusion, 99
Convalescence, 99
Conventional orthoses, 197
Conversion disorder, 99
Convulsion, 99
Cooney procedure, 333
Cooper test, 150
Coopernail sign, 138
Coordination extremity test, 156
Copeland and Howard procedure, 244
Coracoacromial veil, 244

Coracobrachialis, 242
Coracobrachialis muscle, 247
Coracoclavicular ligament, 242
Coracohumeral ligament, 242
Coracoid, 241
Coracoid fracture, 8
Coracoid impingement syndrome, 37
Cordotomy procedure, 305
Core decompression, 107
Core protein, 392
Corner fracture, 8
Corner sign, 119
Coronal femoral component angle, 111
Coronal tibial component angle, 111
Coronary artery bypass graft (CABG), 239
Coronoid fracture, 25
Coronoid process, 247
Corpectomy procedure, 305
Corrective cast, 181
Correlation, 379
Corset front, 205
Cortical bone, 211, 393
Cortical desmoid, 53
Cortical fibrous dysplasia, 57
Cortical fracture, 4
Cortical graft, 218
Cortical screw, 220
Corticocancellous graft, 218
Corticotomy, 213
Costectomy, 244
Costo, 286
Costochondral junction, 286
Costoclavicular maneuver, 136
Costophrenic angle, 112
Costoplasty, 279
Costotransversectomy, 244, 300
Costovertebral angle, 112, 286
Costovertebral joint, 286
Cotrel cast, 179
Cotrel-Dubousset, 304
Cotrel traction, 186
Cotting, 359
Cotton
  fracture, 11
  osteotomy, 214
  test, 154, 154
  Cotton roll, 179
Cotton-loader position cast, 180
Couch, DeRosa, and Throop procedure, 260
Counter, 205
Couple, 383
Coventry osteotomy, 214
Cowen and Loftus procedure, 340
Coxa
  adducta, 91
  breva, 90
  magna, 91
  plana, 55, 60, 91
  saltans, 91
  senilis, 91
  valga, 91

Coxa *(Continued)*
  vara, 91
    vara luxans, 91
Coxalgia, 91
Coxarthria, 91
Coxarthritis, 91
Coxarthrocace, 91
Coxarthropathy, 91
Coxarthrosis, 91
Coxitis, 91
Coxotomy, 260
Coxotuberculosis, 91
Cozen test, 138
Cracchiolo procedure, 359
Cram test, 138
Cramp, 99
Craniomandibular cervical syndrome, 294
Crank test, 141
Crankshaft phenomenon, 291
Crawford-Adams pin, 220
Crawford procedure, 359
Crawford small parts dexterity test, 372
C-reactive protein (CRP), 166
Creatine kinase (CK), 166
Creatine phosphokinase (CPK), 166
Creatinine (Cr), 164, 166
Creep, 383
Creeping substitution, 217
Crego, 258
Crego osteotomy, 214
Crepitus, 99
Crescentic osteotomy, 359
Crescent sign, 117
CREST syndrome, 76
Crevice corrosion, 225
Cricoid ring, 285
Cronin technique, 335
Cross-arm flap, 334
Cross-body abduction maneuver, 141
Cross-body adduction test, 140–141
Cross-chest test, 141
Crossed intrinsic transfer, 337–338
Cross-finger flap, 334, 336
Crossing sign, 117
Cross-leg pedicle skin graft, 273
Cross-linked ultra-high-molecular-weight polyethylene (UHMWPE), 225
Cross-over sign, 117
Cross-over syndrome, 37
Cross-over test, 150
Cross-table lateral view, 109
Cross-training, 368
Crossunion, 13
Crouzon disease, 60
Crowe Classification for Percent of Hip Subluxation, 91t
Crucial angle of Gissane, 112
Cruciate
  retaining, 271
  sacrificing, 271
  screw, 220
  substituting, 271

Cruciform anterior spinal hyperextension (CASH) orthoses, 203
Crush fracture, 9
Crutches, 183
Crutchfield tongs, 186
Cryoprecipitate (Cryo), 172
Cryotherapy, 336, 367
Cryptococcus, 169
  latex antigen test, 169
  neoformans, 169
Crystalline arthropathy, 316
C-telopeptide (cross-links, CTx or CTX), 168
Cubbins approach, 274
Cubbins procedure, 244
Cubital tunnel, 249
Cubital tunnel syndrome, 319
Cuboid bone, 344
Culp procedure, 333
Culture and sensitivity (C&S), 169
Cuneiform, 344
Cuneiform osteotomy, 214
Cup arthroplasty, 256
Curettage, 279
Curette, 279
Curly toe, 353
Current life activities, 374
Curtis procedure, 332
Cushing disease, 84
Custom bi-valved (polymer) TLSO, 203
Custom-molded shoes, 205–206
Cutaneous ligament, 313–314
Cutaneous nerve
  of the arm, 248
  of the forearm, 249
Cut-back zone, 211
Cute postpartum sacroiliiti, 292
Cuticle, 314, 350
Cutting cone, 211
Cyanosis, 78, 99
Cyclooxygenase, 390
Cylinder casts, 180
Cylindrical osteotomy, 359
Cyst, 99
Cystic arthrosis, 71
Cystic osteomyelitis, 49
Cytokine, 390
Cytomorphology, 386

D

D/3, distal third, 3–4
Dactylitis, 329, 353
Dactylolysis spontanea, 352
Damage control orthopaedics, 279
Danis-Weber classification, 31
Dark-field microscopy, 387
Darrach-McLaughlin approach, 274
Darrach resection, 332
Das Gupta procedure, 244
Dashboard dislocation, 34
Dashboard fracture, 10

D'Aubigne procedure, 266, 272
Davis arthrodesis, 228
Davis skin graft, 273
Dawbarn sign, 141
De Andrade and MacNab fixation, 301
De Quervain
    disease, 69, 323
    fracture, 8
    release, 339
De Rosa and Graziano prostheses, 251
Debeyre procedure, 244
Debridement, 99, 279
Decalcification, 99
Decompression, 279, 300
Decompressive laminectomy, 300
Decorin, 390
Decreased foot angle, 112
Decubitus ulcer, 182
Dedifferentiated chondrosarcoma, 51
Deep branch posterior tibial artery, 351
Deep compartment, 263
Deep femoral artery, 255, 266
Deep ligament, 264–265
Deep peroneal nerve, 266
Deep space infection, 329
Deep transverse intermetacarpal ligament, 312
Deep transverse metacarpal ligament, 311
Deep transverse metatarsal ligaments, 350
Deep venous thrombosis (DVT), 73
Defensins, 390
Defervescence, 99
Degenerative, 99
Degenerative arthritis, 92–93, 316
Degenerative disease, 43
Degenerative disk disease, 295–296
Degenerative stenosis, 294
Degenerative tear, 92–93
Degloving, 41, 99
Degrees, 382
Degrees of freedom, 383
Dehiscence, 99, 279
Dehne cast, 179
Dejerine disease, 81
Dejerine sign, 138
Dejerine-Sottas syndrome, 81
Dejour Classification for Trochlear Dysplasia, 121t
Deland procedure, 359
Delayed flap skin graft, 273
Delayed-onset muscle soreness (DOMS), 62
Delayed primary closure, 279, 282
Delayed union, 13
Delayed vertebral collapse, 60
Delbert casts, 180
DeLorme exercises, 369
Delta nail, 220
Delta phalanx, 321
Deltoid, 242
    flap, 336
    ligament, 312, 350
    splitting approach, 274
    sprain, 35

Deltopectoral approach, 274
Demarcation line, 115
Demianoff sign, 138
Demineralized bone graft, 217
Denervation, 334
Denis-Browne bar, 197
Denis Classification, 17
Dennison brace, 204
Dennyson and Fulford procedure, 359
Denver metatarsal bar, 206
Deossification, 99
Deoxyribonucleic acid (DNA), 390
Dependent drainage, 280
Dependent variable, 379–380
Depth-Ischemia Classification Foot Ulcers, 357t
Depressed fracture, 4
Derangement, 99
Derby nail, 220
Dermatofibrosarcoma protuberans (DFSP), 53–54
Dermatomal, 295
Dermatomal pain, 43–44
Dermatome, 295
Dermatomycosis pedis, 352
Dermatomyositis, 76
Dermodesis, 340
Derotation osteotomy, 214
Desault dislocation, 326
Desault sign, 147
Descot fracture, 11
Descriptive, 382
Designed after natural anatomy (DANA) total shoulder, 246
Desmalgia, 69
Desmectasis, 69
Desmin stain, 170
Desmitis, 69
Desmocytoma, 69
Desmodynia, 69
Desmoid, 69
Desmo (ligaments), 234
    surgical procedures on, 234
Desmoma, 69
Desmopathy, 69
Desmoplasia, 69
Desmoplastic, 69
Desmoplastic fibroma of bone, 53
Desmo-root diseases, 69
Desmorrhexis, 69
Desmosis, 69
Desmotomy, 234
Destot sign, 147
Devascularized neuropathies, 206
Developmental dysplasia, 33
    of the hip (DDH), 34, 91
Dewar and Barrington procedure, 244
Dextrorotoscoliosis, 292
Deyerle
    maneuver, 147–148
    pin, 220
    test, 138
Diabetes, 84

Diabetic cheiroarthropathy, 316
Diabetic foot disease, 74, 353
Diabetic foot infection classification (PEDIS grade), 353t
Diabetic neuropathies, 206
Diacondylar fracture, 4
Diagnosis, 99
Dial lock, 199
Dial osteotomy, 214
Dial test, 150, 153
Diamond inlay graft, 218
Diaphragm, 287
Diaphysectomy, 213
Diaphysis, 211, 393
Diaplasis, 213, 279
Diarthrodial cartilage, 229
Dias and Giegerich procedure, 359
Dias-Tachdjian classification, 17
Diastasis, 2, 11
Diastematomyelia, 291, 298
Diastole, 238
Diastrophic dwarfism, 65
Diastrophic dysplasia, 65
Diathermy, 367
Dickson-Diveley procedure, 359
Dickson osteotomy, 214
Differential interference contrast (DIC) microscopy, 387
Differential WBC (diff), 164
Diffuse, 99
Diffuse idiopathic sclerosing hyperostosis (DISH), 71
Digital artery and nerve, 351
Digital color Doppler, 105
Digital fibrokeratoma, 328
Digital fossa, 254
Digital prosthesis, 359
Digital retinaculum, 313
Digital subtraction angiography (DSA), 129
1,25-dihydrocholecalciferol, 394
24,25-dihydroxycholecalciferol, 394
1,25-dihydroxyvitamin D3, 394
1,25-dihydroxyvitamin D, 1,25 hydroxycholecalciferol 1,25(OH)2D, 167
Dillwyn-Evans procedure, 359
Dimon and Hughston procedure, 260
Dimon osteotomy, 214
Dimple sign, 154, 158
Diplegic, 79
Direct Coombs test, direct anti–human globulin test (DAT), 173
Direct electric stimulation, 224
Direct fracture, 4
Direct head rectus femoris, 262
Direct injury dislocation, 33
Direct lateral approach, 275
Directed donor, 171
Dirty wound, 282
Disappearing bone disease, 46
Disarticulation, 277
Discectomy, 300
Discitis, 296
Discogenic pain, 296

Discoid meniscus, 93
Discondylar fracture, 4
Disease, 43
  incidence, 382
  prevalence, 382
Disk replacements, 304
Disk space
  infection, 296
  narrowing, 295
Diskogram, 107
Diskography, 107
Dislocations, 32–34
  ankle, 34
  defined, 2
  elbow, 33–34
  foot, 34
  general, 33
  hip, 34
  knee, 34
  patella, 34
  shoulder, 33
  specific, 33–34
  spine, 34
  terminology, 2–3
Dismemberment, 279
Disorganized disk, 295–296
Displacement, 383
Dissection, 279
Distal approach, 274
Distal bypass, 239
Distal clavicle fractures
  Neer classification for, 24
  stability of, 24
Distal coated stem, 256
Distal dystrophy muscular dystrophy, 63
Distal end pad, 195
Distal finger amputation revision, 333
Distal interphalangeal (DIP)
  fusion, 359
  joint, 344
Distal metatarsal articular angle, 351
Distal palmar crease (DPC), 313
Distal phocomelia, 95
Distal pulp, 314
Distal thigh band, 199
Distal tibial pilon fracture, 28
Distal tingling on percussion (DTP) sign, 157
Distance/time^2, 382
Distraction lengthening, 335
Distraction osteogenesis, 213
Divergent dislocation, 33
Diver's disease, 57
Diverticulum, 99
Dobs bar, 197
Dolichostenomelia, 95
Doll's eye sign, 156
Dome fracture, 10–11
Dome plunger, 220
Dominant inheritance, 100
Donning sleeve, 195
Dooley nail, 220

Doppler ultrasound, 129
Dorrance voluntary-opening hand, 192
Dorr ratio, 115
Dorsal and plantar ligaments
   cuneocuboid, 350
   cuneonavicular, 350
   intercuneiform, 350
   metatarsal, 350
   tarsometatarsal, 350
Dorsal approach, 341
Dorsal bunion, 352
Dorsal capsulectomy, 332
Dorsal capsulodesis, 331
Dorsal column, 287
Dorsal digital artery and nerve, 314
Dorsal expansion, 314
Dorsal extensor compartments, 312
Dorsal intercalated segment instability (DISI), 327
Dorsal intercarpal ligament, 312
Dorsal interossei, 310
Dorsal lateral column, 288
Dorsal lumbar corset, 203
Dorsal lumbar support, 203
Dorsal radial ligament, 312
Dorsal radiocarpal ligament, 312
Dorsal scapular nerve, 243
Dorsal spine, 284
Dorsalis pedis artery, 351
Dorsalis pedis flap, 334
Dorsal-V osteotomy, 359
Dorsal wedge osteotomy, 359
Dorsiflexed metatarsal, 353
Dorsolateral approach, 306
Double-action ankle joint, 200
Double adjustable ankle joint (DAAJ), 197
Double bubble, 256
Double-bundle repair, 267
Double camelback sign, 151
Double cast, 180
Double crush syndrome, 81, 319
Double curve, 293
Double density sign, 117
Double fracture, 4
Double major curve, 293
Double PCL sign, 151
Double pedicle, 273
Double popliteus tendon sign, 117
Double posterior cruciate ligament sign, 117
Double thoracic curve, 293
Douglas skin graft, 272
Dowager's hump, 99
Dowel procedure, 301
Down syndrome, 84
Dragstedt skin graft, 272
Drainage, 280
Drawer sign, 151, 154
Drawer test, 141
Drennan procedure, 359
Dressings, 178, 183–184, 373
   accessories, 183
   materials, 184

Dressings *(Continued)*
   specialized, 184
   types of, 183–184
Drez procedure, 267
Dripping candle wax sign, 117
Drop-arm test, 141
Drop-back phenomenon, 151
Drop finger, 9, 316
Drop foot, 182, 353
Drop foot gait, 159
Drop-lock ring, 200
Drop out cast, 179
DRUJ, 307
Drummond interspinous segmental spinal, 305
Dry dressing, 183
Du Toit and Roux procedure, 244
Dual-energy x-ray absorptiometry (DXA, DEXA), 386
Dual geometry, 256
Dual onlay graft, 218
Dual photon absorptiometry (DPA), 107
Dual photon densitometry (DPD), 107, 125–126
Dual x-ray absorptiometry (DEXA), 107
Duchenne
   disease, 81
   muscular dystrophy, 63
   sign, 145
Ductile deformation, 384
Dugas sign, 141
Dugas test, 141
Dunlop traction, 186
Dunn-Brittain procedure, 359
Dunn-Brittain triple arthrodesis, 359
Dunn procedure, 260, 305
Dunn view, 109
Duplay disease, 69
Duplex Doppler, 129
Duplex ultrasound, 129
Dupuytren
   contracture, 70, 328, 340
   exostosis, 328
   fibromatosis, 353
   fracture, 9, 11
   sign, 148, 158
Dural ectasia, 79
Dura mater, 287
Durham procedure, 359
Durkan test, 145
Duverney fracture, 10
DuVries
   arthroplasty, 359
   plantar condylectomy, 359
   procedure, 362
   procedures, 359
Dwyer, 304
   osteotomy, 214
   procedures, 359
Dwyer-Hartsill fixation, 302
Dye punch fracture, 8, 325
Dynamic-compression plate (DCP), 220
Dynamic finger splint, 201
Dynamic hinged elbow fracture brace, 201

Dynamic hip screw (DHS), 220
Dynamic load, 383
Dynamic orthoses, 198
Dynamic response foot, 194
Dynamic splint, 182, 374
Dynamic tendon transfer, 338
Dynamometer, 370
-dynia, 99
Dys-, 99
Dysautonomia, 79
Dyschondroplasia, 64
Dyscollagenosis, 76
Dyscrasic fracture, 12
Dysesthesia, 99, 317
Dysfunction, 99
Dysmelia, 94
Dysplasia, 99
  epiphysealis capitis femoris, 91
  epiphysealis hemimelia, 65
  epiphysealis hemimelica, 52
  epiphyseal multiplex congenita, 65
Dysraphism, 291
Dyssegmental dysplasia, 84
Dystonia, 99
Dystrophin, 63
Dystrophinopathy muscular dystrophy, 63
Dystrophy, 99

E

Eagle-Barrett syndrome, 88
Earle sign, 148
Early growth response gene EGR2, 81
East Baltimore maneuver, 148
Eaton and Littler procedure, 333
Eaton and Malerich procedure, 334
Eaton procedure, 332
Eaton volar plate arthroplasty, 332
Ebonation, 213, 280
Eburnation, 99
Eccentric contraction, 369
Ecchymosis, 99
Echogenic, 106
Ecker, Lotke, and Glazer procedure, 271
Ecthyma contagiosum, 329
Ectromelia, 94–95
Edema, 99–100
Eden-Hybbinette procedure, 244
Eden-Lange procedure, 244
Edgarton-Grand procedure, 339
Edinburgh method, 121
Edwards, 304
Effleurage, 369
Effort thrombosis, 89
Effusion, 100
Eggers plate and screw, 220
Eggers procedure, 271
Eggshell procedure, 305
Egyptian foot, 353
Ehlers-Danlos syndrome (EDS), 84
Eichenholtz Classification for Foot Charcot Arthropathy, 352t

Elastic, 383
Elastic cartilage, 229–230, 392
Elastic orthoses, 197
  knee, 198
Elastic stable intramedullary nailing (ESIN), 220
Elastic twister orthoses, 199
Elastofibroma, 54
Elastohydrodynamic lubrication, 384
Elbow
  anatomy, 246–250
  blood vessels of, 248
  bones, 246–247
  conditions, 89–90
  disarticulation (ED), 190
  dislocations, 33–34
  extension splint, 201
  flexion test, 143
  hinges, 191
  ligaments of, 249–250
  nerves of, 248–249
Electrical stimulation, 367
Electrical switch control, 191
Electrical testing, 371
Electrocardiogram (ECG), 129, 174
Electrocauterization, 280
Electrocautery, 280
Electroencephalogram (EEG), 174
Electromyography (EMG), 371, 388
Electrophoresis and blotting, 386
Elementary acetabular fracture, 22
Eleventh cranial nerve, 286
Elliott plate, 220
Ellis Jones procedures, 359
Ellis prostheses, 251
Ellison procedure, 267
Ellis-Van Crevel syndrome, 321
Elmslie-Cholmely procedures, 359
Elmslie procedures, 359
Elmslie-Trillat procedure, 268
Elongation, 383
Elson middle slip test, 145
Ely sign, 156
Ely test, 139, 148, 156
Emaciation, 100
Embolus, 74
Emery-Dreifuss muscular dystrophy, 63
Emission frequency, 387
Employment seeking and acquisition, 374
Encephalocelec spina bifida, 299
Encerclage, 220
Enchondral bone, 211
Enchondroma, 52
Enchondromatosis, 52
Endarterectomy, 239
Ender nail, 220
Endochondral ossification, 393
Endocrine fracture, 12
Endoskeletal prosthesis, 196
Endosteum, 211
Endovascular grafting, 239
Endovascular therapy, 239

End-to-end anastomosis, 239
End-to-side anastomosis, 239
Endurance limit, 383
Endurance training, 369
Energy
  conservation, 374
  to failure, 385
  measures, 383
  storing feet, 194
  to yield, 385
Engebretsen procedure, 267
Engelmann disease, 58, 60
Enneking procedure, 267
Enthesis, 70
Enthesitis, 70
Enthesopathy, 70
Entrapment syndrome, 79
Enucleate, 280
Enzyme-linked immunosorbent assay (ELISA), 386
Eosinophilia-myalgia syndrome, 63
Eosinophilic granuloma, 52, 61
Ependymoma, 297
Epiarticular osteochondroma, 52
Epiarticular osteochondromatous dysplasia, 52
Epicondylar fracture, 8
Epicondylitis, 70
Epidemiology, 378–382
Epidermoid cyst, 328
Epidural block, 273
Epigenetics, 390
Epilepsy, 79
Epineural fibrosis, 79
Epineural repair, 333
Epineurotomy, 333
Epiphyseal
  aseptic necrosis, 55
  cartilage, 212
  dysplasia, 67
  exostosis, 52
  fracture, 4
  hyperplasia, 65
  ischemic necrosis, 55
  line, 115
  osteochondroma, 52
  plate, 211–212
  shaft angle, 114
  slip fracture, 6
Epiphysiodesis, 65, 213
Epiphysiolysis, 65, 213
Epiphysiopathy, 65
Epiphysis, 211, 393
  abnormalities, 65–67
  distal tibia fracture, 16–17
  fracture, 27
Epiphysitis, 65
Epithelioid sarcoma, 54
Epitrochlea, 246
Eponychia, 329
Eponychium, 314, 350
Eponymic joint diseases, 72
Eponymic ligamentous diseases, 69

Equatorial contact, 256
Equilibrium, 383
Equinovarus outflare shoes, 207
Equinus, 353
Equinus gait, 159
Erb
  disease, 63
  palsy, 81
  paralysis, 63
Erb-Goldflam disease, 61
Ergometer, 370
Ergotism, 76
Eriacetabular osteotomy (PAO), 215
Erichsen sign, 138
Ericksson procedure, 267
Erosion, 100
Erythema, 100
Erythrocyte sedimentation rate (sed. rate, sedimentation rate, ESR), 166
Eschar, 100
Escharotomy, 336
Escherichia coli (E. coli), 48, 169
Esmarch bandage, 184
Esophagus, 286
Esser skin graft, 273
Essex-Lopresti Classification, 18
Essex-Lopresti fracture, 8
Essex-Lopresti procedures, 359
Established osteoporosis, 83
Esthesia, 100
Etiologic factors, 100
Eurotaper (12/14), 226
Evacuate, 280
Evans procedures, 359
Evans-Wales classification, 18
Ewing's sarcoma, 52
Exacerbation, 100
Exchange nailing, 220
Excise, 280
Excitation frequency, 387
Excursion amplifier sleeve, 191
Exostectomy, 360
Exostosis, 52, 57, 353
Exotic scoliosis, 293
Experimental/interventional, 382
Exploration, 280
Exploratory surgery, 280
EXT, 57
EXT2Extended counter, 57, 206
Extended steel shank, 200
Extension aid, 195
Extension body cast, 179
Extension lag, 151
Extensor carpi radialis brevis (ECRB), 248, 310
Extensor carpi radialis intermedius, 310
Extensor carpi radialis longus (ECRL), 248, 310
Extensor carpi ulnaris (ECU), 310
Extensor digiti quinti proprius (EDQP), 310
Extensor digitorum brevis, 349
Extensor digitorum brevis manus muscle, 310
Extensor digitorum communis (EDC), 310

Extensor digitorum longus, 263, 349
Extensor hallucis brevis, 349
Extensor hallucis longus, 263, 349
Extensor hood, 314
Extensor indicis proprius (EIP), 310
Extensor pollicis brevis (EPB), 310
Extensor pollicis longus (EPL), 310
Extensor wad of three, 247–248
External knee prosthetic components, 195
External malleolus sign, 155
External oblique muscles, 288
External rotation
   drawer test, 151
   injuries, 15
   recurvatum test, 151
External rotators, 254–255
Externally powered tenodesis orthoses, 201
Extirpation, 280
Extraabdominal desmoid, 54, 69
Extraabdominal fibromatosis, 54
Extraanatomic bypass, 239
Extraarticular arthrodesis, 228
Extraarticular fracture, 4
Extracapsular ankylosis, 72
Extracapsular fracture, 4, 10, 16
Extracranial-intracranial bypass (ECIC), 239–240
Extraction, 280
Extra-depth shoes, 206
Extreme lateral interbody fusion (XLIF), 302
Extrinsic muscles, 308–310
Extrinsic tightness test, 145
Extruded disk, 300
Extruded fragment, 300
Extrusion, 296
Extubation, 280
Exudate, 100
Ex vivo, 386
Eycle-Shymer approach, 275
Eyler flexorplasty, 252
Eyler procedure, 245
Eylon procedure, 360
Eyring and Guthrie procedure, 360

F

Fabellofibular ligament, 264
FABERE test, 138–139, 148
Face climbing, 37
Facet, 211
   joint, 283–284
   subluxations, 34
   tropism, 291
Facetectomy procedure, 305
Facial nerve, 286
Factitious edema, 325
Factitious injury, 100
Factor IX, 173
Factor of safety, 383
Factor VIII, 170, 173
Fracture of necessity, 1, 9
FADIRE sign/test, 139

Fahey and O'Brien procedure, 272
Fahey approach, 275
Failure of segmentation, 298
Failure point, 385
Fairbanks and Sever procedure, 245
Fairbanks changes, 121–122
Fairbanks sign, 151
Fajersztajn crossed sciatic sign, 138
False ankylosis, 73
False profile view, 109
Familial dysautonomia, 79
Familial expansile osteolysis, 46
Familial interstitial hypertrophic neuritis, 81
Familial lymphedema, 88
Familial periodic paralysis, 63
Fanconi anemia, 100, 321
Fanconi syndrome, 83
Fan sign, 156
Farmer procedure, 360
Farmer's hook, 192
Fasciae, 234–235
   surgical procedures on, 235
Fasciaplasty, 235
Fascia-related diseases, 70
Fasciectomy, 235, 336
Fasciitis, 70, 329
Fasciodesis, 235
Fascioplasty, 235
Fasciorrhaphy, 231, 235
Fascioscapulohumeral muscular dystrophy, 63
Fasciotomy, 235, 336
Fasting blood sugar (FBS), 166
Fatigue, 383
Fatigue fracture, 12–13
Fatigue limit, 383
Fat pad, 351
Fat pad sign, 117
Fat sat, 126
Fat saturation, 126
Fat suppression, 126
Febrile, 100
Feeding and eating, 373
Feiss line, 115, 351
Feldon 2-pin wrist arthrodesis, 331
Feldon wafer resection, 251
Feller patellar score, 159–160
Felon, 330
Felt padding, 179
Felty syndrome, 76
Femoral Classification for Congenital Deficiencies, 92t
Femoral-femoral bypass (fem-fem bypass), 240
Femur/femoral, 254, 261
   acetabular impingement (FAI), 91
   arteriography, 107
   artery, 255, 266
   condylar shaving, 269
   condyles, 261
   cortical index, 115
   deficiencies, 91–92
   distal, 15
   floating knee fracture, 23

Femur/femoral *(Continued)*
　fracture, 20–21
　　head, 27, 29–30, 115, 254, 256–258
　　intertrochanteric fracture, 18, 20, 29
　　neck, 10, 254
　　nerve, 139, 156, 253, 255
　　offset, 115
　　popliteal bypass (FPB), 240
　　proximal, 16
　　ring allograft (FRA), 302–303
　　shaft fracture, 23, 31
　　shaft line, 115
　　subtrochanteric fracture, 18
　　tibial angle, 112
　　trochanteric fracture, 21
　　vein, 266
Fenestrate, 181
Fenestration, 213
Ferguson procedure, 258
Ferguson's angle, 112
Ferguson-Thompson-King-Moore osteotomy, 214
Fergusson method, 122
Ferkel-Cheng arthroscopic classification, 18
Ferkel-Sgaglione classification, 18
Fernandez procedure, 334
Fernandez prostheses, 251
Ferrari orthoses, 199
FGFR3, 89
Fiber, 392
Fiber bone, 213
Fiberglass cast, 179
Fibermetal, 225
Fibril, 392
Fibrillation, 100
Fibrillin-1, 88
Fibrillin-2, 88
Fibrin clot glue, 334
Fibroblast growth factor 23 receptor (FGFR23), 83
Fibroblast growth factor receptor 3 gene (FGFR3), 89
Fibroblast growth factor receptors 1 and 2 (FGFR 1 & FGFR 2), 59–60, 88
Fibroblasts, 231
Fibrocartilage, 226–227, 230, 392
Fibrocytes, 231
Fibrodysplasia ossificans progressiva, 57
Fibrogenesis imperfecta ossium, 57
Fibroma, 54
Fibromatosis, 54
Fibromodulin, 390
Fibromuscular dysplasia (FMD), 74
Fibrosarcoma, 53, 69
Fibrosis, 68
Fibrositis, 68
Fibrositis ossificans progressiva, 57
Fibrous ankylosis, 73
Fibrous histiocytoma, 68
Fibrous tumors, 53
Fibroxanthoma, 53
Fibroxanthosarcoma, 54
Fibula, 261
Fibular collateral sprain, 35

Fibular facet, 261
Fibular neck, 261
Fick angle, 112, 159
Fielding-Magliato classification, 18
Figure 8, 183
Figure of 4 test, 138–139, 151
Film lubrication, 384
Filum terminale, 287
Finacetto sign, 151
Fine woven bone, 213
Fingers
　benders, 201
　extension procedure, 338
　extensors, 310
　flaps, 334
　flexion procedure, 338
　flexors, 310
　nail, 314
　to nose test, 156
Finite element analysis (FE, FEA), 383
Finite element modeling (FEM), 383
Finkelstein sign, 145
First dorsal interosseous assist, 202
First-generation cementing, 258
First-generation technique, 225
Fisher exact test, 379
Fishmouth incision, 340
Fish osteotomy, 214
Fish procedure, 260
Fisk-Fernandez volar wedge, 334
Fissures, 4, 100
Fistula, 74–75
Five-in-one repair, 267
Fixateurs, 2, 223–224
Fixation, 280
Fixators, 2
External, 223–224
Fixed anatomic, 271
Fixed curve, 292
Flaccid, 100
Flaccid cerebral palsy (CP), 79
Flag flap, 336
Flail, 100
　foot, 354
　joint, 71
Flail-elbow hinge, 202
Flat bones, 211
Flatfoot, 351, 354, 357
Flattening of normal lumbar curve, 293
Flexible flatfoot, 354
Flexible hinge implant, 332
Flexible hinges, 191
Flexible orthoses, 197
Flexible pes planus, 356
Flexion body cast, 179
Flexion contracture, 93
Flexion control orthoses, 203
Flexion exercises, 370
Flexion rotation drawer test, 151
Flexor and extensor retinacula, 312–313
Flexor carpi radialis (FCR), 310–311

Flexor carpi ulnaris (FCU), 310–311
Flexor digiti quinti brevis (FDQB), 310
Flexor digitorum longus and brevis, 263, 349
Flexor digitorum profundus (FDP), 310
Flexor digitorum sublimis (FDS), 310
Flexor digitorum superficialis (FDS), 310
Flexor hallucis longus and brevis, 263, 349
Flexor origin syndrome, 37, 328
Flexor pollicis brevis (FPB) deep and superficial head, 310
Flexor pollicis longus (FPL), 310
Flexor pronator slide, 338
Flexor tendons of the wrist, 310–311
Flexor tenolysis, 338
Flexor wad of five, 248, 310
Flipper hand, 322
Flipping technique, 334
Floating cartilage, 230
"Floating knee,", 15, 23
Floating ribs, 287
Floating shoulder, 35
Floating thumb, 322
Floor reaction orthoses, 197
    ankle foot, 200
Florid reactive periostitis, 59
Flow cytometry, 170, 386
Fluid-controlled knee (hydraulic or pneumatic), 195
Fluidotherapy, 368
Fluorescence microscopy, 387
Fluorescent treponemal antibody (FTA), 169
Fluoroscopy, 107
Flush metatarsal bar, 206
Flynn prostheses, 251
Focal disease, 43
Focal dystonia, 319
Focal fibrocartilaginous dysplasia, 93
Focal scleroderma, 76
Foot/feet, 343–364
    anatomy, 343–351
    arteries of, 357
    athlete's, 352
    bones of, 344–349
    components, 194–195
    conditions, 351–357
    cramps, 354
    diseases, 351–357
    dislocations, 34
    drop, 353
    fracture, 24
    ligaments of, 350
    muscles of, 349–350
    nails, 350
    nerves of, 357
    prostheses for, 364
    surgery, 357–364
    tendons of, 349–350
    veins of, 357
Foot slap gait, 159
Football ankle, 37
Football finger, 37
Foramen, 284
Foramina, 283, 294

Foraminotomy, 300
Forbes procedure, 272
Force plate, 386
Forced adduction test, 141
Forearm
    anatomy, 246–250
    blood vessels of, 248
    bones, 246–247
    lift assist, 191
    ligaments of, 249–250
    muscles of, 247–248
    nerves of, 248–249
    surgery of, 250–252
Forefoot, 344
    equinus, 354
    valgus, 354
    varus, 354
Foreign body, 100
Forestier disease, 291
Forestier test, 138–139
Forged components, 225
Fork strap, 194
Formication sign, 157
Fossae, 307
Foster frame, 187
Foucher technique, 340
Fouchet sign, 151–152
Four-bar linkage, 195
Four-flap Z-plasty, 334
Fourier transform infrared spectroscopy and microscopy (FTIR), 387
Fournier test, 156
Four-poster orthoses, 204
Four-strand cruciate procedure, 337
Four-tendon sign, 117
Fovea centralis, 254
Fowler
    manuever, 145
    metacarpophalangeal arthroplasty, 332
    procedure, 338, 339, 360, 363
    release, 341
    tenodesis, 338
    test, 141, 143
Fowler-Phillip angle, 112
Fowles prostheses, 251
Fox-Blazina procedure, 267
Foxing, 205
Fractures
    ankle, 11–12
    apophyseal, 4
    arm, 8
    articular, 4
    bone involved in, 3–4
    classification, 3–7
    closed, 3, 31
    by compression in long axis of leg, 15
    configuration, 7
    contributing factors, 12–13
    D/3, distal third, 3–4
    defined, 2
    diastasis, 2

Fractures *(Continued)*
  dislocation, 2
  elbow, 8
  extent, 7
  femur, 10–11
  fibula, 11
  foot, 11–12
  forearm, 8–9
  general appearacne, 4–6
  hand, 9
  healing, 13
  hip, 10
  knee, 11
  line, 115
  long bone, 13–14
  M/3, middle third, 3–4
  names, classic and descriptive, 8–12
  of necessity, 1, 9
  open, 3, 19
  P/3, proximal third, 3–4
  pelvis, 10
  shoulder, 8–12
  site, 7
  spine, 9–10
  terminology, 2–3
  tibia, 11
  trauma registry system, 13–14
  wrist, 8–9
Fragile-X syndrome, 95
Fragilitas ossium congenita, 46
Fragility fracture, 4
Fragments
  alignment, 6–7
  defined, 6
  displaced, 7
  position, 6–7
  specific fixation, 325
  undisplaced, 7
Frank dislocation, 33–34
Fränkel
  line, 115
  neurologic assessment, 160
  scale, 160
  sign, 156
Frantz-O'Rahilly classification, 94
FRAX, 18
Free-body diagram (FBD), 383
Free flaps, 334
Free fragment, 300
Free graft, 218
Freeman-Sheldon syndrome, 321, 323
Free pyridinium cross-links, 168
Free-revascularized autograft, 217
Freeze-dried grafts, 217
Freiberg disease, 55, 60
Freiberg infraction, 355
Freid-Green procedure, 360
Frejka orthoses, 199
French osteotomy, 214
French prostheses, 251
Fresh-frozen grafts, 217

Fresh frozen plasma (FFP), 172
Fretting, 100
Fretting corrosion, 226
Frey procedure, 360
Friable, 100
Friddle low-profile neck rings, 205
Friedreich ataxia, 81
Frog-leg lateral view, 109
Frog splint, 182
Fröhlich adiposogenital dystrophy, 60
Froimson and Oh prostheses, 251
Froimson arthroplasty, 332
Froment sign, 145
Frostbite, 75
Frost procedure, 360
Frozen shoulder, 69, 71–72
Frykman Classification, 19
Fulcrum test, 141
Fulford procedure, 360
Fulguration, 280
Fully constrained, 271
Functional capacities assessment, 372
Functional fracture bracing using thermoplastics, 374
Functional mobility, 373
Functional scoliosis, 293
Funiculectomy, 333
Fusiform, 100
Fusion, 280

G

Gadolinium (Gd)–enhanced MRI, 126
Gadopentetate dimeglumine, 126
Gaenslen
  sign, 139
  spikes, 220
  split-heel procedure, 360
Gage procedure, 267
Gage sign, 117
Gaille prostheses, 251
Gait training, 369
Galeazzi
  fracture, 9
  procedure, 268, 271
  sign, 148
Gallie fixation, 301
Gallie procedure, 360
Gallium-67 (67Ga) scan, 126
Galvanic electrical stimulation, 367
Galveston metacarpal brace, 201
Gamekeeper's thumb, 37, 325, 327
Gamma camera, 126
Gamma-glutamyltransferase (gamma-GGT), 164
Gammaglutamyltranspeptidase (GGT), 164
Gamma nail, 220
Ganglia, 284
Ganglion, 329, 354
Ganglion cyst, 68
Ganglionectomy, 340
Ganglioneuroma, 79
Gangrene, 75, 100

Gant osteotomy, 214
Gantzer's muscle, 248
Ganz osteotomy, 214–215
Garceau approach, 364
Garceau-Brahms procedure, 360
Garceau procedure, 360
Garden classification, 19
Garden screws, 220
Gardner syndrome, 60
Gardner-Wells tongs, 186
Gargoylism, 67
Garrod fibromatosis, 68
Garrod pads, 68
Garth view, 109
Gartland, 20
Gartland classification, 19
Gas, 60
Gas gangrene, 330
Gastrocnemius, 263
Gastrocnemius equinus, 354
Gastrocsoleus muscle, 263
Gatellier and Chastang approach, 364
Gaucher disease, 60
Gauntlet cast, 180
Gauze dressing, 183
Gear-stick sign, 148
Gelatinase, 391
Gel casts, 180
Gelman procedure, 360
Gene expression, 390
Genetic code, 390
Genome chip, 387
Genotype, 390
Genu recurvatum, 92
Genu valgum, 92
Genu varum, 92
Gerber classification, 19
Gerber test, 142
Gerdy tubercle, 261
Germinal matrix, 314
Getty procedure, 305
Geyser sign, 117
Ghormley arthrodesis, 228
Ghormley osteotomy, 214
Giannestras procedure, 360
Giant cell reparative granuloma, 57
Giant cell tumor, 53
Gibbus, 293
Gibney bandage, 184
Gibraiel flap, 334
Gibson approach, 275
Giebel blade plate, 220
Gilbert procedure, 272
Gill
  arthrodesis, 228
  fixation, 302
  procedure, 245
  procedure, 272, 360
  prostheses, 251
Gill, Manning, and White fixation, 302
Gillies flap, 335–336
Gillies procedure, 341
Gill-Stein arthrodesis, 331
Gillespie Classification for Longitudinal Deficiency of the Femur, Partial, 96t–97t
Girdle resection, 245
Girdlestone procedure, 360
Girdlestone resection, 260
Glasgow Coma Score (GCS), 160
Gledhill classification, 49
Glenoid
  fossa, 241
  fracture, 20
  labrum, 241–242
Glenosphere, 246
Glickel procedure, 334
Glioma, 79
Global rigidity with associated deformities, 321
Glomus tumor, 79, 329
Glucosamine, 392
Glucose tolerance test (GTT), 166
Gluteal gait, 159
Gluteal lines, 252
Gluteal lurch, 159
Gluteus maximus gait, 159
Gluteus maximus muscle, 255
Gluteus medius and minimus muscles, 255
Gluteus medius gait, 159
Glycocalyx, 100
Glycogen phosphorylase, 67
Glycosaminoglycan (GAG), 392
Gobies, 37
Godfrey test, 151
Godoy-Moreira stud-bolt, 220
Goldfarb and Stern arthrodesis, 330
Goldner procedure, 338
Goldstein procedure, 305
Goldthwait sign, 139
Golfer's elbow, 37, 70, 328
Goniometry, 388
Gordon approach, 274
Gordon reflex, 156
Gore AO screw, 220
Gorham disease, 46, 60
Gosselin fracture, 11
Gouffon pin, 220
Gould modification, 358
Gould procedure, 360
Gout, 82, 85, 316, 354
  arthritis, 85
  node, 85
Gouty arthritis, 70
Gower sign, 158
Graber-Duvernay procedure, 260
Gracilis, 261
Grafts, 215–218
  classification, 216–218
  preservation procedures, 216–217
  revascularization of, 217
  terminology, 216
Gram stain, 169
Grand mal epilepsy, 79

Grand piano sign, 151
Grant, Surrall, and Lehman procedure, 267
Granulation, 100, 280
Granuloma, 280
Grashey view, 109
Gravity stress test, 143
Gray, 107
Gray matter, 288
Grayson ligament, 314
Greater and lesser trochanters, 254
Greater and lesser tuberosity, 241
Greater sciatic notch, 252
Greater tuberosity fracture, 8
Great multangular, 307
Greek foot, 354
Green procedure, 245
Green transfer, 338
Green-Anderson growth chart, 160
Greene procedure, 360
Greenfield filter, 240
Green-Seligson-Henry (GSH) nail, 220
Greenstick fracture, 4, 6
Grenade arm, 36
Grice-Green procedure, 360
Grice procedure, 360
Griefer prosthesis, 191
Grimace test, 151
Grind test, 316
Grip-strength test, 145
Grisel syndrome, 291
Gristina and Webb prosthesis, 246
Grommet, 220
Gross-Kemph nail, 220
Gross Motor Function Classification System (GMFCS), 79t
Ground reaction AFO, 197
Group fascicular repair, 333
Groves and Goldner transfer, 338
Groves procedure, 338
Growth-arrest line, 115
Growth plate, 212
Gruca procedure, 272
Gruen zones, 122
GS alpha protein of adenylate cyclase (GNAS-1), 59, 68
Gschwind classification, 351
GSU nail, 220
Guillain-Barré syndrome, 82
Guilland sign, 156
Guilliatt tourniquet test, 145
Guillotine amputation, 278
Guleke-Stookey approach, 275
Gull wing sign, 117
Gunslinger orthoses, 202
Gustilo classification, 19
Gutter splint, 182
Guyon canal, 313
Gymnast's wrist, 37

H

Haas disease, 60
Habitual dislocation, 33
Haboush universal nail, 220
Haddad and Riordan arthrodesis, 330–331
Haddad procedure, 360
Hagie pin, 220
HAGL, 37
Haglund
 deformity, 351, 354, 356
 process, 351
 syndrome, 354
Hair tourniquet syndrome, 100
Hairline fracture, 4
Hair-on-end sign, 117
Hairpin splint, 182
Hajdu-Cheney syndrome, 60
Half-ring Thomas splint, 185
Half shell, 182
Halifax fixation, 301
Hall and Pankovich prostheses, 251
Hallux, 346
 abductovalgus, 352
 abductus, 352, 354
 adductus, 354
 elevatus, 354
 extensus, 354
 flexus, 354
 malleus, 354
 rigidus, 354
 varus, 354
Hallux valgus, 350–352, 354
 angle, 112, 351
 interphalangeus, 354
 orthoses, 197
Halo brace, 204
Halo cast, 179
Halo-femoral traction, 186
Halo-pelvic traction, 186
Halo traction, 204
Halstead maneuver, 317
Halstead test, 136
Halsted procedure, 337
Hamada Fukuda Classification, 89t
Hamartoma, 329
Hamate, 307
Hamblen Classification of Heterotopic Ossification, 57t
Hamilton-Russell, 187
Hamilton test, 142
Hammer toes, 354
Hammond procedure, 336, 340
Hamstring
 knee, 93
 muscle, 261
 tendon, 234
Hamulus, 307, 313
Hand, 307–342
 anatomy, 307–316
 arteries, 314–316
 bones, 307–308
 fingers, 313–314
 joints, 308
 nails, 314
 nerves, 314–316

Hand *(Continued)*
  structural anomalies, 316–330
  tendons, 310–311
Hand diseases
  congenital, 320–323
  dislocations, 326–327
  infections, 329–330
  muscles, 323–324
  nails, 327–328
  neuropathies, 317–320
  skin disorders, 327–328
  tendons, 323–324
  traumatic disorders, 325–326
  vascular disorders, 324–325
Hand-foot syndrome, 329
Hand ligaments
  collateral, 312
  digital collateral, 312
Hand muscles, 308–311
  extrinsic, 310
  fascia, 311–312
  flexor zones, 311
  forearm, 310–311
  intrinsic, 310
  ligaments, 311–312
  pulleys, 311
Hand-Schüller-Christian disease, 52
Hand surgery, 330–341
  approaches, 341
  arthrodesis, 331
  arthroplasties, 331–333
  congenital deformity repairs, 335
  fingers, 330–331
  microvascular procedures, 334–335
  muscle, 336–337
  neurological procedures, 333
  skin, nails, and fascia procedures, 335–336
  tendon grafts and transfers, 337–339
  tendon repair techniques, 337
  tenosynovectomy, 339
  trauma procedures, 333–334
Handlebar palsy, 37
Hanging arm cast, 180
Hanging hip procedure, 260
Hangman's fracture, 10
Hansen disease, 330
Hansen pin, 220
Hansen-Street nail, 220
Hard clavus, 354
Hard corn, 354
Hardinge approach, 275
Hardinge expansion bolt, 220
Hare traction, 188
Hark procedure, 360
Harmon approach, 274, 276
Harmon procedure, 245
Harrington rod, 221, 304
Harris
  approach, 275
  hip scale, 160
  line, 115

Harris *(Continued)*
  nail, 221
  view, 109
Harris-Beath footprinting mat, 154
Harris-Beath procedure, 360
Harris-Park line, 115
Hassman, Brunn, and Neer prostheses, 251
Hass osteotomy, 214
Hatchet head deformity, 33
Hatchet head shoulder, 65
Hauser metatarsal bar, 206
Hauser procedure, 268, 360
Haversian canals, 211
Haversian system, 393
Hawkins Classification, 19–20
Hawkins impingement sign, 142
Hawkins sign, 117–118
Hay approach, 275
HB_sAg, 173
Head halter traction, 186
Head-shaft angle, 112
Head tilt sign, 136
Healed bone, 13
Healing stages, 13
Heart-hand syndrome, 322
Heat and cold testing, 371
Heberden nodes, 60, 329
Hebosteotomy, 260
Heel
  cord, 349
  counter, 205
  height difference, 151
  pad, 206
  pain syndrome, 355
  spur, 37, 355
  tendon, 231–234
Heel-bisector method, 156
Heel-cord sign, 154
Heel-to-buttocks difference, 151
Heffington frame, 187
Heifetz procedure, 360
Height and weight, 174
Helbing sign, 154
Helft test, 151–152
Helical axis of motion, 383
Helical CT, 125
Heloma durum, 354
Heloma molle, 353
Hemangioendothelioma, 54
Hemangioma, 54
Hemangiomatosis, 46
Hemangiopericytoma, 54
Hemangiosarcoma, 54
Hemarthrosis, 71
Hematocrit and hemoglobin (H&H), 164
Hematocrit cell volume (HCV), 164
Hematoma, 100
Hematomyelia, 297
Hematopoiesis, 210
Hematorrhachis, 297
Hematoxylin and eosin staining (H&E), 170

Hemiarthroplasty, 226
Hemicylindric graft, 218
Hemilaminectomy, 300
Hemimelia, 95, 322
Hemimelic progressive osseous heteroplasia, 58
Hemipelvectomy, 193, 195
Hemiphalangectomy, 360
Hemiplegia, 80
Hemiplegic, 79
Hemi-pulp flap, 333
Hemiresection interposition arthroplasty, 332
Hemivertebra, 298
Hemodilution technique, 171
Hemodynamic test, 158
Hemoglobin (Hb, Hgb), 164
Hemoglobin electrophoresis, 166
Hemolymphangiomatosis, 46
Hemophilia, 85
Hemophilic arthritis, 70
Hemorrhage, 100
Henderson arthrodesis, 229
Henderson fracture, 11
Henderson-Jones chondromatosis, 45, 65
Henderson lag screw, 221
Henry approach, 274–276, 306, 341, 364
Herbert screw, 221
Herbert screw osteosynthesis, 334
Herbert and Fisher Classification, 20
Herbert's of Scaphoid Fractures, 325
Hereditary, 100
Hereditary areflexic dystasia, 82
Hereditary disease, 43
Hereditary multiple exostosis, 322
Hermodsson fracture, 8
Herndon-Heyman procedure, 360
Herndon osteotomy, 214
Herniated intervertebral disk (HID), 296
Herniated nucleus pulposus (HNP), 296, 300
Herniation, 100
Herniation pit, 115
Herpetic whitlow, 330
Herring Lateral Pillar Classification, 122t
Hertz (Hz), 388
Hessel-Nystrom pin, 221
Hetero-digital flaps, 333
Heterograft, 216
Heterotopic ossification, 57
Heuter approach approach, 275
Hex screw, 221
Hey-Groves procedure, 267
Heyman-Herndon procedure, 260
Heyman procedure, 271, 360
Hibbs
 angle, 112
 approach, 306
 arthrodesis, 229
 procedure, 360
 spinal fixation, 302
Hibernoma, 54, 101
Hickory-stick fracture, 4
High Dye dressing, 184

High flex design, 271
High proximal femoral fracture, 28–29
Highest genicular artery, 266
High-grade pleomorphic undifferentiated sarcoma (HGPUS), 54
High-performance liquid chromatography (HPLC), 386
High-pressure liquid chromatography, 386
High-riding patella, 94
High-riding scapulae (Sprengel deformity), 243
High-tide walker, 181
High-voltage pulsed galvanic electrical stimulation, 367
Higley side plate, 221
Hilgenreiner
 angle, 112
 epiphyseal angle, 112
 line, 115–116
Hill-Sachs fracture, 8
Hill-Sachs lesion, 33
Hindfoot, 346
Hindfoot equinus, 355
Hinge joint, 227
Hinged knee, 271
Hip, 253
 abductors, 255
 anatomy of, 254–255
 arteries, 255
 bones, 254
 disarticulation, 193, 195
 diseases, 90–91
 dysplasia of, 258
 fracture, 10
 joint, 195, 199
 ligaments, 255
 muscles, 254–255
 nerves, 255
 other procedures, 259–261
 pointer, 37
 spica, 180
 spica cast, 180
Hip dislocation, 34
 Pipkin classification for, 27
 Stewart and Milford classification for, 29–30
 Thompson and Epstein classification for, 30
Hip surgery
 arthrodesis, 259
 arthroplasty, 255–256
 closed hip reduction, 258
 iliopsoas transfers, 258
 joint replacement, 256–258
 open hip reduction, 258
 osteotomies, 259
Hirayama prostheses, 251
Hirose and Johnson procedure, 360
Hiroshima procedure, 360
Hirschberg sign, 156
His-Haas procedure, 245
Histiocytes, 231
Histiocytosis X, 52
Histocompatibility, 216

Histomorphometry, 387
Histoplasma, 169
Histoplasmosis, 48
Hitchcock procedure, 245
Hitchcock prostheses, 251
Hobb view, 109
Hockey player's hip, 37
Hockey-stick incisions, 330
Hodgkin tumor, 52
Hodgson approach, 306
Hodgson procedure, 305
Hoffa fat, 266
Hoffa fracture, 11
Hoffer procedure, 360
Hoffman-Clayton procedure, 360
Hoffmann sign, 156
Hohl-Moore Classification, 20
Hohmann prostheses, 251
Hoke-Kite procedure, 361
Hoke procedure, 361
Hollenhorst plaque, 75
Holmberg view, 109
Holstein-Lewis fracture, 8, 325
Holt nail, 221
Holt-Oram syndrome, 101, 322
Homan sign, 149
Home, 374
Homogentisic acid, 58
Homograft, 216
Hook, 192
   of hamate, 313
   nail, 327
   test, 143–144, 155
Hooked acromion, 89–90
Hook-pin fixation, 221
Hoop stress fracture, 12
Hoover test, 139
Hop test, 152
Hornblower sign, 142
Horner syndrome, 317
Horseback rider's knee, 34, 37
Horseshoe abscess, 330
Horwitz and Adams arthrodesis, 229
Hotchkiss fracture, 325
Hot packs, 368
Hounsfield unit, 106
House procedure, 335
House reconstruction, 336–337
Housemaid's knee, 93
Houston and Akroyd procedure, 269
Hovanian procedure, 245
Hovanian prostheses, 251
Howmedica compression screw, 221
Howorth procedure, 258
Howship lacuna, 211–212, 393
Hsu and Hsu procedure, 272
Hubbard side plate, 221
Hubbard tank, 368
Huber procedure, 338
Huber transfer, 338
Huckstep nail, 221

Hueter line, 115
Hueter-Mayo procedure, 361
Hueter sign, 158
Hueter-Volkmann law, 393
Hughston
   jerk test, 152
   osteotomy, 214
   procedure, 268, 271
   view, 109
Hughston and Degenhardt procedure, 267
Hughston and Jacobson procedure, 267
Hui-Linscheid procedure, 338
Human genome, 390
Human immunodeficiency virus, viral load test (HIV, viral load), 173
Human immunodeficiency virus-1 antigen (HIV-1 antigen), 173
Human leukocyte antigen–B27 (HLA-B27), 166
Humerus/humeral, 241, 246
   fracture, 21, 24
   head, 24–25, 241
   lateral condylar fracture, 15
   physeal fracture, 25
   proximal, 19
   supracondylar fracture, 19
Hunter rod, 339
Hunter-Scheie syndrome, 67
Hunter syndrome, 67
Huntington
   approach, 276
   chorea, 79
   sign, 156
Hurler syndrome, 67
Hutchinson fracture, 8
Hutchinson sign, 145
Hyaline, 226–227
Hyaline cartilage, 230, 392
Hyaluronic acid, 392
Hybrid fixation, 224, 226
Hybrid knee, 195
Hydrarthrosis, 71
Hydrodynamic lubrication, 384
Hydrostatic bed, 368
Hydrotherapy treatments, 368
25-α-hydroxycholecaliferol receptor 84, 84
25-hydroxycholecalciferol, 394
Hydroxyproline (HYP), 168
25-hydroxyvitamin D, 25-hydroxycholecalciferol (25[OH]D), 167
Hyoid bone, 285
Hypalgesia, 101
Hyperabduction test, 136–137
Hyperalgesia, 101
Hypercholesteremia, 78
Hypercholesterinemia, 78
Hypercholesterolemia, 78
Hyperechoic, 106
Hyperesthesia, 317
Hyperextension, 101
Hyperextension test, 137
Hyperglycemia, 101
Hyperlordosis, 297

Hyperosteoidosis, 44
Hyperparathyroidism, 44, 83
Hyperpathia, 317
Hyperphalangism, 322
Hyperplasia, 101
Hyperplasia fascialis ossificans progressiva, 57
Hypersensitivity reaction, 226
Hypertension, 78, 101
Hyperthyroidism, 44, 84
Hypertonia, 101
Hypertrophic arthritis, 71
Hypertrophic exostosis, 57
Hypertrophic zone, 212
Hypertrophy, 101
Hypochondrodysplasia, 65
Hypoechoic, 106
Hypoglycemia, 101
Hyponychium, 314, 350
Hypoparathyroidism, 83
Hypophosphatasia, 58, 83
Hypoplasia, 101
Hypoplastic thumb, 322
Hypotension, 78, 101
Hypothenar eminence, 313
Hypothenar hammer syndrome, 324–325
Hypothenar muscles, 310
Hypothenar space, 313
Hypotheses, 377
Hypothesis, 377
Hypothyroidism, 84
Hypovolemia, 78
Hypoxia, 78
Hysteresis, 383

I

Iatrogenic, 101
Iatrogenic osteomyelitis, 49
Ideberg classification, 20
Idiopathic, 101
Idiopathic disease, 43
Idiopathic osteoporosis, 83
Idiopathic refractory anemia, 100
Idiopathic scoliosis, 293
Ikuta prostheses, 251
Ilfeld splint, 198–199
Iliac crest, 252–253
Iliac fossa, 253
Iliac screws, 303
Iliacus muscle, 288
Ilioinguinal approach, 274
Iliopectineal line, 253
Iliopsoas muscle, 255, 288
Iliotibial band syndrome, 37
Ilium, 253
Illarramendi and De Carlit procedure, 340
Imaging. *See also* specific modalities
  radiation therapy, 130
  radiologic terminiology, 106–107
  techniques, 105–130
  vascular diagnostic studies, 128–130
Imbrication, 280
Immediate operative prosthesis (IPOP), 196
Immovable joint, 227
Immune serum globulins, 173
Immunoelectrophoresis, 167
Immunologic tests, 173–174
Immunosuppression, 216
Impacted fracture, 4
Impedance plethysmography, 129
Impingement, 101
  sign, 142
  syndrome, 37, 90
  test, 142
Implant, 216, 280
Impulse, 383
Incision and drainage (I&D), 280
Inclan-Ober procedure, 245
Inclinometer, 292
Inclusion cyst, 328–329
Incomplete dislocation, 33
Incomplete fracture, 4
Incomplete paraxial hemimelia, 95
Incorporation, 217
Increased foot angle, 112
Independent variable, 379
Indian hedgehog (IHH), 84
Indirect costs, 378
Indirect head rectus femoris, 262
Indium leukocyte scan, 126
Indium scan, 126
Individual indices, 381–382
Induration, 101
Inertia, 383
Infantile cortical hyperostosis, 58
Infantile hypophosphatasia, 58, 88
Infantile scoliosis, 293
Infarct, 75, 101
Infection, 101
Infectious arthritis, 70
Infectious bone disease, 48–49
Inferior gluteal artery, 255
Inferior pubic ramus, 253
Infiltration, 280, 340
Inflammation, 101
Inflammatory arthritis, 316
Inflammatory fracture, 12
Inflammatory joint disease, 76
Inflammtory disease, 43
Inflare last shoes, 207
Inflatable splint, 188
Infraction fracture, 5
Infrapatellar fat pad, 266
Infrapatellar ligament, 264
Infrapatellar straps, 200
Infrapatellar tendon, 264
Infraspinatus muscle, 242, 287
Infusion, 280
Ingram osteotomy, 214
Ingram procedure, 361
Ingrown nail, 355
Inguinal, 254

Injection, 280
Inlay graft, 218
Inlet view, 109
Innervation, 235
Innominate bone, 253
Innominate osteotomy, 215
Input variable, 379
Insall and Hood procedure, 268
Insall procedure, 268
Insall ratio, 115
Insall-Salvati ratio, 115
Insidious, 101
In situ, 280
In situ bypass, 240
Instantaneous axis of rotation, 383–384
Institute of Sports Medicine and Athletic Trauma (ISMAT) muscle testing, 371
Institutional Animal Care and Use Committee (IACUC), 378
Institutional Review Board (IRB), 378
Instrumental activities of daily living (IADLs), 373–374
Insufficiency fracture, 5, 12
Integrated-shape imaging system (ISIS), 126
Integumentary injury, 14
Intercalary graft, 218
Intercarpal arthrodesis, 331
Intercompartmental supraretinacular arteries, 314
Intercondylar eminence fracture, 24
Intercondylar notch, 261
Intercostal muscle, 287
Intercostal nerves, 314
Interdigital commissure, 314
Interdigital contracture, 325
Interdigital granuloma, 330
Interdigital neuroma, 355
Interdigital pilonidal sinus, 329
Interdigital space, 351
Interferential current, 368
Interleukins, 390
Intermediate bursa, 313
Intermediate ligament, 312
Intermediate phalangectomy, 361
Intermediate prosthesis, 196
1–2 intermetatarsal angle, 350
1–5 intermetatarsal angle, 350
Intermittent claudication, 74
Intermittent compression, 368
Intermittent hydrarthrosis, 77
Internal, 2
Internal derangement
  of joint, 71
  of the knee (IDK), 92–93
Internal fixators, 2
Internal neurolysis, 333
Internal oblique muscles, 288
Internal-rotation drawer test, 152
Internal rotators, 254–255
International Classification for Osteonecrosis of the Femoral Head, 55t
International Classification for Surgery of the Hand in Tetraplegia, 145t, 324t
International Classification System, 13–14

International Federation of Societies for Surgery of the Hand Classificaton System for Anomalies Affecting Hand Function, 320t
International Normalized Ratio (INR), 166
International Organization for Standardization (IOS), 94
International System (SI) units, 388
Interosseous cartilage, 229
Interosseous membrane, 249, 266
Interosseous muscles, 349
Interperiosteal fracture, 4
Interphalangeal arthrodesis, 330
Interphalangeal (IP) joint, 346
Interposition graft, 334
Interscalene block, 340
Interscalene triangle, 314
Interscapulothoracic (forequarter amputation), 190
Intersection syndrome, 323
Interspinal disk, 287
Interspinous ligament, 286
Interspinous pseudarthrosis, 291, 298
Intertrochanteric, 254
Intertrochanteric fracture, 10
  Evans-Wales classification for, 18
  Jensen classification for, 20
  Tronzo classification for, 30–31
Intervertebral disk, 284, 287, 296
Intervertebral vacuum, 60
Intima, 238
In toto, 280
Intraarticular, 4
  arthrodesis, 228
  fracture, 4
  osteochondroma, 52
Intracapsular ankylosis, 73
Intracapsular fracture, 4, 10
Intracortical fibrous dysplasia, 57
Intractable, 101
Intractable plantar keratosis (IPK), 355
Intradural, 287
Intralesional resection, 276
Intramedullary, 284
Intramedullary graft, 218
Intramedullary nail, 221
Intramembranous ossification, 393
Intraneural fibrosis, 80
Intraoperative autologous transfusion (IAT), 171
Intraosseous lipoma, 58
Intraosseous lipomatosis, 58
Intraosseous pneumatocyst, 58
Intraosseous venography, 107
Intraspongy nuclear herniation, 296
Intravenous block, 273
Intravenous (IV)-type basic frame, 187
Intrinsic minus deformity, 319
Intrinsic minus hand, 319
Intrinsic muscles, 308–310, 349
Intrinsic plus hand, 319
Intrinsic tightness test, 145
Intubation, 280
Invasive spine surgery, 299
Inversion ankle stress view, 109

Inverted Napoleon's hat sign, 118
Inverted radial reflex, 139
In vitro, 280, 386
In vivo, 280, 386
Involucrum, 49
Inyo nail, 221
Iodoform dressing, 183
Iodophenylundecylic acid, 106
Iontophoresis, 367
Iowa hip scale, 160
Irradiation, 171–172
Irradiation-sterilized grafts, 217
Irrigation, 280
Irwin osteotomy, 215
Irwin procedure, 272
Ischemia, 75, 101, 390
Ischemic contracture, 63
Ischemic ulcer, 357
Ischial containment sockets, 194
Ischial spine, 253
Ischial tuberosity, 253
Ischial weight-bearing ring or band, 200
Ischiectomy, 260
Ischiopubiotomy, 260
Ischium, 253
Iselin disease, 55, 60
Ishihara cervical spine curve index, 122
Isischiohebotomy, 260
Island flaps, 340
Isler Classification, 20
Isoantibodies, 173–174
Isogenic, 216
Isograft, 216
Isokinetic exercises, 369
Isola, 304
Isolated dislocation, 324
Isometric exercises, 369
Isotonic exercises, 369
Isotropy, 384
Isthmus, 211
Ivory vertebra sign, 118

J

J. R. Moore procedure, 245
J sign, 118, 152
Jaccoud syndrome, 77
Jacksonian epilepsy, 79
Jacob test, 153
Jacobs locking hook, 304
Jaffe-Campanacci disease, 60
Jaffe disease, 57
Jaffe-Lichtenstein disease, 60
Jahss maneuver, 325
Jahss procedure, 361
Jaipur foot, 193
Jamar dynamometer, 372
Janecki and Nelson procedure, 245
Jansen disease, 65
Jansen test, 148
Jansey procedure, 361

Japas osteotomy, 215
Japas procedure, 361
Jarcho-Levin syndrome, 299
Javelin thrower's elbow, 36
Jeanne syndrome, 317
Jeanne test, 146
Jebsen-Taylor hand function test, 373
Jefferson fracture, 10
Jendrassik maneuver, 139, 156
Jensen classification, 20
Jerk test, 142, 153
Jersey finger, 37
Jewett nail, 221
Jobe and Kvitne procedure, 245
Jobe test, 142
Jockey cap patella, 93
Jogger's heel, 37
Jogger's toe, 37
Johansson classification, 20–21
Johansson nail, 221
John C. Wilson arthrodesis, 229
Johnson and Alexander procedure, 331
Johnson and Barington procedure, 359
Johnson and Spiegl procedure, 361
Johnson Classificaiton of Adult Acquired Flatfoot Associated with Posterior Tibial Tendon Insufficienty, 354t
Joint, 226–230
 anatomy of, 226–227
 arthrodesis, 228–229
 fracture, 4
 general surgery, 227–228
 leveling procedures with ulnar lengthening and radial shortening, 340
 of Luschka, 286
 manipulation, 369
 mice, 71
 mobilization, 369
 motions, 406–409
 play, 369
 protection, 374
 stabilizer, 202
 types of, 227
 weight-bearing, 227
Joint capsule, 263
Joint Commission on Accreditation of Healthcare Organizations (JCAHO), 395
Joint diseases
 ankylo-root, 72–73
 arthro-root diseases, 70–71
 capsulo-related, 72
 eponymic, 72
 other, 71
 synovio-related, 72
Jones
abduction frame, 187
 fracture, 11–12
 procedure, 268, 361
 transfer, 338
Jones, Barnes, and Lloyd-Roberts Classification for Tibial Deficiency, 96t–97t

Joplin procedure, 361
Joules, 383
JS Speed prostheses, 251
Judet quadricepsplasty, 269
Jugular vein, 286
Juliano procedure, 361
Jumper's knee, 37, 93
Jump pedicle, 273
Juncturae tendinum, 311–312
Juvara procedure, 361
Juvenile hyaline fibromatosis, 68
Juvenile idiopathic arthritis, 77
Juvenile osteoporosis, 83
Juvenile scoliosis, 293

K

Kager triangle, 113
Kalamchi and Dawe Classification for Tibial Deficiency, 96t–97t
Kalamchi and MacEwen Classification, 122t–123t
Kanavel sign, 146, 330
Kanavel spaces, 313
Kanaya procedure, 340
Kaneda, 304
Kapandji fixation, 334
Kapandji thumb opposition score, 146
Kapel prostheses, 251
Kaplan procedure, 334
Kappis disease, 55, 60
Karakousis and Vezeridis procedure, 260
Karlsson procedure, 361
Kashin-Beck disease, 88
Kashiwagi procedure, 361
Kates-Kessel-Kay procedure, 361
Kaufer procedure, 361
Kawai and Yamamoto procedure, 334
Kawasaki disease, 72
Keel, 226
Keen sign, 155
Kelikian procedure, 271
Keller procedure, 361
Kellgren osteoarthritis grade, 123
Kellogg Speed procedure, 305
Kelly approach, 306
Ken nail, 221
Kendrick procedure, 361
Kenny-Howard splint (A/C harness), 184
Keratin sulfate, 392
Keratins stain, 170
Keratoma, 352
Keratosis, 328
Kerlix dressing, 183
Kernig sign, 156
Kerr sign, 156
Kessel-Bonney procedure, 361
Kessler procedure, 335
Key and Conwell classification, 21
Key arthrodesis, 229
Key pinch, 146, 333
Key to Manual Muscle Evaluation, 370t

Keyhole prostheses, 251
Kickaldy and Willis arthrodesis, 229
Kidner procedure, 361
Kidneys, ureters, bladder (KUB), 107
Kiehn-Earle-DesPrez procedure, 361
Kienböck disease, 55, 60, 324
Kilfoyle classification, 21
Kim test, 142
Kinematics, 384
Kineplastic amputation, 277
Kinesiology, 384
Kinetic apraxia, 78
Kinetic energy (KE), 384
Kinetics, 384
King and Richards procedure, 260
King maneuver, 148
King procedure arthrodesis, 229
Kinking, 75
Kirner deformity, 322
Kirschner wire (K-wire), 186, 221, 334
Kissing spine, 291
Kite flap, 340
Klebsiella organisms, 48
Klebsiella pneumoniae, 169
Kleinert-Atosoy, 335
Kleinert procedure, 337
Klein line, 115
Kleinman shear test, 146
Klemm nail, 221
Klenzak orthoses, 200
Klinefelter syndrome, 88
Kling dressing, 184
Klippel-Feil sign, 156
Klippel-Feil syndrome, 60
Klumpke palsy, 80, 317
Knee
    bearing (K/B), 193
    disarticulation, 193, 195
    dislocations, 34
    disorders, 92–94
    joint, 199
    prosthetic components, 195
Knee Society clinical rating system, 160
Knee Society total-knee arthroplasty roentgenographic evaluation and scoring system, 123
Knee surgery, 267–271
    chronic subluxation of patella, 268–269
    internal derangment, 267–268
    patellar, 269
    prostheses, 269–271
    quadricepsplasty, 269
    total knee, 269
Kniest dysplasia, 67
Knight-Taylor orthoses, 203–204
Knockins, 389
Knock-knee, 92
Knockouts, 389
Knodt distraction rod, 304
Knowles pin, 221
Knuckle pad, 314
Knuttson view, 109

Kocher
 approach, 274–275, 364
 fracture, 8–9
 maneuver, 142
Kochler approach, 364
Koch-Mason dressing, 184
Kocker-Langenbeck approach, 275
Koenig and Schaefer approach, 364
Köhler disease, 55, 60, 355
Kohler fracture, 12
Kohler line, 115
Koman procedure, 361
König disease, 60
Konstram angle, 113
Kortzeborn procedure, 339
Kostuick-Harrington, 304
Krag, 305
Kramer, Craig, and Noel osteotomy, 215
Kramer, Craig, and Noel procedure, 260
Krause-Wolfe skin graft, 273
Kristiansen and Kofoed procedure, 245
Krukenberg procedure, 335
Kujala score, 160
Kumar procedure, 361
Kummel Classification for Longitudinal Ulnar Deficiency at Elbow Joint, 96t–97t
Kümmell disease, 55, 60, 289
Küntscher modified arthrodesis, 229
Küntscher nail, 221
Küntscher rod, 221
Kurosaka screw, 221
Kutler procedure, 334
Kyle classification, 21
Kyphectomy procedure, 305
Kyphoplasty, 300
Kyphoscoliosis, 292–293
Kyphosis, 293

L

Laboratory abbreviations
 blood components and clotting, 174
 other, 175
 serology, 175
 serum chemistries, 174
 urine, 175
Laboratory evaluations, 163–176
 annotated units, 175–176
 bacteriologic studies, 168–169
 blood bank, 171–174
 blood tests, 165–167
 histologic techniques, 170–171
 laboratory abbreviations, 174–175
 musculoskeletal tumors, 171
 notes, 176
 pathologic techniques, 170–171
 pysiologic parameters, 174
 routine, 163–165
 serum tests, 165–168
 special studies, 169–170
 urine tests, 167–168

Laboratory medicine, 163
Labrum, 255
Laced splint, 182
Laceration, 101
Lacertus fibrosus, 250
Lachman test, 152
Lactate dehydrogenase (LDH), 165
Lacuna, 392
Lacunae, 393
Lag screw, 221
LaGuerre test, 138–139
Laing H-beam nail, 221
Lam modification, 268
Lambrinudi procedure, 361
Lamellar bone, 211, 393
Lamey and Fernandez procedure, 334
Lamina, 284
Laminectomy, 300
Laminoplasty, 300
Laminotomy, 300
Lamparski method, 123
Lance disease, 55, 60
Landouzy-Dejerine disease, 63
Landsmeer ligament, 313
Landsmeer test, 323
Lane plate, 221
Lange, 258
Lange procedure, 361
Langenbeck approach, 275
Langenskiöld osteotomy, 215
Langenskiöld procedure, 272
Langerhans cell histiocytosis, 52
Langer line, 158
Langoria sign, 148
Laparotomy, 240
Lapidus procedure, 361
Laquesna and Deseze angle, 113
Larmon procedure, 361
Larsen index, 123
Larsen syndrome, 95
Laryngeal nerve, 286
Lasègue sign, 139–140
Laser Doppler fluximetry, 334–335
Laser scalpel, 276
Lasso procedure, 338
Lateral approach, 341, 364
Lateral arm flap, 335
Lateral bands, 314
Lateral capsule sign, 11
Lateral circumflex artery, 255
Lateral collateral ligament, 264, 350
Lateral collateral sprain, 35
Lateral column, 346
Lateral compartment, 263
Lateral condylar fracture
 Badelon classification for, 15
 Milch classification for, 24
Lateral cutaneous nerve of forearm, 315
Lateral distal femoral angle, 113
Lateral epicondyles, 246
Lateral epicondylitis, 38

Lateral facet, 261
Lateral femoral condyles, 261
Lateral femur approach, 275
Lateral heel wedge, 206
Lateral hip approach, 275
Lateral key pinch sign, 144
Lateral knee approach, 275
Lateral ligament, 234
Lateral malleolus, 261
Lateral mass, 286
Lateral mass screws, 304
Lateral meniscus, 266
Lateral monopodal stance view, 109
Lateral patella tendon conflict, 93
Lateral patellofemoral angle, 113
Lateral plica, 94
Lateral spring-loaded lock, 200
Lateral talo-first metatarsal angle, 351
Lateral view, 109
Latissimus dorsi, 242
    flap, 340
    muscle, 287
Lauenstein procedure, 332
Laufman approach, 276
Lauge-Hansen classification, 21
Laugier fracture, 8–9
Laugier sign, 144
Laurin angle, 113
Lavage, 280
Lead line, 115, 158
Lead pipe fracture, 9
Leadbetter maneuver, 148
Leather gauntlet orthoses, 197
Leeds procedure, 305
Lee procedure, 272
Lefkowitz maneuver, 148
Le Fort fracture, 12
Legg-Calvé-Perthes disease, 55, 60, 198
Legg-Perthes disease, 55, 60, 91
Legg procedure, 260
Lehman procedure, 260
Lehmer approach, 306
Leichtenstern sign, 156
Leinbach screw, 221
Leiomyoma, 54
Leiomyosarcoma, 54
Length, 176
Lenke Scoliosis Classification of Adolescent Idiopathic Scoliosis, 123t, 292t–293t
Lennox Fritschi technique, 338
Lenteneur's fracture, 9
L'Episcopo Zachary procedure, 245
Leprosy, 330
Leptin, 393
Leptomeningitis, 297
Leptomeningopathy, 297
Léri sign, 156
Lesion, 101
Less invasive spine surgery (LISS), 300
Less invasive stabilization system (LISS) plate, 221–222
Lesser multangular, 307

Lesser trochanter, 16
Lesser tuberosity fracture, 8
Letournel and Judet classification, 21–23
Letterer-Siwe disease, 52, 61
Letts Classification for Fibular Deficiencies, 96t–97t
Letts-Vincent-Gouw classification, 23
Leukocyte reduction, 172
Leukonychia, 328
LeukoScan, 126
Levator scapula, 242
Levine Drennan angle, 113
Levine-Edwards classification, 23
Levorotatory scoliosis, 292
Lewis and Chekofsky procedure, 267
Lewis nail, 221
Lhermitte sign, 156
Lichman Classification for Keinböck Disease, 324t–325t
Lichtblau osteotomy, 361
Lichtman Classification for Osteonecrosis of the Lunate in the Wrist, 55t
Lichtman test, 146
Liebig approach, 274
Liebolt
    arthrodesis, 331
    procedure, 361
    prostheses, 251
Lift off test, 142
Ligament, 234
    of ankle, 350
    of arm, 249
    of Struthers, 250
Ligament reconstruction tendon interposition (LRTI) procedure, 332
Ligament replacement devices, 304
    Ligaments of Henry and Wrisberg, 264
Ligamentotaxis, 234
Ligamentous advancement, 268
Ligamentous ankylosis, 73
Ligamentous control orthoses, 198
Ligamentum flavum, 287
Ligamentum mucosa, 264
Ligamentum mucosum, 94
Ligamentum subcruentum, 313
Ligamentum teres, 255
Ligation, 280
Ligatures, 280
Light amplification by stimulated emission of radiation (laser), 280–281
Limb
    casts, 179–180
    girdle muscular dystrophy, 63
    salvage, 39–40, 240
Limb deficiencies
    congenital, 95–97
    intercalary longitudinal, 95
    intercalary transverse, 95
    terminal longitudinal, 95
    terminal transverse, 95
Limbus annulare, 291
Limited-contact dynamic-compression plate (LC/DCP), 221
Limited- or free-motion ankle joint, 200

Limited scleroderma, 76
Lindeman procedure, 268
Linder sign, 139
Lindholm procedure, 361
Line, 212
   defined, 114
   of demarcation, 101
Linea aspera, 261
Linear acceleration, 382
Linear elastic region, 385
Linear fracture, 5
Linear momentum, 384
Linebacker's arm, 37
Linen bone, 213
Link protein, 392
Linsheid instability, 326
Lipid, 238
Lipid reticuloendotheliosis, 88
Lipid storage disease, 88
Lipoblastoma, 54
Lipocalcinogranulomatosis, 88
Lipochondrodystrophy, 67–68
Lipodystrophy, 68
Lipofibroma, 54
Lipoma, 54
Lipoma arborescens, 71
Liposarcoma, 54
Lipping, 101, 119
Lippman screw, 221
Lipscomb procedure, 361
Lisfranc, 193
   amputation, 361
   dislocation, 34
   fracture, 12, 24
   injury, 37–38
   joint, 349
   ligaments, 350
List, 139
Lister tubercle, 247, 313
Little leaguer's elbow, 38
Little leaguer's shoulder, 38
Littler modified tendon revision, 339
Littler procedure, 338, 339, 341
Littler's boutonnière reconstruction, 338
Lloyd-Roberts procedure, 362
Load, 384
Load and shift test, 141–142
Lobstein disease, 46
Lobstein syndrome, 46
Lobster-claw hand, 321
Lobster foot, 355
Local anesthesia, 273
Localio procedure, 305
Location
   specific, 406
   surface, 405
Locked intramedullary osteosynthesis (LIFO), 221
Locked scapula, 33
Locking plates, 221–222, 281
Locomotor ataxia, 80–81
Logistic regression, 379

Long-arm cast (LAC), 180
Long-arm splint, 182
Long Beach pedicle screw, 305
Long finger extension test, 146
Longissimus colli, 286
Longitudinal deficiency of the femur, partial (LDFP), 91
Longitudinal epiphyseal bracket, 58
Long-leg cast (LLC), 180
Long-leg splint, 182
Long-leg walking cast (LLWC), 180
Long ligament, 312
Long opponens orthoses, 201
Long plantar ligaments, 350
Long thoracic nerve, 243
Long tracts, 288
Long tract sign, 156
Loose bodies, 92–93
Loose procedure, 268
Lopamidol (Isovue) myelography, 108
Lordoscoliosis, 293
Lordosis, 297
Lorenz, 258
   osteotomy, 215
   sign, 139
Lorenzo screw, 222
Lorry driver's fracture, 8
Loss of extension test, 152
Losse test, 152
Lottes nail, 222
Lou Gehrig disease, 78
Loughheed and White procedure, 305
Louisiana State University reciprocating gait orthoses, 199
Lovett test, 146
Low bone mass, 47
Low Dye dressing, 184
Lowenstein view, 109
Lower limbs, 261–272
   anatomy of, 261–266
   arteries, 265–266
   bones, 261
   casts, 180
   ligaments, 263–265
   muscles, 261–262
   nerves, 266
   radiologic views, 110
   veins, 265–266
Lower limbs orthoses, 197–199
   ankle, 197
   ankle-foot, 197–198
   components, 199–200
   foot, 197
   hip, 198–199
   hip-knee-ankle-foot, 199
   knee, 198
   knee-ankle-foot, 198
Lower limbs surgery, 266–267, 272
   femur, 266–267
   knee, 267–271
   tendon transfers, 271–272
   tibia, 266–267
Lower motor neuron disease, 80

Lower obstetrical palsy, 80
Lower scapular nerve, 243
Lower spine
  arteries, 288
  bones, 287
  disk and spinal canal, 287–288
  muscles, 288
Low-friction arthroplasty, 258
Lowman procedure, 362
Low-tide walker, 181
Loxoscelism, 101
Lubrication, 384
Lubricin, 392
Lucas and Cottrell osteotomy, 215
Lucas and Murray arthrodesis, 229
Luck
  classification of Dupuytren disease, 329
  nail, 222
  procedure, 340
Ludington sign, 142
Ludloff
  approach, 275
  procedure, 362
  sign, 148
Lumbar curve, 293
Lumbar kyphosis, 293
Lumbar lordosis, 289
Lumbar pad, 205
Lumbar plexus, 253
Lumbar spine, 284, 287
  arteries, 288
  bones, 287
  disk and spinal canal, 287–288
  muscles, 288
Lumbar stabilization, 369
Lumbar thecoperitoneal shunt syndrome, 80
Lumbarization, 291
Lumbodorsal support, 203
Lumbosacral angle, 113
Lumbosacral corset, 202
Lumbosacral curve, 293
Lumbosacral joint angle, 289
Lumbosacral juntion, 20
Lumbosacral kyphosis, 289
Lumbosacral series, 109
Lumbrical plus finger, 324, 327
Lumbricals, 310
Lumen, 238
Lunate bone, 307
Lunate dislocation, 327
Lundholm screw, 222
Lunotriquetral dissociation, 325
Lunula, 314, 350
Lupus erythematosus, 77
Luque, 305
Luque ISF, 305
Luxatio coxae congenita, 34
Luxatio erecta, 33
Luxatio perinealis, 34
Luxation, 2
Lyden procedure, 260

Lyman-Smith traction, 187
Lyme disease, 72
Lymphangiography, 108
Lymphangiomatosis, 46
Lymphoma, 52
Lynholm knee-scoring scale, 160
Lynne and Katcheria procedure, 260
Lynn procedure, 362
Lyonnaise orthoses, 203
Lyophilized grafts, 217
Lysosomal protease, 391
Lytic, 101

M

M/3, middle third, 3–4
MacAusland prostheses, 251
MacCarthy procedure, 305
Maceration, 101
Macewen and Shands osteotomy, 215
Macindo procedure, 336
MacIntosh test, 153
MacIntosh procedure, 268
Macrodactyly, 322, 355
Macronychia, 328
Maddigan, Wissinger, and Donaldson procedure, 269
Madelung deformity, 322
Madura foot, 355
Maffucci's disease, 52
Maffucci syndrome, 65
Mageri fixation, 301
Magerl fixation, 301
Magnetic resonance angiography (MRA), 126
Magnetic resonance imaging (MRI), 105, 126, 386
Magnetic resonance spectroscopy, 127
Magnetic stimulation, 224
Magnuson procedure, 269
Magnuson test, 139
Magnuson-Stack procedure, 245
Ma-Griffith procedure, 362
Main ligament, 312
Maisonneuve fracture, 12
Maisonneuve sign, 146
Majestro-Ruda-Frost procedure, 362
Major histocompatibility complex, 216
Malacoplakia, 58
Malaise, 101
Malawer procedure, 272
Malgaigne fracture, 8, 10
Malignant, 101
Malignant disease, 43
Malignant fibrous histiocytoma, 53–54, 68
Malignant fibrous xanthoma, 54
Malignant giant cell tumor of soft tissue, 54
Malignant peripheral nerve sheath tumor (MPNST), 54
Malignant Schwannoma, 54
Malingering, 101
Malleolar artery, 351
Malleolar osteotomy, 362
Malleolus, 346–347

Mallet finger, 36, 316
  deformity, 9
  revision, 340–341
Mallet fracture, 9
Mallet toes, 355
Mallory classification, 23
Malmo splint, 199
Malrotation, 325
Malta and Saucedo procedure, 260
Malum coxae senilis, 91
Malum deformans, 355
Malunion, 13
Malunited fracture, 13
Mammon procedure, 362
Mancini plate, 222
Maneuver, 131
Mangled extremity severity score (MESS), 40
Manipulation, 281
Manktelow prostheses, 251
Mann procedure, 362
Manske and McCarroll opponensplasty, 335
Manual locking knee, 195
Manual lymphatic drainage, 369
Manual therapy, 369
Manubrium, 287
Maquet line, 113
Maquet procedure, 269
Marathoner's toe, 38
Marble bones, 59
Marchetti and Bartolozzi Classification of spondylolisthesis, 289t
March fracture, 12–13
Marcove, Lewis, Horos procedure, 245
Marcus, Balourdas, Heiple arthrodesis, 229
Marfan-like syndrome, 88
Marfan syndrome, 88, 322
Marginal osteophyte, 289, 291
Marginal resection, 276
Marie-Bamberger disease, 61
Marie-Charcot-Tooth disease, 81
Marie-Foix sign, 155
Marie-Strümpell disease, 77, 294
Marks and Bayne procedure, 341
Maroteaux-Lamy syndrome, 67
Marquardt technique, 278
Marshall knee-scoring scale, 160
Marshall procedure, 268
Marsupialization, 281, 336
Marsupial pedicle, 273
Martin
  bandage, 184
  osteotomy, 215
  procedure, 260, 269
  screw, 222
  Vigorimeter, 373
Martin-Gruber anastomosis, 315
Martin-Gruber connection, 315
Marvel test, 141
Mason Classification, 23
Masses sign, 146
Massie nail, 222

Massive osteolysis, 46
Massive sliding graft, 218
Mass MOI, 384
Masson trichrome, 170
Mastocytosis, 49
Mast-Spiegel-PappasClassification, 23–24
Matched ulnar resection, 332
Materials and methods, 377
Matev procedure, 334
Matev sign, 118
Matles test, 155
Matricectomy, 362
Matrilin 3, 65
Matrix metalloprotease (MMP), 391
Matrix seating system, 205
Matrix unguis, 314, 350
Matrix vesicle, 393
Matte finish, 258, 281
Mauck procedure, 268
Mauclair disease, 61
Mau procedure, 362
Maximum surgical blood order schedule (MSBOS), 172
Mayer procedure, 362
Mayo classification, 24
Mayo metatarsal bar, 206
Mayo procedure, 362
Mazur ankle rating, 160
McAfee fixation, 301
McArdle syndrome, 67
McBride procedure, 362
McBride test, 155
McCarthy sign, 148
McCarty procedure, 260
McCash procedure, 340
McCauley procedure, 362
McConnell taping, 369
McCune-Albright syndrome, 59
McElvenny maneuver, 148
McElvenny procedure, 362
McFarland approach, 275
McGregor line, 115
McKay osteotomy, 215
McKeever and Buck prostheses, 251
McKeever procedure, 245, 362
McKenzie extension exercises, 369
McKusick-type metaphyseal chondrodysplasia, 65
McLaughlan approach, 275
McLaughlin plate or screw, 222
McLaughlin procedure, 245, 269
McMurray
  osteotomy, 215
  sign, 152
  test, 152
McRae line, 115
McReynolds procedure, 362
McShane, Leinberry, and Fenlin procedure, 245
McWhorter approach, 274
Mean corpuscular hemoglobin concentration (MCHC), 164
Mean corpuscular hemoglobin (MCH), 164
Mean corpuscular volume (MCV), 164

Meary angle, 113, 351
Mechanical axis, 113
Mechanical testing, 387
Medial and lateral contoured knee joints, 198
Medial and lateral plantar nerves, 351
Medial approach, 341, 364
Medial arteriosclerosis, 77
Medial circumflex artery, 255
Medial collateral ligament, 264–265
Medial collateral sprain, 35
Medial column, 347
Medial condylar fracture
  Kilfoyle classification for, 21
  Milch classification for, 24
Medial elbow approach, 274
Medial epicondylectomy, 333
Medial epicondyles, 246
Medial epicondylitis, 37, 328
Medial facet, 261
Medial femoral condyles, 261
Medial heel wedge, 206
Medial hip approach, 275
Medial knee approach, 275
Medial ligament, 234
Medial malleolus, 261
Medial meniscus, 266
Medial proximal tibial angle, 113
Medial shelf/medial plica, 94
Medial subluxation test, 152
Medial swivel dislocation, 34
Medial tibial stress syndrome, 38
Medialization ratio, 115
Median basilic vein, 248
Median cephalic vein, 248
Median nerve, 243, 315
Medical antishock trousers (MAST), 188
Medical Research Council (MRC) sensory grade, 156–157
Medoff sliding plate, 222
Medullary canal, 212
Medullary graft, 218
Medullary rod, 222
Megahorn meniscus, 93
Meisenbach procedure, 362
Meissner corpuscles, 315
Meleney infection, 330
Melioidosis, 101
Mellesi cable graft, 235
Melone classification, 325
Melorheostosis, 58
Membranous bone, 212
Mendel-Bekhterev reflex, 156
Meninges, 287
Meningioma, 297
Meningism, 297–298
Meningismus, 297–298
Meningitis, 298
Meningocele, 298
Meningocele spina bifida, 299
Meningoencephalomyelitis, 298
Meningomyelitis, 298
Meningomyelocele, 299

Meniscal bearing, 271
Meniscal flounce, 93
Meniscectomy, 268
Meniscitis, 92–93
Meniscofemoral ligament, 265
Meniscotibial ligament, 265
Meniscus, 227
Meniscus tear, 92–93
Menkes kinky-hair syndrome, 88
Mennell sign, 139
Mennen opponensplasty, 338
Menson and Scheck procedure, 260
Mental reflexes, 157
Meralgia, 80
Merchant angle, 113
Merchant view, 109
Merke sign, 152
Merle d'Aubigne and Postel hip scale, 161
Meryon sign, 158
Mesenchymal chondrosarcoma, 52
Mesenchymal stem cells, 391
Mesenchymoma, 102
Mesh skin graft, 272
Messenger ribonucleic acid (mRNA), 391
Metabolic diseases, 43
  bone formation, 168
  bone resorption, 168
  general bone turnover markers, 167–168
  osteomalacia, 83–84
  osteoporosis, 84
  other, 84–89
  urine chemical tests, 168
Metacarpal lengthening, 334
Metacarpals, 307
Metachondromatosis, 88
Metal foot plate, 200
Metal orthoses, 198
Metalloproteases, 391
Metalloproteinases, 391
Metallosis, 88
Metal-metal bearing, 226
Metaphyseal chondrodysplasia, 65
Metaphyseal-diaphyseal angle, 113
Metaphyseal fibrous defect, 53
Metaphyseal osteotomy, 362
Metaphysis, 212, 393
Metastasis, 102
Metastasize, 102
Metastron, 130
Metatarsalgia, 355
Metatarsals, 347
  bars, 206
  cuneiform exostosis, 355
  head resection with prosthesis, 362
  pads, 206
  supports, 206
Metatarsophalangeal joint dislocation, 34
Metatarsus abductus, 355
Metatarsus adductocavus, 355
Metatarsus adductus, 355
Metatarsus atavicus, 355

Metatarsus equinus, 355
Metatarsus latus, 355
Metatarsus primus varus, 350, 355
Metatarsus valgus, 355
Metatarsus varus, 355
Method, 131
Meyer
　dysplasia, 91
　fixation, 301
　line, 351
Meyer-Burgdorff osteotomy, 215
Meyers-McKeever classification, 24
Meyn and Quigley maneuver, 144
MGHL cord, 69
Michael Reese prosthesis, 246
Michele buckling sign, 139
Michele flip sign, 139
Microamperage electrical nerve stimulation (MENS), 367
Microarray, 387
Micro CT, 386
Microfracture, 230
Microgeodic disease, 102
Micromotion, 226
Micronychia, 328
Microradiography, 387
MicroRNAs (miRNA), 391
Microscopy, 387–388
Microsphere, 388
Microsurgery, 300
Mid-coated stem, 258
Midfoot, 347
Midnight fracture, 12
Midpalmar crease (MPC), 313
Midpalmar space, 313
Midshaft, 13
Midtarsal joint, 347
Midvastus approach, 275
Migration index, 118
Mikulicz angle, 113
Milch
　maneuver, 142
　prostheses, 251
　shortening prostheses, 251
Milch classification, 24
Milgram test, 139
Military brace maneuver, 136, 139
Milk-alkali disease, 58
Milk-alkali syndrome, 83
Milkmaid's dislocation, 33
Milkmaid's elbow, 33
Milkman syndrome, 61
Miller procedure, 362
Mills test, 144
Milroy disease, 88
Milwaukee
　cervicothoracolumbosacral orthosesaxillary sling, 205
　orthoses, 204
　shoulder syndrome, 90
Mimocausalgia, 79
Mimori test, 142
Minerva cast, 179

Minimally invasive percutaneous plate osteosynthesis (MIPPO), 2
Minimally invasive plate osteosynthesis (MIPO), 222
Minimally invasive spine surgery (MISS), 300
Minimally invasive surgery (MIS), 226
Minnesota rate of manipulation test, 373
Minor sign, 139
Mirels Scoring System, 51
Mirror hand, 322
Mital prostheses, 252
Mitchell procedure, 362
Mitochondrial myopathy, 63
Mitogen-activated protein kinase (MAP) kinase, 391
Miyakawa procedure, 269
Mizuno, Hirohata, and Kashiwagi prostheses, 252
Moberg
　dowel graft, 330
　flap, 336, 341
　procedure, 245, 333, 361
Mobile arm support (MAS), 202
Modeling, 393
Modic intervertebral disk changes on MRI, 123
Modified Elmslie procedure, 358
Modified Frankel Classification for Cord Damage Due to Any Cause, 297t
Modified French osteotomy, 214
Modified Kessler suture, 337
Modified lift-off test, 142–143
Modified Mallet classification, 82
Modified Ollier approach, 275
Modified Westergren method, 166
Modular components, 226
Modularity, 226
Modular prosthesis, 196
Modulus (Pa), 385
Moe plate, 222
Mold arthroplasty, 256
Molded Thomas collar, 204
Moleskin, 179
Molesworth approach, 274
Moment of inertia (MOI), 384
Momentum, 384
Mönckeberg sclerosis, 77
Mongensen procedure, 364
Monkey paw, 319
Monoblock, 271
Monodactyly, 322
Mononeuritis multiplex, 80
Monoplanar fixators, 2
Monoplegia, 63, 80
Monostotic fibrous dysplasia, 68
Monteggia Classification, 24
Monteggia dislocation, 34
Monteggia fracture, 9, 34
Montercaux fracture, 12
Moore
　approach, 275
　fracture, 9
　osteotomy, 215
　plate or pin, 222
　procedure, 267

Morbid, 102
Morbidity, 102
Morcellation, 281
Morcellized graft, 218
Morel-Lavallée lesion, 41
Morel syndrome, 61
Moro reflex sign, 156
Morquio sign, 156
Morquio syndrome, 45, 67
Morrey approach, 274
Morrisay procedure, 260
Morscher plate, 222
Morselized graft, 302
Morse taper, 226
Mortise view, 109
Morton
　foot, 355
　neuroma, 355
　syndrome, 355
　test, 155
Mosaicplasty, 230
Mose concentric rings, 123
Motion analysis, 388
Motor apraxia, 78
Motor neuron disease, 80
Mouchet fracture, 9
MPS I H, 67
MPS I H/S, 67
MPS I S, 67
MPS II, 67
MPS III A, 67
MPS III B, 67
MPS III C, 67
MPS III D, 67
MPS IV A, 67
MPS IV B, 67
MPS VI, 67
MPS VII, 67
Mucopolysaccharides, 168, 392
Mucopolysaccharidoses, 67
Mucopolysaccharidosi, 68
Mucopurulent, 102
Mucosanguineous, 102
Mucous cyst, 68, 329
Mulder sign, 155
Müller
　arthrodesis, 229
　osteotomy, 215
　plate, 222
Muller procedure, 268
Multiaxial ankle, 195
Multidirectional instability, 33
Multifragmentary fracture, 4
Multiplanar fixators, 2
Multiplanar frame fixation, 224
Multiplane fixation, 224
Multiple comparison test, 380
Multiple crush syndrome, 319
Multiple epiphyseal dysplasia, 65
Multiple fracture, 5

Multiple hereditary exostosis, 52, 57
Multiple myeloma, 52
Multiple osteochondromatosis, 52
Multiple sclerosis, 80
Mumford-Gurd procedure, 245
Munster cast, 180
Münster prosthetic socket, 190
Murphy
　approach, 275
　nails, 222
　sign, 146, 155
Muscle
　abdominal, 288
　of ankle, 349–350
　of arm, 247
　atrophy, 63, 182
　contracture, 63
　cramps, 38, 63
　diseases, 61–62
　energy technique, 369
　guarding, 63
　insertion, 231
　ischemia, 63
　loss, 27
　origin, 231
　spasm, 63
　transfers, 244
　wasting, 63
Muscle/tendon (MT) injury, 14
Muscular dystrophy, 63
Musculocutaneous nerve, 243
Musculoskeletal diseases, 43–104
　acetabulum deficiencies, 91–92
　anatomic area, 89–91
　bursa-related disease, 69–70
　cartilage diseases, 64–67
　congenital limb absences, 94
　fascia-related disease, 69–70
　femur-related deficiencies, 91–92
　joint disease, 70–73
　knee disorders, 92–94
　ligament-related disease, 69–70
　limb deficiencies, 95–97
　metabolic diseases, 82–89
　muscle diseases, 61–64
　neurologic diseases, 78–82
　soft tissue, 53–54, 67–68
　tendon disease, 69–70
　terminiology, 97–104
　vascular, 73–78
Musculoskeletal Tumor Society Grading System, 49
Mustard procedure, 258
Myalgia, 62
Myasthenia, 61
Myasthenia gravis, 61
Myatrophy, 61
Mycobacterium avium, 169
Mycobacterium marinum, 169
Mycobacterium tuberculosis, 48, 169
Myectomy, 231

Index

Myelalgia, 296
Myelanalosis, 296
Myelapoplexy, 296
Myelasthenia, 296
Myelatelia, 298
Myelatrophy, 296
Myelauxe, 296
Myelencephalitis, 296
Myeleterosis, 296
Myelin protein 0, 81
Myelin protein 22, 81
Myeloblastoma, 52
Myelocele, 298
Myelocele spina bifida, 299
Myelocystocele, 298
Myelocystomeningocele, 298
Myelodiastasis, 298
Myelodysplasia, 298
Myeloencephalitis, 296
Myelofibrosis, 58
Myelogram, 108
Myelography, 108, 299
Myelomalacia, 296
Myelomeningitis, 296
Myelomeningocele, 291, 298
Myeloneuritis, 296
Myeloparalysis, 296
Myelopathy, 296
Myelophthisis, 297
Myeloplegia, 297
Myeloproliferative disease, 52
Myeloradiculitis, 297
Myeloradiculopathy, 297
Myelorrhagia, 297
Myelosclerosis, 297
Myelosyphilis, 297
Myelotomy procedure, 305
Myerson classification, 24
Myoblastoma, 54
Myoblasts, 231
Myobradia, 61
Myocardial infarction (MI), 78
Myocele, 61
Myocelialgia, 61
Myocelitis, 61
Myocellulitis, 61
Myocerosis, 61–62
Myoclasis, 231
Myoclonia, 61
Myoclonus, 61
Myocoele, 61
Myocytes, 231
Myocytoma, 54, 62
Myodegeneration, 62
Myodemia, 62
Myodiastasis, 62
Myodynia, 62
Myodystonia, 62
Myoedema, 62
Myoelectric control, 191

Myofascial release, 369
Myofascitis, 62
Myofibroma, 54
Myofibrosis, 62
Myogelosis, 62
Myoglobinuria, 62
Myohypertrophia, 62
Myoischemia, 62
Myokerosis, 62
Myolipoma, 54, 62
Myolysis, 62
Myoma, 62
Myomalacia, 62
Myomatectomy, 231
Myomatosis, 62
Myomectomy, 231
Myomelanosis, 62
Myo-(muscle), 231
    surgical procedures on, 231
Myoneuralgia, 62
Myoneurasthenia, 62
Myoneurectomy, 231
Myoneuroma, 62
Myoneurosis, 62
Myopachynsis, 62
Myopalmus, 62
Myoparalysis, 62
Myoparesis, 62
Myopathy, 62
Myopathy hand, 80
Myophagism, 62
Myoplasty, 231
Myopsychopathy, 62
Myorrhaphy, 231
Myorrhexis, 62
Myosalgia, 62
Myosclerosis, 62
Myoseism, 62
Myositis, 62
Myositis fibrosa generalisata, 57
Myositis ossificans, 62
Myositis ossificans circumscripta, 62
Myositis ossificans progressiva, 57
Myospasia, 62
Myospasm, 62
Myospasmia, 62
Myosteoma, 62
Myosuture, 231
Myosynizesis, 62
Myotenontoplasty, 231
Myotenositis, 62
Myotenotomy, 231
Myotomic distribution, 295
Myotomy, 231
Myotonia, 62
Myotonia intermittens, 63
Myotonic muscular dystrophy, 63
Myxedema, 102
Myxofibrosarcoma, 54
Myxoma, 54

N

Nachlas knee flexion test, 148
Nachlas test, 140
Naffziger syndrome, 82, 296
Naffziger test, 140
Nail-patella syndrome, 61
Nail plate, 314, 350
Nails
  ankle, 350
  Badgley, 219
  Bailey-Dubow, 219
  bed, 314, 350
  horn, 327
  matrix, 314, 350
N-Alber II, 192
Nalebuff arthrodesis, 331
Namaqualand hip dysplasia, 91
Nancy nail, 222
Napolean test, 141–142
Natatory ligament, 312–313
National Association of Orthopaedic Nurses (NAON), 177
National Board for Certification of Orthopaedic Technologists, 177–178
National Diabetes Data Group (NDDG), 166
National Institute of Arthritis and Musculoskeletal and Skin Diseases (NIAMS), 377
National Institutes of Health Consensus DevelopmentPanel on Osteoporosis, 83
National Institutes of Health (NIH), 377
National Research Council, 196
Nature of the question to be addressed, 380–381
Naughton-Dunn procedure, 362
Navicula cast, 180
Navicular, 347
Navicular bone, 307
Navicular pads, 206
Neal-Robertson litter, 188
Neck
  anatomic, 241
  femoral, 19, 27
  ring, 205
  shaft angle, 113
  sign, 155
  talar, 19–20
Necropsy, 279
Necrosis, 78, 102
Necrotizing fasciitis, 70
Needle biopsy, 279
Neer
  classification, 24–25
  impingement, 142
  lateral view, 109
  procedure, 245
  prosthesis, 246
  staging system, 37
  transscapular view, 109
Neer-Horowitz classification, 25
Negative predictive value, 381
Negative pressure therapy, 325
Negative variance, 323

Negative work, 369
Neibauer prosthesis, 332
Neisseria gonorrhoeae, 48, 169
Nélaton dislocation, 34
Nélaton line, 115, 148
Neoadjuvant therapy, 276
Neoplasm, 102
Neoplastic fracture, 12
Neri bowing sign, 140
Nerves
  of ankle, 357
  of arm, 248–249
  of Bell, 243
  conduction study, 371
  resection, 281
  root sleeve, 287
Nested nails, 222
Neufeld
  nail, 222
  pin, 222
  roller traction, 187
Neuralgia, 80
Neuralgic amyotrophy, 82
Neural tube defect, 80
Neurapraxia, 82t
Neurectomy, 235, 333, 362
Neuritis, 80, 295
Neurofibroma, 54, 68, 295
Neurofibromatosis, 61
Neurofibrosarcoma, 54
Neurofilament stains, 171
Neurogenic, 80
Neurogenic arthropathy, 81
Neurologic diseases, 80
  eponymic, 81–82
  general, 78–81
Neurolysis, 80, 235
Neuroma, 80
Neuromuscular scoliosis, 293
Neuro-(nerves), 235
  orthopaedic surgical procedures on, 235
Neuropathic foot, 352
Neuropathic fracture, 12, 355
Neuropathic ulcer, 357
Neuropathy, 80
Neuropeptides, 391
Neuroplasty, 235
Neuropraxia, 80
Neurorrhaphy, 235
Neurosyphilis, 81
Neurotization, 333
Neurotmesis, 80, 82t
Neurotomy, 235
Neurotripsy, 235
Neurovascular island transfer, 336
Neurovascular (MT) injury, 14
Neutron radiography, 127
Neviaser procedure, 245
Neviaser test, 142
Nevus, 102
Newington orthoses, 198

Newman fixation, 301
Newton meter, 382–383
New York orthopedic front-opening orthoses, 203
New York University (NYU) insert, 200
NEXUS cervical spine criteria, 124
Nicholas procedure, 267
Nicola procedure, 245
Nicoll procedure, 272
Nidus, 102
Niemann-Pick disease, 61
Night splint, 182
Nightstick fracture, 9
Nirschl prostheses, 252
NISSSA Score, 40–41
Node, 102
Nodular fasciitis, 70, 329
Nodule, 102
No-man's land, 311, 324
Nomarski microscopy, 387
Nondisjuction, 391
Noninfectious disease, 43
Nonionic contrast agents, 106
Nonossifying fibroma, 53
Nonparametric test, 379
Nonphyseal fracture, 4
Nonpitting edema, 102
Nonplantigrade foot, 355
Nonrigid stabilization devices, 304
Nonsuppurative osteomyelitis, 49
Nonunion, 13
    of a vertebral compression fracture, 60
Nora tumor, 53
No reflow phenomenon, 335
Normal distribution, 379
Normal flora, 169
Normal last shoes, 207
Normotensive, 78
Northern blot, 386
Norton-Brown orthoses, 202
Norton scoring system, 161
Notch view, 109
No touch test, 152
Noulis test, 152
Noyes test, 151
N-telopeptide (NTx or NTX), 168
Nuchal ligament, 286
Nuchocephalic reflex, 157
Nuclear medicine studies, 105
Nucleus pulposus, 287, 295
Nucleus replacement, 304
Nudge control, 192
Nurick Classificaiton Scale for Spinal Cord Compression Due to Spondylosis, 296t
Nursemaid's elbow, 33
Nutritional index, 102

O

Ober-Barr procedure, 245, 260
Ober procedure, 362
Ober test, 148

Obesity, 102
Objective sign, 158
Oblique fracture, 5
Oblique ligament, 250
Oblique retinacular ligament, 313
Oblique view, 109
O'Brien procedure, 245
O'Brien test, 140, 143
Observation hip, 91
Observational/effectiveness, 382
Obturator artery, 255
Obturator/brim line, 115
Obturator foramen, 253
Obturator nerve, 253, 255
Obturator sign, 148
Occipital nerve, 286
Occipital pads, 205
Occipital screws, 304
Occiput, 286
Occlusion, 78, 102
Occlusive dressing, 184
Occult, 102
Occult fracture, 6
Occupational therapy
    assessment, 372–373
    interventions, 372
    interventions, 373–375
Ochronosis, 58
O'Connell test, 140
O'Connor finger dexterity test, 373
Ocular muscular dystrophy, 63
Oculopharyngeal muscular dystrophy, 63
Oculoplethysmography (OPG), 129
Odds ratio (OR), 379
O'Donoghue procedure, 268, 364
Odontoid fracture, 14–15
Odontoid process, 285
Odontoid view, 109
O'Driscoll classification, 25
O'Driscoll superior labrum anterior to posterior (SLAP) test, 143
-odynia, 102
Ogden Classification, 25–26
    for Ulnar Longitudinal Deficiency, 96t–97t
Ogden fractures, 25–26
Ogden plate, 222
Ogston line, 115
Old dislocation, 33
Olecranon, 247
Olecranon fossa, 246
Olecranon fracture, 26
    Colton classification for, 17
    Mayo classification for, 24
Oligomeric protein of cartilage (cartilage oligomeric matrix protein [COMP]), 65
Olisthy, 291
Olive wire, 222
Ollier approach, 275, 364
Ollier disease, 52, 61, 65
Ollier-Thiersch skin graft, 272
Ombrédanne line, 116

Onco-, 102
One-legged hop test, 152
One-way ANOVA, 379, 381
Onlay graft, 218
Onychalgia, 328
Onychauxis, 355
Onychectomy, 336
Onychia, 328
Onychocryptosis, 355
Onychogryphosis, 328, 355
Onychogryposis, 328
Onycholysis, 328
Onychomadesis, 328
Onychomycosis, 328, 355
Onychophagia, 328
Onychoptosis, 328
Onychorrhexis, 328
Onychotomy, 336, 362
Op Site, 184
Open amputation, 278
Open biopsy, 279
Open book fracture, 10
Open chain exercises, 369
Open dislocation, 33
Open fractures, 3
Opening abductory wedge osteotomy (OAWO), 362
Opening wedge
  cast, 181
  free graft, 334
  osteotomy, 362
Open integumentary injury, 14
Open kinetic chain exercises, 369
Open management, 1
Open-mouth view, 109
Open reduction, 213
Open reduction and internal fixation (ORIF), 218–219
Open-wedge osteotomy, 215
Opera-glass hand, 317
Oppenheim disease, 62
Oppenheim sign, 157
Opponens bars, 202
Opponens digiti minimi (ODM), 310
Opponens digiti quinti (ODQ), 310
Opponens pollicis (OP), 310
Opponensplasty, 338
Orbicular ligament, 250
Organic contracture, 63
Oriental prayer sign, 147
-orrhagia, 102
-orrhea, 102
-orrhexis, 102
Orthopaedic Allied Professionals, 177–178
Orthopaedic oxford, 205–206
Orthopaedic radiography
  procedures, 107–108
  techniques, 107–108
Orthopaedic research, 377–394
  reporting results, 378
  research proposals, 377–378
  terminology, 378–394
Orthopaedic Research Society, 378

Orthopaedic surgeon, 343
Orthopaedic surgery
  amputations, 277–278
  anatomy and, 209–282
  aponeuroses, 231
  arthro-(joints), 226–230
  desmo-(ligaments), 234
  by location, 240–272
  myo-(muscle), 231
  osteo-(bones), 209–226
  replantation microsurgery, 276
  skin grafts, 272–273
  surgical approaches, 273–276
  surgical blocks, 273
  teno-(tendons), 231–234
  terminiology, 278–282
  tissues, 230–235
  tumor treatments, 276
  vascular (blood vessels) system, 235–240
Orthopaedic Trauma Association (OTA) Classification, 26–27
Orthopaedic Trauma Association Registry System, 1
Orthopaedics tests, signs, and maneuvers, 131–136
  ankles, 154–155
  back, 138–140
  elbow, 143–144
  feet, 154–155
  gait, 158–159
  hands, 144–147
  hips, 147–149
  knees, 149–154
  lower limbs, 149
  metabolic tests, 157–158
  neck, 136–138
  neurological examination, 155–157
  observations, 158
  physical examinations, 161
  ratings, 159–161
  scales, 159–161
  shoulder, 140–143
  upper limbs, 143–144
Orthoroentgenogram, 108
Orthoroentgenography, 108
Orthoses, 196–205
  abduction, 198–199
  accommodative, 197
  lower-limb, 197–199
  shoe modifications, 205–207
  upper-limb, 200–202
Orthotics, 374–375
Ortolani click, 148
Ortolani test, 148
Os calcis fracture, 18
Osborne and Cotterill prostheses, 252
Osborne approach, 275
Osborne fascia, 250
Oscilloscope, 106
Osgood osteotomy, 215
Osgood-Schlatter disease, 55, 61
Oshsner clasping test, 146

Os intercuneiforme, 347
Os intermetatarseum, 347
 osis, 102
Os magnum, 307
Os peroneum, 347
Os sustentaculum, 347
Os talocalcaneus, 347
Os tibiale externum, 344, 347, 356
Os trigonum, 347
Os vesalianum, 347
Osmone-Clarke procedure, 362
Ossa tarsi, 347
Osseous, 212
Ossicles, 44
Ossiferous, 212
Ossific, 212
Ossification, 209, 212
Ossification center, 212
Ossifying fibroma of long bone, 46, 57
Ossifying fibroma of the jaw, 58
Ostealgia, 44
Ostectomy, 213
Osteitis
 condensans, 44
 deformans, 44, 61
 fibrosa cystica, 44
 fragilitans, 46
 ossificans, 44
 pubis, 44
Ostemia, 44
Ostempyesis, 44
Osteoaneurysm, 44
Osteoarthritis, 44, 70–71
Osteoarthropathy, 44
Osteoarthrosis, 44–45
Osteoarthrotomy, 213
Osteoarticular, 45
Osteoarticular graft, 218
Osteoblast, 212, 392
Osteoblastoma, 51
Osteo-(bone), 209–226
 anatomy of, 209–226
 fractures, 218–224
 general surgery, 213–214
 grafts, 215–218
 internal prostheses, 224–226
 osteosyntheses, 218–223
 osteotomies, 214–215
Osteocachexia, 45
Osteocalcin, 393
Osteocalcin or bone Gla protein (OC, ON, BGP), 168
Osteocartilaginous exostosis, 353
Osteochondral graft, 218
Osteochondral lesions
 Ferkel-Cheng arthroscopic classification for, 18
 Ferkel-Sgaglione classification for, 18
Osteochondritis, 45
Osteochondritis dissecans, 16, 46
Osteochondrodesmodysplasia, 45
Osteochondrodystrophy, 45
Osteochondrofibroma, 45

Osteochondrolysis, 45
Osteochondroma, 52, 353
Osteochondromatosis, 45, 65
Osteochondropathy, 45
Osteochondrophyte, 45
Osteochondrosis, 45–46, 355
Osteochondrosis deformans tibia, 59
Osteochondrosis dissecans, 46
Osteoclasia, 46
Osteoclasis, 213
Osteoclast, 212, 392
Osteoclastoma, 53, 57
Osteoconductive grafts, 217
Osteoconductive material, 302
Osteocope, 46
Osteocystoma, 46
Osteocyte, 212, 393
Osteodiastasis, 46
Osteodynia, 46
Osteodystrophy, 46
Osteofibrochondrosarcoma, 46
Osteofibroma, 46
Osteofibromatosis, 46
Osteofibrous dysplasia, 46
Osteogenesis imperfecta, 46
Osteogenesis imperfecta congenita, 46
Osteogenesis imperfecta tarda, 46
Osteogenic sarcoma, 50
Osteohalisteresis, 46
Osteoid, 212, 392
Osteoid osteoma, 51
Osteoinductive grafts, 217
Osteoinductive material, 302
Osteokinetic movement, 371
Osteolipochondroma, 46
Osteolipoma, 46
Osteolysis, 46–47
Osteoma, 51
Osteomalacia, 47, 83–84
Osteomatosis, 52
Osteomesopyknosis, 47
Osteomyelitis, 47–49
Osteomyelodysplasia, 47
Osteon, 212, 393
Osteonal bone, 212
Osteonecrosis, 47
Osteonectin, 393–394
Osteoneuralgia, 47
Osteopathia striata, 47
Osteopathy, 47
Osteopenia, 47, 82–83
Osteoperiosteal graft, 218
Osteoperiostitis, 47
Osteopetrorickets, 47
Osteopetrosis, 47
Osteophlebitis, 47
Osteophyte, 47, 119
Osteoplastica, 44, 47
Osteoplasty, 213
Osteopoikilosis, 47
Osteopontin, 393

Osteoporosis, 47, 83–84
Osteoprotegerin (OPG), 394
Osteopsathyrosis idiopathica, 46
Osteoradionecrosis, 47
Osteo-root disease, 44–48
Osteosarcoma, 51
Osteosclerosis, 47
Osteosclerosis fragilis, 47
Osteosis, 47
Osteospongioma, 47
Osteosynovitis, 47
Osteosynthesis, 1, 214
Osteotabes, 47
Osteotelangiectasia, 51
Osteothrombophlebitis, 48
Osteothrombosis, 48
Osteotripsy, 362
Otto pelvis, 34
Outerbridge-Kashiwagi prostheses, 252
Outflare last shoes, 207
Outlet view, 109
Output variable, 379–380
Outrigger, 202
Outside locking hinge, 192
Overhead exercise test, 137
Overhead suspension, 185
Overlapped upright or growth extensions, 200
Overlapping toe, 356
Overlap syndrome, 329
Over-the-top procedure, 268
Overton fixation, 301
Oxidized zirconium, 226

P

P/3, proximal third, 3–4
P value, 380
PA view, 109
Pachydysostosis, 58
Pachyonychia, 356
Packed cell volume (PCV), 164
Packing, 184
Paddle, 281
Pads, 184
Pagddu procedure, 268
Paget disease, 44, 61
Paget-Schroetter syndrome, 89
Painful arc syndrome, 90
Palindromic rheumatism, 77
Palliative, 281
Pallor, 75
Palmaris longus (PL), 310
Palm/palmar, 312–313
　advancement flaps, 341
　bursa, 313
　fascia, 313
　fasciectomy, 341
　fasciotomy, 341
　fibromatosis, 328
　palmar fascial compartments, 312–313
　skin crease, 313

Palm/palmar *(Continued)*
　space infection, 329
　wrist splint, 201
Palmer Classification
　for Triangular Fibrocartilage Complex (FTCC) Injury, 325t–326t
Palpitation, 78
Panels, 164
Panmetatarsal head resection, 362
Panner disease, 55, 61
Panniculitis, 102
Pannus, 71
Pantalar fusion, 362
Pantopaque, 106
Panty cast, 180
Paracentesis, 281
Parachute jumper's dislocation, 34
Paraffin bath, 368
Parallel pitch lines, 351
Paralysis, 80
Paralysis agitans, 80, 82
Parametric test, 380
Parapatellar approach, 275
Paraplegia, 80
Parasympathetic nervous systems, 283
Parathyroid hormone (PTH), 167, 394
Paratonia, 157
Paratrooper fracture, 12
Paravertebral muscle spasm, 291
Parenteral, 281
Paresis, 80
Paresthesia, 80, 102
Parham band, 222
Parkinson disease, 80, 82
Paronychia, 330, 356
Paronychium, 314
Parosteal chondrosarcoma, 52
Parosteal osteosarcoma, 51
Parosteitis, 48
Parosteosis, 48
Parrot-beak tear, 92–93
Parrot pseudoparalysis, 82
Pars interarticularis defect, 289
Pars interarticularis, 284
Parsonage-Andrew-Turner syndrome, 82
Parson's third tubercle, 93
Partial adactylia, 95
Partial aphalangia, 95
Partial dislocation, 33
Partial hand amputation, 190
Partial hemimelia, 95
Partial laminotomy, 300
Partial meniscectomy, 268
Partial ostectomy, 363
Partial patellectomy, 269
Partridge band, 222
Parvin maneuver, 144
Passive range of motion (ROM) exercise, 369
Passive tendon implant, 339
PASTA, 38
Patch angioplasty, 240

Patella/patellar, 261
 alta, 94
 apprehension test, 152
 baja, 94
 button, 271
 clunk syndrome, 94
 condylar shaving, 269
 cubiti, 90
 dislocations, 34
 fracture, 11
 glide test, 152
 grind test, 152
 pad, 200
 retraction test, 152
 subluxation, 34, 115–116
 tendon, 234
 tilt test, 152
Patellar tendon bearing (PTB) cast, 180
Patellar tendon–bearing (PTB) orthoses, 197–198
Patellectomy, 269
Patellofemoral syndrome, 94
Patency, 238
Pathologic, 289
Pathologic dislocation, 33
Pathologic fracture, 12
Patrick test, 138–139, 148
Pauciarticular, 71
Paulos procedure, 268
Pauwels angle, 113
Pauwels Classification, 27
Pauwels osteotomy, 215
Pauwels-Y osteotomy, 215
Pavlik harness, 199
Pavlov ratio, 116
Payr sign, 149
Peabody procedure, 363
Pearson attachment, 185
Pectoralis major and minor, 242
Pectoralis muscle, 287
Pectus carinatum, 102
Pectus excavatum, 102
Pedicle, 285
  flap, 336
  graft, 218, 336
  screws, 304
Pedorthist, 343
Peer reviewers, 378
Peg graft, 218
Pelkan spur, 118
Pellagra, 80
Pellegrini-Stieda disease, 69
Pelvic band, 195
Pelvic femoral angle, 113
Pelvic fracture
 Key and Conwell classification for, 21
 Tile classification for, 30
 Torode and Zieg classification for, 30
 Young-Burgess classification for, 31–32
Pelvis/pelvic
 anatomy of, 252–254
 blood vessels, 253

Pelvis/pelvic *(Continued)*
 bones, 252–253
 girdle, 205, 252–253
 ligaments, 253
 muscles, 253
 nerves, 253–254
 obliquity, 293
 other procedures, 259–261
 ring, 253
 rock test, 140
 sling, 187
 surgery of, 255–261
 traction, 187
Pemberton osteotomy, 215
Pencil-in-cup deformity, 118
Pennsylvania bimanual work sample, 373
Percutaneous biopsy, 279
Percutaneous transluminal angioplasty (PTA), 239
Perdriolle torsiometer, 124
Perforating arteries, 266
Perfusion imaging, 127
Periacetabular osteotomy (PAO), 214
Periarticular fibrositis, 68
Periarticular fracture, 4
Perichondral autografts, 332
Perichondrium, 392
Perilunate dislocation, 327
Perinatal hypophosphatasia, 58
Perineal loops, 205
Perionychium, 314
Periosteal chondroma, 52
Periosteal desmoid, 69
Periosteal fibroma, 68
Periosteal osteosarcoma, 51
Periosteotomy, 214
Periosteum, 212, 394
Periostitis, 58
Periostitis ossificans, 59
Periostomy, 214
Peripheral arterial occlusion (PAO), 75
Peripheral nerves, 283
Peripheral neuropathy, 80, 319
Periprosthetic fracture hip, 31
Peritendinitis stenosans/digitus saltans, 324
Peritendinous fibrosis, 326
Peritoneum, 254
Perkin line, 116
Peromelia, 94
Peroneal artery, 266
Peroneal nerve palsy, 353
Peroneal spastic flatfoot, 356
Peroneus brevis, 263
Peroneus brevis tendon, 349
Peroneus longus, 263
Peroneus longus tendon, 349
Peroneus quartus, 350
Peroneus tertius, 263, 349
Per primam, 281
Perry procedure, 272, 363
Persian slipper foot, 356
Personal hygiene and grooming, 373

Perthes-Bankhart lesion, 33
Perthes disease, 55, 60–61
Pertrochanteric fracture, 10
Pes, 356
Pes anserinus, 262
Pes calcaneocavus, 357
Pes calcaneus, 357
Pes cavovalgus, 357
Pes cavovarus, 351, 357
Pes cavus, 206, 356
Pes equinovalgus, 357
Pes equinovarus, 357
Pes planovalgus, 351, 357
Pes planus, 206, 356–357
Petaling edges, 181
Petechiae, 102
Petit mal epilepsy, 79
Petrie spica cast, 180
Pétrissage, 369
-pexy, 281
Pfeiffer syndrome, 88
PGP nail, 222
Phalangectomy, 341
Phalanges, 307
Phalanx, 347
Phalen maneuver, 146
Phalen-Miller procedure, 338
Phalen test, 146
Phantom bone disease, 46
Phantom limb pain, 281, 317
Phantom limb syndrome, 102
Phase contrast microscopy, 387
Phelps, 245
Phemister approach, 276
Phemister osteotomy, 215
Phenolization, 363
Phenomenon, 131
Phenotype, 391
Philadelphia collar, 204
Phillips screw, 222
Phlebitis, 73
Phlebogram, 129
Phlebography, 129
Phlebothrombosis, 73
Phlegmasia cerulea dolens, 78
Phocomelia, 322
Phonophoresis, 368
Phosphate, 164
Phosphate endopeptidase homolog (PHEX), 84
Phosphorus (P), 164
Photogrammetry, 388
Photon densitometry, 107
Photoplethysmography (PPG), 129
Phrenic nerve, 286
-phyma, 102
Physeal
  angle, 113
  bar, 67
  cartilage, 392
  fracture, 6
  slope, 113

Physiatrist, 365
Physical medicine and rehabilitation, 365–371
  occupational therapy, 371–375
Physical medicine and rehabilitation (PM&R)
  physical therapy modalities, 367–368
  physical therapy procedures, 368–370
  physical therapy services, 366–367
  tests and measurements, 370–371
Physical sign, 158
Physical therapist, 365
Physical Therapy Evaluation (General), 366t
Physical Therapy Treatment Techniques, 366t–367t
Physiolysis, 335
Physis, 29, 211–212, 394
Pia, 287
Piano key sign, 146
Pidcock pin, 222
Piedmont fracture, 9
Pierrot-Murphy procedure, 363
Piezoelectric potential, 388
Pigeon toe, 356
Pigmented villonodular synovitis, 72
Pillion fracture, 11
Pillow orthoses, 199
Pilon, 23–24
Pin tract infection, 182
Pina bifida occulta (SBO), 299
Pincer deformity, 328
Pincer impingement, 91
Pinch, 373
Pinched nerve, 295
Pink sheets, 378
Pinprick test, 371
Piotrowski sign, 157
Pipkin classification, 27
Piriform sclerosis ilium, 44
Pisiform, 307
Piriformis fossa, 254
Piriformis syndrome, 298
Piston sign, 148
Pitch angle, 113
Pitres-Testut sign, 146
Pitres-Testut syndrome, 317
Pitted nail, 328
Pittsburgh for Osteonecrosis of the Femoral Head, 55t
Pivot-jerk test, 153
Pivot shift of elbow, 144
Pivot shift test, 153
Plafond fracture, 12
Plan for data analysis, 377
Planck, 384
Plantar aponeurosis, 351
Plantar arch, 351
Plantar arch support, 206
Plantar artery, 351
Plantar axial view of foot, 109
Plantar calcaneonavicular ligaments, 350
Plantar fascia, 3
Plantar fasciitis, 355–356
Plantar flexed metatarsal, 356
Plantar wart, 356

Plantaris, 263
Plantigrade foot, 356
Plasmacytoma, 52
Plastazote, 206
Plastazote collar, 204
Plaster rolls, 179
Plastic bowing fracture, 6
Plastic collar, 204
Plastic deformation, 384
Plastic region, 385
Plastizote inserts, 206
Platelet gels, 303
Platelets (Plt), 164, 172
Plates and screws, 304
Platou osteotomy, 215
Platysma, 286
Play or leisure, 374
Pleomorphic, 102
Plethysmography, 129
Plexiform, 102
Plexiform bone, 394
Plica, 266
Plica syndrome, 94
Plication, 281
Pneumatic compression boot or sleeve, 183
Pneumoarthrogram, 108
Pneumoarthrography, 108
Podagra, 356
Podiatrist, 343
Poisson ratio, 384
Poland classification, 27
Poland syndrome, 63, 322
Polar contact, 258
Polar MOI, 384
Polarized light microscopy, 170, 387
Poliomyelitis, 81
Polka-dot sign, 118
Pollicization, 341
Pollock sign, 146
Pollock syndrome, 317
Polyacetyl rod, 281
Polyarteritis nodosa, 77
Polyarthritis, 71
Polydactyly, 322, 356
Polymerase chain reaction (PCR), 169, 388
Polymethylmethacrylate (PMMA), 225–226
Polymyalgia rheumatica, 77
Polymyositis, 77
Polyneuritis, 81
Polyostotic fibrous dysplasia, 59, 68
Polyps, 100
Polysyndactyly, 322, 356
Polytetrafluoroethylene (PTFE), 240
Ponsetti bar, 197
Ponte osteotomy procedure, 305
Popeye deformity, 144
Popliteal artery and vein, 75, 266
Popliteal cyst, 72, 94
Popliteal entrapment, 75
Popliteal pterygium syndrome, 94
Popliteus muscle, 262

Population indices, 381
Portal, 281
Port wine hemangioma, 77
Posada fracture, 8
Positions/directions, 374
  anatomic planes, 405–406
  joint motions, 406–409
  location, 405–406
  terminology, 409–412
Positive predictive value, 381
Positive variance, 323
Positive work, 368
Postaxial deficiency, 323
Posterior approach, 306
Posterior bone block elbow, 244
Posterior cervical spinal fixation, 302
Posterior compartment, 263
Posterior cruciate ligament, 263
Posterior cruciate sprain, 35
Posterior dislocation, 34
Posterior drawer test, 153
Posterior elbow approach, 274
Posterior element fracture, 10
Posterior femur approach, 275
Posterior forearm approach, 274
Posterior fracture, 34
Posterior hiatal sign, 118
Posterior hip approach, 275
Posterior horns, 288
Posterior humerus approach, 274
Posterior inferior iliac spine, 253
Posterior intraosseous nerve syndrome, 249, 318–319
Posterior knee approach, 275
Posterior leg approach, 276
Posterior lift-off test, 143
Posterior lip, 254
Posterior longitudinal ligament, 287
Posterior lumbar spinal fixation, 302
Posterior malleolus, 11, 261
Posterior neck muscles, 286
Posterior oblique ligament sprain, 35
Posterior shoulder approach, 274
Posterior shoulder dislocation, 33, 243
Posterior slip angle, 114
Posterior spinal fixation, 302
Posterior spinal muscle segments, 288
Posterior splint, 188
Posterior superior iliac spine, 252–253
Posterior talofibular ligaments, 350
Posterior tibial artery, nerve, and vein, 266, 351
Posterior tibial spine, 261
Posterior tibial tendon insufficiency, 350, 356
Posterior vertebral scalloping sign, 118
Posterior wall sign, 118
Posterolateral approach, 364
  elbow, 274
  femur, 275
  knee, 275
  leg, 276
Posterolateral fixation, 302

Posterolateral forearm approach, 274
Posterolateral instability of elbow, 144
Posterolateral interbody fixation (PLIF), 302
Posteromedial approach, 364
   knee, 275
   leg, 276
Posteromedial impingement, 36
Post-hoc tests, 380
Postphlebitic syndrome, 73
Postpoliomyelitic contracture, 63
Post-total hip internal rotation test, 149
Posttourniquet syndrome, 317
Posttraumatic reflex dystrophy, 79
Posttraumatic vertebral osteonecrosis, 60
Postural fixation, 140
Postyield region, 385
Potential energy (PE), 384
Potenza arthrodeses, 330
Pott
   disease, 61, 294
   eversion osteotomy, 215
   fracture, 12
   paraplegia, 82
Potter arthrodeses, 229
Pouce flottant, 322
Poupart inguinal ligament, 253
Power, 380
Power Doppler, 105, 129
Prader-Willi syndrome, 95
Prake tenodesis, 338
Prayer view, 109
Precision, 380
Precocious osteoarthritis, 65
Predictive salvage index, 40
Predictor variable, 379
Prehallux, 356
Prehensile, 369
Prehension test, 146
Preiser disease, 329
Preliminary data, 378
Prepatellar bursa, 266
Press fit, 226
Pressure
   dressing, 184
   epiphyseal, 211
   epiphysis, 45
   sore, 182
   testing, 371
Preston screw, 222
Prevention and minimization of debilitation, 374
Pridie-Koutsogiannis procedure, 363
Primary center of ossification, 212
Primary closure, 281
Primary lymphoma of bone, 52–53
Primary osteon, 393
Primary spongiosa, 213
Primary subacute osteomyelitis, 49
Prime movers, 231
Primitive dislocation, 33
Procollagen, 392
Procollagen propeptide, 168

Procurvatum, 100
Profiles, 164
Profundus, 248
Profundus artery, 255
Prognosis, 100
Progressive diaphyseal dysplasia, 58
Progressive dystrophic ophthalmoplegia, 63
Progressive osseous heteroplasia, 58
Progressive systemic sclerosis (PSS), 77, 316
Proliferating zone, 212
Proliferative fasciitis, 68
Proliferative myositis, 62
Pronation, 356
Pronation sign, 157
Pronator quadratus (PQ), 248, 310
Pronator syndrome, 318
Pronator teres (PT), 310
Prone external rotation test, 153
Prone hanging test, 151, 153
Proper volar digital nerve and artery, 315
Prophylaxis, 100
Proprioception, 100
Proprioceptive testing, 371
Prospective, 382
Prostate-specific antigen (PSA), 165
Prosthesis, 281
   of antibiotic-loaded acrylic cement (PROSTALAC), 226
Prosthetics, 190–196, 375
   components, 195–196
   lower limb, 193–195
   materials, 195–196
   specialized systems, 196
   techniques, 195–196
   upper limb, 190–191
Protective dressing, 184
Proteoglycan, 67, 392
Proteomics, 391
Prothrombin time (pro time, PT), 166
Proton density, 127
Protrusio acetabuli, 91
Protrusion, 296
Proximal coated stem, 258
Proximal focal femoral deficiency (PFFD), 91
Proximal interphalangeal (PIP) fusion, 347, 363
Proximal phocomelia, 95
Proximal row carpectomy, 332
Proximal thigh band, 200
Proximal tibial fracture, 29
Proximal tibiofibular facet, 261
Proximal tibiofibular joint, 26
Proximal tibiofibular ligament, 265
Prune belly syndrome, 88
Pseudo acetabulum, 254
Pseudo deficiency rickets, 84
Pseudoachondroplasia, 89
Pseudoaneurysm, 75
Pseudoarthrosis, 13
Pseudoarthrosis, 71
Pseudo-Babinski sign, 157
Pseudoclaudication, 291

Pseudoclawing, 326
Pseudofracture, 13
Pseudogout, 89, 316
Pseudohypertrophic muscular dystrophy, 63
Pseudohypoparathyroidism (PHPT), 83
Pseudomalignant fibroosseous tumors, 59
Pseudomonas aeruginos, 169
Pseudomonas organisms, 48
Pseudoreplication, 380
Pseudosarcomatous fibromatosis, 68
Pseudostability test, 146
Psoriatic arthritis (PA), 316
Pterygium, 328
Pubic bone, 253
Pubic osteolysis, 46–47
Pubiotomy, 260
Pubis, 253
Puddu plate, 222
Pudendal nerve, 253
Pugh nail, 222
Pulley exercises, 369
Pulmonary embolism (PE), 73
Pulmonary osteodystrophy, 58
Pulp pinch, 146
Pulse volume recorder (PVR), 130
Pulsed Doppler, 105, 129
Pulver-Taft procedure, 338
Pulver-Taft weave, 337
Pump bumps, 356
Punctum ossificationis, 212
Punctum ossificationis primarium, 212
Punctum ossificationis secundarium, 212
Purdue pegboard, 373
Purpura, 100
Purulent, 100
Push-pull ankle stress view, 109
Push-pull test, 141, 143
Pustulotic osteoarthropathy, 71
Putti
 arthrodeses, 229
 procedure, 245
 screw, 222
 sign, 143
Putti-Mayer procedure, 363
Putti-Platt procedure, 245
Pyarthrosis, 71
Pyknodysostosis, 58
Pylon, 195
Pyoderma gangrenosum, 77, 100
Pyogenic, 100
Pyogenic arthritis, 316
Pyogenic flexor tenosynovitis, 330
Pyogenic granuloma, 330
Pyomyositis, 63
Pyramidal tract, 288
Pyrexia, 100
Pyridinium collagen cross-links (PYD), 168
Pyridinoline (PYD) and deoxypyridinoline (Dpd, DPYD), 168
Pyrocarbon implant, 340
Pyrophosphate deposition disease (CPPD), 89

Q

Q angle, 113
Quadratus lumborum muscle, 288
Quadratus plantae, 350
Quadregia, 324
Quadriceps
 active test, 152–153
 muscle, 262
 reflexes, 157
 test, 158
Quadricepsplasty, 269
Quadrilateral brim, 200
Quadrilateral fixation, 224
Quadrilateral ischial weight-bearing socket, 194
Quadrilateral space syndrome, 90
Quadriplegia, 81
Quadriplegic, 79
Quad snip approach, 275
Quad sparing approach, 275
Quantitative computed tomography (QCT), 107, 386
Queckenstedt sign, 157
Quengle cast, 180
Quenu and Kuss Modified classification, 27
Quenu procedure, 363
Quiescence, 100
Quigley traction, 187

R

R value, 379
Rachialgia, 289
Rachicentesis procedure, 305
Rachiocampsis, 289
Rachiochysis, 289
Rachiodynia, 289
Rachiokyphosis, 289
Rachiomyelitis, 289
Rachioparalysis, 291
Rachiopathy, 291
Rachioplegia, 291
Rachioscoliosis, 291
Rachiotomy procedure, 305–306
Rachisagra, 291
Rachischisis, 291
Rachitomy procedure, 305
Racket nail, 328
Rad, 106, 130
Radial head, 9, 247
 dislocation, 15, 24
 fracture, 9, 23
Radialis sign, 157
Radialization, 335
Radians/time^2, 382
Radiation therapy, 130, 276
Radical resection, 276
Radicotomy, 235
Radicular pain, 295
Radiculectomy procedure, 235, 305
Radiculitis, 81, 295
Radiculoneuritis, 81
Radiculopathy, 295

Radioactive tracers, 388
Radiocarpal arthrodeses, 331
Radiography, 106–107
    angles, 110–114
    indices, 114–116
    lines, 114–116
    methods, 119–125
    ratios, 114–116
    routine views, 108–110
    signs, 116–119
    views, 110
Radiohumeral synostosis, 323
Radioisotope imaging (RII), 105
Radiologist, 106
Radiology, 106
Radiolucent, 106
Radiopaque, 107
Radio-photogrammetry, 388
Radioulnar arthrodeses, 331
Radioulnar subluxations, 34
Radio-ulnar synostosis, 322
Radius/radial, 246–247
    artery, 248, 315
    bursa, 313
    clubbed hand, 322
    collateral ligament, 250, 312
    deficiency, 322
    distal, 19
    drift, 317
    forearm flap, 334
    inclination angle, 113
    lunate angle, 313
    nerve, 243
    sagittal bands, 311
    sensory nerve entrapment, 319
    styloidectomy, 326, 332
    styloid fracture, 9
    tunnel syndrome, 81, 319
    vein, 248
Radley approach, 274
Radley, Liebig, and Brown procedure, 260
Raimiste sign, 157
Raman spectroscopy and microscopy, 387
Ram's horn deformity, 328
Random pattern flaps, 341
Range of motion (ROM) exercises, 369–370
Ranney technique, 338
Rarefaction, 102
RASL procedure, 341
Ratchet tenodesis orthoses, 201
Ray, 351
Ray amputation, 341
Raynaud disease, 77, 329
Raynaud phenomenon, 77, 158, 329
Reactive oxygen species, 391
Real-time polymerase chain reaction (qPCR), 388
Rear foot, 346
Recent dislocation, 33
Receptor activator of nuclear factor kappa B ligand (RANKL), 394
Receptor activator of nuclear factor kappa B (RANK), 394

Recessive inheritance, 100
Reciprocal finger prehension, 201
Reciprocating gait orthoses (RGO), 199
Recrudescence, 100
Rectus abdominis muscles, 288
Rectus femoris muscle, 255, 262
Rectus femoris syndrome, 74
Recurrent dislocation, 33
Recurrent laryngeal nerve, 286
Recurvatum, 6, 101
Red blood cells (RBCs), 172
Red blood count (RBC), 164
Redirection osteotomy, 215
Redlund-Johnell, 291
Reedy nail, 328
Reefing, 281
Referred pain, 43–44, 295
Reflect, 281
Reflex sympathetic dystrophy (RSD), 79, 317–318
Refsum syndrome, 82
Regenerated meniscus, 92–93
Regimen, 281
Regional anesthesia, 273
Regional flaps, 341
Regional migratory osteoporosis, 58
Registered Orthopaedic Technologists, 177–178
Regression, 380
Regression analysis, 379
Regressive remodeling, 103
Reichenheim-King prostheses, 252
Reimers index, 118
Reinforcement maneuver, 139
Reiter syndrome, 72
Release, 281
Release test, 143
Relocation test, 143
REM, 130
Remelting, 226
Remodeling, 394
Remplissage procedure, 245
Renal osteodystrophy, 83
Renshaw Classification for Sacral Agenesis, 298t–299t
Replantation, 341
Replantation microsurgery, 276
Request for applications (RFA), 377
Resection, 281
Resection arthroplasty, 226
Residual limb-compression garment, 195
Residual nerve root irritability, 295
Resistant tennis elbow, 319
Resistive exercise table, 370
Rest, ice, compression, and elevation (RICE), 368
Rest pain, 75
Resting zone, 212
Reston, 179
Resurfacing arthroplasty, 226
Resurfacing procedures, 258
Reticular cartilage, 229–230
Reticulocyte count, 166–167
Retinacula, 70
Retinacular ligament, 311

Retraction, 281
Retrocalcaneal bursitis, 352
Retrocalcaneal exostosis, 354
Retrolisthesis, 288, 291
Retropatellar fat pad, 266
Retrospective, 382
Retroversion, 116
Rett syndrome, 81
Reverdin-Green procedure, 363
Reverdin skin graft, 273
Reversal line, 393
Reversal of cervical lordosis, 293
Reverse Bankhart lesion, 33
Reverse Barton fracture, 9
Reverse Bigelow maneuver, 149
Reverse Colles fracture, 9
Reverse Hill-Sachs lesion, 33
Reverse last shoes, 207
Reverse Mauck procedure, 268
Reverse Monteggia fracture, 9
Reverse pivot-shift test, 153
Reverse shoulder, 246
Reverse tennis elbow, 37
Reverse transcriptase polymerase chain reaction (RT PCR), 388
Reversed vein bypass graft, 240
Review papers, 378
Revised carpal height ratio, 114
Revision, 281
Revision polydactyly, 341
Rhabdomyolysis, 64
Rhabdomyosarcoma, 54
RHAGL, 38
RhBMP-2, 303
RhBMP-7, 303
Rheology, 384
Rheumatoid arthritis, 70, 77
Rheumatoid factor (RF), 167
Rheumatoid nodule, 356
Rheumatoid spondylitis, 77
Rheumatologist, 76
Rheumatology, 76
Rhizomelic, 96
Rhizotomy procedure, 235, 305
Rhomboideus major and minor, 242
Rhomboid fossa, 241
Rib belt, 203
Ribbing disease, 61
Rice bodies, 71
Richardson procedure, 363
Richards screw, 222
Riche-Cannieu connection, 315
Rickets, 58, 83
Ridlon, 258
Rigid corrective orthoses, 197
Rigid dressing, 195
Rigid pes planus, 356
Rigidus, 103
Ring fracture, 10
Ring frame fixation, 224
Ring man shoulder, 38
Ring sign, 118

Riordan procedure, 338, 341
Riseborough and Radin Classification, 28
Risser
  localizer, 179
  procedure, 305
  sign, 118
RMRP, 65
Roaf, Kirkaldy-Willis, and Cattero procedure, 305
Roaf approach, 306
Robert Jones bandage, 184
Robert view, 109
Roberts approach, 274
Robinson and Riley fixation, 301
Robinson approach, 306
Rocker-bottom foot, 356
Rocker sole modification, 206
Rockwood classification, 28
Rockwood procedure, 245
Rod pin, 223
Roentgen (R), 107, 130
Roentgen absorbed dose, 130
Roentgen-equivalent-man (rem), 130
Roentgen ray, 107
Roentgen stereophotogrammetry, 108
Roentgenography, 107
Roentgenology, 106
Roger fixation, 302
Roger procedure, 245
Rogozinski, 305
Rolando fracture, 9, 326
Romberg test, 157
Rongeur, 281
Roo classification, 318
Roo test, 318
Roos test, 137
Root and Siegel procedure, 260
Root procedure, 260
Root sleeve fibrosis, 295
Roper-Day prosthesis, 246
Rose gardener's disease, 71
Rose procedure, 363
Rosenberger orthoses, 203
Rosenberg view, 109
Rotary click test, 147
Rotary control, 205
Rotating, 271
Rotating platform knee, 271
Rotational flap skin graft, 273
Rotational instability, 92–93
Rotator cuff, 242
  injury, 38
  muscle, 287
  tendon, 234
Rotator interval, 242
Rotator unit, 195–196
Rothmund-Thomson syndrome (RTS), 58
Rotter-Erb syndrome, 45
Round cell tumors, 52–53
Rounding of the cranial border, 289
Roussy-Lévy syndrome, 82
Routine and microscopic (R&M) urinalysis, 165

Routine evaluations
  basic chemistry profiles, 164–165
  complete blood count (CBC), 163–164
  urinalysis, 165
Roux-Goldthwait procedure, 269
Roux sign, 149
Rowe and Lowell classification, 28
Rowe and Zarins procedure, 246
Rowe approach, 274
Roy-Camille, 305
Roy-Camille fixation, 301
Royle-Thompson procedure, 339
Rubber band sign, 143
Rubor, 75, 103
Rudimentary, 103
Rudimentary ribs, 291
Ruedi and Allgower classification, 28
Rugger jersey finger, 37
Rugger jersey spine, 118–119
Ruiz-Mora procedure, 363
Runner's bump, 38
Runner's knee, 38
RUNX2, 57
Rupture, 103
Ruptured disk, 296
Rush nail, 223
Rush rod, 223
Russe bone graft, 334
Russell procedure, 272
Russell-Taylor classification, 28–29
Russell-Taylor nail, 223
Russell traction, 187
Rust sign, 137
Rydell nails, 223

S

Saber-cut approach, 274
SACH foot, 195
Sacral agenesis, 298
Sacral ala, 287
Sacral base angle, 112
Sacral belt, 202
Sacral cyst, 295
Sacral fracture, 17, 20
Sacral inclination, 289
Sacral screws, 304
Sacral spine, 284, 287
Sacralgia, 291
Sacralization, 291
Sacralized transverse process, 291
Sacrodynia, 292
Sacrohorizontal angle, 289
Sacroiliac, 253
Sacroiliac belt, 202
Sacroiliac joint, 287
Sacroiliac line, 116
Sacroiliac subluxations, 34
Sacroiliac/symphysis line, 116
Sacroiliitis, 292
Sacrospinous ligament, 253

Sacrotuberous ligament, 253
Sacrovertebral angle, 113
Sacrum, 284, 287
Safety knee, 195
Safety pin orthoses, 201
Safe zone of Lewinnek, 258
Safranin O fast green staining, 171
Sage procedure, 267
Sage rod, 223
Sager traction splint, 188
Sagittal control orthoses, 202, 204
Sagittal coronal control orthoses, 202–203
Sagittal femoral component angle, 113
Sagittal roll, 289
Sagittal rotation, 289
Sagittal stress sign, 155
Sagittal tibial component angle, 113
Sag sign, 151, 153
Sag test, 151
Saha procedure, 246
Sailboarder's injury, 38
Salicylates, 167
Saline dressing, 184
Salmonella, 89
Salmonella organisms, 48, 169
Salter
  fracture, 6
  osteotomy, 215
  sling, 198
Salter-Harris Classification, 29
Salter-Harris fracture, 6
Salter-Thompson Classification for Legg-Calvé-Perthes Disease, 124t
Salvage procedure, 226, 337
Samilson-Preito Classification, 29
Samilson procedure, 363
Sample population, 382
Sample size, 380
Sample size analysis, 378
Sanfilippo syndrome, 67
Sanguineous, 103
Saphenous flap, 341
Saphenous nerve, 266
Saphenous vein, 266
Saponification, 103
Sarbó sign, 157
Sarcoidosis, 103
Sargent procedure, 269
Sarmiento
  cast, 180
  nail, 223
  osteotomy, 215
  procedure, 260
Sartorius muscle, 255
Saturday night palsy, 319
Saucerization, 282
Sauvegrain skeletal age, 124
Sauve-Kapandji prostheses, 252
Scaffold, 282
Scaglietti procedure, 258
Scalar, 384

Scalene block, 273
Scalenus, 286
Scalenus anticus syndrome, 296
Scanning electron microscopy (SEM), 387
Scanogram, 108
Scanography, 108
Scaphoid, 347
 bone, 307
 cast, 180
 fracture, 20
 pads, 206
 ring sign, 326
 shift test, 326
 test, 146
Scapholunate advanced collapse (SLAC) procedure, 316, 331
Scapholunate ballottement test, 326
Scapula/scapular, 241
 assistance test, 143
 dyskinesis sign, 143
 flap, 335
 glenoid fracture, 20
 sign of Putti, 143
 spine, 241
Scapulectomy, 246
Scapulopexy, 281
Scarf procedure, 363
Schanz pins, 223
Schatzker Classification, 29
Scheie syndrome, 67
Scheuermann disease, 55, 61, 294
Schlesinger sign, 149
Schmid disease, 65
Schmid type, 65
Schmorl nodes, 294
Schneider arthrodeses, 229
Schneider nail or rod, 223
Schollner costoplasty, 305
Schreiber maneuver, 157
Schrock procedure, 246
Schultze-Chvostek sign, 157
Schwann tumor, 54, 68
Schwannoma, 54, 82
Sciatica, 292, 295
Sciatic nerve, 253–255, 266
Sciatic plexus, 254
Scissors gait, 159
SCIWORA, 298
Sclerodactyly, 328
Scleroderma, 77, 328
Sclerostin, 394
Sclerotherapy, 129
Sclerotomal pain, 43–44
Sclerotomal pain, 295
Scoliorachitis, 292
Scoliosis, 292
Scoliosis cast, 179
Scotch terrier sign, 119
Scott procedure, 246, 305
Scottish-Rite orthoses, 199
 hip, 198

Scotty dog sign, 119
Scout film, 107
Scout radiograph, 107
Scranton and McDermott Classification of Ankle Osteophytes, 355t
Screw-home mechanism, 153
Screws, 303–304
Scudari procedure, 269
Seatbelt fracture, 10
Sebaceous, 103
Second cervical vertebra, 14–15
Second-generation cementing, 258
Second-generation technique, 225
Second hit, 282
Secondary center of ossification, 212
Secondary chondrosarcoma, 52
Secondary closure, 279, 282
Secondary fracture, 6
Secondary gain, 101
Secondary osteon, 393
Secondary osteosarcoma, 51
Secondary union, 13
Secretan edema, 325
Secretan syndrome, 326
Secreted protein, acidic, rich in cysteine (SPARC), 393–394
Seddon arthrodeses, 331
Seddon Classification, 82t
Seddon procedure, 305
Segmental fracture, 6
Segmental graft, 218
Segmental instability, 294
Segmental spinal dysgenesis, 299
Segond fracture, 11
Seidel nail, 223
Seimon sign, 137
Seinsheimer classification, 29
Selectivity, 381
Selig procedure, 260
Semicircular fixation, 224
Semiconstrained knee, 271
Semi-Fowler position, 187
Semilunar bone, 307
Semilunar cartilages, 266
Semimembranosus, 261
Semirigid collar, 204
Semispinalis muscles, 286
Semitendinosus, 261
Semmes-Weinstein monofilament test, 161, 318, 373
Senegas approach, 275
Senile osteoporosis, 83
Sensitivity, 381
Sensorimotor skills, 374
Sensory testing, 371
Sentinel fracture, 10
Sepsis, 103, 282
Septa, 314
Septae, 313
Septic, 282
Septic arthritis, 70
Septicemia, 103

Sequela, 103
Sequestered disk, 300
Sequestered disk herniation, 296
Sequestration, 296
Sequestrectomy, 214
Sequestrum, 49
Serendipity view, 109–110
Serial cast, 181
Seropurulent, 103
Serosanguineous, 103
Serous, 103
Serratus anterior, 242
Serratus muscle, 288
Serum, 164
Serum calcium (Ca), 167–168
Serum lead, 167
Serum protein electrophoresis (SPE, SPEP), 167
Serum tests
  general, 165–167
  metabolic disease, 167–168
Sesamoid, 212, 307–308, 347
Seventh cranial nerve, 286
Sever disease, 55, 355
Severe osteoporosis, 83
Severin hip dysplasia scale, 124
Sex chromosome, 171
Sex-linked inheritance, 100
SGOT, 164
SGPT, 164
Shaffer plate, 206
Shaft fracture, 10
Shands dressing, 184
Shands dressing, 184
Shank, 205
Shapiro Classification System, 46t
Sharp angle, 113
Sharp dissection, 279
Sharpey fibers, 234
Sharp-Purser test, 137
Sharrard procedure, 258
Shear, 384
Sheath, 196
Sheer testing for lunotriquetral dissociation, 326
Sheet wadding, 179
Sheffield rod, 223
Shelf procedure, 256
Shell osteochondral allograft, 230
Shenton line, 114, 116
Shepherd fracture, 12
Shepherd's crook deformity, 61
Sherk and Probst prostheses, 252
Sherman plate, 223
Shin splints, 38
Shirt-stud abscess, 329
Shock wave therapy, 363
Shoe cookies, 206
Shoe modifications
  callosities, 206–207
  children, 207
  flat feet devices, 206
  high arches, 206

Shoe modifications (Continued)
  infants, 207
  insensitive feet devices, 206
  metatarsal supports, 206
Shoemaker approach, 275
Shoemaker's swan, 206
Shooter's abscess, 330
Short-arm cast (SAC), 180
Short-arm splint, 183
Short CAM walker or boot, 181
Short-leg cast (SLC), 180
Short-leg splint, 183
Short-leg walking cast (SLWC), 180
Short ligament, 312
Short opponens orthoses, 201
Short plantar ligaments, 350
Short tau inversion recovery (STIR), 127
Shoulder
  anatomy of, 240–243
  apprehension, 38
  archer's, 36
  arteries of, 242–243
  bones, 240–241
  branches of, 242–243
  conditions, 89–90
  disarticulation (SD), 190
  dislocation, 29, 33
  girdle, 242
  harness, 192, 195
  ligaments, 242
  muscles, 241–242
  nerves, 243
  pointer, 38
  ring, 205
  separation, 35, 240
  spica cast, 180
  sprain, 35
  stabilization, 244
  subluxations, 34
  veins of, 242–243
Shoulder-hand syndrome, 318
Shuffling gait, 159
Shwachman syndrome, 89
SI belt, 202
Sickle cell anemia, 82, 89
Side joint and thigh laser (joint and corset), 194
Sideswipe fracture, 8
Sierra voluntary-opening hand, 192
Siffert-Foster-Nachamie procedures, 363
Sigmoid notch, 308
Sign, 131
Silesian bandage or belt, 195
Silfverskiöld
  disease, 55, 61
  procedure, 269, 337
  test, 155
Silicone gel socket insert, 196
Sillence Classification System (Modified), 46t
Silver procedures, 363
Silverskold test, 354
Simmonds test, 155

Simmons
    fixation, 302
    procedure, 305
    test, 149
Simple, effective, rapid, and inexpensive (SERI) procedures, 363
Simple dislocations, 33
Sinding-Larsen-Johansson disease, 61
Singh index, 124
Single axis ankle, 195
Single axis knee, 195
Single-hip spica cast, 180
Single localized deformity, 321
Single nucleotide polymorphism (SNP), 391
Single photon emission computerized tomography (SPECT), 127
Sinography, 108
Sinus, 49
Sinus tarsi, 351
Sinus tarsi syndrome, 356
Sitting hip, walking hip, standing hip (SWASH) brace, 199
Sjögren syndrome, 77
Skeletal amyloidosis, 58
Skeletal traction, 187
Skew flap amputation, 278
Skew foot, 356
Skier's injury, 11
Skier's thumb, 37, 326–327
Skillern fracture, 9
Skin creases, 314
Skin grafts, 272–273
    full-thickness, 272–273
    pedicle, 273
    rotational flaps, 273
    split-thickness, 272
Skin laceration, 26
Skiving, 269
Slap foot gait, 159
SLAP lesion, 38
Sleeve fracture, 11
Slice fracture, 10
Slide plate, 223
Slider crank mechanism, 313
Sliding arthrodeses, 229
Sliding inlay graft, 218
Sling, 374–375
Sling and swathe, 183
Slip angle, 114, 289
Slipped capital femoral epiphysis (SCFE), 59
Slipped disk, 296
Slipped epiphysis, 67
Slipper cast, 180
Slocum procedure, 268
Slocum test, 153
Slomann view, 110
Slope, 380
Slough, 103
Sly syndrome, 67
Small interfering RNA (siRNA), 391
Small-patella syndrome, 94
Smillie nail, 223

Smith
    dislocation, 34
    fracture, 9
    maneuver, 149
Smith and Ross test, 146
Smith-Petersen
    approach, 275, 341
    approach, 275
    arthrodeses, 229, 331
    nail, 223
    procedure, 305
    test, 140
Smith physical capacities evaluation (PCE), 373
Smith-Robinson procedure, 301
Smyth pin, 223
Snapping hip, 91
Snapping knee syndrome, 94
Snapping scapula, 90
Snapping tendons, 329, 339
Snapping tendon release, 339
Snowstorm knee, 94
Sock test, 195–196
Socket, 196
Sofield osteotomy, 215
Soft callus, 353
Soft collar, 204
Soft corn, 353
Soft cosmetic cover, 196
Soft socket insert, 196
Soft tissue
    classification, 14
    injury, 31
Soft tissue diseases
    fibro-root diseases, 68
    lipo-root diseases, 68
    muco-root diseases, 68
    myxo-root diseases, 68
Soft voluntary-closing hand, 192
Sole inserts, 206–207
Soleus, 263
Solitary fibromatosis of bone, 59
Solitary fibrous tumor, 54
Somatic sign, 158
Somatization disorder, 103
Somerville procedure, 258
Sonography, 105, 128
Soto-Hall sign, 140
Sourcil, 116
Southern blot, 386
Southwick
    angle, 112, 114
    approach, 306
    fixation, 302
    osteotomy, 215
    slide procedure, 269
Soutter procedure, 260
Space of Poirer, 312
Space shoes, 205–206
Spasm, 103
Spastic cerebral palsy (CP), 79
Spear tackler's spine, 38

Specific Regional Classification Systems for Congenital Limb Absences, 96t–97t
Specific aims, 377
Specificity, 381
Speed
　osteotomy, 215
　procedure, 246, 305
　test, 143
Speed and Boyd prostheses, 252
Spencer osteotomy, 214
Spetzler fixation, 302
Sphincter ani, 253
Spica casts, 179
Spicular bone, 213
Spike osteotomy, 215
Spilled teacup sign, 146–147
Spina bifida, 80, 299
Spinal cord, 287–288
Spinalis muscles, 286
Spine orthoses, 202–204
　cervical, 204
　cervicothoracolumbosacral, 204
　components, 205
　lumbosacral, 202–203
　sacroiliac, 202
　thoracic, 203
　thoracolumbosacral, 203–204
Spine/spinal, 283–306
　accessory nerve, 286
　anatomy, 283–285
　anterior inferior iliac, 252
　anterior superior iliac, 252–253
　anterior tibial, 261
　bamboo, 116
　block, 273
　board, 188
　canal, 283, 287
　cervical spine, 285–286
　dislocations, 34
　lower spine, 287–288
　lumbar spine, 287–288
　region radiologic views, 110
　sign, 140
　stenosis, 294
　structural anomalies, 288–299
　surgery, 299–306
　thalamic tract, 288
　thoracic spine, 286–287
Spine/spinal diseases
　back and neck, 288
　bone, 288–292
　congenital disorders, 298–299
　disk, 295–296
　nerve root, 294–295
　spinal cord, 296–298
　spinal deformities, 292–294
Spine/spinal surgery
　approaches to, 306
　instrumentation, 303–305
　nonfusion devices, 304
　spinal fusions, 301–303

Spinoglenoid cyst, 90
Spinoglenoid notch, 241
Spino-Pelvic Tumor Resection Classification for Reconstruiction Following Combined Resection of Spinal and Pelvic Segments, 301t
Spinous process, 285
Spiral CT, 125
Spiral fracture, 6
Spiral groove, 246
Spira procedure, 246
Spittler prostheses, 252
Splay foot, 350, 356
Splaying, 103
Splenius muscles, 286
Splintered fracture, 4
Splints, 182–183, 374–375
　accessories, 183
　defined, 178
　emergency stabilization, 188
　frames, 184–187
　suspensions, 184–187
　tractions, 184–187
Split stirrup, 200
Spoiled grass (SPGR), 127
Spondylalgia, 288
Spondylarthritis, 288
Spondylarthrocace, 288
Spondylexarthrosis, 288
Spondylitis, 288
Spondylizema, 288
Spondylocace, 288
Spondylocostal dysostosis, 288
Spondylodesis, 306
Spondylodynia, 288
Spondyloepiphyseal dysplasia, 67, 288
　congenita, 67
　of Maroteaux, 67
　tarda, 67
Spondylolisthesis, 34, 288–289
Spondylolysis, 34, 289
Spondylolysis and Spondylolisthesis Classification System, 289t
Spondylomalacia, 289
Spondylopathy, 289
Spondyloptosis, 10
Spondylopyosis, 289
Spondyloschisis, 289
Spondylosis, 289
Spondylosyndesis, 306
Spondylotomy procedure, 306
Sponge test, 140
Spongiosa, 213
Spontaneous fracture, 13
Spontorno index, 116
Spoon nail, 328
Sporotrichosis, 71
Sportman's hernia, 38
Sprain-ligament rupture, 3
Sprains, 35–36
　ankle, 15, 35–36
　knee, 35
　shoulder, 35

Spray and stretch, 370
Spreader bar, 200
Spring ligaments, 350
Spring-loaded crutches, 183
Spring swivel thumb, 202
Spring wire orthoses, 198
Sprinter's fracture, 10
Spur, 119
Spurious ankylosis, 73
Spurling test, 137, 318
Spurs, 103
Spur sign, 119
Squamous cell carcinoma in situ, 327
Squatter's talus, 356
Squeeze film lubrication, 384
Squinting patella, 94
St. Vitus dance, 79
Staheli procedure, 260
Stahl index, 124
Stairs sign, 157
Stamm arthrodeses, 229
Standard deviation (SD), 381
Standard error (SE), 381
Standard estimate of the mean (SEM), 381
Standard orthoses, 199
Standing apprehension test, 153
Standing frame orthoses, 199
Stanisavljevic procedure, 269
Stanitski and Stanitski Classification for Fibular Hemimelia, 96t–97t
Staphylococcus aureus (Staph. aureus), 48, 169
Staples arthrodesis, 229, 252
Staples-Black-Broström procedures, 363
-stasis, 282
Stasis, 78, 282
-stasisstasis, 282
Static exercise, 369
Static orthoses, 202
Static orthoses, 198
Static progressive splints, 375
Static splints, 374
Static tendon transfer, 338
Station test, 157
Statistical errors, 381
Statistics, 378–382
Statue of liberty cast, 180
Statue of liberty orthoses, 201–202
Steele osteotomy, 215
Steeper advanced reciprocating gait orthoses, 199
Stee procedure, 260
Steffee thumb arthroplasty, 332
Steffee plate, 305
Steffe prosthesis, 331
Steinberg Classification for Ostenecrosis of the Hip, 55t
Steinberg Classification Hip Osteonecrosis, 124t
Steindler
    arthrodesis, 229, 252
    effect, 90
    flexorplasty, 252
    matricectomy, 363
    procedure, 246, 363

Steinmann pin, 187, 223
Steinmann test, 153
Stellate fracture, 6
Stem cell, 391
Stener and Gunterberg procedure, 260
Stener lesion, 326
Stenosing tenosynovitis, 329
Stenosis, 78, 103
Stent, 282
Step down osteotomy, 363
Sternal angle, 114
Sternal attachment, 205
Sternal occipital mandibular immobilizer (SOMI) orthoses, 204
Sternoclavicular joint, 241
Sternoclavicular joint separation, 33
Sternoclavicular ligament, 242
Sternocleidomastoid, 242, 286
Sternum, 287
Stewart and Harley arthrodeses, 229
Stewart and Milford classification, 29–30
Stewart-Morel syndrome, 61, 64
Stewart procedure, 246
Stewart prostheses, 252
Stickler syndrome, 65
Stieda fracture, 11
Stiff man syndrome, 64
Stiffness, 384
Stiff ray, 356
Stigma, 103
Stiles-Bunnell procedure, 338
Still disease, 77
Stimson maneuver, 149
Stint skin graft, 273
Stippled epiphysis, 67
Stirrup, 200
Stockinettte, 179
Stone arthrodeses, 229
Stone procedure, 363
Stoop test, 140
Stoppa approach, 275
Straddle fracture, 10
Straight last shoes, 207
Straight leg raising (SLR) test, 139–140
Strain, 35–36, 384
    defined, 3
    gauge, 388
Strap muscles, 286
Strayer procedure, 363
Streaming potential (zeta), 388
Streeter bands, 71, 320
Streeter dysplasia, 320
Street medullary pin, 223
Street nail, 223
Strength, 384
Strength training, 370
Streptococcus organisms, 48, 169
Stress
    fracture, 12–13, 30
    reaction to bone, 13
    relaxation, 384
    shielding, 226

Stress-generated potentials (SGP), 388
Stress-strain curve, 384
Stripe wear, 226
Stroke, 75
Stromelysin, 391
Strontium-89, 130
Strontium-85 resorption rate, 127
Structural curve, 293
Structural graft, 302
Strümpell confusion test, 157
Strümpell sign, 149, 157
Strunsky sign, 155
Strut graft, 218
Stryker frame, 187
Stryker notch view, 110
Stubbies, 193
Student's elbow, 90
Student's t test, 381
Study design, 382
Study groups, 382
Stulberg method, 124
Stump revision, 278
Styloid process, 247
Styloids, 308
Suave Kapanje procedure, 332
Subastragalar dislocation, 34
Subaxial Injury Classificaion Scale, 297t
Subcapital fracture, 10
   Garden classification for, 19
Subchondral bone, 213, 227
Subchondral plate, 227
Subclavian artery, 243
Subclavian carotid bypass, 239
Subclavian steal syndrome, 75
Subclavian vein, 242–243
Subcoracoid dislocation, 33
Subcutaneous, 282
Subcutaneous pseudosarcomatous fibromatosis, 68
Subcuticular, 282
Subglenoid dislocation, 33
Subliminal, 103
Subluxations, 3, 34
Subluxing patella, 92–93
Subperiosteal ABC, 59
Subperiosteal fracture, 6
Subperiosteal giant-cell reparative granuloma, 59
Subscapularis, 242
Subscapularis muscle, 287
Substitution bone, 211
Subtalar arthrodesis, 363
Subtalar arthroereisis, 363
Subtalar joint, 349
Subtrochanteric, 254
Subtrochanteric fracture, 10
   Fielding-Magliato classification for, 18
   Seinsheimer classification for, 29
   Zickle classification for, 32
Subungual abscess, 330
Subungual exostosis, 328
Subungual hematoma, 328
Subungual space, 314

Subungual tissue, 314
Succinylcholine test, 158
Suction socket, 194
Suction socket suspension, 194
Sudeck atrophy, 75, 79, 318
Sugar tong splint, 183
Sugiuka osteotomy, 215
Sulcus, 282
Sulcus angle, 114
Sulcus sign, 143
Sulfoiduronate sulfatase, 67
Sunderland Classification for Grades of Nerve Injury, 82t, 318t
Sunrise view, 110
Sunset view, 110
Superficial and deep palmar arterial arches, 315
Superficial branch of radial nerve, 315
Superficial ligament, 264–265
Superficial peroneal nerve, 266
Superficial radial nerve, 249
Superficial transverse intermetacarpal ligament, 312
Superior dome, 254
Superior gluteal artery, 255
Superior labrum anterior to posterior (SLAP) lesions, 90
Superior mesenteric artery syndrome, 182
Superior pubic ramus, 253
Superior radial head dislocation, 33
Superior suspensory complex, 242
Supernumerary, 103
Supernumerary digits, 322
Superstructure, 205
Supination, 356
Supinator, 310
Supinator muscle, 248
Supinator syndrome, 81
Suppan procedure, 363
Suppurative, 103
Suppurative arthritis, 71
Suppurative osteomyelitis, 49
Supracondylar (PTB-SC), 194
Supracondylar-suprapatellar (SC-SP), 194
Supracondylar cast, 180
Supracondylar cuff, 194
Supracondylar fracture, 8, 11
   Gartland classification for, 19
Suprapatellar plica, 94
Suprapatellar pouch, 266
Suprapatellar straps, 200
Suprascapular nerve, 243
Supraspinatus, 242
Supraspinatus isolation test, 142
Supraspinatus muscle, 287
Supraspinatus outlet view, 109
Sural nerve, 266
Surface electrodes, 2
Surface finish, 258
Surfer's knots, 38
Surgical approaches, 273–276
   to elbow, 274
   to femur, 275
   to forearm, 274
   to hip, 275

Index **497**

Surgical approaches *(Continued)*
  to humerus, 274
  to knee, 275
  to lower limbs, 275–276
  to pelvis, 274–275
  to shoulder, 274
Surgical blocks, 273
Surgical corset, 202–203
Surgical neck, 241
Surgical neck fracture, 8
Surgical procedures
  for ankle, 357–364
  on aponeuroses, 231
  on capsulo-(capsule), 230
  chondro-(cartilage), 230
Surgical shoe or boot, 206
Suspension, 185, 282
Suspensionplasty procedure, 332
Suspension sleeve, 196
Sustained clonus, 155
Sustentaculum tali, 349
Sutherland procedure, 260, 267, 271
Suture, 282
Swafford and Lichtman procedure, 246
Swallow-tail sign, 136
Swan-neck deformity, 317
Swan-neck revision, 339
Swanson
  arthroplasty, 332
  prosthesis, 331–332
  revision, 339
Swede-o, 182
Swedish knee cage, 198
Swimmer's shoulder, 38
Swimmer's view, 110
Swing and stance knee (S n' S), 195
Swiss ball exercises, 370
Symbrachydactyly, 322
Syme, 193
Syme amputation, 278, 363
Symmetrical extension test, 151, 153
Symmetric fusion, 299
Sympathectomy, 240, 335
Sympathetic maintained pain syndrome (SMPS), 318
Sympathetic nervous system, 283
Symphysis pubis, 253
Synarthrosis, 71
Synchondrosis, 65
Synchondrotomy, 230
Syncope, 103
Syndactylization, 363
Syndactyly, 322, 356
Syndesmectomy, 234
Syndesmopexy, 234
Syndesmoplasty, 234
Syndesmorrhaphy, 234
Syndesmosis, 234
Syndesmotomy, 234
Syndrome, 43
Synergists, 231
Synergy, 231
Syngraft (syngeneic), 216
Synostosis, 13, 214, 322
Synovectomy, 341
Synovial cell sarcoma, 54
Synovial cyst, 72
Synovial fluid evaluation, 170
Synovial joint, 227
Synovial membrane, 227
Synovial osteochondromatosis, 45, 65, 72
Synoviochondromatosis, 65, 72
Synovioma, 54
Synovitis, 72, 92–93
Synovitis-acne-pustulosis-hyperostosis osteomyelitis (SAPHO) syndrome, 49
Synovium, 227
Synphalangism, 323
Synpolydactyly, 323
Syringomyelia, 81, 298
Systemic connectivitis, 76
Systemic disease, 43
Systemic lupus erythematosus (SLE), 77, 316
Systole, 238

T
T fracture, 8, 28
T test, 381
Tabes dorsalis, 80–81, 296
Table top test, 147
Taboparesis, 81
Tachdjian orthoses, 198
Tachdjian procedure, 267, 271
Tachycardia, 78
Tackler's arm, 37
Tailbone, 287
Tailor's bunion, 352, 356
Tait pedicle, 273
Tajima procedure, 337
Talar fracture, 16
Talar tilt test, 155
Talectomy, 363
Talipes, 357
Talipes calcaneocavus, 357
Talipes calcaneovalgus, 357
Talipes calcaneovarus, 357
Talipes calcaneus, 357
Talipes cavovalgus, 357
Talipes cavovarus, 357
Talipes equinovalgus, 357
Talipes equinovarus, 357
Talipes planovalgus, 357
Talipes planus, 357
Talipomanus, 322
Talocalcaneal angle, 351
Talocalcaneal bar, 349
Talocalcaneal ligaments, 350
Talocrural angle, 114
Talonavicular ligaments, 350
Talus, 349
  dome of, 16
  osteochondral lesions, 18

Tamai procedure, 272
Tamponade, 282
Tangent-delta, 385
Tangential view, 110
Tantalum, 226, 258
Taper, 226
Taper slip design, 258
Tapotement, 370
Tardy, 103
Tardy ulnar palsy, 319
Target population, 382
Tarsals
   coalition, 349
   dislocation, 34
   ligaments, 350
   pronator shoes, 207
   sinus, 351
   tunnel, 351
Tarsometatarsal articulation
   dislocation, 27
   fracture, 27
   Quenu and Kuss Modified classification for, 27
Tarsometatarsal joint, 349
Tarsus, 347
Tarsus osseous, 347
TAR syndrome, 103, 323
Tartrate-resistant acid phosphatase (TRAP), 168
Task Force on Standardization of Prosthetic-Orthotic Terminology of the Committee on Prosthetic-Orthotic Education, 196
Taylor
   orthoses, 204
   procedure, 272
   spatial frame fixation, 224
Taylor, Townsend, and Corlett procedure, 260
Teardrop, 116
Teardrop fracture, 10
Technetium-99m, 128
Technetium scan, 128
Technique, 131
Tegaderm, 184
Telangiectatic osteosarcoma, 51
Teleroentgenogram, 108
Teleroentgenography, 108
Telfa dressing, 184
Temporary prosthesis, 196
Temporomandibular joint (TMJ) syndrome, 294
Tendinocutaneous flaps, 341
Tendinoplasty, 234
Tendinosuture, 234
Tendo-/teno-root diseases, 69–70
Tendocalcaneus, 231–234, 349
Tendolysis, 234, 338
Tendon, 313
Tendon Achilles lengthening (TAL), 363
Tendon advancement, 338–339
Tendonitis, 69
Tendonitis ossificans traumatica, 69
Tendon reflex examination, 157, 371
Tendon release, 234
Tendoplasty, 234

Tendotomy, 234
Tendovaginitis, 324
Tenectomy, 234
Tennis elbow, 38, 70
Tennis leg, 38
Tennis toe, 38
Teno-(tendons), 231–234
   surgical procedures on, 234
Tenodesis, 234
Tenodesis test, 147
Tenodynia, 69
Tenolysis, 234
Tenomyoplasty, 234
Tenomyotomy, 234
Tenonectomy, 234
Tenonitis, 69
Tenontagra, 69
Tenontitis, 69
Tenontomyoplasty, 234
Tenontomyotomy, 234
Tenontophyma, 69
Tenontoplasty, 234
Tenontothecitis, 69
Tenoperiostitis, 69
Tenophyte, 69
Tenoplasty, 234
Tenorrhaphy, 234, 339
Tenositis, 69
Tenostosis, 69
Tenosuspension, 234
Tenosuture, 234
Tenosynovectomy, 234
Tenosynovitis, 69, 330
Tenotomy, 234, 339
Tenovaginotomy, 339
Tensilon test, 158
Tension, 385
Tension fracture, 13
Tensor fascia lata muscle, 255
Tenth cranial nerve, 286
Teres major and minor, 242
Teres minor muscle, 287
Terminal devices, 192
Terminal devices, hands, 192
Terry Thomas sign, 119, 147
Test
   defined, 131
Tetany, 103
Tethered cord, 299
Tethered patellar tendon syndrome, 94
Tetracycline labeling, 171
Tetraplegia, 324
Texas Scottish Rite Hospital, 305
TGF β2 receptor, 60
Thalassemia, 89
Thanatophoric dysplasia, 89
Thawed plasma, 172–173
Thenar eminence, 313
Thenar flap, 334, 336
Thenar muscles, 310
Thenar palmar crease (TPC), 313

Thenar space, 313
Therapeutic massage, 370
Therapeutic modifications, 374–375
Thermal injuries, 74
Thermography, 128
Thermoplastic/metal orthoses, 199
Thermoplastic orthoses, 198
Thessaly test, 153
Thiemann disease, 55, 61
Thigh atrophy, 94
Third-body wear, 226
Third-generation cementing, 258
Third-generation ceramic, 226
Third-generation technique, 225
Thomas
   heel, 206
   procedure, 363
   ring, 200
   sign, 149, 157
   splint, 185
   squeeze test, 155
   test, 149
Thomas, Thompson, and Straub procedure, 260
Thompson
   approach, 274–275
   nail, 223
   quadricepsplasty, 269
   telescoping V osteotomy, 215
   test, 149
Thompson and Epstein classification, 30
Thompson and Henry approach, 274
Thomsen disease, 62
Thoracic curve, 293
Thoracic extension, 205
Thoracic outlet syndrome, 294, 319–320
Thoracic pad, 205
Thoracic region radiologic views, 110
Thoracic spine, 284
Thoracodorsal nerve, 243
Thoracolumbar curve, 294
Thoracolumbar Injury Classification and Severtiy Score, 298t
Thoracolumbosacral anterior control corset, 203
Thorax, 287
Thornton nail, 223
Three-finger spica, 179
Three-phase bone scan, 125
Throat mold, 205
Thromboangiitis obliterans, 324
Thrombocytopenia, absent radius (TAR) syndrome, 323
Thrombolytic therapy, 240
Thrombophlebitis, 73
Thrombosis, 73
Thrower's elbow, 36–37, 70
Thumb
   abduction procedure, 339
   abductors, 310
   adduction procedures, 29
   adductors, 310
   extensors, 310
   interphalangeal (IP) extension assist, 202

Thumb (Continued)
   post, 202
   spica cast, 180
Thumbnail test, 153
Thumb-to-forearm test, 158
Thurston-Holland sign, 119
Thyroid cartilage, 286
Thyroid gland, 286
Thyroid-stimulating hormone (TSH), 167
Thyroxine (T4), 167
Tibia/tibial, 261
   bolt, 223
   collateral ligament, 264
   distal, 16–17, 23–24
   dysplasia, 96
   eminence, 261
   floating knee fracture, 23
   fracture, 24
   gaiter, 181
   proximal, 15
   vara, 59
Tibialis anterior, 263, 349
Tibialis posterior, 263, 350
Tibialis sign, 157
Tibial phenomenon, 157
Tibial plafond, 23–24
Tibial plateau, 261
Tibial plateau fracture, 11, 20, 29
Tibial sag sign, 153
Tibial tuberosity fracture, 26, 31
Tibiofibular cyst, 72
Tibiofibular ligament, 265
Tibiofibular sprain, 36
Tibiotalar Joint and Distal Tibial Morphology Classification System, 96t–97t
Tic, 81
Tic douloureux, 81
Tidemark, 392
Tieman-Jewett nail, 223
Tietze syndrome, 61
Tikhofr-Linberg procedure, 246, 341
Tillaux Kleiger fracture, 12
Tile classification, 30
Tilt test, 154
Tincture of benzoin, 184
Tinea pedis, 352
Tinel sign, 157
Tiotribology, 385
Tissue inhibitor of metalloproteinases (TIMP), 391
Tissues, 230–235
Toddler fracture, 11
Toe region, 385
Toes
   box, 205
   region, 385
   spica cast, 180
   spread sign, 155
Toe-thumb transfer, 335
Toggle, 223
Tohen procedure, 363
Toilet hygiene, 374

-tome, 282
Tommy John prostheses, 252
Tomogram, 108
Tomography, 108
Tomosynthesis, 128
Tongue, 205
Tongue fracture, 12
Tönnis
    angle, 114
        osteoarthritis grade, 124–125
        system for hip dysplasia, 125
Tonus, 103
Too many toes sign, 155
Tophus, 317
Torn meniscus, 92–93
Torode and Zieg classification, 30
Toronto orthoses, 198
Torque, 382
Torque heels, 207
Torsion unit, 195–196
Torticollis, 103–104
Torus fracture, 4, 6
Total bilirubin, 165
Total contact, 196
Total hip arthroplasty, 161, 258
Total hip replacement, 20–21, 23
Total joint replacement, 226
Total serum protein, 165
Total wrist arthrodeses, 331
Tourniquet, 282
Tourniquet test, 149
Towel clip test, 154
Toxic, 104, 282
Trabecula, 213
Trabecular bone, 393
Trabecular metal, 303
Trabecular pattern, 213
Trachea, 286
Traction, 90, 185–187, 211, 368
    bow, 187
    devices, 178
    epiphyseal, 211
    epiphysis, 45
    exostosis, 60
    injury, 318
    spur, 294
Transacromial approach, 274
Transchondral fracture, 4
Transcondylar fracture, 4
Transcutaneous electrical nerve stimulation (TENS), 367
Transcutaneous oximetry (TcPO$_2$), 130
Transect, 282
Transfemoral, 193–194
Transfemoral suspension, 195
Transforaminal lumbar interbody fixation (TLIF), 302
Transforming growth factor (TGF), 391
Transfusion, 282
Transgenic animals, 389
Transhumeral amputation (TH), 190
Transient ischemic attack (TIA), 75

Transient osteopenia, 59
Transitional vertebra, 294
Translocation, 171
Translucent, 107
Transmetatarsal amputation, 364
Transmission electron microscopy (TEM), 387–388
Transparent dressing, 184
Transplant, 216
Transposition, 282
Transposition flaps, 341
Transradial amputation (TR), 190
Transscaphoid perilunate dislocation, 327
Transthoracic lateral view, 110
Transtibial, 194
Transudate, 104
Transverse approach, 275
Transverse carpal ligament, 312
Transverse fracture, 6
Transverse humeral ligament, 242
Transverse process, 285
Transverse tarsal joint, 347
Transversus muscles, 288
Trapezial hemiarthroplasty, 332
Trapeziectomy, 341
Trapeziometacarpal arthritis, 317
Trapeziometacarpal fusion, 331
Trapeziometacarpal ligament reconstruction, 333
Trapezium, 307
Trapezius, 242
Trapezoid, 307
Trapezoid ligament, 242
Trauma, 104
Traumatic arthritis, 70
Traumatic dislocation, 33
Traumatic neuroma, 80
Trauma view, 110
Tremor, 81
Trendelenburg
    gait, 159
    sign, 149
    test, 149
Triad knee repair, 268
Triangles, 286
Triangular bone, 307
Triangular fibrocartilage complex, 312
Triangular fixation, 224
Triangular ligament, 312
Tribology, 385
Triceps reflexes, 157
Triceps surae, 262–263
Trichorhinophalangeal syndrome, 89
Tricompartmental knee, 271
Trident hand, 323
Trigger finger, 323, 329, 339
Trigger points, 64
Triiodothyronine (T3), 167
Trilateral orthoses, 198
Trillat procedure, 246
Trimalleolar fracture, 12
Triphalangeal thumb, 323

Triplanar control, 204
Triplane fracture, 12
Triple arthrodesis, 364
Triple osteotomy, 215
Triplicate thumb, 323
-tripsy, 282
Triquetrum bone, 307
Triradiate cartilage, 254
Triscaphe arthrodeses, 331
Trisomy 21, 84
Trivector retaining approach, 275
Trochanteric slide, 260–261, 275
Trochanterplasty, 261
Trochlea, 246, 261
Tronzo classification, 30–31
Tronzo nail, 223
Tropocollagen α-chains, 392
Troponin, 167
Trotter bulge test, 154
Trough line, 116
Trough line sign, 119
TRPSII Langer Giedion syndrome, 89
TRPSI Sugio-Kajii syndrome, 89
True ankylosis, 72
True-Flex nail, 223
True knee dislocation, 34
True lateral view, 110
Trumble arthrodeses, 229
Trumpet nail deformity, 328
Trumpet sign, 142
Tscherne classification, 31
Tsuge, 337
Tsuli procedure, 306
Tubercle, 213, 308
  of Tillaux-Chaput, 261
Tuberosity (large), 213
Tuck sign, 147
Tuft, 308
Tuft fracture, 4
Tumbler pedicle, 273
Tumefaction, 104
Tumor, 104
  capsule, 51
  necrosis factor–alpha, 391
  pseudo-capsule, 51
  treatments, 276
Tumoral calcinosis, 89
Tunnel view, 110
Tupper arthroplasty, 332
Turco procedure, 364
Turf-toe, 38–39
Turgid, 104
Turnbuckle, 202
Turnbuckle cast, 179
Turner syndrome, 89
Turret exostosis, 60, 326
Turtle-back nail, 328
Turyn sign, 140
Two-body abrasive wear, 226
Two-incision anterior approach, 275

Two-or four-poster orthoses, 204
Two-point discrimination, 147, 371, 373
Two-way ANOVA, 379
Tyloma, 352
Type and cross-match (T&C), 172
Type and screen (T&S), 172
Type I error, 381
Type II error, 381
Type IX collagen, 65
Type I motor and sensory neuropathy, 81
Type II motor and sensory neuropathy, 81

U

UBE3A, 84
UCBL orthoses, 197
Ulcer, 104, 357
Ullmann line, 116
Ullrich congenital muscular dystrophy (UCMD), 89
Ulna/ulnar, 247
  artery, 248, 315
  bursa, 313
  collateral ligament, 250, 312
  coronoid fracture, 25
  deficiency, 323
  dimelia, 96, 322
  drift, 317
  forearm flap, 341
  fovea sign, 147
  fracture, 15, 19, 24
  impaction syndrome, 326
  nerve, 243, 315–316
  tunnel syndrome, 320
  variance, 323
Ultimate strength (Pa), 385
Ultrasonography/ultrasound, 105, 128, 368
  stimulation, 224
  study, 128
Unciform, 307
Unciform fracture, 9
Uncommitted metaphyseal lesion, 59
Uncompensated rotatory scoliosis, 292
Unconstrained knee, 271
Uncovertebral joints, 286
Underarm orthoses, 204
Undifferentiated pleomorphic sarcoma, 53
Unguis, 314
Unguis incarnatus, 328, 355
Unicameral bone cyst, 59
Unicompartmental knee, 271
Unilateral facet subluxation, 34
Unilateral fixation, 224
Unilateral hip spica cast, 180
Uniplane fixation, 224
Unipolar, 258
Univalve cast, 181
Universal gutter splint, 183
Universal hand dressing, 184
Unna boot, 180
Unsegmented bar, 299

Unstable fracture, 6
Unsustained clonus, 99
Ununited union, 13
Upper limb casts, 179–180
Upper-limb orthoses, 200–202
    componenets, 202
    elbow, 201
    elbow-wrist-hand, 201
    shoulder, 201
    shoulder-elbow-wrist-hand, 201–202
    specialized systems, 202
Upper limbs radiographic views, 110
Upper motor neuron disease, 80
Upper obstetrical palsy, 81
Upper subscapular nerve, 243
Uppsala screw, 223
Upright, 200, 205
Uric acid (UA), 165

V

Vacuum assisted closure (VAC), 184, 325
Vagus nerve, 286
Vainio metaphalangeal interposition, 332
Valgus
    control modifications, 200
    corrective ankle straps, 200
    knee control pads, 200
    stress test, 154
    thrust test, 154
Valpar component work sample series, 373
Valsalva maneuver, 140
Valves, 235
Van Gorder approach, 275
Van Neck disease, 61
Van Ness procedure, 272
Vancouver Classification, 31
Vanishing bone disease, 46
Vanzetti sign, 140
Variability of measurements, 380
Variance (s^2), 381
Varices, 73
Varicose veins, 73
Varus corrective ankle straps, 200
Varus knee control pads, 200
Varus recurvatum test, 154
Varus stress test, 154
Vascular (blood vessels) system, 235–240
Vascular diagnostic studies
    invasive tests, 128–129
    noninvasive tests, 129–130
Vascular diseases and conditions
    associated, 77–78
    blood vessels, 73–77
Vasoconstriction, 77
Vasodilatation, 77
Vasospastic, 77
Vastus intermedius, 262
Vastus lateralis, 262
Vastus medialis, 262, 268
Vastus medialis obliquus (VMO), 262

VATER association, 104
VATER syndrome, 323
Vater-Pacini corpuscle, 316
Vaughn–Jackson syndrome, 324
Vector, 385
Veins, 235, 238
    of ankle, 357
Velcro splint, 183
Veleanu, Rosianu, and Lonescu procedure, 261
Velpeau dressing, 183–184
Velpeau splint, 183
Vena cava, 238
Vena cava filter, 240
Venable screw, 223
Venae communicantes, 266
Venereal Disease Research Laboratory (VDRL), 169
Venn-Watson classification system, 96t–97t
Venogram, 129
Venography, 129
Venous insufficiency, 73
Venous reflux, 73
Venous thromboembolic disease, 75
Ventral inclination angle (VCA), 113
Venules, 235, 238
Verdan
    pedicle, 273
    procedure, 341
    suture, 337
Vermont, 305
Verruca vulgaris, 330, 356
Vertebra/vertibral, 283–284
    artery, 286
    body, 285
    plana fracture, 10
    pseudarthrosis, 60
Vertebroplasty, 301
Vertical patella test, 154
Vertical talus, 357
Vertigo, 81, 104
Veseley-Street nail, 223
Vestigial, 104
Vest-over-pants closure, 282
Viable, 282
Vibration white finger syndrome, 320
Vibrator sense examination, 371
Vickers ligament, 312
Vicular maneuver, 138
Videofluoroscopy, 125
Villous lipomatous proliferation, 71
Villous synovitis, 72
Vimentin stain, 171
Vinculae, 316
Vincula longa and breva, 312
Vinculum brevum, 316
Vinculum longum, 316
Vinke tongs, 187
Virgin screw, 223
Viscoelasticity, 385
Viscosity, 385
Vital signs, 174
Vitamin D, 394

Vitamin D enzyme 25-α-hydroxycholicaliferol-1-hydroxylase, 84
Vitamin D–resistant rickets, 84
Volar approach, 341
Volar Barton fracture, 9
Volar capsular reefing, 339–340
Volar carpal ligament, 312
Volar-flexed intercalated segment instability (VISI), 327
Volar interossei, 310
Volar ligament, 312
Volar plate, 308
Volar splint, 183
Volkmann
 canals, 211, 213
 contracture, 75–76, 324
 deformity, 61
 fracture, 12
 ischemic contracture, 61
 triangle, 12
Voltz arthroplasty, 332
Volume, 176
Volumeter set, 373
Voluntary dislocation, 33
Volz prosthesis, 331
Von Bahr screw, 223
Von Recklinghausen disease, 61, 82
Von Rosen orthoses, 199
Von Rosen view, 110
VonFrey hair test, 373
Voorhoeve disease, 47, 61
Vulpius-Compere procedure, 364
V-Y flaps, 335
V-Y plasty, 364

W

Waddell sign, 140
Waddell triad, 10
Wafer procedure, 341
Wagner
 disease, 55, 61
 osteotomy, 215
 procedure, 267, 272
Wagoner advancement, 338–339
Wagoner approach, 306
Wagoner Classification Foot Ulcers, 357t
Wagon wheel fracture, 11
Wagstaffe fracture, 12
Waist belt, 192, 194
Waldenström
 disease, 61
 sign, 119
 stage, 125
Walker, 180–181, 183
Walker-Mureloch wrist sign, 158
Walking heel, 181
Walther fracture, 10
Ward, Thompson, and Vandergriend procedure, 261
Ward triangle, 114
Warner-Farber procedure, 364

Wartenberg sign, 147
Wartenberg syndrome, 319
Washer woman's sprain, 324
Wassel Classification of Thumb Polydactyly, 96t–97t, 323t
Watanabe Classification for Discoid Meniscus, 93t
Watch crystal nail, 328
Watson-Cheyne procedure, 364
Watson-Jones
 approach, 275
 arthrodeses, 229
 frame, 187
 nail, 223
 procedure, 246, 364
Watson-Jones Classification, 31
Watson test, 146–147
Wear, 385
Wear debris disease, 104
Weaver and Dunn procedure, 246
Weaver's bottom, 59
Webb procedure, 261
Weber
 classification, 31
 osteotomy, 215, 246
 procedure, 272
Weber, Brunner, and Freuler procedure, 261
Weber-Vasey prostheses, 252
Web ligament, 313
Webril, 179
Webspace, 314
Wedge cast, 181
Wedge fracture, 10
Wedging, 294
 of olisthetic vertebra, 289
Weeping lubrication, 384
Weight, 175–176, 385
Weight-lifter's shoulder, 39
Weiland procedure, 272
Weil procedure, 364
Weiss sign, 157
Weiss spring, 223
Well-leg cast, 180
Well-leg traction, 187
Wellmerling maneuver, 149
Werdnig-Hoffmann disease, 62
Wertheim Bohlman fixation, 302
West and Soto-Hall procedure, 269
West Point view, 110
Western blot, 386
Westin procedure, 364
Wet leather sign, 147
Wet reading, 107
Wet-to-dry dressing, 184
Wheatstone bridge, 388
Whiplash, 39
Whirlpool, 368
Whistling face syndrome, 321, 323
White arthrodeses, 229
White blood count (WBC), 164
Whitecloud and Larocca fixation, 302
White procedure, 267

Whitesides approach, 306
White slide procedure, 364
Whitman
  frame, 187
  maneuver, 149
  osteotomy, 215
  plate, 206
  procedure, 246
  talectomy procedure, 364
Whitman-Thompson procedure, 364
Whole blood, 173
Whole upper extremity involvement, 321
WHO Working Group, 83
Wiberg angle, 111
Wickstrom arthrodeses, 331
Wide resection, 276
Williams
  (flexion) exercises, 370
  nail, 223
  rod, 223
Willow fracture, 4
Wilmington jacket, 204
Wilson
  approach, 275
  fracture, 9
  plate, 223
  procedure, 229, 359, 364
  prostheses, 252
  sign, 154
Wilson and Jacobs procedure, 272, 364
Wilson and McKeever procedure, 246
Wiltse Classification of Spondylolisthesis, 289t
Wiltse plate, 305
Wiltse procedure, 306
Wimberger sign, 119
Winberger line, 116
Windblown hand, 321
Window, 181
Windshield wiper sign, 119
Windswept hips, 91
Winged scapula, 90
Wingfield frame, 258
Winograd procedure, 364
Winquist-Hansen classification, 31
Winter procedure, 306
Wire-frame collar, 204
Wirth Jager procedure, 268
Wisconsin interspinous segmental spinal, 305
Wolf blade plate arthrodeses, 229
Wolf procedure, 364
Wolfe
  graft, 334
  skin graft, 273
Wolff's law, 394
WOMAC, 161
Woodward procedure, 246
Work, 385
Work to failure, 385
Work to yield, 385
World Health Organization (WHO), 166
Wormian bone, 213

Wound, 104
Woven bone, 213, 394
Wraparound procedure, 335
Wraparound splint, 183
Wright maneuver, 138
Wrinkle test, 158
Wrist, 307–342
  anatomy, 307–316
  bones, 307–308
  disarticulation (WD), 190–191
  diseases, 316–330
  drop, 319
  extension procedure, 339
  extensors, 310
  fingers, 313–314
  flexion unit, 192
  flexors, 310
  joints, 308
  ligaments, 312
  nails, 314
  nerves and arteries, 314–316
  palm, 312–313
  scaphoid fracture, 20
  structural anomalies, 316–330
  subluxations, 34
  surgery, 330–341
  tendons, 310–311
  units, 193
Wrist diseases
  arthritic deformities, 316–317
  congenital, 320–323
  dislocations, 326–327
  infections, 329–330
  muscles and tendons, 323–324
  nail and skin disorders, 327–328
  neuropathies, 317–320
  traumatic disorders, 325–326
  vascular disorders, 324–325
Wrist-driven tenodesis orthoses (WDWHO), 201
Wrist muscles, 308–311
  extrinsic, 310
  fascia, 311–312
  flexor zones, 311
  forearm, 310–311
  intrinsic, 310
  ligaments, 311–312
  pulleys, 311
Wrist surgery
  approaches, 341
  arthrodeses, 331
  arthroplasties, 331–333
  congenital deformity repairs, 335
  fingers, 330–331
  microvascular procedures, 334–335
  muscle, 336–337
  neurological procedures, 333
  skin, nails, and fascia procedures, 335–336
  tendon grafts and transfers, 337–339
  tendon repair techniques, 337
  tenosynovectomy, 339
  trauma procedures, 333–334

Wryneck, 39, 103–104
Wu procedure, 364
Wu sole opposition test, 155

X

X-axis, 379
Xenogeneic, 216
Xenograft, 216, 303
Xeroform dressing, 184
Xiphoid, 287
X-linked hypophosphatemic rickets, 84
X-ray, 106–107

Y

Y and T fracture, 11
Y fracture, 8
Y-axis, 379–380
Yee approach, 274
Yellow cartilage, 229–230
Yergason test, 143
Y osteotomy, 215
Yield point, 385
Y-line, 116
Y scapular view, 110
Young approach, 275
Young procedure, 364
Young-Burgess classification, 31–32
Yount procedure, 268

Z

Zachary sensory grade, 156–157
Zadik procedure, 363–364
Zanca view, 110
Zancolli
    capsuloplasty, 333
    procedure, 339–340
    prostheses, 252
    static-lock procedure, 333
Zancholli-Lasso procedure, 333
Zaricznyj procedure, 268
Zarins and Rowe, 268
Zeir procedure, 246
Z-foot, 356
Zickle classification, 32
Zickle nail, 223
Zielke, 305
Zirconium, 226
Zone of provisional calcification, 212
Z-plasty, 364
Zuelzer hook plate, 223
Zygapophyseal joint, 284